Core Topics in Cardiac Anesthesia, Second Edition

Core Topics in Cardiac Anesthesia, Second Edition

Edited by

Jonathan H. Mackay FRCP FRCA
Consultant Anaesthetist
Papworth Hospital
Cambridge, UK

Joseph E. Arrowsmith MD FRCP FRCA FFICM
Consultant Anaesthetist
Papworth Hospital
Cambridge, UK
Examiner, Royal College of Anaesthetists

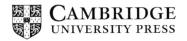
CAMBRIDGE
UNIVERSITY PRESS

CAMBRIDGE UNIVERSITY PRESS
Cambridge, New York, Melbourne, Madrid, Cape Town,
Singapore, São Paulo, Delhi, Mexico City

Cambridge University Press
The Edinburgh Building, Cambridge CB2 8RU, UK

Published in the United States of America by
Cambridge University Press, New York

www.cambridge.org
Information on this title: www.cambridge.org/9780521196857

© Cambridge University Press 2012

First published 2012

Printed in the United Kingdom at the University Press, Cambridge

*A catalogue record for this publication is available from the
British Library*

Library of Congress Cataloging-in-Publication Data

Core topics in cardiac anaesthesia / edited by Jonathan H. Mackay,
Joseph E. Arrowsmith. – 2nd ed.
    p.   cm.
  Includes bibliographical references and index.
  ISBN 978-0-521-19685-7 (Hardback)
1. Anesthesia in cardiology.   2. Heart–Surgery.
I. Mackay, Jonathan H.   II. Arrowsmith, Joseph E.   III. Title.
  RD87.3.H43C67 2012
  617.9′67412–dc23
                                                          2011033949

ISBN 978-0-521-19685-7 Hardback

"Mother stuns medics as she suffers heart failure, gives birth and has life-saving surgery . . . all in one day"

Mail Online, 17 April 2009

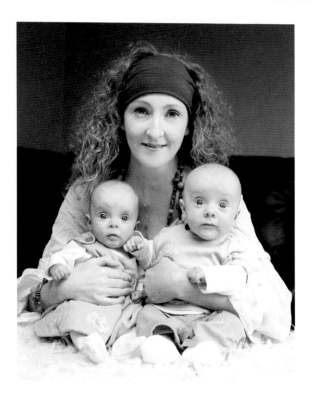

April 2009 Nina Whear (38) and her twins, [left] Evie (birthweight 3lb 11oz/1673 g) and [right] Alfie (birthweight 4lb 10oz/2098 g). In January 2009, while in late pregnancy, Nina presented to her local hospital with acute type A aortic dissection. She was transferred to Papworth Hospital, where she underwent emergency Cesarean section followed by replacement of her ascending aorta under the care of John Kneeshaw (Chapter 36) and Sam Nashef (Chapters 17 and 18). Nina was the first mother of twins in the UK, and one of only a handful worldwide, to survive surgery for this lethal complication of pregnancy without fetal loss. Photograph: Albanpix Ltd/Rex Features, with permission. With thanks and best wishes to Nina, Alfie and Evie.

Contents

vii

Section 9 – Cardiopulmonary bypass

Section 10 – Cardiac intensive care

Section 11 – Miscellaneous topics

Contributors

Yasir Abu-Omar
Registrar in Cardiothoracic Surgery, Papworth Hospital, Cambridge, UK

Matthew E. Atkins
Fellow in Anesthesia, Duke University Medical Center, Durham, NC, USA

Joseph E. Arrowsmith
Consultant Anaesthetist, Papworth Hospital, Cambridge, UK

Alan Ashworth
Consultant Anaesthetist, Wythenshawe Hospital, Manchester, UK

Rubia Baldassarri
Cardiothoracic Department, University Hospital of Pisa, Pisa, Italy

Craig R. Bailey
Consultant Paediatric Anaesthetist, Evelina Children's Hospital, London, UK

David J. Barron
Consultant Surgeon, Birmingham Children's Hospital, Birmingham, UK

Christiana C. Burt
Consultant Cardiothoracic Anaesthetist (LT), The Heart Hospital, London, UK

David Cardone
Consultant Anaesthetist, Royal Adelaide Hospital, Adelaide, South Australia

Coralie Carle
Anaesthetic Specialty Registrar, Lancashire Cardiac Centre, Blackpool, UK

Jose Coddens
Onze Lieve Vrouw Clinic, Aalst, Belgium

Alan M. Cohen
Consultant Anaesthetist, Bristol Royal Infirmary, Bristol, UK

Simon Colah
Senior Clinical Perfusion Scientist, Cambridge Perfusion Services, Cambridge, UK

Sarah Conolly
Consultant Anaesthetist, James Cook University Hospital, Middlesborough, UK

David J. Daly
Consultant Anaesthetist, The Alfred Hospital, Melbourne, Australia

Helen M. Daly
Consultant Paediatric Anaesthetist, Evelina Hospital, London, UK

Stefan G. De Hert
Professor of Anesthesiology, University of Amsterdam, Amsterdam, The Netherlands and Ghent University Hospital, Ghent, Belgium

Ravi J. De Silva
Consultant Cardiac Surgeon (LT), The Oxford Heart Centre, Oxford, UK

Mark Dougherty
Consultant Cardiothoracic Anaesthetist, Royal Victoria Hospital, Belfast, Northern Ireland, UK

John J. Dunning
Consultant Surgeon, Papworth Hospital, Cambridge, UK

Maros Elsik
Fellow in Cardiology, Papworth Hospital, Cambridge, UK

Betsy Evans
Specialty Registrar in Cardiothoracic Surgery, Papworth Hospital, Cambridge, UK

Florian Falter
Consultant Anaesthetist, Papworth Hospital,
Cambridge, UK

Nigel Farnum
Consultant Anaesthetist, Queen Elizabeth Hospital,
Barbados, West Indies

Jens Fassl
Department of Anesthesiology, Penn State College
of Medicine, Penn State Milton S. Hershey Medical
Center, Hershey, PA, USA

Juliet E. Foweraker
Consultant Microbiologist, Papworth Hospital,
Cambridge, UK

Simon P. Fynn
Consultant Cardiologist, Papworth Hospital,
Cambridge, UK

Andrew I. Gardner
Consultant Anaesthetist, Sir Charles Gairdner
Hospital, Perth, Australia

Margaret I. Gillham
Consultant Microbiologist, Papworth Hospital,
Cambridge, UK

Martin J. Goddard
Consultant Pathologist, Papworth Hospital,
Cambridge, UK

Maximilien J. Gourdin
Anaesthetist, Cliniques Universitaires UCL de
Mont-Godinne, Yvoir, Belgium

Jon Graham
Consultant Anaesthetist, Austin and Repatriation
Medical Centre, Melbourne, Australia

Stephen J. Gray
Consultant Anaesthetist, Papworth Hospital,
Cambridge, UK

Cameron Graydon
Fellow in Anaesthesia, Hospital for Sick Children,
Great Ormond Street, London, UK

Fabio Guarracino
Director of Cardiothoracic Anaesthesia and Intensive
Care Medicine, Azienda Ospedaliera Universitaria
Pisana, Pisa, Italy

Roger M. O. Hall
Consultant Anaesthetist, Papworth Hospital,
Cambridge, UK

Michael Haney
Associate Professor of Anesthesia and Intensive Care
Medicine, Umeå University, Umeå, Sweden

Charles W. Hogue
Associate Professor of Anesthesiology and Critical
Care Medicine, The Johns Hopkins Hospital,
Baltimore, MD, USA

Ben W. Howes
Consultant Anaesthetist, Bristol University Hospitals,
Bristol, UK

Bevan Hughes
Consultant Anesthesiologist, Vancouver General
Hospital and Clinical Assistant Professor, University
of British Columbia, Vancouver, Canada

Siân I. Jaggar
Consultant Anaesthetist, Royal Brompton Hospital,
London, UK

David P. Jenkins
Consultant Surgeon, Papworth Hospital,
Cambridge, UK

Jörn Karhausen
Assistant Professor, Division of Cardiothoracic
Anesthesia, Duke University Medical Center,
Durham, NC, USA

Todd Kiefer
Assistant Professor of Medicine,
Division of Cardiovascular Medicine,
Duke University Medical Center,
Durham, NC, USA

Khalid Khan
Consultant Anaesthetist, James Cook University
Hospital, Middlesborough, UK

Andrew A. Klein
Consultant Anaesthetist, Papworth Hospital,
Cambridge, UK

John D. Kneeshaw
Consultant Anaesthetist, Papworth Hospital,
Cambridge, UK

Andrew C. Knowles
Consultant Anaesthetist, Lancashire Cardiac Centre, Blackpool, UK

Catherine V. Koffel
Service d'Anesthésie Réanimation Cardiothoracique, Hôpital Cardiologique Louis Pradel, Lyon, France

R. Clive Landis
Edmund Cohen Laboratory for Vascular Research, Chronic Disease Research Centre, University of the West Indies, Barbados, West Indies

Trevor W. R. Lee
Assistant Professor of Anaesthesia, St Boniface Hospital, Winnipeg, Manitoba, Canada

Clive J. Lewis
Consultant Transplant Cardiologist, Papworth Hospital, Cambridge, UK

Jonathan H. Mackay
Consultant Anaesthetist, Papworth Hospital, Cambridge, UK

Amod Manocha
Anaesthetic Specialty Registrar, Central London School of Anaesthesia, London, UK

Jonathan B. Mark
Professor and Vice Chairman, Department of Anesthesiology, Duke University Medical Center, and Chief, Anesthesiology Service, Principal Investigator, Patient Safety Center of Inquiry, Veterans Affairs Medical Center, Durham, NC, USA

Sarah Marstin
Consultant Anaesthetist (LT), Portsmouth Hospital, Portsmouth, UK

William T. McBride
Consultant Anaesthetist, Royal Victoria Hospital, Belfast, Northern Ireland, UK

Kenneth H. McKinlay
Consultant Anaesthetist, Golden Jubilee Hospital, Glasgow, UK

Alan F. Merry
Professor of Anaesthesia, Auckland University, Auckland, New Zealand

Berend Mets
Eric A. Walker Professor and Chair, Department of Anesthesiology, Penn State College of Medicine, Penn State Milton S. Hershey Medical Center, Hershey, PA, USA

Britta Millhoff
Anaesthetic Specialty Registrar, St George's Hospital, London, UK

Kevin P. Morris
Consultant Paediatric Intensivist, Birmingham Children's Hospital, Birmingham, UK

Samer A. M. Nashef
Consultant Surgeon, Papworth Hospital, Cambridge, UK

Andrew Neitzel
Senior Anesthesiology Resident, University of British Columbia, Vancouver, Canada

Stephane Noble
Chef de Clinique, Department of Cardiology, University Hospital of Geneva, Switzerland

Rabi Panigrahi
Attending Cardiothoracic Anesthesiologist, Hartford Hospital, Hartford, CT, USA

Barbora Parizkova
Consultant Anaesthetist, Papworth Hospital, Cambridge, UK

J. M. Tom Pierce
Consultant Cardiac Anaesthetist, Southampton General Hospital, Southampton, UK

Mihai V. Podgoreanu
Associate Professor of Anesthesiology, Duke University Medical Center, Durham, NC, USA

Hans-Joachim Priebe
Professor of Anaesthesia, University Hospital Freiburg, Freiburg, Germany

Paul Quinton
Consultant Anaesthestist, St George's Hospital, London, UK

C. Ramaswamy Rajamohan
Anaesthetic Specialist Registrar, Papworth Hospital, Cambridge, UK

Doris M. Rassl
Consultant Pathologist, Papworth Hospital, Cambridge, UK

Tom Rawlings
Anaesthetic Specialty Registrar, St George's Hospital, London, UK

Fiona E. Reynolds
Consultant Anaesthetist, Birmingham Children's Hospital, Birmingham, UK

Andrew J. Richardson
Consultant Cardiac Anaesthetist, Southampton General Hospital, Southampton, UK

David Riddington
Consultant Anaesthetist, Queen Elizabeth Hospital, Birmingham, UK

Andrew Roscoe
Assistant Professor in Anesthesia, Toronto General Hospital, Toronto, Canada

Paul H. M. Sadleir
Consultant Anaesthetist, Sir Charles Gairdner Hospital, Perth, Australia

Ving Yuen See Tho
Consultant Anaesthetist, Singapore General Hospital, Republic of Singapore

Herve Schlotterbeck
Chef de Clinique, Academic Anaesthetic Department, University Hospital of Geneva, Geneva, Switzerland

Maura Screaton
Critical Care Practitioner, Papworth Hospital, Cambridge, UK

Shitalkumar Shah
Anaesthetic Specialty Registrar, Royal Victoria Hospital, Belfast, UK

Harjot Singh
Consultant Anaesthetist, Queen Elizabeth Hospital, Birmingham, UK

Jon H. Smith
Consultant Anaesthetist, Freeman Hospital, Newcastle upon Tyne, UK

M. L. Srikanth
Anaesthetic Specialty Registrar, Golden Jubilee Hospital, Glasgow, UK

Yeewei W. Teo
Clinical Fellow in Anaesthesia, Wythenshawe Hospital, Manchester, UK

Kamen P. Valchanov
Consultant Anaesthetist, Papworth Hospital, Cambridge, UK

Jean-Pierre van Besouw
Consultant Anaesthestist, St George's Hospital, London, UK

Isabeau A. Walker
Consultant Anaesthetist, Great Ormond Street Hospital, London, UK

Stephen T. Webb
Consultant Anaesthetist, Papworth Hospital, Cambridge, UK

Francis C. Wells
Consultant Cardiothoracic Surgeon, Papworth Hospital, Cambridge, UK

John Whitbread
Senior Clinical Perfusion Scientist, Cambridge Perfusion Services, Cambridge, UK

Charles Willmott
Director of Cardiothoracic Anaesthesia, Princess Alexandra Hospital, Brisbane, Queensland, Australia

Patrick Wouters
Professor of Anesthesia, University of Gent, Gent, Belgium

Reviews of the first edition

"The book has set itself clear objectives and very largely achieves them. Whilst trying not to be all-encompassing nor the only reference book required for this burgeoning field, it covers all the necessary and relevant areas to provide a sound basis and grounding in good clinical practice."

"The extensive list of abbreviations . . . reduces confusion and enhances the flow of the text."

"There is little cross-over between chapters and each chapter covers the topic in sufficient detail to make it useful as a stand-alone reference text."

". . . a thoughtfully produced and well-written book."

Jonathan J. Ross, Sheffield, UK.
British Journal of Anaesthesia 2005; 94(6): 868

"The book relies heavily on tables and figures, which makes it an effective didactic teaching tool."

"The pharmacology section includes a succinct summary of the drugs used every day in the cardiac operating rooms."

". . . the chapter on signs and symptoms of cardiac disease is one of the best this reviewer has seen."

". . . an excellent introductory text book for the trainee in cardiac anesthesia."

"likely to become a classic in the resident or fellow library."

Pablo Motta MD, Cleveland Clinic Foundation, USA.
Anesthesia & Analgesia 2006; 102(2): 657

". . . the ubiquitous use of well-labeled diagrams, photographs and clinical tracings adds understanding at every level . . . a delight to use as a teaching device."

". . . a rare text that is without institutional bias or personal beliefs."

". . . I would advise curious learners to save their time and money until they have absorbed all that this book has to offer!"

J. Cousins, London, UK
Perfusion 2006; 21(3): 193

Preface

Despite the passage of seven years since the publication of *Core Topics in Cardiac Anaesthesia*, the fundamental principles of cardiac anesthesia remain unchanged. In contrast, the clinical landscape has undergone significant change – the resurgence of primary percutaneous intervention in acute coronary syndromes, new developments in electrophysiology, use of percutaneous devices in patients previously considered inoperable, a reawakening of interest in extracorporeal support in the wake of global influenza pandemics, and the withdrawal of aprotinin.

Although primarily aimed at residents and fellows in anesthesia, *Core Topics in Cardiac Anaesthesia* proved popular with residents and fellows in cardiac surgery, clinical perfusionists and critical care nurses. In preparing the second edition we have carefully considered the advice of our readers and reviewers. Their suggestions were unambiguous; explain complex topics in an easy to digest and a readily accessible manner, use figures and tables in preference to text, and avoid all unnecessary repetition and bias. Above all they were anxious for us to retain the first edition's brevity, clarity and portability. Accordingly, our instructions to contributing authors and editorial aims were unchanged; produce a concise yet comprehensive overview of the subject emphasizing pathophysiology, basic scientific principles and the key elements of practice.

The title, selection of contributors and style of content of the second edition have been carefully adjusted to give it a greater international appeal. The pharmacology section has been changed to present a large volume of data in an accessible and more appealing format. There are new chapters on right heart valves, pulmonary vascular disease, cardiac tumors and cardiac trauma. Acknowledging the changing role of the cardiothoracic anesthesiologist, we have added chapters on catheter laboratory and hybrid operating room procedures, and acute coronary syndromes. Extracorporeal support is now discussed in a separate chapter and antimicrobial prophylaxis, resuscitation and perioperative transesophageal echocardiography (TEE) have been updated to reflect changes in international guidelines. Lastly, we present a eulogy to aprotinin.

Certification and accreditation in perioperative TEE has now become the *de facto* "Board" qualification for cardiothoracic anesthesiologists in many countries. Unfortunately, this merely assures the quality of echocardiography instead of the wide range of knowledge and competencies expected of a well rounded specialist in cardiac anesthesia. Because there are already several excellent TEE books, we have strenuously resisted the temptation to turn our second edition into a "TEE manual".

We would like to thank all of those who have made the publication of this volume possible; our international panel of contributors for taking the time to share their knowledge and expertise; Deborah Russell and Joanna Chamberlin of Cambridge University Press for their encouragement, advice, generosity and seemingly inexhaustible patience; and our Specialist Registrars for their advice and proofreading. Last, we wish to thank our families for their unstinting support during this enterprise.

Jon Mackay
Joe Arrowsmith
May 2011

Preface to the first edition

This book is primarily aimed at anaesthetic trainees in the first 3–6 months of subspecialty training in cardiac anaesthesia and critical care. It is our response to the many trainees who have regularly asked us to recommend a small textbook on cardiac anaesthesia.

We realise that it is impossible to produce a truly comprehensive review of cardiac anaesthesia in ~120,000 words but hope that this book provides a sound grounding in all of the core topics. The content of this book has been very much guided by The Royal College of Anaesthetists' *CCST in Anaesthesia* manual, The Society of Cardiovascular Anesthesiologists' *Program Requirements for Resident Education*, and recent examination papers from the United Kingdom, North America and Australasia.

Our instructions to contributing authors and editorial aims were simple; produce a concise yet comprehensive overview of the subject emphasising pathophysiology, basic scientific principles and the key elements of practice. We hope that the use of a presentation format that relies on figures and tables in preference to text will aid comprehension and recall.

We have endeavoured to avoid repetition of information, long lists of references and institutional bias. We trust that the curious trainee will turn to the larger textbooks and the Internet for more detailed discussions and exhaustive literature reviews. Finally, we hope that many sections of this book will also appeal to those preparing trainees for examinations and to clinical nurse specialists working in the field of cardiothoracic intensive care.

We would like to thank all of those who have made the publication of this volume possible; our international panel of contributors for taking the time to share their knowledge and expertise; Gill Clark and Gavin Smith of Greenwich Medical Media for their encouragement, advice and patience; and our Specialist Registrars for their advice and proof reading. Last, we wish to thank our families for their willing, and occasionally unwilling, support during this enterprise.

Jon Mackay
Joe Arrowsmith
January 2004

Foreword to the second edition

The first edition of *Core Topics in Cardiac Anesthesia* provided a unique collection of short, succinct reviews of key topics in cardiac anesthesia. Purposefully aiming to avoid being encyclopedic, the authors summarized information by effective use of tables, graphs, and brief digestible text, concluding with bulleted key points and a short reference list. This approach proved quite successful, enabling trainees to read an entire short chapter whilst preparing for an upcoming case. By presenting important basic information in a format that can be quickly grasped, as well as additional depth in selected areas, the book answered a critical need for trainees.

This second edition builds on this strong tradition. The editors have kept the excellent format while adding key topics relevant to modern cardiac anesthesiology beyond the conventional operating room and expanding to treatment of patients with cardiopulmonary pathophysiology. Updated and stunning illustrations along with informative tables are another hallmark of this new edition. Carefully selected international authors keep the book free of institutional or country-specific bias. The result is a delightful and effective update that retains all of the original positives while making the book overall more comprehensive and valuable to an expanded audience. Indeed, we predict that many of these concise chapters will be helpful in providing quick reviews to not only trainees, but to all practicing anesthetists and other cardiovascular practitioners who wish an instant refresher before delivering care to a particularly complicated patient with cardiovascular disease. As such, this edition not only addresses an unmet need, it has all the makings of a classic!

Debra A. Schwinn, MD
Professor & Chair, Department of Anesthesiology
Allan J Treuer Endowed Professor in Anesthesiology
University of Washington, Seattle, WA, USA

G. Burkhard Mackensen, MD, PhD
Professor & Chief, Division of Cardiothoracic Anesthesiology
UW Medicine Research & Education Endowed Professor in Anestesiology
Department of Anesthesiology
University of Washington, Seattle, WA, USA

Foreword to the first edition

Cardiac anaesthesia brings many divergent disciplines into one unifying practice, making it one of the most complex anaesthetic subspecialties. It requires an understanding of pathology, physiology, pharmacology, internal medicine, cardiology, cardiac surgery and intensive care. The ever-expanding nature of the specialty presents considerable challenges for both the everyday practitioner and the trainee – for whom this text is particularly targeted.

In this day and age, when a vast amount of information is already available both in print and on-line, one may be forgiven for questioning the need for yet another printed textbook. By way of an answer, the Editors (both of whom have worked in the UK and the USA) have produced a textbook (rather than a *cookbook*) that addresses a relatively unfulfilled need – a source that is specifically directed towards those who represent the future of our specialty. By incorporating contributions from authors from many countries, the Editors have largely avoided national and institutional bias.

Today's anaesthetic trainees are confronted with the seemingly impossible task of assimilating, understanding and memorizing an almost infinite body of information. Those who succeed in this task are invariably those who can confidently identify core principles without getting distracted by minute details. The Editors never intended to produce an exhaustive reference and the need to consult other sources of detailed information has, therefore, not been completely eliminated. This book does, however, provide the trainee with a very convenient framework onto which further knowledge can be added as it is acquired. The manner in which the authors have organized and presented information in this book should help the reader to more quickly see the "bigger picture" and appreciate the subtleties of cardiac anaesthesia.

Hilary P. Grocott, MD, FRCPC
Associate Professor of Anesthesiology

Mark F. Newman, MD
Merel H. Harmel Chair and Professor of Anesthesiology
Duke University, Durham, NC, USA

Abbreviations

A	
AAA	**Abdominal aortic aneurysm**
ABG	**Arterial blood gas**
AC	Adenylyl cyclase
ACA	Anterior cerebral artery
ACC	American College of Cardiology
ACE	**Angiotensin converting enzyme**
ACEI	Angiotensin converting enzyme inhibitor
ACh	Acetylcholine
ACHD	Adult congenital heart disease
ACoA	Anterior communicating (cerebral) artery
ACP	American College of Physicians
ACS	Acute coronary syndrome(s)
ACT	**Activated clotting time**
ACTH	Adrenocorticotrophic hormone
ADP	Adenosine diphosphate
ADQI	Acute Dialysis Quality Initiative
AECC	American-European Consensus Conference
AED	Automatic external defibrillator
AEP	Auditory evoked potential
AF	**Atrial fibrillation**
AHA	American Heart Association
AKI	Acute kidney injury
ALI	Acute lung injury
ALS	Advanced life support
AMVL	Anterior mitral valve leaflet
AMP	Adenosine monophosphate
ANH	Acute normovolemic hemodilution
ANP	Atrial natriuretic peptide
ANS	Autonomic nervous system
AP	Action potential
APD	Action potential duration
APB	Atrial premature (ectopic) beat
APC	Activated protein C
APL	Antiphospholipid
APOE	Apolipoprotein E
APTT	**Activated partial thromboplastin time**

APUD	Amine precursor uptake decarboxylation
AR	**Aortic regurgitation (incompetence)**
ARDS	**Acute respiratory distress syndrome**
ARF	**Acute renal failure**
ARVC	Arrhythmogenic right ventricular cardiomyopathy
ARVD	Arrhythmogenic right ventricular dysplasia
AS	**Aortic stenosis**
ASA	**American Society of Anesthesiologists**
ASD	**Atrial septal defect**
ASE	American Society of Echocardiography
ASH	Asymmetrical septal hypertrophy
AT	Antithrombin
	Atrial tachycardia
AT-I	Angiotensin I
AT-II	Angiotensin II
ATP	Adenosine triphosphate
AV	**Aortic valve**
A-V	Atrioventricular
AVA	Aortic valve (orifice) area
AVN	Atrioventricular node
AVR	**Aortic valve replacement**
AVSD	Atrioventricular septal defect
AXC	**Aortic cross-clamp**
B	
BA	Basilar artery
BAER	Brainstem auditory evoked response
BBB	Bundle branch block
BCPS	Bidirection cavopulmonary shunt
BD	*Bis die* (twice daily) ≡ Q12H (*Quaque 12 hora*)
BIS	Bispectral (index)
BiVAD	Biventricular assist device
BJ	Bezold-Jarisch

BLS	Basic life support
BNF	**British National Formulary**
BNP	Brain natriuretic peptide
BP	**Blood pressure**
BP_D	Diastolic blood pressure
BP_S	Systolic blood pressure
BPEG	British Pacing and Electrophysiology Group
BSAC	British Society for Antimicrobial Chemotherapy
βTG	β-Thromboglobulin
B-T	Blalock–Taussig (shunt)
C	
CABG	**Coronary artery bypass graft**
CAD	Coronary artery disease
cAMP	**Cyclic adenosine monophosphate**
CASS	Coronary Artery Surgery Study
cAVSD	Complete atrioventricular septal defect
CBF	Cerebral blood flow
CBFV	Cerebral blood flow velocity
CCS	**Canadian Cardiovascular Society**
CCU	Critical/coronary care unit
CFAM	Cerebral function analyzing monitor
CFD	Color-flow Doppler
CFM	Cerebral function monitor
cGMP	**Cyclic guanosine monophosphate**
CHARGE	Coloboma, heart, atresia, retardation, genital, ear
CHB	Complete (third degree) heart block
CHD	Congenital heart disease
CI	**Cardiac index**
CICR	Calcium-induced calcium release
CK-MB	Creatinine kinase MB (isoenzyme)
$CMRO_2$	Cerebral metabolic rate (for oxygen)
CNS	**Central nervous system**
CO	**Cardiac output**
CoA	Coarctation of the aorta
COMT	Catechol-o-methyltransferase
COPD	**Chronic obstructive pulmonary disease**
CPAP	Continuous positive airway pressure
CPB	**Cardiopulmonary bypass**
CP	Cavopulmonary
CPP	Cerebral perfusion pressure
CPR	**Cardiopulmonary resuscitation**
CRA	Chronic refractory angina

CRI	Cardiac risk index
CRP	**C-reactive protein**
CRT	Cardiac resynchronization therapy
CSA	Cross-sectional area
CSF	**Cerebrospinal fluid**
CT	**Computed tomogram/tomography**
CTA	CT angiography
CTEPH	Chronic thromboembolic pulmonary hypertension
CVA	**Cerebrovascular accident**
CVD	Cerebrovascular disease Cardiovascular disease
CVP	**Central venous pressure**
CVS	Cardiovascular system
CVVHF	Continuous veno-venous hemofiltration
CWD	**Continuous-wave Doppler**
CXR	**Chest X-ray/radiograph**
D	
2D	Two dimensional
DA	Ductus arteriosus
DAG	Diacylglycerol
DASI	Duke Activity Status Index
D_AvO_2	Arteriovenous oxygen difference
DC	Direct current
DCM	Dilated cardiomyopathy
DDAVP	Desmopressin (1-desamino-8-D-arginine vasopressin)
DFT	Defibrillation energy threshold
DHCA	Deep hypothermic circulatory arrest
DH	Dorsal horn
DIC	**Disseminated intravascular coagulation**
DM	**Diabetes mellitus**
DNA	**Deoxyribonucleic acid**
DNAR	Do not attempt resuscitation
DPTA	Diethylenetriaminepentaacetic acid
DSCT	Dual-source CT
DVT	Deep vein thrombosis
E	
E_A	Arterial elastance
EACA	ε-Aminocaproic acid
EBCT	Electron-beam CT
EC	Ejection click
ECC	Extracorporeal circulation
ECG	**Electrocardiograph**
ECLS	Extracorporeal life support

ECMO	Extracorporeal membrane oxygenation		Gd-ceMRI	Gadolinium contrast-enhanced magnetic resonance imaging
ECT	Ecarin clotting time		Gd-DTPA	Gadolinium diethylenetriaminepentaacetic acid
EDHF	Endothelium-derived hyperpolarizing factor		GFR	Glomerular filtration rate
EDM	Early diastolic murmur		**GI**	**Gastrointestinal**
	Esophageal Doppler monitor		GMP	Guanosine monophosphate
EDPVR	End-diastolic pressure–volume relationship		GP	Glycoprotein
EDV	End-diastolic volume		GPCR	G-protein-coupled receptors
EEG	**Electroencephalograph**		GRE	Glyopeptide-resistant *Enterococcus*
E$_{ES}$	End-systolic elastance		GRK	G-protein-coupled receptor kinase
EF	Ejection fraction		GSW	Gunshot wound
ELISA	Enzyme-linked immunosorbent assay		**GTN**	**Glyceryl trinitrate**
EMD	Electromechanical dissociation		GTP	Guanosine triphosphate
EMI	Electromagnetic interference		GUCH	Grown-up congenital heart
EP	Electrophysiological / electrophysiology			
EPIC	Evaluation & Prevention of Ischemic Complications (study)		**H**	
			Hb	**Hemoglobin**
EPO	Erythropoietin		Hb-SS	Hemoglobin-SS (Homozygous sickle)
ERC	European Resuscitation Council		HCC	Hepatocardiac canal
ERP	Effective refractory period		HD	Hemodialysis
ESBL	Extended-spectrum beta-lactamase		HF	Hemofiltration
ESC	European Society of Cardiology		HFOV	High freq. oscillatory ventilation
ESPVR	End-systolic pressure–volume relationship		5-HIAA	5-Hydroxyindoleacetic acid
			HIT	Heparin-induced thrombocytopenia
ET	Endothelin		HITS	Heparin-induced thrombocytopenia syndrome
ETT	**Endotracheal tube**		HLHS	Hypoplastic left heart syndrome
			HMWK	High-molecular-weight kininogen
F			HOCM	Hypertrophic obstructive cardiomyopathy
FAC	Fractional area change			
FAST	Focused abdominal sonogram for trauma		HPVC	Hypoxic pulmonary vasoconstriction
FDG	Fluorodeoxyglucose		**HR**	**Heart rate**
FDPs	Fibrin(ogen) degradation products		HU	Hounsfield units
FFA	Free fatty acid			
FFP	**Fresh-frozen plasma**		**I**	
FFR	Fractional flow reserve		**IABP**	**Intra-aortic balloon pump**
FO	Fossa ovalis		IAS	Interatrial septum
	Foramen ovale		ICA	Internal carotid artery
FOB	Fiberoptic bronchoscopy		ICAM	Intercellular adhesion molecule
FRC	Functional residual capacity		**ICD**	**Implantable cardiodefibrillator**
FTT	Failure to thrive		ICP	Intracranial pressure
FVL	Factor V Leiden		ICS	Intercostal space
			ICU	**Intensive care unit**
G			ID	Internal diameter
GABA	Gamma aminobutyric acid		**IDDM**	**Insulin-dependent diabetes mellitus**
GCS	Glasgow coma scale			

Ig	Immunoglobulin	LHC	Left heart catheterization
IGF	Insulin-like growth factor	LICA	Left internal carotid artery
IHD	**Ischemic heart disease**	LIJ	Left internal jugular
IHSS	Idiopathic hypertrophic subaortic stenosis	LIMA	Left internal mammary artery
		LLSE	Left lower sternal edge
IJV	Internal jugular vein	LMWH	Low-molecular-weight heparin
IL	Interleukin	LMS	Left main stem (coronary artery)
ILR	Implantable loop recorder	LPA	Left pulmonary artery
INR	International normalized ratio	LPHB	Left posterior hemiblock
IPAH	Idiopathic pulmonary arterial hypertension	LPS	Lipopolysaccharide
		LSC	Late systolic click
IPPB	Intermittent positive-pressure breathing	LSCA	Left subclavian artery
		LSCV	Left subclavian vein
IPPV	Intermittent positive-pressure ventilation	LSPV	Left superior pulmonary vein
		LUSE	Left upper sternal edge
IRI	Ischemia-reperfusion injury	**LV**	**Left ventricle/ventricular**
IRV	Inverse ratio ventilation	LVAD	Left ventricular assist device
ITP	Idiopathic thrombocytopenic purpura	LVEDA	Left ventricular end-diastolic area
		LVEDP	**Left ventricular end-diastolic Pressure**
ITU	Intensive therapy unit		
IV	**Intravenous**	LVEDV	Left ventricular end-diastolic volume
IVI	Intravenous infusion	LVEF	Left ventricular ejection fraction
IVC	**Inferior vena cava**	LVESA	Left ventricular end-systolic area
IVRT	Isovolumic relaxation time	LVESPVR	Left ventricular end-systolic pressure–volume relationship
IVS	Interventricular septum		
IVUS	Intravascular ultrasound	LVESV	Left ventricular end-systolic volume
		LVID	Left ventricular internal diameter
J		LVF	Left ventricular failure
JGA	Juxtaglomerular apparatus	**LVH**	**Left ventricular hypertrophy**
JW	Jehovah's Witness	**LVOT**	**Left ventricular outflow tract**
K		**M**	
KIU	Kallikrein inhibitory units	**MAC**	**Minimal alveolar concentration**
KK	Kallikrein		Membrane attack complex
		MAO	Monoamine oxidase
L		**MAP**	**Mean arterial pressure**
LA	**Left atrium/atrial**	MAPCAs	Major aorta pulmonary collateral arteries
LAA	Left atrial appendage		
LAD	**Left anterior descending (coronary artery)**	MAPK	Mitogen-activated protein kinase
		MCA	Middle cerebral artery
LAHB	Left anterior hemiblock	McSPI	Multicenter Study of Perioperative Ischemia
LAP	Left atrial pressure		
LAST	Left anterior short thoracotomy	MDCT	Multidetector row CT
LAX	Long axis	MDO_2	Myocardial oxygen delivery
LBBB	**Left bundle branch block**	ME	Mid-esophageal
LBP	Lipopolysaccharide binding protein	MEP	Motor evoked potential
LCA	Left coronary artery	MET	Medical emergency team
LCC	Left coronary cusp	METs	Metabolic equivalents
LCOS	Low cardiac output state	**MI**	**Myocardial infarction**

MIBI	Methoxyisobutyl nitrile	**NSAID**	**Non-steroidal anti-inflammatory drug**
MICS	Minimally invasive coronary surgery	**NSR**	**Normal sinus rhythm**
	Minimally invasive cardiac surgery	NSTEMI	Non-ST-elevation myocardial infarction
MIDCAB	Minimally invasive direct coronary artery bypass	NTS	Nucleus tractus solitarius
MOF	Multi-organ (system) failure	**NYHA**	**New York Heart Association**
MPA	Main pulmonary artery		
MPAP	Mean pulmonary artery pressure	**O**	
MPI	Myocardial performance index	OD	Once daily
MR	**Mitral regurgitation (incompetence)**	OPCAB	Off-pump coronary artery bypass
MRI	**Magnetic resonance imaging**	OS	Opening snap
MRSA	**Methicillin-resistant** *Staphylococcus aureus*	**P**	
MS	**Mitral stenosis**	**PA**	**Pulmonary artery**
MSM	Midsystolic murmur	PABD	Preoperative autologous blood donation
MUF	Modified ultrafiltration	PAD	Pulmonary artery diastolic
MUGA	Multiple gated acquisition	**PAFC**	**Pulmonary artery floatation catheter**
MV	**Mitral valve**	PAH	Pulmonary arterial hypertension
MVO$_2$	**Myocardial oxygen consumption**	PAI	Plasminogen activator inhibitor
MVP	Mitral valve prolapse	**PAP**	**Pulmonary artery pressure**
MVR	**Mitral valve replacement**	PAPVD	Partial anomalous pulmonary venous drainage
MW	Molecular weight	pAVSD	Partial atrioventricular septal defect
		PAWP	**Pulmonary artery wedge pressure**
N		PBF	Pulmonary blood flow
N$_2$O	Nitrous oxide	PCA	Patient-controlled analgesia
NAD	Nicotinamide adenine dinuleotide		Posterior cerebral artery
NASPE	North American Society of Pacing and Electrophysiology		Pulse contour analysis
NCC	Non-coronary cusp	PCC	Prothrombin complex concentrate
	Non-compaction cardiomyopathy	PCH	Pulmonary capillary hemangiomatosis
NDMR	Non-depolarizing muscle relaxant	PCI	Percutaneous coronary intervention
NEC	Necrotizing enterocolitis	PCoA	Posterior communicating (cerebral) artery
NG	**Nasogastric**		
NIBP	**Non-invasive blood pressure**	PCR	Polymerase chain reaction
NICE	National Institute for Health and Clinical Excellence	PCV	Pressure-controlled ventilation
		PD	Peritoneal dialysis
NIDDM	**Non-insulin-dependent diabetes mellitus**	PDA	Patent ductus arteriosus
			Posterior descending (coronary) artery
NIH	National Institutes of Health		
NIRS	Near infrared spectroscopy	PDE	Phosphodiesterase
NIV	Non-invasive ventilation	PDGF	Platelet-derived growth factor
NMB	Neuromuscular blockade/blocker	**PE**	**Pulmonary embolus/embolism**
NMDA	*N*-methyl-D-aspartate	PEA	Pulmonary (thrombo) endarterectomy
NO	Nitric oxide		
NOS	Nitric oxide synthetase		
NPV	Negative predictive value		
NR	Nuclear receptors	**PEEP**	**Positive end-expiratory pressure**

PET	Positron emission tomography
PF_3	Platelet factor 3
PF_4	Platelet factor 4
PFO	Patent foramen ovale
PGE_2	Prostaglandin E_2
PGI_2	Prostaglandin I_2 (prostacyclin)
PH-T	Pressure half-time
PHT	Pulmonary hypertension
PISA	Proximal isovelocity surface area
PKA	Protein kinase A
PKC	Protein kinase C
PLB	Phospholamban
PMI	Perioperative myocardial infarction
PMR	Papillary muscle rupture
PO	*Per os* (by mouth)
PONV	**Postoperative nausea and vomiting**
PPAR	Peroxisome proliferator-activated receptors
PPB	Plasma protein binding
PPCI	Primary percutaneous coronary intervention
PPM	Permanent pacemaker
PPHN	Persistent pulmonary hypertension of the newborn
PPV	Pulse pressure variation
	Prone position ventilation
	Positive predictive value
PR	**Pulmonary regurgitation (incompetence)**
PRBC	Packed red blood cells
PS	**Pulmonary stenosis**
PSM	Pansystolic murmur
PSV	Pressure-support ventilation
PT	Prothrombin time
PTCA	Percutaneous transluminal coronary angioplasty
PV	**Pulmonary valve**
	Pulmonary vein
PVC	Polyvinyl chloride
PVd	Pulmonary vein diastolic
PVD	Pulmonary vascular disease
PVF	Pulmonary venous flow
PVOD	Pulmonary veno-occlusive disease
PVR	**Pulmonary vascular resistance**
PVs	Pulmonary vein systolic
PWD	**Pulsed-wave Doppler**

Q	
Q_P	Pulmonary flow
Q_S	Systemic flow
QDS	*Quater die sumendus* (four times daily)
	$\equiv$ Q6H (*Quaque 6 hora*)
R	
RA	**Right atrium/atrial**
RAA	Right atrial appendage
RAD	Right axis deviation
RBBB	**Right bundle branch block**
RBC	**Red blood cell**
RBF	Renal blood flow
RCA	Right coronary artery
RCC	Right coronary cusp
RCP	Retrograde cerebral perfusion
RCCV	Right common cardinal vein
RCRI	Revised cardiac risk index
REMATCH	Randomized evaluation of mechanical assistance for the treatment of congestive heart failure
RHC	Right heart catheterization
RICA	Right internal carotid artery
RIJ	Right internal jugular
RIND	Reversible ischemic neurologic deficit
RMP	Resting membrane potential
RNA	**Ribonucleic acid**
RPA	Right pulmonary artery
RPM	Revolutions per minute
RR	**Respiratory rate**
RRT	Renal replacement therapy
RSCA	Right subclavian artery
RSCV	Right subclavian vein
RTA	Road traffic accident
RV	**Right ventricle/ventricular**
RVAD	Right ventricular assist device
RVEDP	Right ventricular end-diastolic pressure
RVEF	Right ventricular ejection fraction
RVH	**Right ventricular hypertrophy**
RVOT	**Right ventricular outflow tract**
RWMA	Regional wall motion abnormality
S	
S_1	First heart sound
S_2	Second heart sound

S_3	Third heart sound	TCD	Transcranial Doppler
S_4	Fourth heart sound	TCPC	Total cavopulmonary venous connection
SA	**Sinoatrial**	TDI	Tissue Doppler imaging
SACP	Selective antegrade cerebral perfusion	TDS	*Ter die sumendus* (three times daily) $\equiv$ Q8H (*Quaque 8 hora*)
SAM	Systolic anterior motion (of the anterior mitral valve leaflet)	TEA	Thoracic epidural analgesic
SAN	Sinoatrial node	**TEE**	**Transesophageal echocardiography**
SaO$_2$	**Arterial oxygen saturation**	TEG	Thromboelastogram/ thromboelastography
SAX	Short axis	TENS	Transcutaneous electrical nerve stimulation
SC	Subcutaneous	TG	Transgastric
SCA	Society of Cardiovascular Anesthesiologists	TGA	Transposition of the great arteries
SCS	Spinal cord stimulation	TGF	Transforming growth factor
SCUBA	Self-contained underwater breathing apparatus	**TIA**	**Transient ischemic attack**
SERCA	Sarcoplasmic reticulum calcium ATPase	TIVA	Total intravenous anesthesia
		TMF	Transmitral flow
SIRS	Systemic inflammatory response to sepsis	TnC	Troponin C
S$_J$vO$_2$	Jugular venous oxygen saturation	TnI	Troponin I
SLE	Systemic lupus erythematosus	TnT	Troponin T
SNP	**Sodium nitroprusside**	TNF	Tumor necrosis factor
SNS	Sympathetic nervous system	TOF	Tetrology of fallot
SPECT	Single photon emission computed tomography	tPA	Tissue plasminogen activator
		TPG	**Transpulmonary gradient**
SR	Sarcoplasmic reticulum	**TR**	**Tricuspid regurgitation (incompetence)**
SSEP	Somatosensory evoked potential		
SSFP	Steady-state free precession	**TS**	**Tricuspid stenosis**
ST	Sinus tachycardia	TT	Thrombin time
STEMI	ST-elevation myocardial infarction	**TTE**	**Transthoracic echocardiography**
SV	**Stroke volume**	**TV**	**Tricuspid valve**
SVC	**Superior vena cava**	TXA	Tranexamic acid
SVG	Saphenous vein graft		
SvO$_2$	**Mixed venous oxygen saturation**	**U**	
SVR	**Systemic vascular resistance**	UA	Unstable angina
SVT	**Supraventricular tachycardia**	UHF	Unfractionated heparin
		u-PA	Urokinase plasminogen activator
T		UTI	Urinary tract infection
T_3	Triiodothyronine	UV	Umbilical vein
T_4	Thyroxine		
TA	Truncus arteriosus	**V**	
TAPSE	Tricuspid annular plane systolic excursion	VA	Vertebral artery
		VACTERL	(syndrome) Vertebral anomalies, Anal atresia, Cardiovascular anomalies, Tracheoesophageal fistula, Esophageal atresia, Renal, Limb defects
TAPVD	Total anomalous pulmonary venous drainage		
TAVI	Transcatheter aortic valve implantation	VAD	Ventricular assist device
TB	**Tuberculosis**	VALI	Ventilator-associated lung injury

VC	*Vena contracta*	**VSD**	**Ventricular septal defect**
V_D	Volume of distribution	VSR	Ventricular septal rupture
VEP	Visual evoked potential	**VT**	**Ventricular tachycardia**
VF	**Ventricular fibrillation**	V_T	Tidal volume
VHD	Valvular heart disease	VTI	Velocity-time integral
VHF	Very high frequency	VV	Vitelline vein
VIP	Vasoactive intestinal peptide	vWF	Von Willebrand factor
VLM	Ventrolateral medulla	VWR	Ventricular (free) wall rupture
V_{O_2}	Oxygen consumption		
VOT	Ventricular outflow tract	**W**	
VPB	Ventricular premature (ectopic) beat	**WBC**	**White blood cell (count)**
VRE	Vancomycin-resistant *Enterococcus*	WPW	Wolf–Parkinson–White (syndrome)

Cardiac embryology and anatomy

Doris M. Rassl and Martin J. Goddard

An appreciation of the normal development of the heart and great vessels and normal adult cardiac anatomy is essential to the understanding of congenital and acquired heart disease.

Embryology

The heart develops predominantly from splanchnic mesoderm, together with some influx of neural crest cells, which contribute to endocardial cushions. Union of the left and right endothelial channels results in the primitive heart tube, which starts to beat in the third week of gestation. The "arterial" end of the tube lies cephalad while the "venous" end lies caudad. A series of dilatations form the primitive heart chambers (Figure 1.1).

The initially straight heart tube transforms into a helically wound loop, normally with a counterclockwise winding (Figure 1.2). Such cardiac looping

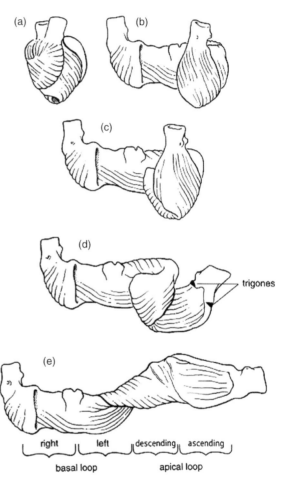

Figure 1.2 Schematic representation of the ventricular myocardial band. (a) Normal position. (b) Pulmonary artery separated. (c) Complete separation of right free wall showing 90° crossing of horizontal fibers with vertical ones. (d) Dismounting of the aorta separates vertical fibers. (e) Extended myocardial band. Reproduced with permission from Buckberg GD. *Semin Thorac Cardiovasc Surg* 2001; 13(4): 320–32.

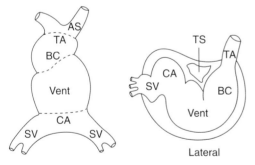

Figure 1.1 The primitive heart at around 3 weeks' gestation. The sinus venosus (SV) has left and right horns, and receives blood from the vitelline and umbilical veins. The common atrium (CA) lies between the SV and single ventricle (Vent). The bulbus cordis (BC) is divided into a proximal and distal portions. The outflow tract, composed of the distal BC and the truncus arteriosus (TA), is in continuity with the aortic sac. The transverse sinus (TS) is the area of pericardial cavity lying between the arterial and venous ends of the heart tube.

Core Topics in Cardiac Anesthesia, Second Edition, ed. Jonathan H. Mackay and Joseph E. Arrowsmith. Published by Cambridge University Press. © Cambridge University Press 2012.

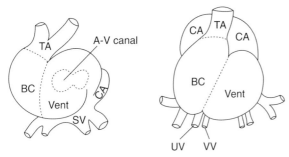

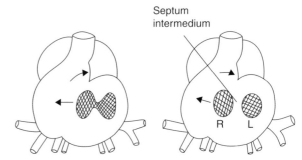

Figure 1.3 The primitive heart during the fourth and fifth weeks of gestation. The left horn of the SV receives blood from the left common cardinal vein. The right horn of the SV receives blood from the hepato-cardiac canal and the right common cardinal, umbilical (UV) and vitelline (VV) veins.

Figure 1.4 Fusion of the dorsal and ventral endocardial cushions forms the septum intermedium that divides the atrioventricular canal into left and right channels.

establishes the basic topological left-right asymmetry of the ventricular chambers, and brings the segments of the heart tube and the developing great vessels into their topographical relationships. This cardiac looping is regarded as an important process in cardiac morphogenesis and several of the well-described congenital cardiac malformations (e.g. topological left-right asymmetry) may result from disturbances in this looping process.

Lengthening of the heart tube and differential growth cause buckling of the tube within the pericardial cavity. As a result the common atrium and sinus venosus come to lie behind the bulbus cordis and common ventricle (Figure 1.3).

Further development consists of division of the atrioventricular (A-V) canal, formation of the interatrial and interventricular septa and partition of the outflow tract. Development and fusion of dorsal and ventral endocardial cushions divide the A-V canal into left and right channels. During this division, enlargement of the endocardial cushions forces the channels apart while the distal bulbus cordis migrates to the left (Figure 1.4).

Partition of the atrium begins with development of the sickle-shaped septum primum, which grows down from the dorsal wall to fuse with the septum intermedium. Before complete obliteration of the foramen primum by the septum primum, degenerative changes in the central portion of the septum result in the formation of the foramen secundum. The thicker septum secundum grows downward from the roof on the right side of the septum primum to overlie the foramen secundum. As the lower edge does not reach the septum intermedium a space between the free margin of the septum

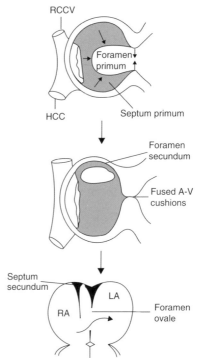

Figure 1.5 Formation of the intra-atrial septum. In the upper diagrams, the developing septum primum (shaded) is viewed from the right side of the common atrium. RCCV, right common cardinal vein (primitive SVC); HCC, hepatocardiac channel (primitive IVC).

secundum and foramen secundum (known as the foramen ovale) persists (Figure 1.5). The right horn of the sinus venosus becomes incorporated into the RA (as the vena cavae) and the left horn becomes the coronary sinus.

The interventricular septum is formed by the fusion of the inferior muscular and the membranous (bulboventricular) septa. The primary interventricular foramen, which is obliterated by formation of the septum, is bounded posteriorly by the A-V canal. The resulting separation of the bulbus cordis

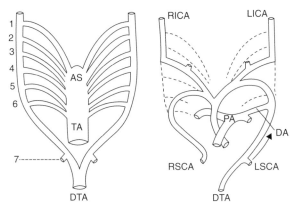

Figure 1.6 The fate of the pharyngeal arch arteries and development of the great arteries. The pharyngeal arch arteries coalesce to form the left and right dorsal aortae, which join to form the primitive descending thoracic aorta (DTA). The aortic sac (AS) becomes the right half of the aortic arch, and brachiocephalic and common carotid arteries. The left dorsal aorta forms the left half of the aortic arch. The third arch arteries form the internal carotid arteries (LICA and RICA). The sixth arch arteries and truncus arteriosus (TA) form the pulmonary arteries (PA). The distal portion of the left sixth arch artery forms the ductus arteriosus (DA). The seventh intersegmental arteries form the subclavian arteries (LSCA and RSCA).

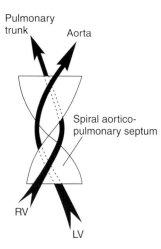

Figure 1.7 Partition of the truncus arteriosus by the helical aorticopulmonary septum into the ascending aorta and main pulmonary trunk.

from the ventricle results in the formation of the RV and LV.

The truncus arteriosus (TA), aortic sac, pharyngeal arch arteries (Figure 1.6) and dorsal aortae develop into the great vessels of the superior mediastinum.

Partition of the outflow tract begins during formation of the interventricular septum as two pairs of ridges grow into the lumen. The left and right bulbar ridges unite to form the distal bulbar septum and the left and right aorticopulmonary ridges fuse to divide the TA into the aorta and main pulmonary trunk (Figure 1.7).

Differentiation of the thick myoepicardial mantle that surrounds the primitive endocardial tube results in formation of the epicardium, myocardium and fibrous tissue of the heart. The myocardium further differentiates into a spongy, trabeculated inner layer and a compact outer layer. In the atria, the trabeculae form the pectinate muscles, whereas in the ventricles they form the chordae tendinae and papillary muscles. The myocardium of the atria remains in continuity with that of the ventricles until separated by the development of fibrous tissue in the A-V canal. The small strand of myocardium that bridges this fibrous tissue differentiates into the cardiac conducting system.

Raised folds arising from the margins of the distal ventricular outflow tracts and A-V channels become excavated on their downstream surfaces to form the pulmonary, aortic, tricuspid and mitral valves.

Fetal circulation

The fetal circulation (Figure 1.8) differs from the adult circulation in the following respects:

- *Umbilical vein* and *ductus venosus* Carries oxygenated placental blood to the IVC via the ductus venosus.
- *Foramen ovale* The opening of the IVC lies opposite the foramen ovale. Oxygenated blood is directed across the foramen by the Eustachian valve into the LA and distributed to the head and arms.
- *Pulmonary circulation* High pulmonary vascular resistance (PVR) results in minimal pulmonary blood flow and physiological RVH.
- *Ductus arteriosus* Venous blood returning from the head and arms enters the RA via the SVC. The majority of blood ejected into the main pulmonary trunk is directed into the descending thoracic aorta via the wide ductus arteriosus.
- *Umbilical arteries* These paired vessels, arising from the iliac arteries, return deoxygenated blood to the placenta.

At birth the cessation of umbilical blood flow, coupled with lung expansion and respiration, yields the so-called transitional circulation. This circulation is inherently unstable and may persist for a few hours or several weeks.

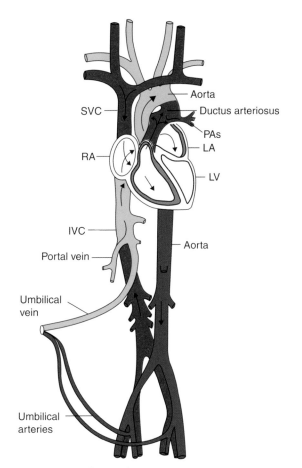

Figure 1.8 The fetal circulation.

- *Umbilical vessels* Close shortly after birth.
- *Ductus venosus* Becomes ligamentum venosum.
- *Foramen ovale* When LA pressure > RA pressure, flow across the foramen effectively ceases. May remain patent into adulthood.
- *Pulmonary circulation* Pulmonary blood flow increases with rapid decline in PVR. PVR ≈ SVR at 24 h. PVR continues to fall for several months.
- *Ductus arteriosus* Functional closure at birth as blood is diverted to the pulmonary circulation. Anatomical closure may take several weeks.

Normal cardiac anatomy

Pericardium

The pericardium is a cone-shaped structure, composed of fibrous and serosal parts, that encloses the heart and the roots of the great vessels. The fibrous part consists of dense connective tissue that merges superiorly with the adventitia of the great arteries, and inferiorly with the central tendon of the diaphragm. The inner surface of the fibrous pericardium is lined by the parietal layer of serous pericardium, which is reflected over the surface of the heart as the visceral layer or epicardium. A thin film of pericardial fluid separates the two serosal layers. The pericardial reflections create the oblique sinus, a blind recess behind the LA bounded by the four pulmonary veins and the IVC, and the transverse sinus between the aorta and PA in front and the SVC and LA behind.

Heart borders

- Right   SVC, RA, IVC
- Left   Edge of LV
- Anterior   RA, RV, small strip of LV
- Posterior   LA, pulmonary veins (× 4)
- Inferior   RV
- Superior   LA appendage.

Right heart chambers

The RA receives the SVC superiorly, and the coronary sinus and IVC, both guarded by rudimentary valves, inferiorly. A superior elongation, the RA appendage, overlies the root of the aorta. The sulcus terminalis is a groove on the surface of the RA running from the junction of the SVC and RA appendage to the IVC. The sulcus is reflected on the inner surface of the RA as a ridge of muscle; the crista terminalis. The character of the inner surface of the RA reflects its embryological origins. The surface posterior to the crista terminalis originates from the sinus venosus and is smooth, whereas that anterior to the crista originates from the primitive atrium and is trabeculated by bands of pectinate muscle. The interatrial septum forms the posteromedial wall of the RA. A shallow depression in the center of the septum, the fossa ovalis, represents that part of the septum primum not covered by the septum secundum (Figure 1.9).

The tricuspid valve separates the RA and RV. The three cusps – septal, inferior and anterior – are attached at their bases to the fibrous A-V ring. The free edges and inferior surfaces of the cusps are attached via chordae tendinae to papillary muscles from the trabeculae of the RV wall.

On the surface of the heart, the RA is separated from the crescent-shaped RV by the right A-V groove in which the right coronary artery lies. The ventricular

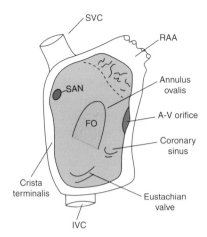

Figure 1.9 The interatrial septum viewed from the right side of the heart. The annulus ovalis is a sickle-shaped ridge of tissue in the septum secundum that surrounds the fossa ovalis (FO). Posterior to the crista terminalis the lining of the atrium is smooth. SAN, sinoatrial node; RAA, right atrial appendage.

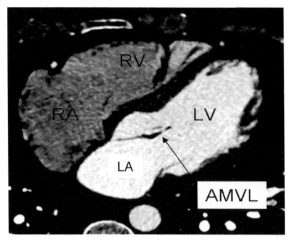

Figure 1.10 CT image showing a four-chamber view of the normal heart. AMVL, anterior mitral valve leaflet.

cavity is lined by a series of ridges known as the trabeculae carnae. One of these trabeculae, the moderator band, lies free within the cavity and carries part of the RV conducting system. The smooth-walled outflow tract or infundibulum leads to the main pulmonary trunk.

The pulmonary valve consists of three semi-lunar cusps, two anterior and one posterior, attached at their bases to a fibrous ring.

Left heart chambers

The LA lies directly behind the RA, from which it is separated by the interatrial septum. The small LA appendage arises from the superior aspect of the LA and overlies the RV infundibulum. The four pulmonary veins, namely – left and right, superior and inferior – drain into the posterior wall of the LA. With the exception of the LA appendage, which is trabeculated by pectinate muscles, the LA cavity is smoothwalled.

The mitral valve is a complex structure composed of both valvular and subvalvular components. The valve apparatus comprises two asymmetrical leaflets attached to a flexible, saddle-shaped annulus. The subvalvular apparatus comprises chordae tendinae, papillary muscles and adjacent LV myocardium.

The LA is separated from the LV by the left A-V groove, in which the left circumflex coronary artery lies. The ventricle is circular in cross section and has a wall thickness three to four times that of the RV. With the exception of the aortic vestibule, which has smooth walls, the lining of the LV cavity has prominent trabeculae carnae.

Structure–function relationships

As a consequence of the looping of the heart tube (Figure 1.2) the ventricular myocardium consists of a continuous muscular band that extends from the PA to the aorta. This band is curled in a helical manner that describes two spirals – a basal loop, with right and left segments, and an apical loop. During the cardiac cycle myocardial contraction begins in the right basal segment, followed by the left segment, so that the basal loop contracts, leading to narrowing of the ventricular mass – the pre-ejection phase. The wave of contractile activity then spreads to the descendant limb, causing the base and apex to rotate in opposite directions. This twisting of the descendant segment causes axial ventricular shortening – the ejection phase. After activation of the ascendant segment there is reciprocal rotation of the base and the apex (Figure 1.2). This "untwisting" leads to axial lengthening of the ventricles, implying a descent of the base of the ventricles, elongation and an associated drop in intra-ventricular pressure – the pre-suction phase. The atrioventricular valves open and the suction phase begins when ventricular pressure falls below atrial pressure. Relaxation of the ventricular myocardium leads to further filling – the drainage phase.

Nerve supply

The heart is innervated by afferents and efferents of both the sympathetic and parasympathetic nervous system. The parasympathetic supply comes from the

5

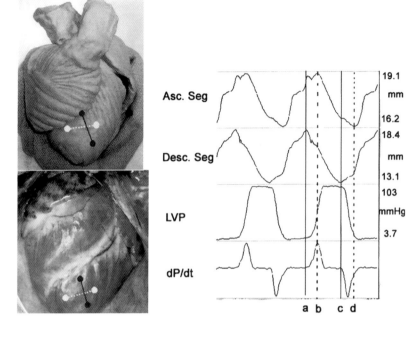

Figure 1.11 Contraction of the myocardium comprises rotary torsion (shortening the ventricular cavity) and thickening (narrowing the ventricular cavity to compress the ventricular contents). At the LV apex, superficial segments ascend toward the base (darker vertical lines) whilst deep segments descend away from the base (lighter horizontal lines). The start (a) and end (c) of contraction of the descending segments precedes the start (b) and end (d) of contraction of the ascending segments. Reproduced with permission from Buckberg GD, *et al. Semin Thorac Cardiovasc Surg* 2001; 13(4): 342–57.

vagus nerves via the cardiac plexuses. Short post-ganglionic fibers pass to the SA and A-V nodes and are only minimally distributed to the ventricles. The sympathetic supply arises from the cervical and upper thoracic sympathetic trunks and supplies both the atria and ventricles. Post-ganglionic fibers arise in the paired stellate ganglia. The right stellate ganglion supplies the anterior epicardial surface and the inter-ventricular septum. The left stellate ganglion supplies the lateral and posterior surfaces of both ventricles. Although the heart has no somatic innervation, stimulation of vagal afferents may reach conscious-ness and be perceived as pain.

Conducting system

This is discussed in Chapter 2.

Blood supply

The right coronary artery arises from the anterior aortic sinus, passes between the pulmonary trunk and RA appendage and descends in the right A-V groove until it reaches the posterior interventricular groove. In 85% of patients the artery continues as the posterior descending artery (i.e. "right" dominance). In its course, it gives off atrial, SA and A-V nodal, and ventricular branches before dividing into the poster-ior descending and RV marginal arteries.

The left coronary artery arises from the left poster-ior aortic sinus and divides into the left anterior (inter-ventricular) descending and circumflex arteries. The LAD descends anteriorly and inferiorly to the apex of the heart. In its course it gives off one or more diagonal branches and a series of septal perforating branches, which supply the anterior interventricular septum. The left circumflex artery runs posteriorly in the left A-V groove until it reaches the posterior interventricular groove, where it may continue as the posterior descend-ing artery in 15% of patients. In its course, the circum-flex artery gives off one or more obtuse marginal branches (Figure 1.12 and Figure 1.13).

Venous drainage

The majority (75%) of venous blood drains via the coronary sinus into the RA. The coronary sinus is 2–3 cm in length and lies adjacent to the circumflex artery in the left posterior A-V groove. Its principal tribu-taries are the great, small, middle and posterior LV cardiac veins (Figure 1.14).

The anterior cardiac veins drain the anterior part of the RV and empty directly into the RA.

The diminutive Thebesian veins may empty into any of the cardiac chambers and account for a small amount of venous drainage. Those draining into the left heart contribute to the "anatomical shunt".

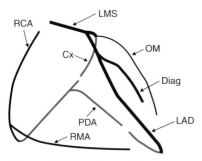

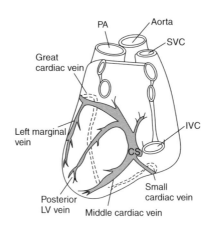

Figure 1.14 Posterior view of the heart showing the anatomy of the coronary sinus (CS) and cardiac veins.

Figure 1.12 The anatomy of the coronary arteries. LMS, left main stem; RCA, right coronary artery; Cx, circumflex; OM, obtuse marginal; Diag, diagonal; LAD, left anterior descending; PDA, posterior descending artery; RMA, right marginal artery.

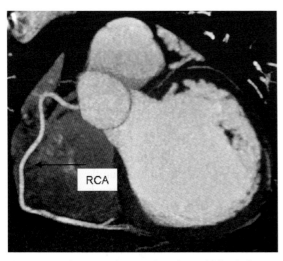

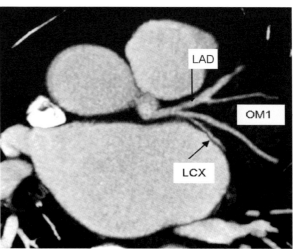

Figure 1.13 CT images showing the right- and left-sided coronary circulation. RCA, right coronary artery; LAD, left anterior descending artery; LCX, left circumflex artery; OM1, first obtuse marginal artery.

Key points

- Knowledge of cardiac embryology is necessary to understand congenital heart disease.
- The spiral pattern of the heart has implications for myocardial structure and function.
- In the fetal circulation, oxygenated blood is directed across the foramen ovale into the LA to supply the head and arms.
- The posterior descending artery arises from the right coronary artery in 85% of patients.
- The venous drainage of the anterior RV does not enter the coronary sinus.

Further reading

Buckberg G, Hoffman JI, Mahajan A, Saleh S, Coghlan C. Cardiac mechanics revisited: the relationship of cardiac architecture to ventricular function. *Circulation* 2008; **118**(24): 2571–87.

Buckberg G, Mahajan A, Saleh S, Hoffman JI, Coghlan C. Structure and function relationships of the helical ventricular myocardial band. *J Thorac Cardiovasc Surg* 2008; **136**(3): 578–89.

Drake RL, Vogl AW, Mitchell AWM (Eds.). *Gray's Anatomy for Students*, 2nd edition. London: Churchill Livingstone; 2009.

Kocica MJ, Corno AF, Carreras-Costa F, *et al.* The helical ventricular myocardial band: global, three-dimensional, functional architecture of the ventricular myocardium. *Eur J Cardiothorac Surg* 2006; **29**(Suppl 1): S21–40.

Männer J. The anatomy of cardiac looping: a step towards the understanding of the morphogenesis of several forms of congenital cardiac malformations. *Clin Anat* 2009; **22**(1): 21–35.

Moorman AF, Christoffels VM. Cardiac chamber formation: development, genes, and evolution. *Physiol Rev* 2003; **83**(4): 1223–67.

Chapter 2

Cardiac electrophysiology

Stefan G. De Hert

Anesthesiologists may witness cardiac arrhythmias either as an existing comorbidity, or as a perioperative complication. In both instances, the occurrence of such arrhythmias may have significant consequences on outcome.

Anatomy

When in sinus rhythm the heart beats in an orderly sequence. Specialized cardiac muscle cells (myocytes) in the sinoatrial (SA) node generate cardiac action potentials (APs), which cause normal myocytes to contract. APs are transmitted through the heart via the conducting system (Figure 2.1).

The cells of the conducting system are modifications of general cardiac myocytes, and classified; as *nodal*, *transitional* and *Purkinje* myocytes (Table 2.1). All myocytes in the conducting system are capable of spontaneous, rhythmic generation of cardiac APs. The anatomy and physiology of this system ensures

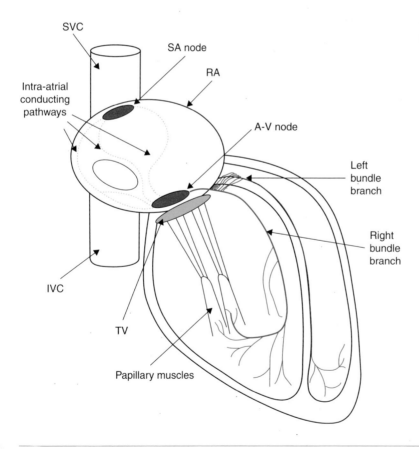

Figure 2.1 The cardiac conducting system.

Core Topics in Cardiac Anesthesia, Second Edition, ed. Jonathan H. Mackay and Joseph E. Arrowsmith. Published by Cambridge University Press. © Cambridge University Press 2012.

Table 2.1 AP conduction velocities in the cardiac conducting system

Tissue	Myocyte type	Conduction rate (m s^{-1})
SA node	Nodal	0.05
Intra-atrial pathways	General and Purkinje	1
AV node	Transitional	0.05
Bundle of His	Transitional and Purkinje	1
Purkinje system	Purkinje	4
Myocardium	General	0.6

that atrial systole precedes ventricular systole. Whichever focus produces an AP most frequently acts as the pacemaker – in sinus rhythm this is the SA node.

SA node

The SA node lies within the right atrial (RA) wall in a groove at the junction of the superior vena cava (SVC) and RA. Macroscopically it is a flattened ellipse possessing a "head", "body" and "tail", measuring $10 \times 3 \times 1$ mm and often covered by a plaque of subepicardial fat.

The SA node is supplied by the right coronary artery (RCA) in 65% of hearts, and by the circumflex branch of the left coronary artery (LCA) in 35%. The largest branch of the SA nodal artery – the *ramus cristae terminalis* – runs through the center of the SA node. It has a large lumen and thick adventitia, knitting firmly with a thick collagenous network of connective tissue within the node. It has been suggested that this structure might function as a baroreceptor for the atrial natriuretic peptide homeostatic system. It might be expected that rhythmically discharging excitable cells have a high oxygen demand, but there are surprisingly few branches within the node. The majority of the blood flows onwards to perfuse the RA.

Pacemaker cells are nodal myocytes lying within the core of the node. Arranged in clusters, each cell has one large nucleus and pale cytoplasm containing few organelles. They are non-contractile, possessing a small number of myofibrils arranged randomly.

Intra-atrial conduction pathways

It was initially thought that the cardiac AP was conducted between the SA node and atrioventricular node (AVN) as a wave of depolarization spreading radially via gap junctions between general atrial myocytes. However, the cardiac AP reaches the AVN more quickly than would be expected had it been passing through ordinary myocardium. In fact there are three specialized conducting pathways consisting of Purkinje fibers in the atria; the *anterior, middle* and *posterior internodal tracts*.

Atrioventricular node

The AVN is an oval structure measuring $8 \times 3 \times 1$ mm. It lies within the atrial septum and has a surface in the RA near the basal attachment of the septal leaflet of the tricuspid valve, and a surface in the LA adjacent to the mitral valve annulus.

Microscopically the center of the AVN contains a small number of nodal myocytes, surrounded by a fibrous network of long transitional myocytes – similar to that of the SA node but less dense. Transitional myocytes provide an electrical link between the nodal P cells and more distal parts of the conducting system. They have a smaller diameter than general cardiac myocytes but possess similar organelles and contractile apparatus. Cardiac APs are conducted slowly in the AVN and are therefore likely to be responsible for normal A-V conduction delay. Under normal circumstances, these cells are the only electrical link between atria and ventricles, as these chambers are electrically insulated from each other by a fibrous annulus.

The first and largest branch of the posterior septal branch of the RCA supplies the AVN in 80% of hearts; otherwise the node derives its blood supply from the left circumflex artery.

Accessory conducting pathways

In addition to the AVN, accessory conducting pathways may form abnormal electrical connections between the atria and ventricles. These pathways are caused by disordered cardiogenesis and consist of normal cardiac myocytes or specialized conducting tissue. In these circumstances there is incomplete formation of the mitral or tricuspid fibrous annuli that electrically insulate the atria from the ventricles. Depending on the relative refractory periods of the normal AV nodal and the accessory conducting pathways, circumstances may arise when excitation passes retrogradely into the atria through the accessory pathway having already traversed the fibrous annulus via the AVN. This may trigger a re-entrant tachycardia,

9

such as that seen in patients with Wolff–Parkinson–White syndrome.

His and Purkinje system

The tracts of transitional myocytes running from the AVN narrow quickly as they pass through the fibrous annulus into the interventricular septum (IVS). The common bundle is then said to branch into the left and right bundles at the crest of the IVS. In fact, it is somewhat misleading to consider the branching as a simple bifurcation.

The right bundle runs as a discrete aggregation of fascicles until it reaches the anterior papillary muscle of the tricuspid valve where it splits into a fine network of subendocardial Purkinje fibers, which form a network throughout the RV.

The left bundle is a flat sheet of fine fascicles, which leave the left margin of the common bundle throughout its course towards the IVS. The sheet passes over the LV aspect of the IVS and runs towards the apex of the LV. After 3 cm it splits into anterior and posterior fascicles, maintaining the sheet-like arrangement. The anterior sheet runs towards the anterior papillary muscle of the mitral valve, and the posterior sheet towards the posterior papillary muscle. After reaching the papillary muscles, both sheets split into fine Purkinje networks penetrating the whole of the LV wall and IVS. The networks consist of Purkinje cells, which are wider and shorter than the surrounding general myocytes.

The cytoplasm of Purkinje cells is packed with mitochondria and glycogen, and there is a large sarcoplasmic reticulum, but very few myofibrils. This apparatus provides the copious amounts of energy needed for the rapid conduction of APs. The Purkinje networks have large and numerous nexuses, interdigitating with general cardiac myocytes, allowing efficient conduction of the AP to the myocardium.

Electrophysiology

The cardiac action potential

The normal resting membrane potential (RMP) of cardiac myocytes varies between -60 and -90 mV. The RMP, which is mainly determined by the equilibrium between intracellular and extracellular potassium. The equilibrium potential for potassium (E_K) is given by the Nernst equation:

$$E_K = -61 \log[K^+]_i/[K^+]_e$$

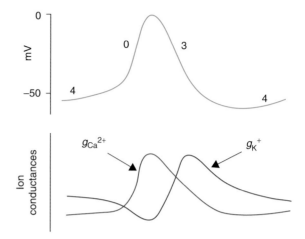

Figure 2.2 The sinoatrial node action potential. Spontaneous diastolic depolarization (the pacemaker potential) is thought to occur as a result of decreasing K^+ conductance and slightly increased Ca^{2+} conductance.

where $[K^+]_i$ and $[K^+]_e$ are the intracellular and extracellular potassium concentrations respectively. For example, if $[K^+]_i = 150$ mM and $[K^+]_e = 4$ mM, then EK $= -96$ mV. The electrophysiological differences between nodal and ventricular myocytes can be explained on the basis of differences in ion channels and mechanisms of polarization.

The unique property of spontaneous depolarization at the level of the SA node cells (cardiac muscle automaticity) allows for the pacemaker activity. Unlike atrial and ventricular muscle, pacemaker tissue is characterized by an unstable RMP, secondary to a decrease in K^+ conductance (gK^+) and a small increase in Ca^{2+} conductance (gCa^{2+}) through transient (T-type) channels thought to underlie the so-called pacemaker potential or pre-potential (Figure 2.2).

The cardiac AP typically consists of five distinct phases (Figure 2.3).

Phase 0: rapid depolarization phase is due to the rapid influx of Na^+ ions into the myocyte via fast Na^+ channels. The slope of phase 0 represents the maximum rate of depolarization of the cell and is steep (almost vertical) in the ventricle. In atrial pacemaker tissue, depolarization is primarily the result of slower Ca^{2+} influx via L-type channels. As a result, the slope of phase 0 in the sinoatrial and the AVN tissue is flatter than in the ventricle.

Phase 1: early repolarization is caused by an increase in K^+ conductance. Complete repolarization is delayed by a simultaneous increase in Ca^{2+}

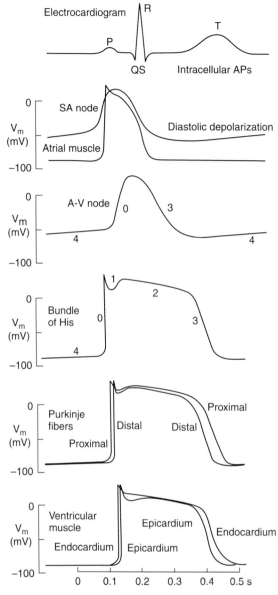

Figure 2.3 Schematic representation of the cardiac conducting system.

conductance. Phase 1 does not occur in the action potential of the SA node and the AVN.

Phase 2: "plateau" phase is the result of a balance between the inward movement of Ca^{2+} through L-type calcium channels and the outward movement of K^+ through the slow delayed rectifier potassium channels. The Na^+-Ca^{2+} exchanger current and the Na^+-K^+ pump current are also involved, but play a minor role. Phase 2 is also absent in the AP of the SA node and the AVN.

Phase 3: repolarization occurs as a consequence of increased K^+ influx and decreased Ca^{2+} efflux.

Phase 4: resting membrane potential is the period between completion of repolarization and the start of the next action potential.

Under normal conditions, cardiac APs are generated in the SA node and then transmitted via atrial Purkinje fibers to the AVN. The pacemaker cells of the heart spontaneously depolarize at a regular rhythm, thereby generating the normal HR. Abnormal spontaneous depolarization results in arrhythmias. Heart block occurs when the activity of the primary pacemaker cells is not propagated to the rest of the heart. In such cases latent pacemaker tissue may spontaneously depolarize, albeit at a rate slower than the SA node.

Neural control

The autonomic innervation of the heart arises from the stellate ganglion (T_{1-4}) and the right vagus nerve. Cholinergic stimulation of muscarinic receptors in the SA node causes membrane hyperpolarization with prolongation of phase 3 and diastolic depolarization. As a result it takes longer for the pacemaker potential to reach its firing threshold and HR slows. Stimulation of left vagus nerve causes hyperpolarization of the cells in the AVN, further slowing conduction between the atria and ventricles. Sympathetic stimulation enhances Ca^{2+} influx in the pacemaker cells of the SA node. The pacemaker potential reaches the firing threshold more quickly, AP conduction velocity becomes more rapid and HR increases. The left stellate ganglion has a similar effect in the AVN, resulting in faster A-V transmission of APs (Figure 2.4).

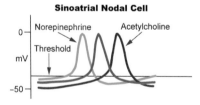

Figure 2.4 The effect of parasympathetic (acetylcholine) and sympathetic (norepinephrine) stimulation on the cardiac action potential in the SA and AV nodes.

Arrhythmias

Many cardiac rhythm disturbances are thought to be caused by disorders of ion channels. In recent years many of these so-called "channelopathies" have been demonstrated to have a genetic basis. Conditions such as the long QT syndromes are discussed elsewhere. See Chapter 40.

One of the most commonly encountered acquired cardiac rhythm disorders is atrial fibrillation (AF). While there is no single unifying etiology, contributing factors include atrial distension, ischemia, electrolyte and endocrine disorders, and old age. In previous years the emphasis for the treatment of AF was ablative therapy. More recently, however, there has been a renewed interest in drug treatment with the introduction of two novel agents that are capable of blocking atrial specific ion channels (vernakalant and dronedarone). While such drugs have the theoretical advantage of reducing or even eliminating the risk of ventricular proarrhythmias, their efficacy and safety profile in different disease states remain to be established.

Key points

- All cardiac myocytes are capable of spontaneous depolarization.

- The SA node normally generates APs at the highest frequency and therefore acts as the cardiac pacemaker.
- The autonomic nervous system acts on the conducting system, influencing HR and rhythm.
- Knowledge of the normal anatomy, physiology and blood supply of the conducting system allows an understanding of the origins of arrhythmias and heart block.

Further reading

Barrett KE, Barman SM, Boitano S, Brooks HL (Eds.). *Ganong's Review of Medical Physiology*, 23rd edition. London: McGraw Hill Medical, 2009.

Levick JR. *An Introduction to Cardiovascular Physiology*, 5th edition. London: Hodder Arnold, 2009.

Lynch C III (Ed.). *Clinical Cardiac Electrophysiology. Perioperative Considerations* (Society of Cardiovascular Anesthesiologists Monograph). Baltimore, MD: Williams & Wilkins, 1994.

Cardiac excitation–contraction coupling

M. L. Srikanth and Kenneth H. McKinlay

Excitation–contraction coupling is the mechanism by which membrane depolarization leads to myocardial contraction.

Morphology

Cardiac muscle cells (cardiomyocytes) are elliptical; typically 50–100 μm in length and 10–25 μm in diameter. Unlike skeletal muscle, which is composed of separately innervated motor subunits, cardiomyocytes may be branched and interdigitate with surrounding cardiomyocytes to form a syncytium (Figure 3.1).

Cardiomyocytes comprise a bi-layer lipid membrane (sarcolemma), cytoplasm, which contains mitochondria and several cytoskeletal proteins (desmin, integrin, talin and α-actinin), and bundles of myofibrils containing contractile (actin and myosin)

and regulatory proteins (tropomyosin, tropinin, titin). The basic contractile unit is the sarcomere (Greek; sárx = "flesh", méros = "part") surrounded by sarcoplasmic reticulum (SR). Mitochondria are prominent in cardiomyocytes to provide the steady supply of ATP required to sustain cardiac contraction.

The sarcolemma displays regular invaginations that permit the extracellular space to penetrate deep into the cardiomyocyte. These invaginations constitute the transverse (T) tubular system. The lumen of the T tubule is continuous with the extracellular fluid surrounding the cell and action potential (AP) is propagated down the T tubule.

The boundaries of the sarcomere are demarcated by Z-lines (German; Zwischenscheibe), a band of structural protein to which the thin filaments are anchored (Figure 3.2). These filaments are composed

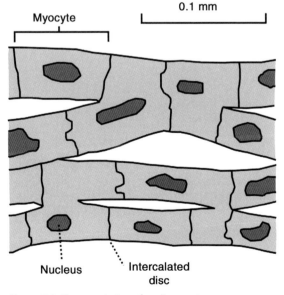

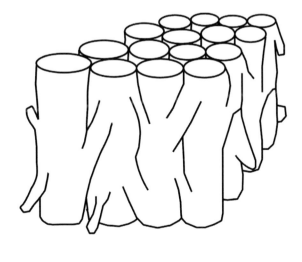

Figure 3.1 The organization of cardiomyocytes.

Core Topics in Cardiac Anesthesia, Second Edition, ed. Jonathan H. Mackay and Joseph E. Arrowsmith. Published by Cambridge University Press. © Cambridge University Press 2012.

(a)

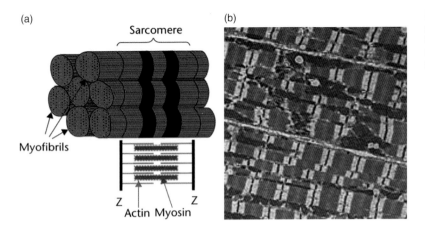

(b)

Figure 3.2 (a) The structure of the sarcomere. The sarcomere lies between two Z-lines. (b) Transmission electron micrograph showing characteristic striated pattern.

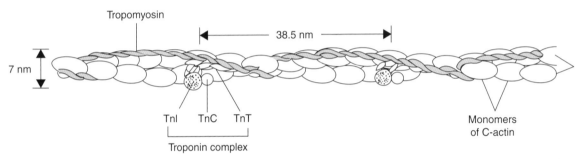

Figure 3.3 A thin filament consisting of two strands of actin polymer entwined with tropomyosin. Tropinin (Tn) complexes are sited at regular intervals along the filament.

of two helically arranged strands of actin polymer intertwined with a strand of tropomyosin–troponin complexes at regular intervals (Figure 3.3).

Thick filaments are composed of bundles of up to 300 molecules of myosin. Each molecule comprises two heads (which extend towards the thin filaments), a hinge and a tail, which is anchored to the M-line. Each thick filament is surrounded by a hexagonal array of thin filaments.

Individual myofibrils are connected via specialized interdigitating areas of cell membrane known as intercalated discs, which coincide with the Z-line. These anchor myocytes together and allow force to be transmitted between them. Within the discs, areas of fused cell membrane called gap junctions provide a low-resistance pathway for propagation of electrical activity within the myocardium. Paired hexameric (~26 kDa) proteins span the sarcolemma and intervening intracellular space (Figure 3.4). These connections permit the transmission of ions such as Ca^{2+} and small (<1 kDa) secondary messengers, such as inositol triphosphate.

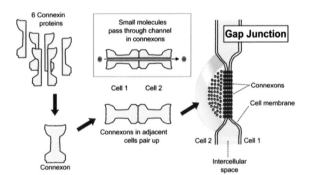

Figure 3.4 The structure of cardiomyocyte gap junctions. Each connexon comprises six connexin proteins. Reproduced with permission from O'Day H. www.utm.utoronto.ca/~w36io315.

A third filament system exists, consisting mainly of the giant (30,000 kDa) protein titin, which serves to impart structural integrity and elasticity to the stretched muscle.

Molecular mechanisms

Force production depends upon the interaction between actin and myosin. The myosin heads contain

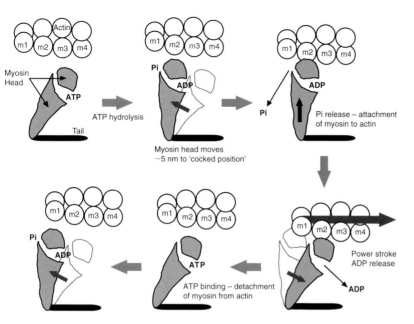

Figure 3.5 The cycle of actin-myosin interaction and force generation. From Lynch C. The Biochemical and cellular basis of myocardial contractility. In Waritier DC (Ed.). *Ventricular Function*. Baltimore: Williams & Wilkins; 1995.

an actin-binding site and an enzymatic site (myosin-ATPase) that hydrolyzes adenosine triphosphate (ATP). During contraction, the myosin head binds to actin at a 90° angle and, with the hydrolysis of ATP, produces movement of myosin on actin by swivelling. Relaxation of this actin–myosin bond only occurs when a new ATP molecule binds to the enzymatic site. The myosin head then disconnects and reconnects at the next linkage site and the process is repeated in serial fashion. The force generated by a single sarcomere is proportional to the number of actin–myosin bonds and the degree of muscle shortening depends on repetitive cycling of the above process.

The troponin–tropomyosin complex regulates actin–myosin interactions. The troponin complex comprises tropomyosin-binding (TnT), calcium-binding (TnC) and inhibitory (TnI) subunits. Under resting conditions TnI is tightly bound to actin and tropomyosin, obscuring the actin–myosin binding site. When Ca^{2+} binds to TnC, TnI binding is weakened, inducing a conformational change in tropomyosin that reveals actin–myosin binding sites. The subsequent binding of myosin to actin is the fundamental basis of force production.

The role of calcium

As fluctuations in the cytosolic concentration of Ca^{2+} modulate the actin–myosin interaction, the control of intracellular Ca^{2+} is central to excitation–contraction coupling (Figure 3.6).

Contraction

Depolarization of the sarcolemma by the cardiac AP results in activation of voltage-gated L-type Ca^{2+} channels and a passive influx of Ca^{2+} down a huge electrochemical gradient. This in turn leads to the greater release of Ca^{2+} from the larger pool of Ca^{2+} in the SR. Although this calcium-induced calcium release (CICR) is well described, its control has not been fully elucidated. The T-tubules bring the sarcolemmal L-type channels into close proximity to the calcium-release channels (CaRC) – the so-called ryanodine (RyR_2) receptors – that conduct Ca^{2+} from the lumen of the SR to the cytoplasm.

Relaxation

Relaxation is an active process that is dependent on the removal of Ca^{2+} from the cytosol to the SR and extracellular space. In contrast to Ca^{2+} release, which occurs down a concentration gradient, this is an active energy-consuming process. The principal mechanism of re-sequestration is via the sarco-endoplasmic reticulum Ca^{2+}-ATPase (SERCA); for each mole of ATP hydrolyzed, two moles of Ca^{2+} are returned to the SR. This pump is regulated by the phosphorylation status of another SR protein, phospholamban (PLB). In the phosphorylated state,

15

Movement of calcium during excitation–contraction coupling in cardiac muscle and the positive inotropic effect of catecholamines

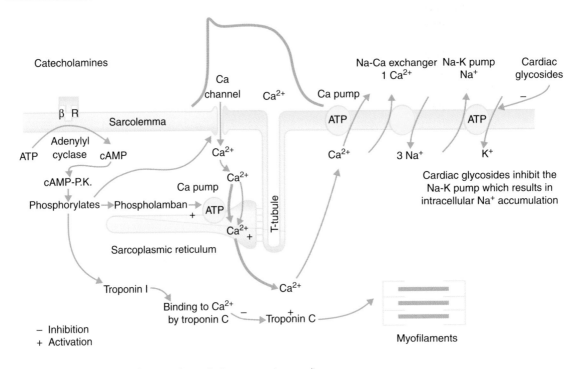

Figure 3.6 The role of calcium during cardiac excitation–contraction coupling.

PLB facilitates Ca^{2+} re-uptake by SERCA while in the dephosphorylated state it inhibits re-uptake of Ca^{2+}. Other mechanisms of Ca^{2+} re-uptake include the Na^+-Ca^{2+} exchanger, sarcolemmal Ca^{2+}-ATPase and cytosolic Ca^{2+} binding proteins, such as calmodulin and calsequestrin. Once the cytosolic Ca^{2+} concentration falls below the 0.1 μM threshold for activation, the interaction between actin and myosin ceases.

Regulation of contraction force

Systolic function

Any process that elevates cytoplasmic Ca^{2+} will increase the force of myocardial contraction. Catecholamines activate β_1-adrenergic receptors to produce a G-protein-mediated increase in cAMP and enhanced activity of a cAMP-dependent protein kinase. This leads to phosphorylation of sarcolemmal L-type calcium channels, enhancing Ca^{2+} entry into the cell. Phosphorylation of myosin also occurs, increasing the rate of cross-bridge cycling.

Cardiac glycosides inhibit Na^+-K^+-ATPase activity in the sarcolemma, leading to increased intracellular Na^+. This results in a reduction in the transmembrane Na^+ concentration gradient which in turn reduces the driving force for the Na^+-Ca^{2+} exchanger. This leads to reduced Ca^{2+} extrusion, increased intracellular Ca^{2+} and hence increased force of contraction.

Impairment of Ca^{2+} influx, signal transduction or TnC binding affinity may result in systolic dysfunction.

Diastolic function

β_1-Adrenergic receptor activation by catecholamines accelerates relaxation. Phosphorylation of PLB by cAMP-dependent protein kinase enhances Ca^{2+} reuptake by the SR. Relaxation is facilitated by the phosphorylation of TnI, which inhibits the binding of calcium to TnC. Impaired SR Ca^{2+}-ATPase function and enhanced Ca^{2+} binding to TnC may reduce the rate of relaxation, leading to diastolic dysfunction.

Key points

- Excitation–contraction coupling refers to the process by which electrical depolarization of the cardiac cell leads to myocardial contraction.
- Force production is dependent upon the interaction between actin and myosin, which is modulated by tropomyosin and the action of Ca^{2+} on the troponin complex.
- Catecholamines increase myocardial contractility by increasing intracellular Ca^{2+}.

Further reading

Kirkman E. Electromechanical coupling and regulation of force of cardiac contraction. *Anaesth Intens Care Med* 2009; 7(9): 310–12.

Klabunde R E. Cardiovascular physiology concepts. http://www.cvphysiology.com.

Chapter

4

Ventricular performance

Fabio Guarracino and Rubia Baldassarri

Ventricular performance is dependent on both systolic and diastolic function. Diastole and systole rhythmically alternate to respectively store and eject the stroke volume (SV) and thus generate the cardiac output (CO). Impaired ventricular performance may occur as a result of isolated systolic dysfunction, isolated diastolic dysfunction, or both.

Preload, afterload and intrinsic myocardial contractility are considered the essential determinants of the volume of blood ejected during systole.

Preload

Preload is a passive force that stretches muscles fibers and determines the resting length of individual

sarcomeres at the end of diastole. The "Otto Frank and Ernest Starling Law of the Heart" states that the force of myocardial contraction is determined by the initial muscle fiber length – the "force-length" relationship. As preload increases, both stroke volume and the force of the myocardial contraction increase (Figure 4.2). This relationship is not linear, and beyond a certain point – the maximum isometric force – further increases in preload may actually reduce SV.

Afterload

Afterload can be defined as the load opposing muscle shortening during ventricular ejection. The rate of muscle shortening is therefore inversely proportional

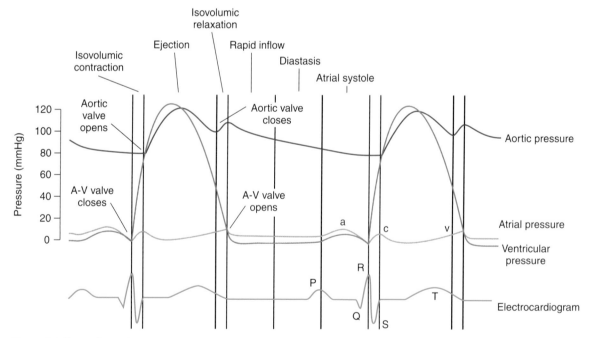

Figure 4.1 The cardiac cycle.

18 *Core Topics in Cardiac Anesthesia, Second Edition*, ed. Jonathan H. Mackay and Joseph E. Arrowsmith. Published by Cambridge University Press. © Cambridge University Press 2012.

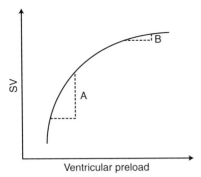

Figure 4.2 The Frank-Starling Law. A: small change in preload produces a large increase in SV. B: large change in preload produces minimal change in SV.

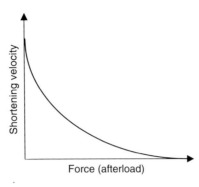

Figure 4.3 The force–velocity relationship. The greater the afterload the slower the rate of muscle shortening.

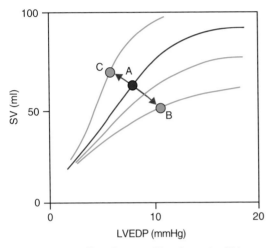

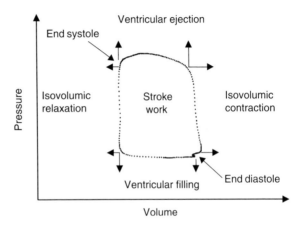

Figure 4.4 The effect of positive (C) and negative (B) inotropy on the normal (A) Frank-Starling relationship. Preload is represented by left ventricular end-diastolic pressure (LVEDP).

Figure 4.5 The left ventricular pressure–volume relationship during a single cardiac cycle. The area within the pressure volume loop is the stroke work. Note that in respiratory physiology, the axes are typically reversed.

to afterload – the "force–velocity" relationship (Figure 4.3). In contrast, shortening velocity is directly proportional to preload.

Contractility

Contractility or inotropy is the intrinsic property of cardiomyocytes to contract independently of preload and afterload. For any given combination of preload and afterload, an increase in contractility increases the force generated during isometric contraction, and increases both the extent and velocity of muscle shortening during isotonic contraction. The net effect is an upwards and leftward shift of the Frank-Starling relationship (Figure 4.4).

Pressure–volume relationship

Plotting ventricular pressure against ventricular volume throughout the cardiac cycle yields a

pressure–volume loop (Figure 4.5). While ventricular pressure can be readily measured, measuring ventricular volume during the cardiac cycle is more problematic. Conventional techniques such as ventriculography, echocardiography, and radionuclide and magnetic resonance imaging have largely been replaced by the conductance catheter, which allows beat-to-beat measurement of ventricular volume in real time.

The relationship between LV pressure and LV volume during the cardiac cycle has four phases.

- *Isovolumic relaxation:* the period between AV closure and MV opening (normal duration 90–120 ms), when pressure decreases without any change in LV volume.
- *Ventricular filling* has three components: early rapid passive filling, slow filling (diastasis) and active filling during atrial contraction. The rate of filling is proportional to LV compliance and MV

19

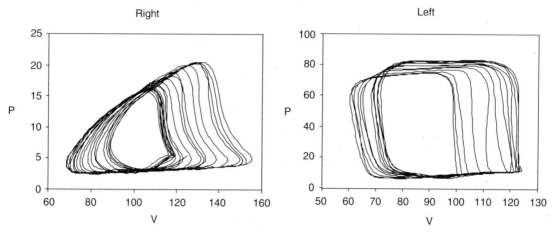

Figure 4.6 Comparison of left and right ventricular pressure volume loops. Pressure in mmHg, Volume in ml.

pressure gradient, and inversely proportional to MV orifice area.

- *Early:* the MV opens when LA pressure > LV pressure. This phase, which is thought to be augmented by LV "suction", accounts for 75% of LV filling in young, healthy adults.
- *Diastasis:* the slow filling phase that generally contributes less than 5% to LV filling. LA and LV pressures are almost equal.
- *Active:* atrial contraction contributes about 20% of the total LV filling. This phase is characterized by an increase in LA pressure with retrograde blood flow into the pulmonary veins and by an increase in LV pressure. The relative contribution to LV filling during this phase increases as LV compliance falls, for example in the early stages of LV diastolic dysfunction.
- *Isovolumic contraction* during which ventricular pressure increases. The LV volume remains constant between MV closure and AV opening.
- *Ventricular ejection:* the AV closes when aortic pressure exceeds LV pressure (end-systole). A relatively load-independent measure of LV performance is the so-called myocardial performance index (MPI), which is defined as the sum of isovolumic contraction time and isovolumic relaxation time divided by the ejection time.

The width of the pressure–volume loop represents SV, the difference between end-diastolic volume and end-systolic volume. The area contained within the loop represents the stroke work which is generally expressed as SV × (MAP − LVEDP).

Unlike the LV, ejection from the RV begins earlier in systole and, due to the high capacitance of the pulmonary vascular bed, RV pressure is not sustained throughout systole. These two factors account for the triangular RV loop morphology (Figure 4.6). For this reason and because right-heart pressures are around one-fifth those in the left, RV stroke work is less than LV stroke work. Although ejection during the pressure rise is mechanically efficient it is dependent on the low impedance of the pulmonary vasculature. As RV afterload increases, the RV pressure volume relationship begins to resemble that of the LV.

By altering preload (fluid administration) and afterload (vasoconstrictor administration) a series of pressure–volume loops can be obtained from which two important relationships can be derived (Figure 4.7).

- The slope of the end-diastolic pressure–volume relationship (EDPVR) is a measure of ventricular compliance. The relationship between pressure and volume at end-diastole is generally curvilinear.
- The slope of the end-systolic pressure–volume relationship (ESPVR) – also known as the end-systolic elastance (EES) – is a load-independent measure of ventricular contractility. The ESPVR is linear within the normal physiological range. EES can be calculated as end-systolic pressure/(end-systolic volume − V_0), where V_0 is the point at which the EES line crosses the x-axis.

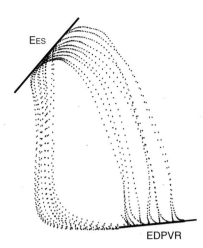

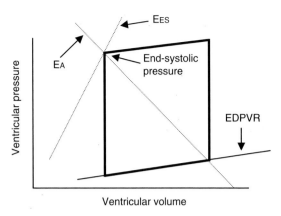

Figure 4.7 A series of LV pressure volume loops showing the slope of the end-systolic pressure volume relationship (E_{ES}) and the slope of the end-diastolic relationship (EDPVR).

Figure 4.8 Ventriculo-arterial coupling: The relationship between end-systolic elastance (E_{ES}) and arterial elastance (E_A). Arterial elastance can be thought of as the combination of arterial resistance, impedance, capacitance and inductance. The ventricle delivers maximal (stroke) work when the E_A:E_{ES} ratio approaches 1.0.

Ventriculo-arterial coupling

Ventricular performance depends on the interaction between ventricle and vasculature. The ratio between arterial elastance and E_{ES} defines ventriculo-arterial coupling, and reflects the mechanoenergetic performance of the heart. Arterial elastance (E_A) is an integrative index of the main determinants of afterload – resistance, impedance, inductance and compliance. Derived from the pressure–volume loop, E_A is the slope of the line joining the end-diastole and end-systolic points (Figure 4.8). It can be approximated by the ratio of end-systolic pressure to SV.

Key points

- Ventricular performance is dependent on both systolic and diastolic function, which are in turn dependent on preload, afterload and contractility.

- Cardiac output is a crude, load-dependent index of ventricular function.
- The ventricular pressure–volume loop allows assessment of ventricular function (E_{ES}) and arterial elastance (E_A).
- The end-systolic pressure–volume relationship is a load-independent measure of ventricular function.

Further reading

Andrews DT, Royse AG, Royse CF. Functional comparison of anaesthetic agents during myocardial ischaemia-reperfusion using pressure-volume loops. *Br J Anaesth* 2009; **103**(5): 654–64.

Coronary physiology

Michael Haney

An adequate coronary circulation and supply of oxygen to myocardial cells is necessary for maintenance of normal heart function. The coronary circulation is unique in that the organ supplied generates the perfusion pressure for the whole circulation. The heart relies almost entirely on aerobic substrate metabolism and, in comparison to other tissues, myocardial oxygen extraction (75%) and oxygen consumption are high.

Coronary blood flow

Myocardial perfusion is dependent on the left and right coronary arteries. Typical resting coronary blood flow is $70–80$ ml min^{-1} 100 g^{-1}. Rearranging Ohm's law (Electromechanical coupling and regulation of force of cardiac contraction = Electromechanical coupling and regulation of force of cardiac contraction) gives:

$$Coronary\ blood\ flow = Coronary\ perfusion\ pressure/$$
$$Coronary\ vascular\ resistance$$

It follows, therefore, that coronary blood flow can be increased by increasing coronary perfusion pressure or by reducing coronary vascular resistance. Coronary perfusion pressure is the difference between the pressure at the coronary ostia (i.e. aortic root diastolic pressure) and the pressure at the end of the coronary circulation (i.e. LVEDP).

$$Coronary\ perfusion\ pressure \approx$$
$$Aortic\ root\ diastolic\ pressure - LVEDP$$

Coronary vessels can be described as being either epicardial or intramural. Intramural vessels can be subepicardial or subendocardial, and branch into the substance of the ventricles or penetrate and communicate with a subendocardial network of branching

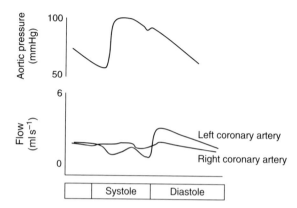

Figure 5.1 Schematic representation of flow in left and right coronary arteries.

vessels. During the cardiac cycle, mechanical ventricular forces exert pressure on the outside of intramural vessels. For this reason, regional coronary blood flow is phasic – the variation during the cardiac cycle based on the result of dynamic "driving" pressure and resistance. "Driving" pressure is strongly influenced by changes in intracardiac pressures during the cardiac cycle where tissue pressures generated by cardiomyocyte contraction are transmitted to imbedded coronary vessels. This leads to phasic variations in coronary flow with significant coronary flow occurring during diastole (Figure 5.1).

In the absence of significant coronary artery disease, the majority of coronary vascular resistance lies in small arterioles and the microvasculature (vessel diameter <150 μm). Unlike other tissues, the myocardial microcirculation has high capillary density and short diffusion distances in order to meet the exacting metabolic demands of the myocardium.

The process whereby coronary blood flow is regulated by myocardial oxygen consumption (MVO_2)

Core Topics in Cardiac Anesthesia, Second Edition, ed. Jonathan H. Mackay and Joseph E. Arrowsmith. Published by Cambridge University Press. © Cambridge University Press 2012.

independently of coronary perfusion pressure is termed autoregulation and is common to a number of vascular beds. Despite quite marked alterations in coronary perfusion pressure, coronary blood flow remains relatively constant between coronary perfusion pressures from 50 to 140 mmHg. If coronary perfusion pressure falls outside these limits, flow becomes directly dependent on perfusion pressure.

Autoregulation principally occurs in vessels of diameter >150 μm. Myogenic control mechanisms play an important role; however, metabolic and endothelial factors, particularly nitric oxide (NO), are primarily involved in the control of vascular resistance during autoregulation. When NO levels are reduced or NO production is inhibited the lower limit of autoregulation is increased and the myocardium becomes more vulnerable to hypoperfusion.

Myocardial O_2 delivery

Myocardial oxygen delivery (MDO$_2$) is the product of coronary blood flow and oxygen content.

Myocardial DO_2 = Coronary blood flow ×
Coronary blood O_2 content

Acute, physiological increases in MDO$_2$ can only be generated by increasing coronary blood flow. If arterial oxygen saturation $\approx100\%$, increasing coronary blood O_2 content requires red cell transfusion.

Myocardial O_2 demand

Relative to other tissues, MVO$_2$ is high (8–10 ml 100 min^{-1} g^{-1} at rest). Under normal conditions the myocardium relies almost entirely on aerobic metabolism. The five- to six-fold increase in MVO$_2$

that occurs during maximal exertion therefore requires a corresponding increase in MDO$_2$ (Figure 5.2).

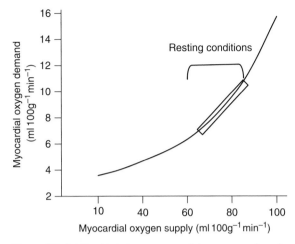

Figure 5.2 Relationship between myocardial oxygen supply and demand. At rest the relationship between myocardial oxygen delivery (MDO$_2$) and consumption (MVO$_2$) is near-linear.

Demand versus supply

The determinants of MDO$_2$ and MVO$_2$ are shown in Figure 5.3. MVO$_2$ is directly proportional to ventricular wall tension, myocardial contractility and heart rate. MDO$_2$ is directly proportional to aortic pressure and inversely proportional to LVEDP, coronary vascular resistance and HR. As HR increases, the time for diastole coronary blood flow shortens.

Coronary blood flow is the critical determinant of total myocardial metabolism. If MDO$_2$ is unable to match MVO$_2$, myocardial cells temporarily shift to anaerobic substrate metabolism. When these limited resources become exhausted, subsequent cellular energy depletion leads to disruption of cellular

Determinants of myocardial oxygen demand	Determinants of myocardial oxygen supply
• Wall tension	• Aortic pressure
• Myocardial contractility	• LVEDP
• HR	• Coronary vascular resistance
	• HR

Figure 5.3 Determinants of myocardial oxygen demand and supply.

function. The scope for increasing MDO$_2$ through an increase in coronary perfusion pressure is limited. Alterations in MDO$_2$ under physiological conditions are therefore primarily achieved by alterations in the coronary vascular resistance.

Coronary vascular resistance

In health, the close coupling of MDO$_2$ and MVO$_2$ is largely achieved by changes in coronary vascular resistance (Figure 5.2). While the local effective perfusion pressure is largely influenced by extravascular compressive forces, local vasodilatory effects also increase coronary blood flow. At the same time, some degree of coronary vasoconstriction may be important in maintaining the distribution of coronary flow to vulnerable regions such as the subendocardium.

Coronary vascular tone represents the balance of a large number of endothelium-derived, neurohumoral and metabolic vasoactive mediators. There is no single final mediator or final common pathway that determines local coronary vascular tone. Similarly, no single factor or cofactor is essential for coronary vasodilatation to occur. The systems involved in regulation of local coronary vascular tone seem to be somewhat redundant, and appear to be able, in health, to compensate for each other to a large degree.

Metabolic regulation

While there is presumption of a direct link between local metabolism and local vascular tone, no single chemoreceptor or final common link has been identified. Close coupling of metabolism and vascular tone is demonstrated by the very consistent (high) degree of oxygen extraction and low coronary venous oxygen tension. A low myocardial oxygen tension has not been proved to be, by itself, strongly vasoregulatory.

Increased metabolic activity leads to local accumulation of metabolic intermediates such as adenosine and hydrogen ions. When MVO$_2$ > MDO$_2$, cardiac myocytes generate adenosine as a result of adenosine triphosphate (ATP) metabolism. Most of the adenosine leaves the cell to reach the extracellular space, where it acts to dilate vascular smooth muscle cells. It is chiefly the small arterioles (25–100 μm diameter) that are the major target of adenosine-induced vasodilatation. Once in the circulation, adenosine is broken down by adenosine deaminase. Adenosine only has a role in the maintenance

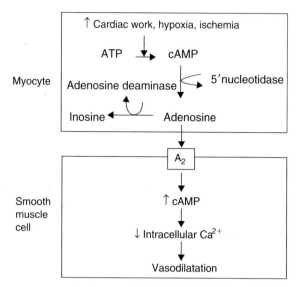

Figure 5.4 Schematic representation of the production and action of adenosine.

of coronary vascular tone when MVO$_2$ > MDO$_2$, for instance during hypoxemia, ischemia, or periods of increased heart work.

Adenosine acts at purinergic (P$_1$) receptors. These receptors are further subdivided into myocardial (A$_1$) and vascular (A$_2$) receptors. Activation of A$_2$ receptors increases the intracellular concentration of cyclic adenosine monophosphate (cAMP), leading to a reduction in intracellular Ca^{2+} and the binding affinity of vascular myosin light-chain kinase. This leads to relaxation of vascular smooth muscle and coronary vasodilatation (Figure 5.4). Part of the action of adenosine may also involve endothelial NO production leading to increased intracellular cyclic guanosine monophosphate (cGMP) concentration and vasodilatation in vascular smooth muscle. Adenosine may also act via ATP-sensitive potassium (K$_{ATP}$) channels to cause smooth muscle hyperpolarization and vasodilatation. Interestingly, adenosine receptor blockade does not seem to limit the capacity for local vasodilatation.

Endothelial regulation

Nitric oxide – generated by NO synthetase – is continuously released from coronary endothelial cells under resting conditions and is the most important endothelial mediator of resting coronary artery and arteriolar tone. NO leads to local vascular smooth muscle relaxation via cGMP and calcium-activated

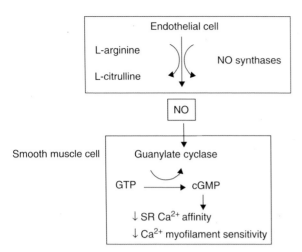

Figure 5.5 Schematic representation of the production and action of endothelial-derived nitric oxide.

potassium (Kca) channels, and possibly K_{ATP} channels. NO release is triggered by both local receptor systems (e.g. muscarinic, histaminergic and bradykininergic) and local mechanical shear forces on endothelial cells. This is termed *flow-mediated* vasodilatation – the response to shear or drag on the endothelial surface. NO also seems to be involved in coronary vasodilatation in response to increased MVO_2. However, blocking NO production does not appear to interfere with local vasoregulatory response to changes in local MVO_2 (Figure 5.5).

Prostanoids, such as prostacyclin, appear to play a role in local coronary vasodilatation. Inhibition of the enzyme cyclooxygenase, however, does not block coronary vasoregulation.

A group of endothelium-derived hyperpolarizing factors (EDHF) hyperpolarize smooth muscle through opening sarcolemmal Kca channels, though their clinical significance is not yet clear.

Autonomic and neurohumoral regulation

Epicardial and intramyocardial coronary arteries are densely innervated by sympathetic and parasaympathetic nerve fibers. Sympathetic stimulation occurs via both vasoconstrictory alpha (α_1 and α_2) receptors and vasodilatory beta (β_1, β_2 and β_3) receptors. Under *physiological* conditions both norepinephrine and epinephrine mediate coronary vasodilatation due to their β receptor effects, in contrast to their peripheral effect of vasoconstriction, which is α-mediated.

α_1-Adrenergic receptors are predominantly located in vessels $>100\ \mu m$ in diameter, whilst α_2 receptors are located in the smaller arterioles. The magnitude of vasoconstriction produced by activation of α_2 receptors is approximately double that of the α_1 receptors. In the presence of coronary disease and a dysfunctional endothelium, α_2 receptors may have a greater functional significance. When MVO_2 is increased, α_1 receptors appear to be primarily involved in vasoconstriction, and this has been interpreted as possibly a means by which subendocardial perfusion is improved, perhaps by reducing compliance in larger vessels.

The β_1 receptors predominate in coronary arteries and arterioles $>100\ \mu m$ in diameter, whereas β_2 receptors are located in vessels $<100\ \mu m$ in diameter. Under normal physiological conditions, β-adrenergic stimulation causes vasodilatation of healthy coronary arteries. However, this is usually masked by increases in HR and myocardial contractility following β-receptor activation. β-Receptor blockade reduces both MVO_2 and coronary blood flow by direct and indirect means.

Acetylcholine (ACh) mediates NO release from the endothelium via muscarinic (M_1, M_2 and M_3) receptors. ACh is, therefore, a potent coronary vasodilator when the endothelium is intact, although vasoconstrictor responses may predominate with endothelium dysfunction due to direct effects on smooth muscle cells.

Endocrine and paracrine regulation

Angiontensin II acts as a weak positive inotrope and weak coronary vasoconstrictor. Histamine and bradykinin can be released locally in the coronary circulation, both promoting vasodilatation, and bradykinin seems to be involved in local influence on other vasodilatory systems. Endothelins – peptides elaborated from endothelium – produce local, regional and systemic vasoconstriction.

Myogenic regulation

Myogenic control refers to the intrinsic properties of vascular smooth muscle which lead to contraction when intravascular pressure is elevated, and relaxation when pressure is reduced. This response to vascular smooth muscle stretching may protect the downstream circulation from a sudden increase in arterial pressure. The myogenic response is independent of any neural or humoral influences, although the effects

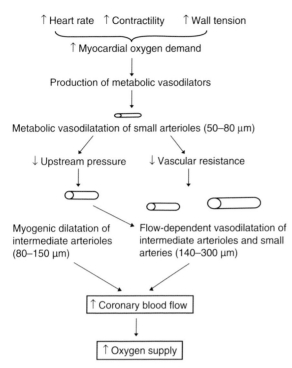

Figure 5.6 Interaction between metabolic, myogenic and endothelial control mechanisms.

may be modulated by the endothelium. The myogenic response remains incompletely understood; however, the primary stimulus is the application of asymmetrical mechanical force to the vessel wall which is subsequently transduced into a signal for muscle contraction via activation of ion channels and length-dependent alterations in contractile protein function. Activation of stretch-sensitive cation channels leads to an increase in intracellular cation concentration, which in turn leads to membrane depolarization, calcium-induced calcium release from the sarcoplasmic reticulum and smooth muscle contraction. Recent data suggest that in conditions of increased oxidative stress reactive oxygen species may also be involved in the myogenic response (Figure 5.6).

Pathophysiology

Vasoregulation distal to coronary stenosis

When there is significant narrowing in a large vessel, there is a reduction in distal pressure. During laminar flow, resistance to flow is inversely proportional to the fourth power of vessel radius (Poiseuille's law).

$$\text{Resistance} = 8 \times \text{Viscosity } (\eta) \times \text{Length}/\pi \times \text{Radius}^4$$

A post-stenotic pressure of 40 mmHg at rest has been suggested as being critical. Below that, if local metabolic demands increase and remaining vasodilatory reserves are not enough to increase flow, then relative hypoperfusion and ischemia results. In this setting, a larger proportion of total coronary vascular resistance is located in larger arteries when the distal vessels are maximally dilated. Extramural pressure and the arterial pressure-drop across penetrating intramyocardial arteries may decrease the margin for adequate coronary flow, particularly in subendocardial regions. Arterioles may retain a degree of responsiveness (vasomotor tone) even when there is a critical coronary stenosis, despite active metabolic vasoregulation.

Ischemia, vasodilatation and persistent vascular tone

While maximum vasodilatation might be expected in hypoxic or ischemic myocardial areas, there may be some persisting small artery tone despite hypoperfusion. Some persisting tone in more proximal arteries mediated by α-adrenergic mechanisms may be beneficial for redistribution and augmentation of subendocardial flow.

Angiontensin II and endothelin, as well as other mediators such as thromboxane A_2 and serotonin, are recognized as having coronary vasoconstrictor effects. They may also promote improved flow in hypoperfused myocardial regions through differential vascular effects in different areas of the coronary circulation.

Collateral blood flow

Collateral, interarterial vessels form in response to chronic myocardial ischemia. If the stimulus for collateral vessel development is gradual, MDO_2 may ultimately be sufficient at rest even in the presence of complete proximal coronary occlusion. Collateral vessels are subject to the same extramural forces and vasoregulatory mechanisms; their responsiveness can potentially be deleterious by diverting blood flow away from normal myocardium. (see Chapter 7).

Endothelial dysfunction

Endothelial dysfunction commonly occurs as a result of inflammation, atherosclerosis or diabetes mellitus.

Vasospasm – vasoconstriction unrelated to local MVO_2 – may occur as a consequence of autonomic imbalance, impaired local vasodilator mechanisms (endothelial or vascular smooth muscle dysfunction), inflammation or drug effects. Coronary spasm can lead to ventricular dysrhythmias, myocardial ischemia or myocardial infarction.

Interactions between perfusion and myocardium

Increases in coronary blood flow are associated with changes in A-V conduction and ventricular repolarization, as well as an increase in contractile force and MVO_2. This so-called "Gregg effect" is thought to be mediated via stretch-activated ion channels. In contrast, transient periods of coronary hypoperfusion induce transient myocardial contractile dysfunction that persists after reperfusion; a phenomenon known as "stunning". Myocardial stunning, hibernation and ischemic preconditioning are discussed further in Chapter 20.

Key points

- Coronary blood flow is coupled to MVO_2 and highly dependent on coronary vascular resistance.
- Under physiological conditions microcirculatory autoregulation controls vascular resistance and blood flow.
- Autoregulatory mechanisms include endothelial, metabolic, neurogenic and myogenic responses.
- Critical coronary stenosis impairs autoregulation and causes ischemia when MVO_2 is increased.

Further reading

Barbato E. Role of adrenergic receptors in human coronary vasomotion. *Heart* 2009; **95**(7): 603–8.

Camici PG, Crea F. Coronary microvascular dysfunction. *N Engl J Med* 2007; **356**(8): 830–40.

Duncker KJ, Bache RJ. Regulation of coronary blood flow during exercise. *Physiol Rev* 2008; **88**(3): 1009–86.

Liu Y, Gutterman DD. Vascular control in humans: focus on the coronary microcirculation. *Basic Res Cardiol* 2009; **104**(3): 211–27.

Spaan J, Kolyva C, van den Wijngaard J, *et al.* Coronary structure and perfusion in health and disease. *Philos Transact A Math Phys Eng Sci* 2008; **366**(1878): 3137–53.

Stern S, Bayes de Luna A. Coronary Artery Spasm. *Circulation* 2009; **119**(18): 2531–4.

Tune JD, Gorman MW, Feigle EO. Matching coronary blood flow to myocardial oxygen consumption. *J Appl Physiol* 2004; **97**(1): 404–15.

Chapter

6

Cardiovascular control mechanisms

Patrick Wouters

Introduction

Through evolution, higher organisms have developed complex cardiovascular control mechanisms to:

- preserve the internal milieu of cells, tissues and organs within a narrow range (homeostasis),
- adapt its performance to varying internal and external demands (allostasis).

These mechanisms exert their control in three areas: myocardial performance, vascular tone and blood volume (Table 6.1).

Table 6.1 Cardiovascular control mechanisms

Pump performance	Cardiac pump function: SV, HR
Vascular tone	Arteries, veins
Intravascular content	Blood volume, hematocrit

Some adaptive cardiovascular control mechanisms act within seconds (immediate), while others take minutes to hours (intermediate) or even weeks to months (long-term) to become fully operational. Furthermore, these mechanisms can be considered according to the level at which they operate: those that act within the isolated anatomical structures that comprise the cardiovascular system (intrinsic), and those that act remotely (extrinsic).

Table 6.2 Levels of cardiovascular control

Intrinsic	Heart: coronary blood flow, Frank-Starling relationship Vasculature: autoregulation
Extrinsic	Neural: autonomic, baroreceptor, chemoreceptor Humoral: renin/angiotensin, ADH, aldosterone, ANP

Intrinsic mechanisms

The heart

Heterometric autoregulation: the Frank-Starling relationship

An increase in preload causes myocardial contraction more forcefully. This fundamental property allows the heart to match venous return and cardiac output. In contrast to skeletal muscle, heterometric autoregulation cannot be explained by the sliding filament theory. Cardiac sarcomeres, which demonstrate a steeper length–tension relationship, nearly always function at optimal actin-myosin alignment. It is more likely that a direct relationship between sarcomere length and Ca^{2+} sensitivity (length-dependent activation) is the basic mechanism underlying the Frank-Starling relationship.

Homeometric autoregulation: the Anrep effect

An abrupt increase in afterload causes myocardial contraction more forcefully. This rise in contractility allows the heart to overcome increased resistance to ejection while keeping end-diastolic volume unchanged; hence the term homeometric. The precise mechanism is unclear but probably involves activation of sarcolemmal stretch receptors. The clinical significance of the Anrep effect is limited because of its narrow operating range. Indeed a progressive increase in afterload will ultimately reduce SV and lead to an increase in end-diastolic volume. Recent data suggest that the Anrep effect may play a more significant role in the right ventricle in the setting of pulmonary hypertension.

The force–frequency relationship: the Bowditch, treppe or staircase effect

An increase in HR increases myocardial contractility. Conversely, a decrease in HR has a negative effect on

Core Topics in Cardiac Anesthesia, Second Edition, ed. Jonathan H. Mackay and Joseph E. Arrowsmith. Published by Cambridge University Press. © Cambridge University Press 2012.

contractile performance. This is due to proportionally higher Ca^{2+} entry in comparison to Ca^{2+} removal in myocytes with increasing heart rates. The hemodynamic benefits of tachycardia are achieved at the expense of an increase in MVO_2 and are limited by reduced diastolic coronary blood flow and ventricular filling time.

The vascular system

Autoregulation of blood flow refers to the intrinsic capacity of organ systems to couple perfusion to metabolic requirements despite changes in arterial blood pressure. It is mediated by small arteries and arterioles by means of:

- *A myogenic mechanism*: an increase in blood pressure causes arteriolar vasoconstriction, while a decrease in blood pressure causes vasodilatation. Electrophysiological studies have shown that stretch depolarizes vascular smooth muscle cells and causes pacemaker cells to spontaneously depolarize and repolarize.
- *A metabolic mechanism*: any imbalance between substrate (e.g. O_2, glucose, etc.) supply and demand results in the accumulation of vasoactive metabolites. A number of substances (e.g. adenosine, CO_2, K^+) have been shown to contribute to this local autoregulatory mechanism. K_{ATP} channels have recently assumed a prominent role as mediators of local metabolic flow regulation.

Allostasis, the adaptation of regional blood flow to increased metabolic demands, is also partially regulated at the local level. The endothelium participates in this vasodilatory response by releasing NO during shear stress (see Chapter 5).

Control of circulating volume

There is no intrinsic hemodynamic mechanism for acute regulation of blood volume. However, the kidneys operate independently to regulate circulating volume and blood pressure by a mechanism called "pressure diuresis". This refers to the direct relationship between arterial blood pressure and urine output, and contributes to the autoregulation of volume status over a period of hours or days.

Extrinsic mechanisms

Superimposed on the local (intrinsic) adaptive mechanisms, extrinsic control is executed over the

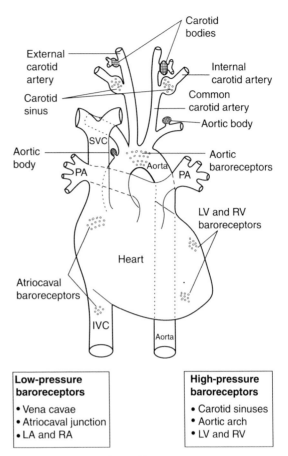

Low-pressure baroreceptors	High-pressure baroreceptors
• Vena cavae • Atriocaval junction • LA and RA	• Carotid sinuses • Aortic arch • LV and RV

Figure 6.1 Aortic and carotid baroreceptors.

cardiovascular system by the autonomic nervous system (ANS) and by hormonal feedback mechanisms.

The autonomic nervous system

Immediate cardiovascular control is predominantly under the influence of the ANS. The principal afferents arise from mechanoreceptors (high and low pressure sensors) and chemoreceptors in the major vessels and heart (Figure 6.1).

Information on pressure and the chemical composition of blood is continuously transmitted via vagal and spinal afferents to the vasomotor center in the brain stem. The nucleus of the solitary tract (NTS) is the first relay station for visceral afferents and is involved in all medullary autonomic reflexes.

Several areas in the brainstem and forebrain are reciprocally interconnected to form the central autonomic network. This network is also influenced by somatosensory input and behavior. From the NTS, neurotransmission continues via the ventral medulla to excitatory neurons in the rostral ventrolateral medulla (VLM), inhibitory neurons in the caudal VLM and the vagal cardiomotor neurons in the nucleus ambiguus (Figure 6.2). Excitatory connections are mediated by L-glutamine while inhibition is mediated by GABA and glycine.

The efferent components of ANS cardiovascular control comprise both the sympathetic and parasympathetic systems. Cardiac sympathetic efferents arising from the thoracic segments (T_1–T_4) cause positive chronotropy (increased heart rate), dromotropy (increased conduction velocity), inotropy (increased contractility) and lusitropy (better relaxation) primarily via the β_1-adrenergic effect of norepinephrine. Blood vessels receive postganglionic sympathetic efferents from the thoracolumbar region (T_1–L_3). Preganglionic sympathetic neurons originating in the thoracic spinal cord also innervate the adrenal medulla.

The parasympathetic efferents arise from the brain stem and sacral spinal segments. Postganglionic cardiac parasympathetic efferents are located primarily at the atrial level where the release of acetylcholine produces negative chronotropy and dromotropy.

Arterial baroreceptor reflex

This is the single most important immediate homeostatic mechanism regulating arterial pressure. High-pressure mechanoreceptors, located in the carotid sinus and aortic arch, encode the level and rate of change of arterial blood pressure. An increase in blood pressure causes a depressor reflex, i.e. an inhibition of sympathetic output and an increase in parasympathetic output. The net result is bradycardia, reduced cardiac performance and vasodilatation. A decrease in blood pressure has the opposite effect, i.e. a withdrawal of parasympathetic tone and an increase in sympathetic output.

Cardiopulmonary baroreceptor reflex

Stretch receptors located in the atria and pulmonary arteries operate at a lower pressure range but have

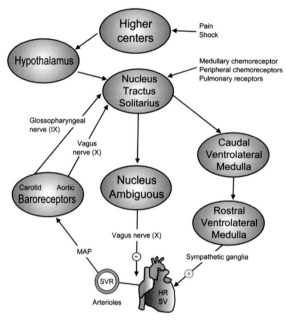

Figure 6.2 Baroreceptor reflexes. Reproduced from Arrowsmith JE, Falter F. Cardiovascular support: pharmacological. In: Griffiths M, Cordingley J, Price S (Eds.). *Cardiovascular Critical Care*. Oxford: Wiley Blackwell; 2010. pp. 100–19.

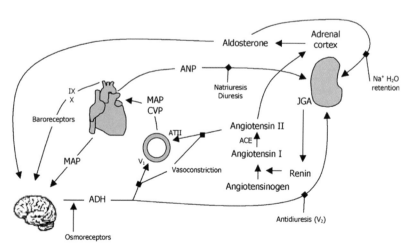

Figure 6.3 Control of intravascular volume. Reproduced from Arrowsmith JE, Falter F. Cardiovascular support: pharmacological. In Griffiths M, Cordingley J, Price S (Eds.). *Cardiovascular Critical Care*. Oxford: Wiley Blackwell; 2010. pp. 100–19.

a similar negative feedback loop. Hemodynamic responses are particularly powerful when these pressure receptors are activated at the same time as arterial mechanoreceptors. Atrial stretch receptors also play a role in volume regulation by stimulating the release of atrial natriuretic peptide (ANP), inhibiting the release of arginine-vasopressin from the hypothalamus, and decreasing renal renin release.

The Bezold–Jarisch reflex

Originally described as a hypotensive and bradycardic response to the injection of veratrine, this reflex is now recognized to originate from high-pressure mechanoreceptors and chemoreceptors in the ventricular wall. Afferent signals travel via unmyelinated C fibers. The Bezold–Jarisch (B-J) reflex is another negative feedback system, i.e. an increase in ventricular pressure inhibits sympathetic output from the vasomotor center. The B-J reflex operates in concert with the arterial baroreflex; the latter being the dominant regulator of blood pressure. The sympatho-inhibitory response of the B-J reflex, however, has a more pronounced effect on renal blood flow.

The Bainbridge reflex

Stimulation of low-pressure atrial sensors (innervated by dorsal root ganglion neurons) can cause an increase in sympathetic outflow with resultant tachycardia, vasoconstriction and inotropy. Conversely, low atrial pressure (volume) causes bradycardia – effectively opposing the high-pressure baroreceptor reflex. Teleologically speaking, the heart benefits from a positive feedback mechanism that counters volume overload. The reduction in HR associated with hypovolemia would allow more time for diastolic ventricular filling. The reflex is weak and in reality a direct relationship between filling status and HR is rarely observed. In contrast, tachycardia is mostly indicative of hypovolemia in adult patients, because the baroreceptor reflex is the dominant control mechanism. Exceptions, where the Bainbridge reflex may predominate, include neonates and infants, who often develop a tachycardia in response to acute volume overload and a bradycardia when hypovolemic. The paradoxical and sometimes life-threatening bradycardia in hypotensive patients recovering from spinal anesthesia has also been attributed to the Bainbridge reflex.

Arterial chemoreceptor reflex

Chemoreceptors in the carotid and aortic bodies respond primarily to a decrease in O_2 partial pressure. Stimulation results in a reflex increase in minute ventilation and an increase in sympathetic activity.

The sympathetic and parasympathetic nervous systems have been considered reciprocal components of the ANS with directionally opposite activity. Recent data question this simplified view and show that co-activation of both systems occurs frequently. Current research also focuses on the role of non-cholinergic, non-adrenergic transmitters which are co-localized in presynaptic vesicles, and released from the postganglionic autonomic (mainly parasympathetic) efferents.

Hormonal control

The adrenal medulla releases epinephrine and norepinephrine into the circulation. The concentration of norepinephrine in blood is three to five times higher than that of epinephrine; however, the majority represents spill-over from sympathetic nerve endings. In normal conditions neither circulating levels of epinephrine nor norepinephrine affect the cardiovascular system. The only exception is β_2-mediated vasodilatation by epinephrine in skeletal muscles during defense behavior or emotional excitation. Under physiological conditions, metabolic effects of epinephrine predominate. In pathophysiological conditions, such as denervation and receptor sensitization of the heart and vessels, circulating catecholamines assume a more prominent role in cardiovascular control.

Renin-angiotensin system

Hypotension causes the release of renin by the juxtaglomerular apparatus, which in turn triggers the hepatic production of angiotensin I. After conversion to angiotensin II, principally in the lungs, this potent vasoconstrictor contributes to blood pressure regulation. The renin-angiotensin vasoconstrictor system is unidirectional – it has no role in correcting increases in blood pressure. Angiotensin II also decreases the renal excretion of salt and water and stimulates aldosterone secretion.

Antidiuretic hormone and aldosterone

Antidiuretic hormone (ADH) is secreted by the posterior pituitary gland in response to an increase in plasma osmolality, and by hypotension and hypovolemia. It produces vasoconstriction and increases water retention in the kidney. The role of ADH in volume control is probably inferior to the mechanism of pressure diuresis. Together with the thirst mechanism, ADH provides a very precise control of body fluid osmolality and plasma sodium concentration. Aldosterone also contributes to sodium homeostasis, albeit to a lesser extent. Its primary function in the intact organism is to regulate potassium.

Atrial natriuretic peptide

Atrial natriuretic peptide is released by atrial myocytes in response to stretch. It produces vasodilatation, inhibits the release of renin and aldosterone, and increases renal sodium and water excretion.

Further reading

Armour JA. Cardiac neuronal hierarchy in health and disease. *Am J Physiol Regul Integr Comp Physiol* 2004; **287**(2): R262–71.

Campagna JA, Carter C. Clinical relevance of the Bezold-Jarisch reflex. *Anesthesiology* 2003; **98**(5): 1250–60.

Jänig W. *The Integrative Action of the Autonomic Nervous System: Neurobiology of Homeostasis.* Cambridge: Cambridge University Press; 2006. pp. 106–67.

Low PA, Benarroch EE. Cardiovascular and respiratory reflexes: physiology and pharmacology. In *Clinical Autonomic Disorders*, 3rd edition. Philadelphia: Lippincott Williams & Wilkins; 2008. pp. 43–56.

Paton JF, Boscan P, Pickering AE, Nalivaiko E. The yin and yang of cardiac autonomic control: vago-sympathetic interactions revisited. *Brain Res Brain Res Rev* 2005; **49**(3): 555–65.

Triposkiadis F, Karayannis G, Giamouzis G, Skoularigis J, Louridas G, Butler J. The sympathetic nervous system in heart failure physiology, pathophysiology, and clinical implications. *J Am Coll Cardiol* 2009; **54**(19): 1747–62.

Chapter

7

Anesthesia and the cardiovascular system

Ben W. Howes and Alan M. Cohen

Central nervous system (CNS) depression is the goal of general anesthesia, but it is accompanied by effects on the cardiovascular system (CVS). The various mechanisms involved are summarized in Table 7.1.

Volatile agents

Volatile agents depress sympathetic activity directly, with the exception of desflurane, which produces hyper-activity at 0.5–2.0 MAC. CNS depression and slowed action potential (AP) conduction reduce the reflex tachycardia resulting from reduced SVR and contractility. All fluorinated agents directly depress myocardial contractility by reducing Ca^{2+} influx into cardiac myocytes. The depressant effects of volatile agents result in decreased myocardial O_2 demand (MVO_2). Evidence suggests that this may improve myo-cardial oxygen balance during myocardial ischemia.

Most studies indicate that inhalational anesthetics can cause coronary vasodilatation. Isoflurane pro-duces dose-dependent vasodilatation, primarily in the small, high-resistance vessels (similar to sodium

Table 7.1 Mechanisms of action of anesthesia on the cardiovascular system

Direct pharmacological	Depression of cardiomyocyte contractility and action potential conduction Reduction of vasomotor tone in coronary and systemic circulations
Indirect pharmacological	Release of vasoactive substances (e.g. histamine) Sensitization of the heart to endogenous catecholamines Autonomic nervous system depression
Non-pharmacological	Tracheal intubation and extubation – increased HR, increased contractility and vasoconstriction via the sympathetic nervous system; or vagally mediated bradycardia Intermittent positive-pressure ventilation – impaired venous return Hypercarbia – increased HR, contractility and vasoconstriction via central chemoreceptors Patient positioning – changes in venous return

Table 7.2 Effects of volatile agents on the cardiovascular system

Properties	HR	MAP	CO	SVR	PVR	Catecholamine sensitization
Halothane	↓↓	↓↓	↓↓	↓	↓	↑↑↑
Nitrous oxide	–	–	–	–	↑/–	↑/↓
Enflurane	↑	↓↓	↓	↓	↓	↑
Isoflurane	↑↑	↓↓	↓	↓↓	↓	↑
Desflurane	↑	↓↓	↓	↓↓	↓/–	↑
Sevoflurane	↑/↓	↓↓	Slight ↓	↓	↓	↑

Core Topics in Cardiac Anesthesia, Second Edition, ed. Jonathan H. Mackay and Joseph E. Arrowsmith. Published by Cambridge University Press. © Cambridge University Press 2012.

33

nitroprusside), while halothane exerts its vasodilatory effects on large, low-resistance vessels (similar to glyceryl trinitrate). With the exception of isoflurane and desflurane, changes in coronary blood flow are in proportion to MVO_2 – autoregulation is maintained.

It has long been known that volatile anesthetic agents may induce dysrhythmias in the presence of circulating catecholamines. Direct laryngoscopy, surgical stimulation and conditions such as acidosis, hypokalemia and hypocalcemia may, therefore, provoke malignant dysrhythmias. Halothane, in particular, slows pacemaker APs by binding to sarcolemmal Ca^{2+} channels and permits other pacemaker tissue to predominate. This concern is largely historical as modern volatile agents (isoflurane, desflurane and sevoflurane) are generally unlikely to cause dysrhythmias at concentrations used in routine clinical practice.

Coronary steal

"Steal" is defined as an increase in blood flow to a normally perfused area following coronary arteriolar vasodilatation at the expense of a decrease in perfusion to a collateral dependent area. The prerequisite conditions for this phenomenon are (Figures 7.1 and 7.2):

- total occlusion of the artery supplying the "steal-prone" area
- perfusion of "steal-prone" area dependent on collateral vessels
- >90% stenosis in the artery supplying the collaterals.

Although isoflurane-induced coronary steal has been demonstrated in animal models there is limited evidence for its existence as a clinically relevant phenomenon in humans.

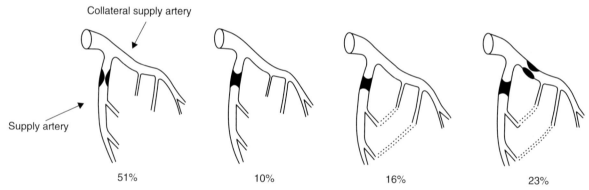

Figure 7.1 The four angiographic anatomical variants defined by the Coronary Artery Surgery Study (CASS) Registry. Total occlusion of a vessel associated with ≥50% stenosis in the collateral supply vessel was demonstrated in 23% of angiograms. However, only 12% of the 16 249 angiograms studied met the criteria for steal-prone anatomy – i.e. ≥90% stenosis of the collateral supply artery.

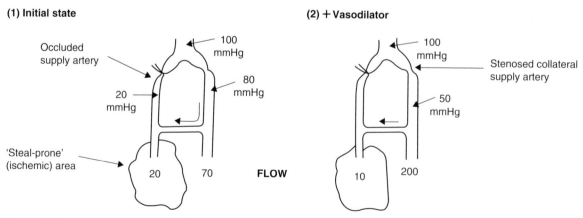

Figure 7.2 Proposed mechanism of vasodilator-induced coronary steal. In the initial state a collateral supply vessel pressure of 80 mmHg (distal to the stenosis) generates a perfusion pressure of 20 mmHg in the steal-prone (ischemic) area. Following vasodilator administration increased blood flow to the non-ischemic area reduces flow to the steal-prone area from 20 to 10 arbitrary units.

Table 7.3 Effects of intravenous anesthetic agent on the cardiovascular system

	HR	MAP	Contractility	SVR	PVR	Notes
Propofol	↓ or →	↓	↓	↓		
Thiopental	↑ or →	↓	↓	↓	↓	Effects depend on patient baroreceptor compensation
Etomidate	→	→	→	→		Adrenocortical suppression
Ketamine	↑	↑	↓	↑	↑	Sympathetic stimulation may precipitate CVS collapse
Benzodiazepines	→	↓	↓	↓	→	Less marked effects than propofol/thiopental

Anesthetic cardiac preconditioning

In addition to their indirect hemodynamic and cardio-protective effects (described above), recent research has suggested that inhalational anesthetic agents also provide direct protection against the adverse consequences of myocardial ischemia. This effect mimics ischemic preconditioning, where minor episodes of myocardial ischemia can result in protection from a subsequent severe ischemic episode (see Chapter 20). Research into the clinical usefulness of this phenomenon, by assessing release of cardiac troponin or early postoperative cardiac function, is ongoing. A systematic review, published in 2006, found that volatile anesthetic agents provided myocardial protection in patients undergoing coronary surgery, although no mortality benefit was demonstrated. The use of volatile anesthetic agents is now recommended by the American Heart Association for patients at risk of myocardial infarction undergoing non-cardiac surgery.

Nitrous oxide

Nitrous oxide (N_2O) produces modest dose-dependent cardiac depression. Unlike other inhalational agents, this effect is offset by an increase in SVR secondary to sympathetic stimulation. The addition of N_2O to a volatile anesthetic agent has been shown to result in less depression of arterial pressure than with volatile agents alone.

Intravenous anesthetic agents

The most commonly used agents, propofol and thiopental, are CVS depressants. Etomidate has minimal cardiovascular effects but its use is limited by significant suppression of the adrenocortical axis. Ketamine is a sympathomimetic which may cause ischemia in

Table 7.4 Effects of neuromuscular blocking drugs on the cardiovascular system

	CVS effects	Notes
Suxamethonium	↑HR, ↑SVR. ↓HR in children and in repeat dosing	Sympathetic mediated. ↑oxygen demand may worsen ischemia
Aminosteroids e.g. vecuronium, rocuronium	Usually no effects. ↓HR in combination with fentanyl	Profound neuromuscular block is rapidly reversible with sugammadex
Atracurium	↑HR, ↓SVR can occur due to histamine release	
Pancuronium	↑HR (due to atropine-like antimuscarinic effect)	Can be used to prevent fentanyl-induced bradycardia

the presence of coronary disease if not used carefully. Whichever agent is used, experience and careful titration are required to prevent CVS instability. Intravenous sedative agents such as benzodiazepines (e.g. midazolam) are commonly used as adjuncts to intravenous anesthetic drugs to limit the required dose and minimize their adverse cardiovascular effects.

Neuromuscular blocking drugs

Currently used neuromuscular blocking drugs generally have few cardiovascular effects although

Table 7.5 Effect of local anesthetics on the cardiovascular system

	Maximum dose	CVS effects in toxicity	Notes
Lidocaine	3.0 mg kg^{-1} (plain) 7.0 mg kg^{-1} (with adrenaline)	Pro-dysrhythmic	CNS effects of toxicity (e.g. tinnitus) occur earlier than CVS effects
Bupivacaine	2.0 mg kg^{-1}	Pro-dysrhythmic	CVS effects may be first sign of toxicity
Levobupivacaine[a]	2.5–3.0 mg kg^{-1}	↓↓contractility, CVS collapse at high concentration	

[a] Maximum safe dose undetermined.

individual drugs may have their own effects, such as vasodilatation due to histamine release caused by atracurium.

Regional anesthesia

The CVS effects of regional anesthetic techniques result either from sympathetic blockade or from inadvertent IV injection of local anesthetic drugs. Neuraxial blockade with local anesthetics causes sympathetic block, resulting in ↓SVR, ↓MAP and compensatory ↑HR to maintain cardiac output. Neuraxial anesthesia should be used with particular caution in conditions such as severe AS, where CO is limited ("limited" being a preferable term to the more commonly used "fixed"), since adequate compensation may be impossible and lead to CVS collapse. An inadvertently high neuraxial block (e.g. "high spinal") may result in cardiac sympathetic blockade. This initially manifests as bradycardia, but may progress to malignant dysrhythmias and, ultimately, cardiac arrest.

Sub-toxic doses of local anesthetic drugs in the circulation do not have clinically significant hemodynamic or dysrhythmogenic effects. However, toxic doses resulting from inadvertent IV injection can lead to severe cardiovascular effects and, in the case of bupivacaine, a potentially fatal reduction in cardiac contractility. Life-threatening local anesthetic toxicity has been successfully treated with intravenous administration of lipid emulsion.

Opioids

Opioids have formed an important part of anesthetic techniques for cardiac surgery since Lowenstein first advocated the use of high-dose morphine (1–3 mg

Table 7.6 Effects of opioids on cardiovascular system

Fentanyl

Part of balanced anesthesia at 10–15 µg kg^{-1}. Occasional ↓HR, generally stable.

Morphine

Unpredictable effect on diseased heart.
Histamine release and direct action causes ↓SVR.
May cause ↓HR via vagus. Used mainly post-operatively.

Alfentanil

Shorter half-life than fentanyl. Given by loading dose and infusion.
No advantage over fentanyl for cardiac surgery and possibly less CVS stability.

Remifentanil

Ultra-short-acting, extra-hepatic metabolism. Given by infusion.
Rapidly administered high doses cause muscle rigidity and bradycardia.
Cessation only in the presence of an alternative analgesic technique.

Sufentanil

5–10 times more potent than fentanyl.
High-dose sufentanil (15 µg kg^{-1}) is virtually indistinguishable from high-dose fentanyl (100 µg kg^{-1}).

kg^{-1}) for patients undergoing valve surgery in 1969. Morphine was superseded by high-dose fentanyl (50–150 µg kg^{-1}), which provided greater hemodynamic stability – primarily due to the absence of histamine release. Intermediate-dose fentanyl (10–15 µg kg^{-1}) is common in current practice as it causes less bradycardia and muscle rigidity at induction, as well as facilitating earlier postoperative tracheal extubation.

Opioids have relatively few effects on the CVS in comparison to other agents and reduce the dose of induction and maintenance agents required. At high doses they reduce the stress response and provide postoperative analgesia. Hemodynamic autoregulation is preserved and there are few toxic effects. Opioids must be given as part of a balanced anesthetic technique to reduce side effects: respiratory, CNS and GI depression, nausea, vomiting and pruritis.

CPB significantly alters opioid pharmacodynamics. The effects of hemodilution and sequestration are balanced, in part, by a reduction in plasma protein binding and a reduction in elimination. The overall effect is a reduction in opioid concentration at the onset of CPB. During prolonged hypothermic CPB, however, the impact of reduced clearance tends to predominate when opioids are administered by infusion.

The effect of CPB on the pharmacokinetics of anesthetic drugs is discussed in Chapter 12.

Key points

- The CNS effects of general anesthesia are mirrored in other organ systems.
- The CVS effects of anesthetic agents are dependent on patient age and physiological status.
- Anesthetics have both direct and indirect actions on the CVS.

- Direct myocardial and vascular depression is often compensated for or obscured by autonomic reflexes.

Further reading

Agnew NM, Pennefather SH, Russell GN. Isoflurane and coronary heart disease. *Anaesthesia* 2002; **57**(4): 338–47.

Ebert TG, Muzi M. Sympathetic hyperactivity during desflurane anesthesia in healthy volunteers. A comparison with isoflurane. *Anesthesiology* 1993; **79**(3): 444–53.

Fleisher LA, Beckman JA, Brown KA, *et al.* ACC/AHA 2007 Guidelines on perioperative cardiovascular evaluation and care for noncardiac surgery. *J Am Coll Cardiol* 2007; **50**(17): 1707–32.

Landoni G, Biondi-Zoccai GG, Zangrillo A, Bignami, *et al.* Desflurane and sevoflurane in cardiac surgery: a meta-analysis of randomized clinical trials. *J Cardiothorac Vasc Anesth* 2007; **21**(4): 502–11.

Lowenstein E, Hallowell P, Levine FH, Daggett WM, Austen WG, Laver MB. Cardiovascular response to large doses of intravenous morphine in man. *N Engl J Med* 1969; **281**(25): 1389–93.

Priebe H-J. Isoflurane and coronary hemodynamics. *Anesthesiology* 1989; **71**(6): 960–76.

Rusy BF, Komai H. Anesthetic depression of myocardial contractility: a review of possible mechanisms. *Anesthesiology* 1987; **67**(5): 745–66.

Symons JA, Myles PS. Myocardial protection with volatile anaesthetic agents during coronary artery bypass surgery: a meta-analysis. *Br J Anaesth* 2006; **97**(2): 127–36.

Appendix

Table 7.7 Summary of pharmacokinetic data for opioids commonly used in cardiac anesthesia

	Morphine	Alfentanil	Fentanyl	Sufentanil	Remifentanil
pKa	7.93,9.63	6.5	8.43	8.01	7.07
Solubility: ethanol	1:250	1:5	1:140	–	–
Solubility: water	1:5000	1:7	1:40	–	–
Octanol/H_2O partition coefficient	6.03	145	955	1.75	17.9
Ditribution half-life (min)	–	3.5	5–12	1.4	1
Elimination half-life (h)	2	1.2	1–4	3.5	0.15
Clearance (ml kg^{-1} min^{-1})	11.5	7.5	12.8	11.3	40–60
V_D (l kg^{-1})	1.5–4	0.28	3–4	2.9	0.1–0.2
V_D – steady state (l kg^{-1})	1–3	0.996	2.2	1.7	0.3
Protein binding (%)	35	89	80	91	70

V_D = volume of distribution.

Cardiac receptors

Todd Kiefer and Mihai V. Podgoreanu

Homeostatic regulation of the cardiovascular system relies on the ability of the heart to recognize and respond to many extracellular signaling molecules, including peptides, biogenic amines, steroid hormones, fatty acid derivatives and a variety of other classes of small molecules (Table 8.1). These extracellular messengers reach their cellular targets by four different signaling routes: *endocrine* (carried in the bloodstream), *neurotransmitter* (released from nerve endings), *paracrine* (diffused from an adjacent cell), and *autocrine* (released by the same cell).

The response to a given extracellular messenger (*ligand*, "first" messenger) is mediated by receptors, which are proteins that recognize and bind high-affinity specific ligands. After a ligand binds to a receptor, a multi-step signal transduction cascade is set in motion that eventually results in a functional response within the cell. This may be a change in intracellular ion concentration or gene expression, for example. However, the biological pathways that make up the *signal transduction cascade* generally branch at multiple steps, involve both positive and negative feedback loops, and often interconnect with other receptor signaling pathways to affect disparate pathways in a manner independent of the native ligand. This allows regulatory control to be exercised on signal transduction, which may take the form of amplification of the response, its integration with other responses, or its termination to prevent uncontrolled signaling after receptor binding. Such signal diversification explains how, during hemodynamic stress, neurohormonal-regulatory mediators

Table 8.1 Extracellular messengers involved in regulation of cardiac function

Peptides	Purines	Catecholamines	Steroids	Fatty acid derivatives	Other molecules
Growth factors	Adenosine	Epinephrine	Aldosterone	Eicosanoids (prostaglandins, leukotrienes, lipoxins)	Nitric oxide (NO)
Cytokines	ATP, ADP	Norepinephrine	Estrogen	Circulating free fatty acids	Acetylcholine
Angiotensin-II		Dopamine	Cortisol		Histamine
Arginine vasopressin (antidiuretic hormone, ADH)					Thyroxine
Bradykinin					1α-25-dihydroxy-vitamin D_3
Natriuretic peptides (ANP, BNP)					Bile acids
Erythropoietin					Oxysterols

Core Topics in Cardiac Anesthesia, Second Edition, ed. Jonathan H. Mackay and Joseph E. Arrowsmith. Published by Cambridge University Press. © Cambridge University Press 2012.

(catecholamines, endothelin, angiotensin-II and vasopressin) may cause both short-term *functional responses* (positive inotropic, lusitropic, chronotropic effects, vasoconstriction and fluid retention), and also slower *proliferative responses* and programmed cell death (*apoptosis*), which play important (often maladaptive) roles in chronic heart disease.

Classification

There are four broad classes of receptors: *plasma membrane receptors* (bind ligands at the cell surface, Table 8.2), *intracellular receptors* (bind ligands that enter the cytosol), *nuclear receptors* (ligand-activated transcription factors that bind to target genes in the nucleus), and *adhesion molecules* (involved in cell-cell and cell-matrix interactions).

The most physiologically and pharmacologically relevant receptors involved in regulation of cardiac function interact with heterotrimeric guanyl nucleotide-binding proteins (*G-proteins*), and are part of one of the largest family of receptors in biology commonly called *G-protein-coupled receptors* (GPCRs). The receptors contain a conserved structure of seven hydrophobic α-helices that lie within the lipid bilayer of the cell membrane, and so are often referred to as *seven-transmembrane-spanning* or *heptahelical* receptors. The G-protein subunits amplify and propagate signals in the cytoplasm by modulating the activity of effector molecules such as adenylyl cyclase (AC), phospholipases and ion channels. In turn, these *effector molecules* regulate the production of *second messenger molecules* (cyclic adenosine monophosphate, cAMP; cyclic guanosine monophosphate, cGMP; inositol-1,4,5-triphosphate, InsP3; diacylglycerol, DAG; and Ca^{2+}), in a highly complex pathway that ultimately activates *serine/threonine protein kinases* (protein kinase A, PKA; protein kinase C, PKC; and Ca^{2+}-calmodulin complex, CaM kinase) responsible for both the *functional* and *proliferative* cellular responses (Figure 8.1, Table 8.3).

Table 8.2 Plasma membrane receptors

GPCRs	Ion-channel receptors	Enzyme-linked receptors
$\alpha_{1A, 1B, 1D}$ receptor subtypes $\alpha_{2A, 2B, 2C}$ receptor subtypes	L-type Ca^{2+} channels	Tyrosine kinase receptors Fibroblast growth factor (FGF) receptors Platelet-derived growth factor (PDGF) receptors Insulin-like growth factor (IGF) receptors Vascular endothelial growth factor (VEGF) receptors Erythropoietin (EPO) receptors
$\beta_{1,2,3}$ receptor subtypes	Ach receptors	Cytokine receptors Tumor necrosis factor α (TNFα) receptors Interleukin receptors Growth hormone receptors Transforming growth factor (TGF) receptors Bone morphogenetic protein receptors
M_2 muscarinic receptors	Serotonin receptors	Other receptors Atrial natriuretic peptide (ANP) receptors Brain natriuretic peptide (BNP) receptors
Adenosine receptors		
Arginine vasopressin (ADH) receptors		
Bradykinin receptors		
Endothelin receptors		
Histamine receptors		
Dopaminergic receptors		
APJ receptors (apelin)		

Table 8.3 Important GPCRs

Receptor	Tissue distribution	Ligand	Primary G-protein	Primary effector	Second messengers
β_1-AR	Heart	Norepinephrine, epinephrine, β-agonists	G_s	L-type Ca^{2+} channel hyperpolarization-activated cyclic nucleotide-gated channels, phospholamban, troponin I and myosin binding protein-C, phospholemman	↑ cAMP/PKA
β_2-AR	Heart, lung, vessels, kidney	Norepinephrine, epinephrine, β-agonists	G_s, G_i	L-type Ca^{2+} channel hyperpolarization-activated cyclic nucleotide-gated channels, phospholamban, troponin I and myosin-binding protein-C, phospholemman	↑ cAMP/PKA
β_3-AR	Heart, brain, adipose, liver, myometrium, bladder	Norepinephrine, epinephrine	G_i	Adenylate cyclase	↑ cGMP ↓ cAMP
$\alpha_{1A, 1B, 1D^-}$ AR AT_1, ET	Heart, vessels, smooth muscle	Norepinephrine, epinephrine, α-agonists, angiotensin-II, endothelin	G_q	PLC_b	↑ DAG/InsP$_3$, PKC, AKT
α_2-AR	Coronary vessels, CNS, pancreas, platelet	Norepinephrine, epinephrine	G_i	Adenylate cyclase	↓ cAMP/PKA
M_2	Heart	Acetylcholine	G_i	Adenylate cyclase, K^+ channels	↓ cAMP/PKA, ↑ outward K^+ current
A_2	Coronary vessels, heart, PA	Adenosine	G_s	Adenylate cyclase, K_{ATP} channels, N-type Ca^{2+} channels	↑ cAMP/PKA, ↑ outward K^+ current
APJ	Heart, vessels	Apelin	G_i, G_q	Adenylate cyclase, PLC	↓ cAMP/PKA, ↑ DAG/InsP$_3$, PKC

Regulation

The ligand-receptor interaction is determined by two properties of the receptor: the *binding affinity* (expressed as the dissociation constant, K_d), and the receptor *density*. Regulation of GPCR function is mediated by a process called *desensitization*, which reduces the receptor responsiveness to its extracellular messengers (Figure 8.2). Two important examples with clinical implications for the cardiac anesthesiologist include the desensitization of β-adrenergic receptors (β-ARs), which can be *chronic* in the failing heart (due to chronic activation of the sympathetic nervous

41

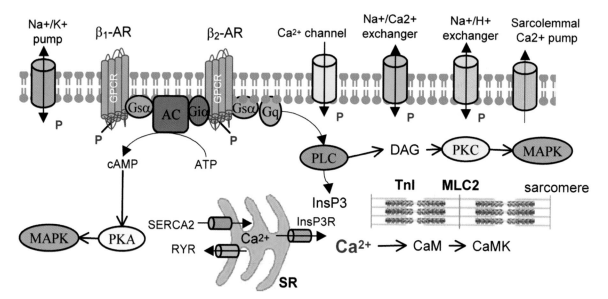

Figure 8.1 The β-adrenergic signal transduction cascade in cardiomyocytes leading to Ca^{2+}-mediated Ca^{2+} release. Agonist binding to either $β_1$- or $β_2$-AR stimulates $G_{sα}$ protein, which binds to AC, catalyzing the production of cAMP from ATP, and activation of PKA. PKA phosphorylates the voltage-dependent L-type Ca^{2+} channels, Na^+/H^+ exchange channels and Na^+/K^+ pump at the sarcolemma, the ryanodine receptor (RYR) and phospholamban (PLB) at the sarcoplasmic reticulum (SR), and troponin-I (TnI) in the sarcomeres, resulting in increased inotropic and lusitropic effects. The $β_2$-AR is also able to bind $G_{iα}$- or G_q-proteins; G_q activates phospholipase C (PLC), which causes the release of DAG and InsP3. InsP3 binds to the InsP3 receptor (InsP3R) and releases Ca^{2+} from the SR. Ca^{2+} combines with calmodulin (CaM), which activates the CaM-dependent protein kinases (CaMK) and the sarcolemmal Ca^{2+} pump, which ultimately results in the phosphorylation of PLB, myosin light chain 2 (MLC2), and Na^+/Ca^{2+} exchanger. DAG and CaM activate PKC, which in turn phosphorylates MLC2. The dephosphorylated regulatory protein PLB binds to the SR Ca^{2+} pump (SERCA2), inhibiting its activity; phosphorylation by PKA and/or CaMK causes PLB to dissociate from SERCA2, relieving the inhibitory effect. Note the activation of proliferative responses by both PKA and PKC via the MAPK pathways.

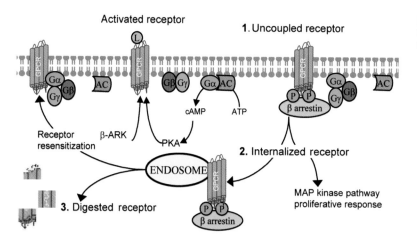

Figure 8.2 Mechanisms of β-AR desensitization: L, ligand; $G_{αβγ}$, G-protein subunits.

system) and *acute* after CPB (due to associated catecholamine surges). One mechanism for desensitization is receptor *down-regulation*, which refers to a decrease in the number of receptors expressed on the cell surface. This occurs when there is decreased transcription of the gene that encodes the receptor, destabilization of receptor messenger RNA that diminishes translation into the receptor protein, or increased receptor degradation (operates over hours). In general, receptor desensitization occurs by a sequential three-step process: *uncoupling* (phosphorylation), *internalization* (sequestration) and *digestion* (degradation). Uncoupling is a rapid process (seconds to minutes) that occurs when a protein kinase called *β-adrenergic receptor kinase* (β-ARK) phosphorylates a ligand-bound β-AR, thereby preventing it from activating a G-protein. β-ARK is one of a family of protein kinases called *G-protein receptor kinases* (GRKs). β-ARK-mediated desensitization requires a co-factor called *β-arrestin*, which binds to the phosphorylated C-terminal intracellular peptide chain. β-Arrestin also functions to attract phosphodiesterase (which metabolizes cAMP to an inactive state) to the β-AR receptor complex to further regulate the intracellular signaling process. As GRKs phosphorylate only agonist-occupied GPCRs, this process is known as "agonist-specific" or *homologous desensitization*. In contrast, second messengers can be phosphorylated by protein kinases activated by other signal transduction systems (e.g. PKA by cAMP and PKC by DAG), in a process called "non-agonist-specific" or *heterologous desensitization*. Likewise, PKA has been shown to phosphorylate the β-AR thereby switching receptor coupling from Gs to Gi in a feedback loop process to decrease signaling after the initial wave of biochemical activation. Uncoupling is a fully reversible step, as the receptors can be dephosphorylated by *GPCR phosphatases* in a process called *resensitization*. Another level of control in the redundant mechanisms designed to tightly regulate signaling pathways involves receptor trafficking. The two identified destinations for β-ARs are *recycling* and *degradation*. Receptor internalization occurs when the phosphorylated β-arrestin-bound uncoupled receptors are removed from the plasma membrane and transferred inside the cell, in a process that is still reversible. Internalized β2-AR-β-arrestin complexes can act as scaffolds that activate mitogen-activated protein kinase (MAPK)-mediated proliferative pathways, with significant implications in pressure-overload hypertrophy and ventricular remodeling. Manipulating myocardial β-ARK activity to improve functional responsiveness to catecholamines in cardiomyopathy and heart failure is the focus of intense research. After a prolonged exposure to an agonist, proteolytic enzymes within the cell digest the internalized receptors, which is the final, irreversible step of the desensitization process.

A reverse process, of enhanced sensitivity, can be seen after the heart is denervated or more commonly after prolonged administration of β-adrenergic blockers (*denervation sensitivity*). This appears to be the result of increased numbers of β-ARs by a process of externalization. Increased β-AR density on the cell surface makes abrupt withdrawal of β-blocker therapy dangerous and may be implicated in the etiology of atrial dysrhythmias after cardiac surgery.

The complexity of this elegant biological signaling system has been further delineated with research demonstrating that GPCRs may transmit intracellular signals in a G-protein-independent manner. This process relies on the activation of β-arrestin and its interaction with a different program of cellular signaling than that which occurs in response to G-protein-mediated signaling. Future research will explore the disparate signaling pathways linked to the β-AR and potential ways to pharmacologically alter the activation of the pathways through the use of biased ligands, which are discussed below in the section on receptor blockade.

Recent studies have demonstrated a *genetic basis* for the regulation of many GPCRs. Genetic heterogeneity in the structure of both $β_1$- and $β_2$-ARs in the human population has been identified and associated with various degrees of receptor down-regulation or altered coupling to Gs. Genetic polymorphisms in the β-ARs and other receptors and signaling molecules may lead to an understanding of the inter-individual differences in the pathophysiology of congestive heart failure, responses to treatment for heart failure and the hemodynamic response to CPB among other cardiovascular processes. In the future, it is anticipated that this line of genomic research will contribute to the identification of high-risk individuals and the design of appropriate personalized therapeutic strategies (Table 8.4).

Receptor blockade

Classically, ligands that interact with receptors were classified as *agonists* (if binding activates the signal transduction cascade), *antagonists* (no intracellular signal) and *partial agonists* (weak activation of the signal transduction cascade, e.g. intrinsic sympathomimetic activity), with all exhibiting competitive kinetics. Recent research in transgenic animals emphasizes the importance of a two-state model of receptor activation (at least for β-ARs) by competitive ligands. In the absence of a ligand, the receptor can undergo spontaneous transition from the inactivated

Table 8.4 Genetic polymorphisms and associated cardiovascular phenotypes

Polymorphism	Observed phenotype
β_1-AR ARG→GLY 389	Decreased inotropic support post cardiopulmonary bypass in CABG patients treated chronically with metoprolol
	Increased heart rate and myocardial contractility in response to dobutamine
	In patients with HF, higher peak oxygen consumption values
	Improved survival in patients treated with the beta-blocker bucindolol
	Greater ejection fraction improvement in heart failure patients treated with metoprolol or carvedilol
β_1-AR SER→GLY 49	Increased survival and decreased left ventricular end-diastolic diameter in HF patients treated with beta-blockers
β_2-AR GLY→ARG 16	Increased survival in patients treated with beta-blockers following an acute coronary syndrome
β_2-AR GLN→GLU 27	Increased risk of sudden cardiac death
β_2-AR THR→ILE 164	Decreased responsiveness to β_2-AR stimulation
α_{2C}-AR deletion 322–325	Increased risk to develop HF in African-Americans. Risk is even greater if the β_1-AR ARG→GLY 389 polymorphism is jointly present
GRK5 LEU 41	Increased transplant-free survival in patients with congestive heart failure

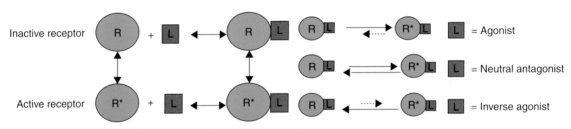

Figure 8.3 Two-state model of β-AR activation: R, inactive receptor; R*, active receptor; L, ligand.

(R) to the activated (R*) state (Figure 8.3). Ligands can be classified into *agonists, neutral agonists* and *inverse agonists* according to their tendency to shift this equilibrium towards the active-state R* (agonists) or inactive-state R (inverse agonists). Although most β-adrenergic blockers act as inverse agonists, some with weak inverse agonist effects may be classified as neutral antagonists. The following β-adrenergic blockers display increasing inverse agonist effects: bucindolol < carvedilol < propranolol < metoprolol. The model explains the inability of neutral antagonists to fully block the effects of receptor over-expression, as they counteract activation by endogenous catecholamines but not by spontaneous transition into the active receptor conformation. This may be of clinical relevance with respect to the tolerability of various

β-adrenergic blockers and the treatment of withdrawal syndrome .

Furthermore, a novel concept termed *biased ligands* has emerged from research involving β-ARs, β-arrestin and GRKs. Biased ligands appear to function as antagonists of the classic β-AR-mediated signaling pathways while activating β-arrestin signaling, leading to activation of various cell survival signaling programs. A more complete understanding of the physiology and pharmacology related to biased ligands is the focus of ongoing research.

Emerging receptor concepts

While β-adrenergic receptors remain the most extensively studied and characterized model of

Table 8.5 Nuclear receptors

Receptor	Ligands	Cardiovascular effects
PPAR ($\alpha,\beta/\delta,\gamma$)	Fatty acids, fibrates, leukotriene B4, thiazolidinediones	Regulation of metabolic activity, blood pressure, myocardial hypertrophy and ischemia-reperfusion injury
Thyroid hormone receptor	Triiodothyronine (T3)	Increased inotropy, chronotropy and cardiac output Decreased systemic vascular resistance Regulation of myocardial metabolism
Estrogen receptor (ERα, ERβ)	17β-estradiol	Endothelial function, vasodilatation, atherogenesis, regulation of lipid metabolism, and myocardial anti-hypertrophic effects
Estrogen receptor related receptor (ERR)	Orphan	Interacts with PGC-1 to alter cellular energy utilization and response to pressure overload
Mineralocorticoid receptor	Aldosterone, spironolactone	Myocardial fibrosis, myocardial hypertrophy, sodium and water retention, hypertension
Vitamin D receptor	1α-25-dihydroxy-vitamin D_3	Inhibition of left ventricular hypertrophy via multiple mechanisms, putative anti-inflammatory, anti-thrombotic and anti-atherosclerotic actions
Glucocorticoid receptor	Cortisol	Associated with accelerated atherosclerosis, hypertension and adverse cardiovascular events
Liver X receptors (LXRα, LXRβ)	Oxysterols	Cholesterol and fatty acid homeostasis, atherogenesis, control of innate immunity and inflammation
Farnesoid X receptor	Bile acids	Metabolic control of lipid, glucose and energy homeostasis, control of inflammatory pathways, atherogenesis

cardiovascular physiology and pharmacology, the importance of *nuclear receptors* (e.g. peroxisome proliferator-activated receptors, PPARs) and *cytokine/growth factor receptors* (e.g. erythropoietin) in cardiac physiology and as therapeutic targets is being rapidly recognized. Several representative examples are discussed in the following sections.

Nuclear receptors

Nuclear receptors (NRs) are transcription factors that respond to hormonal and environmental signals by inducing adaptive transcriptional responses involved in regulation of many biological processes responsible for cardiac and vascular pathobiology, such as metabolic control (both glucose and lipid), inflammation, proliferation in the vascular wall, and regulation of circadian rhythms. The human NR superfamily contains 48 members, all sharing a conserved modular structure that includes a ligand-binding domain and a DNA-binding domain. The first identified, and hence termed "classical" NRs were the hormone (estrogen,

androgen, mineralocorticoid and glucocorticoid) receptors. Members of the "nonclassical" group were originally discovered as so-called "orphan" receptors because they lacked an identifiable ligand; however, several of them had been "de-orphanized" over the last several years (Table 8.5). Many of these are activated by dietary-derived compounds, such as fatty acids and derivatives for the PPARs, oxysterols for the liver X receptors (LXRs), and bile acids for the farnesoid X receptor (FXR).

The classic model of NR receptor activation involves the binding of a lipophilic ligand to the ligand-binding domain of the receptor within the cell (Figure 8.4). This contrasts with the model for G-protein-coupled and tyrosine kinase receptors, where the interaction between receptor and ligand occurs at the interface of the cell membrane and extracellular milieu. Once bound by ligand, the receptor forms a homo- or heterodimer, which varies according to specific NR subtype. Subsequently, this dimerized complex interacts with various DNA response elements in the promoter regions of target

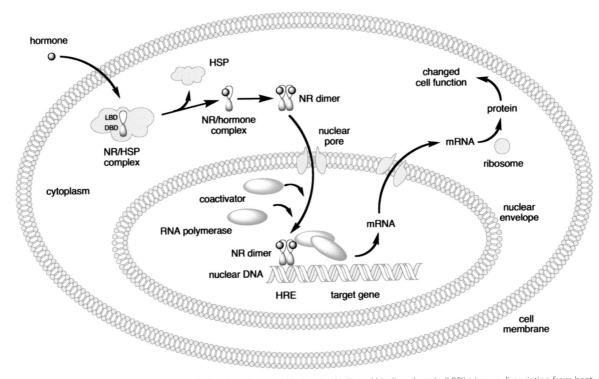

Figure 8.4 Mechanism of nuclear receptor (NR) action. Hormone binding to the ligand binding domain (LBD) triggers dissociation from heat shock protein (HSP), dimerization, and translocation to the nucleus where it binds to a specific DNA sequence known as the NR/hormone response element (HRE), a process regulated by coactivator and corepressor proteins. The NR DNA complex in turn recruits other proteins that are responsible for translation of downstream DNA into RNA and eventually protein, which results in changes in cell function.

genes to both induce and repress the expression of specific genes, leading to an alteration of cellular physiology. The regulation of this process is tightly controlled by the interaction of multiple coactivator and corepressor molecules with the nuclear receptor-DNA complex. An example of one such coactivator is the peroxisome proliferator-activated receptor γ coactivator-1 (PGC-1) that plays a pivotal role in the expression of genes related to cellular metabolism, energy utilization, and mitochondrial functional capacity and biogenesis by several members of the NR superfamily. Moreover, an added layer of complexity has been reported with the ligand-independent activation of NRs via phosphorylation events initiated by intracellular signaling kinases. Thus, the NR signaling model represents another distinct paradigm in the field of signal transduction biology.

In addition to regulating transcription of target genes via binding to NR response elements, many NRs display anti-inflammatory activities. The classic example is the glucocorticoid receptor, which mediates the effects of glucocorticoids. One more recent example of a NR with multiple effects on the cardiovascular system is the PPAR family. There are three PPAR subtypes, PPAR-α, PPAR-β/δ and PPAR-γ, encoded by different genes. Each PPAR subtype (α, β/δ or γ) forms a heterodimer with the retinoid X receptor (RXR) once a ligand binds to the PPAR ligand-binding domain. A number of different ligands for the various PPAR subtypes have been identified. PPAR-α is the target for the fibrate class of pharmacological agents used to treat hypertriglyceridemia. PPAR-γ is activated by the thiazolidinedione class of pharmacological agents used in the treatment of diabetes mellitus. Several experimental synthetic agonists of PPAR-β have also been identified. Currently, scientific evidence suggests that fatty acids are the endogenous agonists for the PPAR family. The actions of the PPARs on cardiovascular function vary with receptor subtype, with a common theme being anti-inflammatory effects mediated by a complex interplay of metabolic actions on adipose tissue, immune cells (macrophages, monocytes), endothelial cells and the myocardium. Furthermore, experimental work in animal models of hypertension has linked PPAR-α and PPAR-γ activation with decreased blood pressures. Similarly, the downregulation of PPAR-α has been implicated in the pathogenesis of myocardial hypertrophy. Another important line of research has investigated the role of PPAR-α and PPAR-γ in models of ischemia-reperfusion injury where agonists of these receptor subtypes were associated with smaller infarct sizes and preservation of left ventricular function. The ultimate role of PPARs in the modulation of the cardio-metabolic axis to prevent and/or treat cardiovascular diseases remains to be determined.

Erythropoietin

Erythropoietin (EPO) is a well-characterized growth factor responsible for stimulating red blood cell development. Along with its traditional role in erythropoiesis, EPO is also involved in various aspects of cardiac function. It exerts its actions on target cells by binding to tyrosine kinase-linked receptors on the cell membrane. The EPO receptor is expressed in cardiac myocytes, cardiac fibroblasts, vascular smooth muscle cells and endothelial cells. In the cardiovascular system, the EPO receptor activates the JAK2, STAT, ERK1/2, Akt and PI3K signaling pathways to initiate a cellular response through changes in gene expression, inhibition of apoptosis and stimulation of endothelial nitric oxide synthase. Experimental evidence from numerous animal studies of myocardial infarction and ischemia-reperfusion injury have demonstrated that EPO administration decreases infarct size and adverse remodeling, and minimizes the loss of left ventricular systolic function. However, small studies in humans have led to equivocal findings. At the present time, several ongoing clinical trials are investigating the potential cardioprotective role of EPO in humans.

Key points

- Regulation of cardiac performance involves changes in cell biochemistry, changes in organ physiology and proliferative responses.
- These functional and proliferative responses are mediated by a large variety of receptors and highly complex signal transduction pathways.
- Understanding the mechanisms involved in receptor desensitization has important clinical applications.
- A two-state model of receptor activation has replaced classic ideas about β-receptor agonists and antagonists. The β-receptor can undergo spontaneous transition between the inactivated and activated states.
- Recent studies have demonstrated genetic polymorphisms in the regulation of β-ARs.
- A greater understanding of genetic polymorphism data could be utilized to predict patients at risk for cardiovascular disease, and to personalize therapy for optimal outcome.

Further reading

Brodde OE. β1- and β2-adrenoreceptor polymorphisms and cardiovascular diseases. *Fund Clin Pharmacol* 2008; **22**: 107–25.

Dorn GW, Liggett SB. Mechanisms of pharmacogenomic effects of genetic variation within the cardiac adrenergic network in heart failure. *Mol Pharmacol* 2009; **76**: 466–80.

Huang W, Glass C. Nuclear receptors and inflammation control: molecular mechanisms and pathophysiological relevance. *Arterioscl Thromb Vasc Biol* 2010; **30**: 1542–9.

Katz AM. *Physiology of the Heart*, 5th revised edition. 2010. Philadelphia: Lippincott Williams & Wilkins.

Patel PA, Tilley DG, Rockman HA. Physiologic and cardiac roles of β-arrestins. *J Mol Cell Cardiol* 2009; **46**: 300–8.

Rockman HA, Koch WJ, Lefkowitz RJ. Seven-transmembrane-spanning receptors and heart function. *Nature* 2002; **415**: 206–12.

Chapter

Inotropes and vasoactive drugs

9

Mark Dougherty and Stephen T. Webb

Numerous drugs are used to manipulate hemodynamics in the perioperative period. This chapter provides a summary of the characteristics of the more frequently used drugs. In order to fully appreciate the mechanisms of action it is necessary to review the molecular biology governing the mechanism of myocardial contraction outlined in previous chapters.

Table 9.1 Definitions of terms used in this chapter

Term	Definition
Inotrope	A positive inotrope produces an increase in contractility
Chronotrope	A positive chronotropic agent produces an increase in the rate of contraction
Lusitrope	A positive lusitrope produces an enhancement of ventricular relaxation
Dromotrope	A positive dromotrope enhances the conduction velocity through the A-V node

In the interests of brevity, much of the information is presented as tables using the following symbols:

⚙ Mechanism of action ⚖ Dose ♥ Hemodynamic effects

℞ Indications and usage ⚠ Adverse effects ? Comments

Table 9.2 Principal cardiovascular distribution and effects of stimulation of adrenoreceptor subtypes

Receptor	Distribution	Stimulation effects
α_1	Systemic arterioles Systemic veins	Vasoconstriction Venoconstriction
α_2	Pre-ganglionic sympathetic nerves Post-ganglionic sympathetic nerves	Vasodilatation ($\downarrow$ norepinephrine release) Vasoconstriction
β_1	Heart Systemic arterioles	+ chronotropy + inotropy + dromotropy Increased automaticity Renal vasodilatation
β_2	Heart Systemic arterioles Systemic veins	+ chronotropy + inotropy + dromotropy Increased automaticity Vasodilatation Venodilatation

Inotropes and vasoconstrictors

Table 9.3 Classification of inotropes by mechanism of action

Class	Characteristics
I	Drugs that increase cAMP via Gs-protein receptor complex-mediated activation of adenylyl cyclase (β-agonists) and inhibition of cAMP metabolism (phosphodiesterase, PDE-3 inhibitors)
II	Drugs that increase intracellular Ca^{2+} via non-cAMP-dependent mechanism mediated by Gq-protein complex activation of phospholipase C (α_1-agonists)
III	Drugs that effect ion channel conductance or ion exchange mechanisms, such as Na^+K^+ ATPase (cardiac glycosides)
IV	Drugs that modulate intracellular Ca^{2+} regulation (levosimendan)
V	Drugs that augment contractility through multiple pathways

Dopamine

 Naturally occurring Precursor of norepinephrine. Low dose DA_1 receptor effects ↑ dose β_1 effects predominate ↑↑ dose α_1 effects predominate

 IVI: 1–10 µg kg^{-1} min^{-1}
Low dose: 1–3 µg kg^{-1} min^{-1}
Intermediate dose: 3–10 µg kg^{-1} min^{-1}
High dose: >10 µg kg^{-1} min^{-1}

♥ Low dose: renal and splanchnic vasodilatation
Intermediate dose: ↑ HR ↑ CO ↓ SVR
High dose: ↑ PVR ↑↓ CO

℞ Intraoperative separation from CPB Post-cardiac surgery augmentation of CO

⚠ Dose-dependent tachycardia and cardiac arrhythmias

? Offset by uptake into nerve terminals and metabolism by MAO and COMT

Catecholamines

Epinephrine/adrenaline

 Naturally occurring Acts at α- and β-adrenoreceptors ↑ Dose → progressive shift from β_1 and β_2 effects to α_1 effects

⚖ IVI: 0.005–0.1 µg kg^{-1} min^{-1}

♥ ↑ CO ↑ HR ↑ MAP Dose-dependent ↑ SVR
At higher doses ↑ SVR → ↓ CO
β_1 effect enhances ventricular relaxation

℞ Cardiac arrest Anaphylaxis Cardiogenic shock Post-cardiac surgery low CO syndrome

⚠ Dose-dependent arrhythmias PA vasoconstriction Renal and splanchnic vasoconstriction ↑ Glucose ↑ Lactate ↓ K^+

? Offset by neuronal uptake and metabolism by monoamine oxidase (MAO) and catechol-*O*-methyl transferase (COMT)

Dobutamine

 Synthetic derivative of isoproterenol Effects mediated predominantly via β_1- and β_2-adrenoreceptors

⚖ IVI: 1–20 µg kg^{-1} min^{-1}

 ↑ HR ↑ CO ↓ SVR ↓ PVR

℞ ↓ CO with ↑ SVR (e.g. cardiogenic shock)

 Dose-dependent arrhythmias ↓ MAP if ↑ SVR not offset by ↑ CO Coronary steal Tachyphylaxis

? Elimination $T_{1/2} \approx 2$ min Offset by redistribution and COMT metabolism

Dopexamine

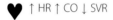 Synthetic dopamine analogue
Direct effects on β_2 and DA_1 receptors
Acts indirectly on β_1 receptors by $\downarrow$ uptake of endogenous catecholamines

⚖ IVI: 1–6 μg kg^{-1} min^{-1}

♥ $\uparrow$ HR $\uparrow$ CO $\downarrow$ SVR

℞ $\downarrow$ CO with $\uparrow$ SVR (e.g. cardiogenic shock)

⚠ Dose-dependent arrhythmias
Tachyphylaxis

? Elimination $T_{1/2}$ = 6–11 min
Clearance is by tissue uptake and hepatic metabolism
Evidence for the perioperative use to improve renal and splanchnic perfusion limited

Norepinephrine (noradrenaline)

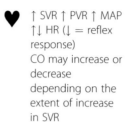 Naturally occurring
Predominantly β_1 and α effects

⚖ IVI: 0.01–0.2 μg kg^{-1} min^{-1}

♥ $\uparrow$ SVR $\uparrow$ PVR $\uparrow$ MAP
$\uparrow\downarrow$ HR ($\downarrow$ = reflex response)
CO may increase or decrease depending on the extent of increase in SVR

℞ $\downarrow$ CO unresponsive to fluids and other inotropes
$\downarrow$ MAP secondary to $\downarrow$ SVR (e.g. post-cardiac surgery vasoplegic syndrome and septic shock)

⚠ $\downarrow$ CO (vasoconstriction → $\uparrow$ afterload)
$\uparrow$ PVR
Renal, hepatic and mesenteric ischemia
Skin, soft tissue and muscle ischemia

? Clearance by redistribution, neuronal uptake and MAO and COMT metabolism

Table 9.4 Relative receptor activity of catecholamines

Drug	Receptor					
	α_1	α_2	β_1	β_2	DA_1	DA_2
Epinephrine	+++	++	+++	++	–	–
Dopamine	++	+	++	+++	+++	+++
Dobutamine	+	–	+++	+	–	–
Dopexamine	–	–	+	+++	++	++
Isoproterenol	–	–	++	++	–	–
Norepinephrine	+++	+++	+	–	–	–

Isoproterenol (isoprenaline)

 Synthetic catecholamine
Predominantly β_1 and β_2 effects

⚖ IV bolus: 1–4 μg
IVI: 1–10 μg min^{-1}

♥ $\uparrow$ HR $\uparrow$ CO
$\downarrow$ SVR $\downarrow$ PVR

℞ Acute bradyarrhythmias (e.g. heart block)
Optimization of HR in the denervated heart (e.g. post-heart transplantation)
Pulmonary hypertension
Torsades des pointes

⚠ Dose-dependent arrhythmias
$\downarrow$ MAP
Coronary steal

? Elimination $T_{1/2}$ < 2 min
Metabolized by COMT and MAO

Metaraminol (Aramine®)

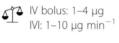 Synthetic catecholamine
Predominantly α_1 agonist
Some nonspecific β-adrenoreceptor agonism

⚖ IV bolus: 3–15 μg kg^{-1}

♥ $\uparrow$ SVR $\uparrow$ MAP (may $\uparrow$ PVR)
Slight $\uparrow\downarrow$ HR
CO may increase or decrease depending on the extent of increase in SVR

℞ $\downarrow$ MAP secondary to $\downarrow$ SVR

Metaraminol (Aramine®)

 ↓ CO
(vasoconstriction →
↑ afterload)
↑ PVR

? Useful alternative
to phenylephrine
in bradycardic or
β-blocked patient

Phenylephrine (Neosynephrin®)

 Synthetic catecholamine
Pure α₁ agonist

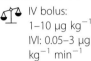 IV bolus:
1–10 μg kg^{-1}
IVI: 0.05–3 μg
kg^{-1} min^{-1}

 ↑ SVR ↑ MAP (may ↑ PVR)
↑↓ HR (↓ = reflex
response)
CO may increase or
decrease depending on the
extent of increase in SVR

Rx ↓ MAP
secondary to
↓ SVR

 ↓ CO (vasoconstriction →
↑ afterload)
↑ PVR

? Elimination
$T_{1/2}$ = 2–3 h
MAO and COMT
metabolism

Non-catecholamines

Phosphodiesterase III inhibitors

 Mediated by
inhibition of PDE-3
isoenzyme
preventing
breakdown of
intracellular cAMP

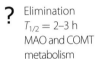 IV loading
dose → IVI
See Table 9.4 for
individual doses

 ↑ HR ↑CO ↓ SVR ↓
PVR
+ lusitropic effect,
+ dromotropic
effect
Tachyphylaxis not a
feature

Rx Separation from CPB
↓ CO post-cardiac
surgery
↓ CO associated with
RV dysfunction and
pulmonary
hypertension
Potentiation of the
inotropic action of
catecholamines

 ↓ MAP
Arrhythmias
Accumulation in
renal dysfunction
Thrombocytopenia
(inamrinone >24 h)

? Concurrent
vasopressor
administration may
be required to
maintain MAP

Table 9.5 Phosphodiesterase III inhibitors – pharmacokinetics
and dosing schedules

Drug	Relative potency	T₁/₂	Dose
Inamrinone	1	5–8 h	IV loading dose: 0.75–1.5 μg kg^{-1} IVI: 5–20 μg kg^{-1} min^{-1}
Milrinone	20	2–3 h	IV loading dose: 25–75 μg/kg IVI: 0.37–0.75 μg kg^{-1} min^{-1}
Enoximone	1.5	6–8 h	IV loading dose: 0.5–1.0 mg kg^{-1} IVI: 3–10 μg kg^{-1} min^{-1}

Renal clearance = 60–80%

Levosimendan

 Ca^{2+} sensitizer:
↓ Ca^{2+} binding
coefficient of
troponin C and
stabilizes
troponin C in
active state
Opens ATP-
dependent K$^+$
channels
↑↑ doses →
↑ PDE-3 effects

 IV loading dose:
12–24 μg kg^{-1}
IVI: 0.1 μg kg^{-1} min^{-1} for
24 h

 ↑ CO ↑ HR
↓ SVR ↓ PVR
Coronary
vasodilatation
Improves
ventricular
arterial
coupling

Rx Acute heart failure,
particularly acutely
decompensated chronic
heart failure in the setting
of long-term β-blocker
therapy
May be beneficial in high-
risk cardiac surgical
patients with severe LV
dysfunction or recent
acute coronary
syndrome (ACS)

51

Levosimendan

  ↑ myocardial contraction without increasing myocardial oxygen demand
Elimination $T_{1/2} = 1$ h – active metabolites prolong duration of action
An oral preparation is under development

Vasopressin (argipressin)

 Endogenous antidiuretic hormone
Acts on V_1 receptors (vasoconstriction), V_2 receptors (anti-diuresis)

 IVI: 0.01–0.1 units min^{-1}

 ↑ SVR
Minimal effect on HR
↑↓ CO depending on extent of ↑ SVR

R$_X$ Catecholamine-resistant ↓ MAP with ↓ SVR (e.g. post-cardiac surgery vasoplegic syndrome and septic shock)
Perioperative ↓ MAP related to preoperative ACE inhibition

 Vasoconstriction-induced ↓ CO
Multi-organ and peripheral ischemia
Caution at doses > 2.4 units h^{-1}

? May be superior to norepinephrine in setting of pulmonary hypertension

Methylene blue

 Highly ionized base with oxidation-reduction properties inhibits activation of guanylate cyclase, preventing the cGMP mediated vasodilatation
May ↓ tumor necrosis factor (TNF) levels → release of endogenous norepinephrine from adrenergic fibers

♥ ↑ MAP ↑ PAP ↑ SVR
CVP/LAP unchanged

⚠ Methemoglobinemia at higher doses
Dizziness, headache, confusion and abdominal pain
Hemolysis in those with glucose 6-phosphate dehydrogenase deficiency

Calcium

 ↑ extracellular Ca^{2+} → ↑ intracellular Ca^{2+}
↑ muscle contraction following binding to troponin C

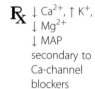 IV bolus: 6.8–13.6 mmol (0.5–1.0 g)

♥ Effects dependent on ionised Ca^{2+}
↑ SVR ↑ MAP, minimal effect on HR
↑ CO in hypocalcemia

R$_X$ ↓ Ca^{2+}, ↑ K^+, ↓ Mg^{2+}
↓ MAP secondary to Ca-channel blockers

⚠ Potentiation of ischemia-reperfusion injury

? 10% $CaCl_2$ 10 ml ≈ 6.8 mmol
10% Ca gluconate 10 ml ≈ 2.2 mmol

Triiodothyronine (T$_3$)

 Independent of intracellular cAMP

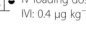 IV loading dose: μg kg^{-1}
IVI: 0.4 μg kg^{-1}

 ↑ HR ↑ CO + lusitropy

R$_X$ Optimization of brain-dead organ donor (widely used but controversial)
Myxedema coma

 Cardiac arrhythmias

? Used as an alternative to oral (levo)thyroxine (T$_4$)

 IVI: 1.5–7.0 μg kg^{-1} depending on indication

R$_X$ Rescue therapy in vasoplegic syndrome
Methemoglobinemia

? Elimination $T_{1/2} = 5.25$ h in volunteers
Turns patient's skin and secretions blue!

Vasodilators and antihypertensives

Nitrovasodilators

Nitrovasodilators (glyceryl trinitrate, sodium nitro-prusside and nitric oxide) produce vasodilatation by a direct effect on vascular smooth muscle. The production of nitric oxide (NO) or S-nitro-sothiols stimulates guanylate cyclase. The resulting elevation in cGMP causes a reduction in intracellular Ca^{2+} and smooth muscle relaxation. The process of producing NO or S-nitrosothiols requires sulfhydryl (-SH) groups. Continuous administration of nitrovasodilators may deplete –SH groups and result in tolerance. Tolerance may be reversed by administration of a sulfhydryl donor (e.g. N-acetylcysteine).

Glyceryl trinitrate (GTN, nitroglycerin, NTG)

 NO donor
↑ cGMP in vascular smooth muscle

 IVI: 0.1–10 µg kg^{-1} min^{-1}
Sublingual: 400–500 µg

 Dilates epicardial and interconnecting coronary arteries → ↑ coronary blood flow, in both normal and stenotic coronary vessels
↑ subendocardium blood flow (↓ LVEDP)
↓ SVR may → ↑ CO
Low doses → ↓ CVP ↓ PAP
Systemic and renal venodilatation predominate
Coronary perfusion pressure maintained if intravascular volume adequate
↑↑ doses → ↑ arteriolar vasodilatation
↓ SVR → ↓ coronary perfusion pressure

R_X Myocardial ischemia (e.g. ACS)
Hypertension
Heart failure
Coronary vasospasm

 Tolerance
Rebound hypertension on withdrawal
Increased intrapulmonary shunt and reversal of hypoxic pulmonary vasoconstriction
Methemoglobinemia

? Metabolized in 1–3 min by hepatic reductase
Inhibits platelet aggregation

Sodium nitroprusside

 NO donor
↑ cGMP in vascular smooth muscle

 IVI: 0.25–10 µg kg^{-1} min^{-1}

 Low doses → arteriolar vasodilatation
↑↑ doses → vasodilatation and venodilatation
Dose-dependent ↓ CVP ↓ SVR ↓ PVR ↓↓ MAP
Reflex ↑ HR → variable effect on CO

R_X Perioperative ↑↑ MAP associated with ↑ SVR
Hypotensive anesthesia
No-reflow phenomenon post-angioplasty

 Coronary steal
Methemoglobinemia, cyanide and thiocyanate toxicity
Tolerance
Rebound hypertension on withdrawal
Increased intrapulmonary
shunt and reversal
of hypoxic
pulmonary vasoconstriction

 ? Duration of action = 1–2 min

Nitric oxide (NO)

 ↑ cGMP in vascular smooth muscle

 ↓ PVR with no change in SVR
Selective vasodilatation of ventilated lung regions improves ventilation–perfusion (V:Q) matching

Methemoglobinemia
NO_2 toxicity
Chronic administration causes terminal bronchiole epithelial hyperplasia

Inhaled: 0.05–20 ppm

℞ Pulmonary hypertension
RV dysfunction
ARDS, transplantation, extracorporeal membrane oxygenation (ECMO), ventricular assist device (with high TPG)

? Elimination $T_{1/2} = 6$ s

Table 9.6 Hemodynamic effects of nitrosovasodilators

Drug	Hemodynamic parameter					
	HR	BP	CO	Preload	SVR	PVR
GTN	↑	↓	↑↔	↓↓	↓	↓
Sodium nitroprusside	↑	↓	↑↔	↓	↓↓	↓
NO	↔	↔	↑↔	↓↔	↔	↓↓↓

Non-nitrate vasodilators

Phentolamine (Rogitine®, Regitine®)

 Potent α_1-adrenoreceptor antagonist
Also acts as antagonist at α_2-adrenoreceptors and 5HT receptors

 ↓↓ MAP
Reflex ↑ HR (baroreceptor, α_2 blockade)

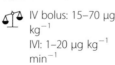 IV bolus: 15–70 µg kg^{-1}
IVI: 1–20 µg kg^{-1} min^{-1}

℞ Hypertension during CPB
Pheochromocytoma
Cocaine-induced hypertension

Prostacyclin (PGI$_2$)

 Product of arachidonic acid metabolism
Acts on vascular smooth muscle receptors
Stimulates adenylyl cyclase resulting in vasodilatation and platelet disaggregation

 IV administration →
↓ SVR ↓ PVR ↑ CO
Aerosolized →
↓ systemic effects

 Systemic hypotension (especially during CPB)
IV administration may ↑ intrapulmonary shunt and impair hypoxic pulmonary vasoconstriction

 IVI: 1–35 ng kg^{-1} min^{-1}
Aerosolized inhalation: 50 ng kg^{-1} min^{-1}

 Pulmonary hypertension
RV dysfunction
Anticoagulation of extracorporeal circuits

? Elimination $T_{1/2} = 2$–3 min

Nicardipine

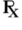 Dihydropyridine Ca-channel blocker
Minimal direct negative inotropic or chronotropic action
Reflex tachycardia may occur

 ↓ SVR ↓ MAP
+ Lusitropy effect
Coronary and cerebral vasodilatation

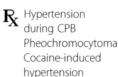 ↓ MAP

Oral: 20–40 mg three times daily
IVI: 1–4 µg kg^{-1} min^{-1}

 Perioperative hypertension
Perioperative myocardial ischemia
Coronary vasospasm

 Onset of action within 1–2 min (IV)
Elimination $T_{1/2} =$ 30 min Hepatic metabolism, renal excretion

Labetalol (Trandate®)

 Selective α_1-adrenoreceptor antagonist
Non-selective β-adrenoreceptor antagonist
Partial β_2-adrenoreceptor agonist
Racemic mixture of four isomers
α:β effect ratio = 1:3 (oral), 1:7 (IV)

Oral: 100 mg twice daily (max 2400 mg daily)
IV bolus: 5–10 mg
IVI: 2 mg min^{-1} titrated to effect

♥ ↓ SVR ↓ MAP
Dose-dependent ↓ HR

℞ Preoperative management in aortic dissection
Perioperative hypertension, particularly in association with myocardial ischemia
Pregnancy-induced hypertension
Pheochromocytoma

⚠ Systemic hypotension
Exacerbation of heart failure

? Elimination $T_{1/2}$ = 6 h
Hepatic metabolism → inactive metabolites

Esmolol (Brevibloc®)

Ultra-short-acting selective β_1-adrenoreceptor antagonist

♥ ↓↓ HR ↓ CO ↓ MAP

IV bolus: 0.25–0.5 mg kg^{-1}
IVI: 50–200 µg kg^{-1} min^{-1}

℞ Perioperative hypertension
Supraventricular tachyarrhythmias
Aortic dissection

⚠ ↓↓↓ HR
↓↓ MAP

? Rapid onset of action
Elimination $T_{1/2}$ = 9 min
Metabolized by red blood cell esterases

Hydralazine

 Activates K_{ATP} channels → predominantly arterial smooth muscle relaxation

Oral: 10–50 mg four times daily
IV bolus: 2.5–5 mg

♥ ↓ SVR ↓ PVR ↓ MAP
May cause a reflex ↑ HR

℞ Perioperative hypertension

⚠ Reflex sympathetic activation may precipitate myocardial ischemia
Coronary steal

? The onset in 5–15 min
Peak effect at 20 min
Metabolism by hepatic acetylation
Elevated plasma levels and a prolonged effect may develop in slow acetylators

Diazoxide

Benzothiadiazine analog
Directly acting K^+ channel opener

Oral: 5 mg kg^{-1} day^{-1}
IV bolus: 0.5–1 mg day^{-1}

 ♥ ↓ SVR → ↓ MAP+ reflex ↑ HR

℞ Hypertensive emergencies
Intractable hypoglycemia

⚠ Na^+ and H_2O retention
Hyperglycemia – inhibits insulin release

? Long duration of action
Not removed by dialysis

Fenoldopam

 Peripheral DA_1 and α_2 receptor agonist

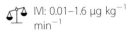 IVI: 0.01–1.6 µg kg^{-1} min^{-1}

♥ Coronary, renal, mesenteric and peripheral arterial vasodilatation
Rapid ↓ BP$_S$ ↓ BP$_D$ ↓ SVR ↑ SV ↑ CO

℞ Hypertensive emergencies
Perioperative use not conclusively shown to preserve renal function

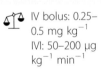

Fenoldopam

 ↑ intraocular pressure
Dose-dependent tachycardia
↓ MAP
↓ K^+

? Elimination
$T_{1/2} = 5$ min
Hepatic conjugated
Eliminated in urine (90%) and feces (10%)
May → ↑ plasma norepinephrine levels

Nesiritide

 Recombinant analog of human B-type natriuretic peptide
↑ vascular smooth muscle guanylate cyclase → arterial and venous relaxation
Natriuresis
↓ effect of endothelin, ↓ rennin, ↓ aldosterone

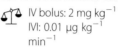 IV bolus: 2 mg kg^{-1}
IVI: 0.01 μg kg^{-1} min^{-1}

 ↓ CVP ↓ SVR ↓ PAP
↓ PVR ↓ MAP

R_X Acute heart failure
Limited evidence of renal protection in cardiac surgery

 Hypotension
Physically incompatible with heparin and heparin-coated central venous catheters

? The clinical effect > elimination $T_{1/2}$ of 18 min
Metabolized by proteolytic cleavage by vascular endopeptidases and by internalization of receptor-drug complexes

Key

 Mechanism of action

Dose

♥ Hemodynamic effects

R_X Indications and usage

⚠ Adverse effects

? Comments

Further reading

Dickstein K, Cohen-Solal A, Filippatos G, *et al.* ESC Guidelines for the diagnosis and treatment of acute and chronic heart failure 2008. *Eur Heart J* 2008; **29**(19): 2388–442. (Dosage corrections in *Eur Heart J* 2010; **12**(4): 416 and *Eur Heart J* 2010; **31**(5): 624).

Elliott P. Rational use of inotropes. *Anaesth Intens Care Med* 2006; 7(9): 326–30.

Gillies M, Bellomo R, Doolan L, Buxton B. Bench-to-bedside review: Inotropic drug therapy after adult cardiac surgery – a systematic literature review. *Crit Care* 2005; **9**(3): 266–79.

Raja SG, Rayen BS. Levosimendan in cardiac surgery: current best available evidence. *Ann Thorac Surg* 2006; **81**(4): 1536–46.

Anti-dysrhythmic drugs

Alan Ashworth and Kamen P. Valchanov

There are several ways to classify anti-dysrhythmic drugs. The most popular and widely used is the Vaughan Williams classification, which characterizes drugs according to their primary pharmacodynamic action on cardiac myocytes and action potential (AP). These drugs can also be classified according to the indication for their clinical use. The selection of an anti-dysrhythmic drug is determined by the origin of the arrhythmia (supraventricular or ventricular), the etiology, the hemodynamic impact, and the desired effect (i.e. cardioversion, prophylaxis or ventricular rate control).

Anti-dysrhythmic drugs generally have a narrow therapeutic window and numerous side effects.

Paradoxically anti-dysrhythmic drugs may be proarrhythmogenic, particularly in the presence of electrolyte abnormalities. There is a need for newer anti-dysrhythmic drugs with equal or greater efficacy and fewer side effects.

Vaughan Williams classification

Class I drugs

Class I drugs reduce the entry of Na^+ ions into myocytes by blocking Na^+ channels in the open or inactivated state. The reduction of Na^+ ion entry results in reduction of the maximum rate of rise of

Table 10.1 Vaughan Williams classification of antiarrhythmic drugs. Classes I and IV act on ion channels, class II acts on receptors and class III has mixed action

Class/action		Drugs	APD	MRD	ERP	AVC	Cont
Ia	APD prolonged	Procainamide	↑	↓↓	↑	↓↓	↓
		Disopyramide	↑	↓↓	↑	↓↓	↓↓↓
		Quinidine	↑	↓↓	↑	↓↓	↓
Ib	APD shortened	Lidocaine	↓	↓	↑↑		
		Mexiletine					
Ic	APD unchanged	Flecainide	–	↓↓↓		↓↓	↓↓
II	Beta blockers	Propranolol				?↓	↓↓
		Metoprolol					↓↓
III	K$^+$ channel blockers; APD and ERP prolonged	Amiodarone	↑↑↑		↑↑↑	↓	
		Sotalol	↑↑↑		↑↑↑	↓	↓↓
		Ibutilide	↑↑				
		Bretylium					
IV	Ca^{2+} channel blockers	Verapamil	↓↓			↓↓	↓↓↓

APD, action potential duration; MRD, maximum rate of depolarization; ERP, effective refractory period; AVC, atrioventricular conduction; Cont, myocardial contractility.

Core Topics in Cardiac Anesthesia, Second Edition, ed. Jonathan H. Mackay and Joseph E. Arrowsmith. Published by Cambridge University Press. © Cambridge University Press 2012.

phase 0 of the AP during depolarization (Figure 2.3). This reduces the rate of diastolic depolarization in abnormal ectopic foci so that the diastolic potential reaches the threshold for depolarization more slowly, thereby allowing the SA node to resume its normal function as the pacemaker.

This class is further divided according to effect on the cardiac AP. Class 1a drugs increase (*Accentuate*) cardiac AP duration, class 1b (*Brief*) drugs decrease cardiac AP duration and class 1c drugs have no effect.

Class Ia

Prolongation of cardiac AP duration is useful for the treatment of re-entrant tachyarrhythmias; increasing AP duration in the accessory (re-entrant) pathway and inhibiting retrograde AP conduction. Procainamide, disopyramide and quinidine have similar pharmacokinetic and pharmacodynamic profiles.

Procainamide (Pronestyl®)

♦ Class Ia
↑ Atrial refractory period
Partially blocks K^+ channels

⚖ IV loading: 15 mg kg^{-1} (slowly)
IVI: 7 mg^{-1} kg^{-1} (30 mins) → 2 mg min^{-1}

♥ Prolong cardiac AP duration
QRS widening
Hypotension

℞ Supraventricular tachycardia
Ventricular tachycardia
Wolff–Parkinson–White syndrome

⚠ Lupus syndrome with prolonged use and in slow acetylators
Proarrhythmic – torsades de pointes

? Limited availability in some countries
Plasma $T_{1/2}$ 2–4 h
Metabolism: 40% hepatic acetylation
Elimination: renal 60% unchanged

Disopyramide (Rythmodan®)

♦ Class Ia
↑ Atrial refractory period

⚖ IV loading: 2 mg kg^{-1} over 5 min
IVI: 400 µg kg^{-1} h^{-1}
Max: 300 mg (1st hour), 800 mg day^{-1}

♥ Prolong cardiac AP duration
QRS widening
Myocardial depression → hypotension

℞ Supraventricular arrhythmias
Ventricular arrhythmias

⚠ Agranulocytosis
Significant hypotension
Ventricular arrhythmias

Class Ib

Reduced cardiac AP duration is useful for the treatment of ventricular arrhythmias. In addition to their phase 0 effects, they suppress the activity of ectopic pacemakers, reducing the slope of the pacemaker potential (phase 4) and increasing the pacemaker excitability threshold (Figure 2.3). Mexiletine, which can be given by mouth, has similar effects to lidocaine, but is no longer widely available.

Lidocaine

♦ Class Ib

⚖ IV loading: 100 mg (over 5 min)
IVI: 4 mg min^{-1} (30 min), 2 mg min^{-1} (2 h), then 1 mg min^{-1}

♥ Myocardial depression → hypotension

℞ Ventricular arrhythmias

⚠ Neurologic: tinnitus, vertigo, paresthesia, seizures, coma
Severe hypotension, bradycardia

✗ A-V conduction block (any grade)
Severe hepatic dysfunction
Cardiac failure
Acute porphyria

? Plasma $T_{1/2}$ = 8 min
Metabolism: 90% hepatic (CYP1A2)
Elimination: renal 10% unchanged

Class Ic

Flecainide, a fluorinated derivative of procainamide, blocks K^+ and Ca^{2+} channels in addition to Na^+ channels. It binds and dissociates from

Na^+ channels slowly, causing prolonged intra-atrial, nodal and intraventricular conduction times and suppression of ectopic pacemakers. It also blocks Na^+ channels in Purkinje fibers, leading to QRS complex broadening and prolongation of the QT interval. Propafenone, which is structurally similar to flecainide and has similar actions, acts on Na^+ channels.

Flecainide (Tambocor®)

 Class Ic: slows intra-atrial, nodal and intraventricular AP conduction

IV: 2 mg kg^{-1} (over 10–30 min, maximum 150 mg)
IVI: 1.5 mg kg^{-1} h^{-1} (1 h) → 100–250 µg kg^{-1} h^{-1} (for up to 24 h, maximum 600 mg)

♥ Significant negative inotropic effects

Rx Wolff–Parkinson–White syndrome and other dysrhythmias associated with accessory pathways
Ventricular tachyarrhythmias resistant to other treatment (IV only)

⚠ Proarrhythmic effects
Reversible hepatotoxicity, dizziness, paresthesia

X Left ventricular dysfunction
Recent MI with ventricular ectopics
Increased mortality in patients post-MI (1989 CAST study)

? Plasma $T_{1/2}$ = 12–27 h
Metabolism: 75% hepatic
Elimination: renal 25% unchanged

Class II drugs

Class II drugs (β-blockers) antagonize the effects of endogenous catecholamines by blocking post-synaptic β-adrenoreceptors. They also reduce the release of norepinephrine from terminal post-ganglionic sympathetic neurons. β-Blockers reduce the rate of diastolic depolarization in the SA node and conduction tissue, and reduce slow Ca^{2+} influx. This reduces the automaticity of the conducting system during diastole and prolongs the effective refractory period of the AVN. β-Blockers should be used with caution in combination with verapamil and in patients with decompensated heart failure or asthma.

Esmolol (Brevibloc®)

 Class II

IV bolus: 10–20 mg (over 1 min)
IVI: 50–200 µg kg^{-1} min^{-1}

♥ Rapid ↓ MAP and ↓ HR

Rx Short-term control of ↑ MAP and ↑ HR
Supraventricular tachycardia

⚠ Severe hypotension and bradycardia – effects short-lived

X A-V conduction block
Severe ventricular dysfunction

? Use with caution in asthmatics
Plasma $T_{1/2}$ = 9 min
Metabolism: red cell esterases

Sotalol (Sotacor®)

Class II
Class III action via K^+ channel blockade

IV: 1–1.5 mg kg^{-1} at 10 mg min^{-1}

♥ ↓ MAP and ↓ HR
Prolongation of PR and QT intervals
Effects magnified by hypokalemia

Rx Prophylaxis in paroxysmal SVT
Atrial fibrillation
Electrophysiological studies
Prevention of AF in cardiac surgery?

⚠ Similar to other β-blockers
Torsades de pointes – limits use for treatment of sustained ventricular tachyarrhythmias

X Prolonged QT interval
Torsades de pointes
Renal dysfunction

? Plasma $T_{1/2}$ = 12 h
Metabolism: negligible
Elimination: 100% renal unchanged

59

Labetalol (Trandate®)

⚙ Class II and α_1-adrenoreceptor blockade
Ratio of $\beta:\alpha$ activity = 3:1

⚖ IVI: 2 mg min^{-1} until satisfactory response
(up to 200 mg)

♥ ↓↓ MAP and ↓ HR (β)
↓ SVR (α_1)

℞ Hypertensive crises – eclampsia,
pheochromocytoma, type A aortic dissection

⚠ Postural hypotension
Drug eruption

✗ Asthma
Heart failure
A-V conduction block

? Plasma $T_{1/2}$ ~ 6 h
Metabolism: hepatic
Elimination: renal

Metoprolol (Lopressor®)

⚙ Class II – relatively β_1 selective

⚖ IV: 5 mg every 2 min (max 15 mg)

♥ ↓ MAP and ↓ HR

℞ Hypertension
Arrhythmias

? Plasma $T_{1/2}$ = 3–7 h
Metabolism: hepatic
Elimination: renal

Class III drugs

Class III drugs exert their anti-dysrhythmic effects by reducing K^+ efflux and Ca^{2+} influx (phase 3). This results in prolongation of the cardiac AP and the refractory period in conduction pathways, which reduces the automaticity of ectopic foci. Drugs in this class also interrupt re-entrant arrhythmias by preventing retrograde conduction in pathways with a prolonged refractory period.

Drugs that prolong the AP duration are of most clinical use in the treatment of supraventricular tachyarrhythmias and arrhythmias due to aberrant conduction pathways (e.g. Wolff–Parkinson–White syndrome). Sotalol, which has mixed class II and class III actions, is discussed above. Bretylium, which blocks neuronal norepinephrine release, is no longer available.

Amiodorane (Cordarone®)

⚙ Class III – K^+ channel blocker
Also blocks Na^+ and Ca^{2+} channels

⚖ IV: 5 mg kg^{-1} (300 mg over 60 min) followed by
15 mg kg^{-1} (900 mg over 23 h)
PO maintenance: 600 mg day^{-1} reducing to
200 mg day^{-1} after 2 weeks
IV following cardiac arrest: 300 mg

♥ Prolongs cardiac AP duration and refractory period
↑ QT interval
Myocardial depression – less than other
anti-dysrhythmic drugs

℞ Paroxysmal atrial, nodal and ventricular
tachyarrhythmias
Atrial fibrillation/flutter
Persistent ventricular fibrillation

⚠ Structural analog of thyroxine → altered thyroid
function
Pulmonary fibrosis
Photosensitivity
Hepatic dysfunction
Corneal microdeposits

✗ Sinus bradycardia
Thyroid dysfunction
Pregnancy and breast feeding
Severe heart failure

? Plasma $T_{1/2}$ = 60 days
Substantial plasma protein binding
Metabolism: hepatic (active metabolites)
Elimination: principally biliary
Not removed by dialysis

Ibutilide (Corvert®)

⚙ Pure class III agent
Acts only on slow Na+ channels
Prolonged AP duration

Ibutilide (Corvert®)

⚖️ IV: 0.01 mg kg^{-1} (over 10 min) repeated once if initial dose unsuccessful

♥ Hemodynamic effects ($\downarrow$ MAP) less pronounced than class I agents

℞ Pharmacological cardioversion of acute atrial fibrillation/flutter

⚠️ Short duration of action
Proarrhythmic in severe LV dysfunction
QT interval prolongation $\rightarrow$ polymorphic VT and torsades de pointes

✗ Asthma
Heart failure
A-V conduction block

❓ Most effective agent for AF of recent onset. Not available in UK
Plasma $T_{1/2} = 6$ h
Metabolism: hepatic oxidation
Elimination: 80% renal

Class IV drugs

Calcium channel blockers exert their anti-dysrhythmic actions by blocking Ca^{2+} influx via voltage-dependent Ca^{2+} channels (phase 2). They are particularly useful in the treatment of re-entrant tachyarrhythmias.

Verapamil (Cordilox®, Isoptin®)

⚙️ Class IV
Potent SA node and AVN blockade

⚖️ IV: 5–10 mg (over 3 min)

♥ $\downarrow$ MAP and $\downarrow$ HR

℞ Supraventricular dysrhythmias
Hypertension
Angina pectoris

⚠️ Bradycardia $\rightarrow$ asystole
Flushing
Constipation

✗ Heart failure
A-V conduction block
Concurrent β-blocker therapy
AF in WPW syndrome

❓ May be preferable to adenosine in asthmatics
High plasma protein binding
Plasma $T_{1/2} = 3$–7 hours
Metabolism: 65–80% hepatic
Elimination: 10% renal
Not removed by dialysis

Diltiazem (Tildiem®, Cardizem®)

⚙️ Class IV

⚖️ IV: 20 mg (over 2 min) repeated after 15 min if HR >110
IVI maintenance: 5–15 mg h^{-1}

♥ $\downarrow$ MAP and $\downarrow$ HR
Less impact on ventricular function than verapamil

℞ Supraventricular dysrhythmias
Hypertension
Angina pectoris

⚠️ Bradycardia
Flushing

✗ A-V conduction block

❓ IV preparation not available in some countries
Plasma $T_{1/2} = 3$–5 h
Metabolism: 60% hepatic
Elimination: 40% renal

Unclassified anti-dysrhythmic drugs

Adenosine (Adenocor®)

⚙️ Endogenous nucleoside composed of a molecule of adenine attached to ribofuranose. Produced during normal metabolic activity
Effects mediated by G_i-protein-coupled adenosine (A_1) receptors causing $\downarrow$ Ca^{2+} influx, $\downarrow$ glutamate release and $\downarrow$ K+ channel activation $\rightarrow$ cell membrane hyperpolarization, $\downarrow$ AP duration and slope of the pacemaker potential

⚖️ IV: 6 mg (over 2 s) followed by 12 mg after 1–2 min if required

♥ Negative inotropy, reduction in SA node automaticity and AVN conduction
↓ MAP and ↓ HR

℞ Paroxysmal SVT – therapeutic and diagnostic

⚠ Bronchospasm
Chest tightness, choking sensation
Flushing

✗ Asthma
Decompensated heart failure
2°/3° A-V conduction block
Prolonged QT interval
Severe hypotension

? Plasma $T_{1/2} < 5$ s
Metabolism: RBC, vascular endothelium
No dose change required in renal or hepatic disease

Digoxin

⚙ Glycoside. Blocks ouabain-sensitive membrane Na^+/K^+ ATPase →
↑ intracellular Na^+ concentration →
↑intracellular Ca^{2+} concentration secondary to
↓ removal Ca^{2+} via the Na^+/Ca^{2+} exchanger
↑ AP duration
↑ effective refractory period in AVN
Direct ↑ vagal activity

⚖ IV loading dose: 10 μg kg^{-1} (over 30 min) repeat after 6 h
Maintenance: 125–250 μg day^{-1}

♥ ↓ HR (↓ A-V conduction)
Positive inotropy
Potentially dangerous interactions with verapamil, amiodarone, erythromycin, and epinephrine

℞ Control of ventricular rate in atrial tachyarrhythmias

⚠ *Side effects common*
CVS: atrial or ventricular extrasystoles, paroxysmal atrial tachycardia with A-V block and ventricular tachycardia or fibrillation
Gastrointestinal: nausea, vomiting, diarrhea
Neurologic: blurred vision, xanthopsia (yellow-green halo), confusion

✗ A-V conduction block
SVT associated with accessory pathway
Ventricular tachycardia/fibrillation
Hypertrophic cardiomyopathy
Constrictive pericardial disease

? Narrow therapeutic window (0.5–2.0 ng ml^{-1}) – specific antidote = anti-digoxin antibody (Digibind®, Digifab®)
Plasma $T_{1/2}$ = 36–48 h (longer in renal dysfunction)
Metabolism: 15% hepatic
Elimination: renal

Magnesium sulfate

⚙ Fourth most common cation in body, 35–40% present in cardiac and skeletal muscle
Anti-dysrhythmic effects due to membrane stabilization
Acts as Ca^{2+} antagonist → ↓ AP duration

⚖ IV bolus: 1–2 g (4–8 mmol)

♥ ↓ MAP and ↓ HR
A-V conduction block → asystole

℞ Arrhythmias – particularly in the presence of hypokalemia
Cardiac arrest
Torsades de pointes

⚠ Inhibition of platelet aggregation
Muscle weakness – potentiates neuromuscular blockers

✗ Severe renal impairment
Severe hypotension

? Potentiates effects of Ca^{2+} channel blockers

Key points

- For any unstable tachyarrhythmia the first-line treatment is electrical cardioversion.
- Proarrhythmic side effects are more likely when more than one drug is used.
- Class III agents cause less hemodynamic instability than Class I agents.
- Many anti-dysrhythmic drugs have narrow therapeutic windows and have many potentially serious side effects.
- Anti-dysrhythmic drugs which prolong the QT interval increase the risk of torsades de pointes.

Key

 Mechanism of action   Dose   ♥ Hemodynamic effects

℞ Indications and usage   ⚠ Adverse effects   ? Comments

Further reading

Ehrlich JR, Nattel S. Atrial-selective pharmacological therapy for atrial fibrillation: Hype or Hope? *Curr Opin Cardiol* 2009; **24**(1): 50–5.

Morrison LJ, Deakin CD, Morley PT, *et al.* 2010 International Consensus on Cardiopulmonary Resuscitation and Emergency Cardiovascular Care Science With Treatment Recommendations. Part 8: Advanced Life Support. *Circulation* 2010; **122**(suppl 2): S345–421.

Riera AR, Uchida AH, Ferreira C, *et al.* Relationship among amiodarone, new class 3 anti-arrhythmics, miscellaneous agents and acquired long QT syndrome. *Cardiol J* 2008; **15**(3): 209–19.

Savelieva I, Camm J. Anti-arrhythmic drug therapy for atrial fibrillation: current anti-arrhythmic drugs, investigational agents, and innovative approaches. *Europace* 2008; **10**: 647–65.

Anticoagulants and procoagulants

Alan F. Merry

Management of coagulation is required for CPB and unfractionated heparin (UFH), reversed by protamine sulfate, is almost always used for this. During CPB, coagulation is affected by hemodilution, damage to platelets, and activation of the coagulation and fibrinolytic pathways. Coagulation may also be affected by preoperative medications (notably aspirin and clopidogrel), and by the administration of antifibrinolytic and other adjunctive agents.

Heparin

Unfractionated heparin

Antithrombin (AT) and heparin co-factor 2 required
Combines with AT, ↑ affinity of AT for thrombin by >1000 fold
Augments activity of factor Xa and several other factors
Thrombin has two exosites; direct thrombin inhibitors bind to one or both (see below); fibrin binds to exosite 1; (paradoxically) heparin binds to exosite 2 and the resulting heparin-thrombin-fibrin complex restricts the action of heparin-AT to the liquid phase
Neutralized by platelet factor 4 (PF4), but the resulting complex may activate platelets and generate antibodies in some people
Endothelium contributes to this process through protease-activated receptors and heparan (which contributes to homeostasis)

Supplied in at least two formulations: 1000 U ml^{-1} and 5000 U ml^{-1}
100 U equates ≈ 1 mg

Standard dose for initiating CPB = 300 U kg^{-1} but the effect on coagulation is variable and must be measured with the activated clotting time (ACT)
Supplementary doses may be needed to maintain an adequate ACT

Heparin resistance
Failure of heparin 500 U kg^{-1} to prolong ACT > 480 s
Usually secondary to ↓ AT levels
Usual treatment is with FFP or AT concentrate
Acquired: (1) Increased hepatic clearance of AT-heparin-thrombin complexes following prior administration of heparin (e.g. patients treated with heparin infusions pre-CPB). (2) AT depletion in hepatic failure, nephrotic syndrome, preeclampsia, shock, disseminated intravascular coagulation and prior heparin administration. (3) Heparin-induced thrombocytopenia
Congenital: incidence 1 in 1000
Heparin-induced thrombocytopenia (HIT)
Type I occurs through direct platelet activation and is mild
Type II is characterized by an otherwise unexplained fall in platelet count of at least 50%, the presence of heparin-PF4 antibodies (predominantly IgG) and a high risk of arterial or venous thrombosis, typically occurring 5–14 days after heparin exposure
Associated with heparin tachyphylaxis
Treatment consists of stopping heparin (including heparin in flushes) and substitution of an alternative anticoagulant
Transient hypotension
Due to histamine release and binding of negatively charged heparin with Ca^{2+}; usually clinically insignificant

Core Topics in Cardiac Anesthesia, Second Edition, ed. Jonathan H. Mackay and Joseph E. Arrowsmith. Published by Cambridge University Press. © Cambridge University Press 2012.

Unfractionated heparin

? Polyanionic mucopolysaccharide, originally identified in 1916 from liver tissue
Now derived from either bovine lung or porcine intestinal mucosa
Contains molecules with molecular weights between 5 and 30 kDa, and its composition and activity is variable
Molecules highly negatively charged because of sulfhydryl ($CH_2OSO_3^-$) groups on side chains
Highly protein-bound

Managing patients with contraindications to heparin

A patient with a history of HIT with no detectable heparin-PF4 antibodies may receive UFH on one occasion – immediately prior to CPB. UFH should be avoided for several months before and after surgery because:

- HIT antibodies are transient, and decline to undetectable levels over approximately 3 months;
- if UFH is given to a patient with a history of HIT, but no detectable antibodies, at least 5 days are required for new antibodies to develop (and the majority do not develop antibodies at all).

Proven allergy is an absolute contraindication to heparin. If heparin-PF4 antibodies are present, options include:

- review of the decision to operate (where indications are marginal)
- deferment of surgery (if possible) to provide time for antibodies to UFH to subside
- use of an alternative to UFH (see below)
- use of UFH in combination with a platelet activation inhibitor.

Alternatives to heparin

Direct thrombin inhibitors

These bind to thrombin at exosite 1 (the "univalent" agents argatroban, efegatran, inogatran) or at both exosite 1 and exosite 2 (hirudin, irreversibly, and bivalirudin, reversibly).

Table 11.1 Advantages and disadvantages of direct thrombin inhibitors

Advantages	Disadvantages
No cross reactivity with heparin	Cost
Active against free and clot-bound thrombin	Difficulty measuring the anticoagulant effect
No cofactors are required	Conventional ACT assays unreliable
	Lack of a reversal agent
	Unfamiliarity (for many clinicians at least)

Table 11.2 Direct thrombin inhibitors

Argatroban

Elimination $T_{1/2} = 40$–50 min
Metabolized in the liver so this may increase substantially in the presence of hepatic impairment
Limited experience in cardiac surgery

Hirudin

Small molecule isolated from leech (*Hirudo medicinalis*) saliva
Largely superseded by recombinant r-hirudin (lepirudin and desirudin)
Acts independently of AT
Actions not neutralized by PF4
Degradation and elimination are primarily renal
Elimination $T_{1/2} \approx 60$ min (severely prolonged in renal failure)
Hemofiltration may ↑ elimination after CPB (plasmapheresis more effective)
Hirudin and r-hirudin used successfully for CPB and for treating HIT
Antibodies are generated in almost half the patients receiving lepirudin, and anaphylaxis has been reported to this agent.

Bivalirudin

Synthetic 20-amino-acid peptide
Amino-terminal segment binds to thrombin active exosite
Carboxy-terminal segment binds to fibrinogen exosite
Binding is reversible via proteolytic cleavage of the amino-terminal segment by plasma enzymes (including thrombin)

65

Table 11.2 (*cont.*)

Plasma $T_{1/2} \approx 25$ min, prolonged in renal failure (but markedly less so than r-hirudin – renal clearance accounts for only 20% of administered bivalirudin)

Hemofiltration may ↑ elimination after CPB (larger pore size filters appear to be more effective)

Experience in cardiac surgery is increasing

Recommended dose for CPB is 1.0 mg kg^{-1} followed by an infusion of 2.5 mg kg^{-1} h^{-1} adjusted to maintain a plasma level >10 μg ml^{-1} and 50 mg added to the CPB pump prime

In one study, graft patency was improved with bivalirudin after off-pump CABG surgery, which is consistent with findings in percutaneous coronary intervention

Clot may form in stagnant blood (e.g. chest cavity, cardiotomy reservoir)

Avoidance of stasis may require CPB circuit modifications

After stopping bivalirudin at the end of CPB, additional drug should be administered to the pump, which should be continuously recirculated and static lines saline flushed

Any blood returned to the patient should be processed with a cell saver to reduce bivalirudin levels

Other alternatives to unfractionated heparin

Table 11.3 Other alternatives to unfractionated heparin

Low-molecular-weight heparins (LMWH)

Short chains (mean MW = 4–5 kDa), which act via factor Xa inhibition

Unsuitable for cardiac surgery because:
– cross reaction to heparin antibodies may occur
– lack of an antagonist
– lack of potency
– long elimination $T_{1/2}$
– difficulty in monitoring effect on coagulation

Ancrod

Purified from venom of Malaysian pit viper (*Calloselasma rhodostoma*)

Causes defibrinogenation over 12–24 h

Can be reversed by cryoprecipitate and platelets

Predicting therapeutic levels and preventing coagulation factor consumption are both problematic

Danaparoid

Heparinoid factor Xa inhibitor

Occasionally used in management of patients with HIT

Unsuitable for cardiac surgery because:
– long elimination $T_{1/2}$
– lack of a point-of-care monitor of anti-Xa activity
– lack of an antagonist

Platelet inhibitors in conjunction with heparin

In patients with HIT, platelet activation and the development of heparin-PF4 antibodies can be completely inhibited by an infusion of iloprost, a stable analog of prostacyclin with a short terminal $T_{1/2}$ (15–20 min) and potential benefits to RV function. Epoprostenol is freeze-dried prostacyclin with a shorter $T_{1/2}$ (6 min), but is unstable at room temperature and in light. Prostacyclins cause vasodilatation and predictable hypotension, manageable with vasoconstrictors.

Tirofibran, a platelet glycoprotein IIb/IIIa antagonist with a $T_{1/2}$ of approximately 2 h, has been used successfully with UFH in CPB in a number of patients with HIT.

Protamine

Protamine

 Cationic protamine reverses anionic heparin by a simple acid-base interaction forming a stable compound without anticoagulant activity

 Numerous dosage regimens advocated, but one typical approach is:

1 mg kg^{-1} for every 100 U of UFH given in the initial dose: thus a 70 kg male patient may receive 21 000 units ("210 mg") UFH before CPB (with or without supplementation) and be given 210 mg of protamine after CPB, in the first instance

Supplementary doses according to ACT, measured over the next 1–2 h: protamine has a short half life (4.5 min), and UHF may be liberated from tissues or administered in blood re-infused from the CPB reservoir

 Transient hypotension
Common if protamine is administered too rapidly
Attributed to direct myocardial depression or to histamine release
Severe anaphylactic reactions
IgE-mediated phenomena may occur infrequently
Incidence increased with fish allergy and vasectomy and previous exposure to protamine-containing insulins and to protamine itself

Protamine

Pulmonary hypertension (PHT)
With RV failure and systemic hypotension (thought to be mediated by thromboxane; rare).
Overdosing
May cause coagulopathic bleeding

? Peptide found in high concentrations in DNA
Carries positive charge due to a high content of arginine amino acids
Pharmacological preparations derived from salmon sperm

Managing patients with contraindications to protamine

A convincing history of protamine allergy precludes its use. In theory one might consider alternatives to protamine, such as heparinase and recombinant PF4, but none has yet become established as a therapeutic option. Other options include:

- review of the decision to operate or of the planned operation (as above)
- heparin without reversal
- review of the planned operation (e.g. for coronary surgery; off-pump surgery without reversal of heparin may be preferable).

Monitoring coagulation during CPB

ACT monitoring is routine with heparin.

- ACT activators are typically diatomaceous earth (celite) or kaolin. Kaolin became widely used after the introduction of aprotinin because aprotinin artifactually increased celite ACT measurements.
- An ACT of >300 s is thought to avoid fibrin deposition on the oxygenator and a "safe" minimum is typically considered to be 480 s. Some clinicians advocate a higher ACT, but the optimal ACT for CPB has yet to be definitively agreed.
- The appropriate ACT for off-pump coronary surgery is even less clear, but an ACT >300 s is often accepted.
- The ACT provides a relatively nonspecific indication of coagulation, and should therefore be supplemented by other indicators of coagulation status as indicated clinically.
- The ACT may be increased by hypothermia, hemodilution, thrombocytopenia, excess

protamine, aprotinin (for celite-activated ACT) and antiphospholipid syndrome (for kaolin-activated ACT)

Monitoring coagulation with direct thrombin inhibitors is more difficult.

- The ACT, prothombin time, activated partial thromboplastin time (APPT) and thrombin time are all prolonged by direct thrombin inhibitors.
- The APPT correlates well at low concentrations of lepirudin and bivalirudin, and can be used when treating HIT; the test is less useful at concentrations required for CPB.
- The ecarin clotting time (ECT) was specifically developed for monitoring direct thrombin inhibitors. Ecarin, which is derived from the venom of the snake *Echis carinatum*, converts prothombin to meizothrombin. The latter binds direct thrombin inhibitors (and has been proposed as a possible reversal agent for bivalirudin), after which clot will form provided adequate levels of fibrinogen and thrombin are present (so plasma must be added to the sample). Unfortunately ECT testing is no longer commercially available.
- The ACT appears to correlate reasonably well with lower concentrations of bivalirudin, but less well at the concentrations needed for CPB.
- A plasma-modified ACT test and a newer modified ACT (the ACTT) test have been described for monitoring direct thrombin inhibitors. These extend the linearity of the measure at doses sufficient for CPB.

Aprotinin

Aprotinin is a 58-amino-acid polypeptide derived from bovine lung. It has nonspecific, serine protease inhibitory properties. It inhibits pro-inflammatory cytokine release and maintains glycoprotein homeostasis. It reduces platelet glycoprotein (GpIb, GpIIb/IIIa) loss and prevents the expression of pro-inflammatory adhesive glycoproteins on granulocytes. After considerable controversy, aprotinin has been withdrawn from the market in many countries, following publication of evidence that its use, while clearly reducing blood loss, may increase overall mortality. Many advocates still argue that it has value in selected patients at high risk of bleeding, notably in

Table 11.4 The aprotinin story

1993	Approved by FDA for use in high-risk patients undergoing CABG surgery
1998	Indications broadened to include any patient undergoing CPB
Aug 2002	Blood conservation using antifibrinolytics: a randomized trial in cardiac surgery patients (BART) study starts recruiting patients at 19 Canadian centers
Jan 2006	Multicenter Study of Perioperative Ischemia (McSPI) propensity-adjusted, multicenter observational study of 4374 patients undergoing coronary revascularization with CPB (1295 received aprotinin) reported that use of aprotinin was associated with: – doubling of the risk of renal failure requiring dialysis – 55% increase in the incidence of myocardial infarction or heart failure – 181% increase in the risk of stroke or encephalopathy Mangano DT, Tudor IC, Dietzel C. The risk associated with aprotinin in cardiac surgery. *N Engl J Med* 2006; 354(4): 353–65
Feb 2007	Observational, multicenter (McSPI) study of mortality after CABG surgery (3786 patients). Use of aprotinin was associated with significantly greater risk of death at 5 years (20.8% vs. 12.7%). Mangano DT, Miao Y, Vuylsteke A, *et al.* Mortality associated with aprotinin during 5 years following coronary artery bypass graft surgery. *JAMA* 2007; 297(5): 471–9
Sep 2007	FDA gain access to McSPI dataset
Oct 2007	BART study terminated on the recommendation of independent data and safety monitoring committee. An interim analysis of 2163 patients reveals a "strong trend" towards higher mortality in the aprotinin group
Nov 2007	Bayer temporarily suspends worldwide marketing of aprotinin (Trasylol®) pending publication of the results of the BART study
May 2008	Multicenter, blinded study of 2331 high-risk cardiac surgical patients randomized to receive aprotinin ($n = 781$), tranexamic acid ($n = 770$) or aminocaproic acid ($n = 780$). Primary outcome was massive postoperative bleeding. Secondary outcomes included death from any cause within 30 days. Use of aprotinin was associated with: – increased 30-day mortality (6% vs. 4%) – 9% decrease in the risk of massive bleeding – no increase in the risk of renal failure requiring dialysis Fergusson DA, Hébert PC, Mazer CD, *et al.* A comparison of aprotinin and lysine analogues in high-risk cardiac surgery. *N Engl J Med* 2008; 358(22): 2319–31
Sep 2008	Reanalysis of McSPI dataset by FDA. Variables known to be associated with adverse outcomes (i.e volume of blood transfused, duration of CPB and duration of DHCA) were not included in the original McSPI analysis. After restratification according to risk of adverse outcome, the use of aprotinin was found to be associated with: – no increase in relative risk of death, heart failure, MI or renal dysfunction Royston D. Aprotinin; an economy of truth? *J Thorac Cardiovasc Surg* 2008; 136(3): 798–9

FDA, US Food & Drug Administration.

pediatric cardiac surgery. In the minds of many cardiac surgeons and anesthesiologists the story is far from over! (Table 11.4)

Antifibrinolytics

The lysine analogs tranexamic acid (TXA) and ε-aminocaproic acid (EACA) bind to plasminogen and prevent tissue-plasminogen activator (tPA)-mediated release of active plasmin. The prevention of plasminogen binding to fibrin via lysine-binding sites results in a fibrin polymer with greater resistance to fibrinolysis. Both drugs are more effective in prophylaxis than in the treatment of fibrinolysis. Use of these agents appears to have increased since the withdrawal of aprotinin. Adverse events include central venous catheter-related thrombosis, deep vein thrombosis (DVT) and pulmonary embolism (PE).

Tranexamic acid

Trans-4-(aminomethyl)-cyclohexanecarboxylic (tranexamic) acid (Cyclokapron®) for parenteral administration is currently licensed for short-term use in patients with hemophilia to reduce or prevent hemorrhage and reduce the need for replacement therapy during and following tooth extraction. TXA is not currently available in the USA. A loading dose of 10–30 mg kg^{-1} followed by an infusion of 5–16 mg kg^{-1} h^{-1} is in line with published data. In some centers, TXA is also added to the CPB prime.

TXA is inexpensive and appears to have a relatively low risk:benefit ratio. The use of higher dosing regimens appears to be associated with an increased risk of generalized seizures.

ε-Aminocaproic acid

6-Aminohexanoic (epsilon-aminocaproic) acid (Amicar®) is licensed for the treatment of fibrinolytic bleeding following cardiac surgery (with or without CPB), hematological disorders such as amegakaryocytic thrombocytopenia, life-threatening placental abruption, hepatic cirrhosis and neoplastic disease. It is currently unavailable in the UK. EACA is reported to be ten times less potent than TXA; a typical dosing regimen comprises a loading dose of 10 g followed by an infusion of 2 g h^{-1}.

Prolonged administration of EACA may cause skeletal muscle weakness and necrosis. The clinical presentation may range from mild myalgias and fatigue to a severe proximal myopathy with rhabdomyolysis, myoglobinuria and acute renal failure.

Desmopressin

Desamino-8-D-arginine vasopressin (DDAVP) is a long-acting analog of vasopressin that has no vasoconstrictor properties. DDAVP increases von Willebrand's factor and factor VIII levels (hence its use to treat hemophilia A and von Willebrand's disease), but studies in cardiac surgery have failed to demonstrate a reduction in blood loss or transfusion requirements in patients who did not have inherited bleeding disorder. It may be of use when bleeding is due to confirmed or suspected platelet dysfunction (e.g. uremia). No "best" dosing regimen has been described but doses of up to 0.3 μg kg^{-1} are usually administered.

Prothrombin complex concentrate

Prothrombin complex concentrate (PCC) contains purified human coagulation factors II, VII, IX and X. It is indicated for reversal of warfarin in the setting of life-threatening bleeding. Despite an absence of evidence from prospective randomized controlled trials, it is also used for refractory bleeding when conventional blood product replacement has failed. Many Jehovah's Witnesses will accept use of PCC.

Recombinant factor VIIa (eptacog alfa, NovoSeven®)

Recombinant activated factor VII (rFVIIa) is currently licensed for the treatment of spontaneous and surgical hemorrhage in hemophilia A and B patients with inhibitory antibodies against factors VIII and IX, respectively. It is thought to generate thrombin and activate platelets at the site of vascular injury. The activated platelet surface then forms a template, on which rFVIIa mediates further activation of coagulation. This in turn generates a "thrombin burst", which leads to the conversion of fibrinogen to fibrin. In recent years, there has been increasing interest in the unlicensed use of rFVIIa in the treatment of uncontrolled hemorrhage following cardiac surgery that has failed to respond to conventional measures. Doses of 90 μg kg^{-1} are reported in the cardiac surgical literature, although doses of up to 270 μg kg^{-1} have been used in hemophiliacs. Despite accumulating evidence of efficacy, there is a significant risk of serious adverse events associated with the use of FVIIa. A recent multicenter randomized controlled trial comparing rFVIIa to placebo for the management of refractory bleeding following cardiac surgery found a non-significant trend to increased 28 day mortality in the rFVIIa group.

Key points

- Unfractionated heparin with protamine reversal is by far the most commonly used strategy for managing anticoagulation for CPB.
- Heparin (including LMWH) may induce immune-mediated thrombocytopenia and thrombosis.
- All heparin substitutes have limitations.
- Although hypotension almost invariably follows protamine administration, life-threatening complications are rare.

- Pharmacological interference with the coagulation system may have serious unintended consequences.

Key

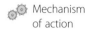 Mechanism of action   Dose    Hemodynamic effects

 Indications and usage   Adverse effects   **?** Comments

Further reading

Gill R, Herbertson M, Vuylsteke A, *et al.* Safety and efficacy of recombinant activated factor VII: a randomized placebo-controlled trial in the setting of bleeding after cardiac surgery. *Circulation* 2009; **120**(1): 21–7.

Koster A, Schirmer U. Re-evaluation of the role of antifibrinolytic therapy with lysine analogs during cardiac surgery in the post aprotinin era. *Curr Opin Anaesthesiol* 2011; **24**(1): 92–7.

Merry AF. Focus on thrombin: alternative anticoagulants. *Semin Cardiothorac Vasc Anesth* 2007; **11**(4): 256–60.

Murkin JM, Falter F, Granton J, Young B, Burt C, Chu M. High-dose tranexamic acid is associated with nonischemic clinical seizures in cardiac surgical patients. *Anesth Analg* 2010; **110**(2): 350–3.

Murphy GS, Marymont JH. Alternative anticoagulation management strategies for the patient with heparin-induced thrombocytopenia undergoing cardiac surgery. *J Cardiothorac Vasc Anesth* 2007; **21**(1): 113–26.

Pifarré R (Ed). *New Anticoagulants for the Cardiovascular Patient.* Philadelphia: Hanley & Belfus, 1997.

Chapter

12

Effects of CPB on drug pharmacokinetics

Jens Fassl and Berend Mets

The institution of CPB has profound effects on the plasma concentration, distribution and elimination of drugs. The major factors responsible for this are hemodilution, altered plasma protein binding, altered regional blood flow, hypothermia, isolation of the lungs from the circulation and sequestration of drugs into components of the extracorporeal circuit. These changes, which are influenced by physicochemical and pharmacokinetic characteristics, result in an alteration in free drug and effector-site concentration.

Factors during CPB affecting drug pharmacokinetics

Hemodilution and plasma protein binding

The CPB circuit is primed with 1500–2000 ml of crystalloid solution corresponding to a potential 30% increase in circulating blood volume with associated hemodilution occurring when CPB is instituted. The immediate effect of this hemodilution is a decrease in circulating drug concentration. The eventual plasma concentration of a drug is dependent on its plasma protein binding, its original volume of distribution and the extent of equilibration between tissue and plasma at the time of institution of CPB. An important consideration is the distinction between the total plasma concentration and the "free" or unbound fraction. The free concentration of the drug is that which moves to the effector site and can be eliminated. The impact of hemodilution on the unbound fraction of drugs tends to be greater for drugs that have high plasma protein binding (PPB). This may result in greater transfer of drug from the blood-prime mixture to the tissues, and thus a lower eventual circulating drug concentration. The volume of distribution (VD) is another factor determining the circulating

concentration of drugs during CPB. Drugs with a large inherent VD tend to be less affected by hemodilution, as there is a large tissue reservoir from which the drug can diffuse back into the circulation to plasma.

Heparin administration can result in the displacement of plasma protein-bound drugs (e.g. propofol). The mechanism appears to be heparin-induced lipase release leading to the hydrolysis of plasma triglycerides to form non-esterified fatty acids, which bind competitively to plasma proteins. The administration of protamine reverses this effect.

The acute effects of hemodilution only (disregarding the effects of altered distributional changes from altered PPB and so increased free fractions) can be established from the formula:

$$\Delta Css = Css \times Vpp/V1 + Vpp$$

where ΔCss is change in drug concentration; Css the drug concentration prior to hemodilution, Vpp the volume of pump prime and $V1$ = the VD of the central compartment or the α phase.

The effects of hemodilution mean that the apparent VD and effective (free) concentration of a drug are greater if administered during rather than before CPB.

Hypotension and altered blood flow

CPB is associated with hypotension and altered regional blood flow, particularly at the onset of CPB, during aortic cross-clamping and declamping, and during cardioplegia administration. This is due to reduced blood viscosity and SVR. Associated alterations in hepatic and renal blood flow may affect the metabolism and elimination of drugs.

Core Topics in Cardiac Anesthesia, Second Edition, ed. Jonathan H. Mackay and Joseph E. Arrowsmith. Published by Cambridge University Press. © Cambridge University Press 2012.

Hypothermia

Hypothermia may affect the hepatic metabolism and elimination of drugs by direct (enzymatic) inhibition and altered intrahepatic blood flow. Moreover, hypothermia may interfere with the binding affinity of some drug receptors and increase the relative potency of volatile anesthetic agents.

Lung isolation

Exclusion of the lungs during CPB interrupts normal pulmonary artery blood flow, although bronchial blood flow remains intact. The lungs act as a reservoir for basic drugs such as lidocaine, propanolol and fentanyl administered prior to CPB and so with re-establishment of the pulmonary circulation, upon separation from CPB, sequestered drug may return to the circulation. This may raise the systemic concentration above earlier levels or re-establish plasma concentrations sufficient to exert a pharmacological effect.

Sequestration in CPB circuit

In vitro experiments have demonstrated that a significant amount of fentanyl and alfentanil can be sequestered in bypass equipment. There was no evidence that this has any clinical relevance, although theoretically there is a possibility of reducing plasma concentration due to circuit uptake.

Specific drugs

Propofol

Propofol exhibits a high degree of PPB (unbound fraction <4%) and has a high hepatic extraction ratio (>0.8). Changes in PPB can lead to clinically significant changes in the anesthetic effects of propofol. The use of propofol infusions (3–6 mg kg^{-1} h^{-1}) during CPB has been extensively studied. There is a decrease in total concentration following the onset of CPB associated with a small increase in the free fraction. Sequestration may decrease the total circulating concentration initially, although plasma concentration may rise during CPB as a result of decreased clearance. The impact of heparin on the concentration of free propofol (as mentioned above) is reversed by protamine. In a recent study, Takizawa *et al.* found a significantly increased anesthetic effect of propofol during normothermic CPB. This was thought to be

due to an increased unbound concentration, rather than a change in total drug concentration. Using two propofol administration regimens (4 mg kg^{-1} h^{-1} and 6 mg kg^{-1} h^{-1}) the total blood propofol concentration was unchanged during CPB relative to the pre-CPB value in both groups (2–5 µg/ml), although the unbound concentration increased 2-fold (0.04 → 0.08 µg/ml – lower propofol infusion rate) during CPB. The enhanced efficacy of propofol may be caused by a reduction in the number of PPB sites during CPB.

Volatile anesthetics

The circulating concentration of volatile anesthetic agents administered via the CPB circuit is governed by three factors:

- The blood:gas solubility coefficient of the agent – hypothermia increases solubility.
- The tissue:gas solubility coefficient of the agent – hypothermia increases tissue uptake.
- Uptake by the oxygenator depends on the agent and the type of oxygenator.

Taking a number of studies together it is evident that there may be a delay in achieving therapeutic partial pressures when volatile agents are first administered during CPB.

Nussmeier *et al.* demonstrated that, after 32 minutes of isoflurane administration (1% at 32°C), blood partial pressure had only reached 51% of inlet partial pressure. Using desflurane, which has lower blood gas solubility, Mets *et al.* demonstrated that initial wash-in was significantly faster. Although the arterial concentration reached 50% of inlet concentration within 4 min, it took a further 28 min to reach 68%. Desflurane wash-out during CPB was also rapid; the arterial concentration fell by 82% within the first 4 min, and by 92% 20 min after discontinuation of desflurane and rewarming the patient.

In contrast to these studies, where the volatile agent was first administered during CPB, Goucke *et al.* examined the effect of enflurane (1%) administration both before and during hypothermic CPB. Compared to pre-CPB, there was a 26% increase in median blood enflurane *concentration* (not partial pressure) upon cooling to 28°C. The blood enflurane concentration returned to within the pre-CPB range after separation from CPB, suggesting that body cooling increased enflurane concentration during CPB.

Benzodiazepines

The plasma concentration of benzodiazepines falls after the initiation of CPB but tends to rise after separation from CPB. This may be explained on the basis of prolonged elimination half-life, redistribution and hemoconcentration in the post CPB period.

Opioids

The effect of CPB on opioids depends on the mode of administration. It has been demonstrated that, following administration of a single bolus dose, plasma concentrations of fentanyl and sufentanil decreased by 53% and 34%, respectively upon initiation of CPB. The extracorporeal and pulmonary sequestration of opiates is directly proportional to lipid solubility. Like benzodiazepines, the elimination half-life of opioids may be prolonged after CPB.

Opiate infusions during hypothermic bypass may lead to significant accumulation due to reduced hepatic clearance. A near constant remifentanil concentration can be achieved by reducing the infusion rate by 30% for every 5°C decrease in temperature.

Muscle relaxants

Plasma concentrations of these typically polar drugs would be expected to fall, as a result of hemodilution, at the onset of CPB. However, altered organ blood flow and hypothermic CPB decrease metabolism and elimination. The net effect is that muscle relaxant requirements fall during CPB. Because of significant inter-patient variability it is suggested that neuromuscular monitoring be used if early tracheal extubation is contemplated.

Key points

- A number of physical and chemical factors account for the alteration of drug pharmacokinetics during CPB.

- Changes in the plasma concentration of drugs, secondary to increased volume of distribution, are often balanced by a reduction in plasma protein binding.
- Hypothermia and altered regional blood flow reduce drug metabolism and elimination.
- Hypothermia increases the solubility of volatile anesthetic agents in blood. This simultaneously increases the concentration of the agent, while reducing its partial pressure.
- Hypothermia reduces the minimum alveolar concentration (MAC) of anesthetic agents.
- Hypothermia may significantly increase the time required to achieve a therapeutic partial pressure when a volatile agent is first administered after the onset of CPB.

Further reading

Goucke CR, Hackett LP, Barrett PH, Ilett KF. Blood concentrations of enflurane before, during, and after hypothermic cardiopulmonary bypass. *J Cardiothorac Vasc Anesth* 2007; **21**: 218–23.

Mets B. The pharmacokinetics of anesthetic drugs and adjuvants during cardiopulmonary bypass. *Acta Anaesthesiol Scand* 2000; **44**: 261–73.

Mets B, Reich NT, Mellas N, Beck J, Park S. Desflurane pharmacokinetics during cardiopulmonary bypass. *J Cardiothorac Vasc Anesth* 2001; **15**: 179–82.

Nussmeier NA, Lambert ML, Moskowitz GJ, *et al.* Washin and washout of isoflurane administered via bubble oxygenators during hypothermic cardiopulmonary bypass. *Anesthesiology* 1989; **71**: 519–25.

Takizawa E, Hiraoka H, Takizawa D, Goto F. Changes in the effect of propofol in response to altered plasma protein binding during normothermic cardiopulmonary bypass. *Br J Anaesth* 2006; **96**: 179–85.

Chapter

13

Symptoms and signs of cardiac disease

Joseph E. Arrowsmith

Despite the widespread availability of investigational tests and imaging techniques for the diagnosis and management of cardiac disease, eliciting a comprehensive history and performing a systematic physical examination remain essential clinical skills.

Table 13.1 Describing patient symptoms

Nature	Description, anatomic site, radiation
Onset	Acute versus chronic
Progression	Static, rapid versus gradual worsening
Modifying factors	Provoking, exacerbating, relieving
Associations	Related symptoms

Symptoms

The presence or absence of specific symptoms should be sought in a systematic fashion. Symptoms should be described in terms of their nature (using the patient's own words), onset, duration and progression, as well any modifying factors or associations.

Overall functional status

Originally published in 1928, the New York Heart Association (NYHA) functional capacity classification provides an assessment of the impact of symptoms (dyspnea, angina, fatigue, palpitation) on physical activity. An objective assessment of severity of cardiovascular disease, added in 1994, recognizes the fact that severity of symptoms

Table 13.2 The New York Heart Association (NYHA) classification of functional capacity (first published 1928) and American Heart Association (AHA) objective assessment. (http://www.americanheart.org)

Functional capacity	Objective assessment
Class I: Patients with cardiac disease but without resulting limitation of physical activity. Ordinary physical activity does not cause undue fatigue, palpitation, dyspnea, or anginal pain	**A**: No objective evidence of cardiovascular disease
Class II: Patients with cardiac disease resulting in slight limitation of physical activity. They are comfortable at rest. Ordinary physical activity results in fatigue, palpitation, dyspnea, or anginal pain	**B**: Objective evidence of minimal cardiovascular disease
Class III: Patients with cardiac disease resulting in marked limitation of physical activity. They are comfortable at rest. Less than ordinary activity results in fatigue, palpitation, dyspnea, or anginal pain	**C**: Objective evidence of moderately severe cardiovascular disease
Class IV: Patients with cardiac disease resulting in inability to carry on any physical activity without discomfort. Symptoms of heart failure or the anginal syndrome may be present even at rest. If physical activity is undertaken, discomfort is increased	**D**: Objective evidence of severe cardiovascular disease

Examples: Class I-D, asymptomatic patient with an aortic gradient >100 mmHg; Class IV-A, angina at rest with normal coronary arteries; Class IV-D, cardiogenic shock.

Core Topics in Cardiac Anesthesia, Second Edition, ed. Jonathan H. Mackay and Joseph E. Arrowsmith. Published by Cambridge University Press. © Cambridge University Press 2012.

(i.e. functional capacity) may not reflect the severity of underlying cardiovascular disease.

Dyspnea

The sensation of uncomfortable breathing. It is essential to make the distinction between cardiac and respiratory causes. Mechanisms include: hypoxia, hypercarbia, bronchoconstriction, bronchial mucosal edema, reduced lung compliance (increased work of breathing), reflex hyperventilation, and reduced vital capacity (hydrothorax, ascites, pregnancy).

Cardiac causes include: elevated pulmonary venous pressure, reduced pulmonary blood flow (right → left shunt), and low cardiac output (RV failure). An acute onset may suggest papillary muscle or MV chordal rupture, whereas a more insidious onset may suggest gradually worsening ventricular function.

- *Associated symptoms:* especially chest pain, palpitation, diaphoresis and (pre-)syncope.
- *Postural:* supine (orthopnea, paroxysmal noctural dyspnea), other (atrial myxoma)

Hemoptysis

Not uncommon in cardiac disease. Frank hemoptysis may occur in MS (bronchial or pulmonary vein rupture) and pulmonary infarction. In pulmonary edema the sputum is frothy and often streaked with blood. Pulmonary causes include TB, bronchiectasis and cancer.

Chest pain

Etiology may be cardiac (ischemic and non-ischemic) or non-cardiac. Enquiry should be made about the quality, location, radiation, timing and duration of pain, as well as any provoking, exacerbating or relieving factors and associated symptoms.

Non-ischemic cardiac causes include; aortic dissection ("tearing" central pain radiating to back), MV prolapse (sharp infra-mammary pain), pericarditis (dull central chest pain worsened on leaning forward), and pulmonary embolus (pleuritic pain worse on inspiration).

Non-cardiac causes include: esophagitis and esophageal spasm (relieved by nitrates), biliary and pancreatic disorders, pleural inflammation and musculoskeletal disorders of the chest wall and spine.

Table 13.3 The Canadian Cardiovascular Society (CCS) angina scale

Grade	Activity
I	*"Ordinary physical activity does not cause angina";* e.g. walking or climbing stairs. Angina occurs with strenuous/rapid/prolonged exertion at work/recreation.
II	*"Slight limitation of ordinary activity";* e.g. angina occurs walking/climbing stairs after meals, in cold, in wind, under emotional stress, or only during the few hours after awakening, walking >2 blocks on the level or climbing >1 flight of stairs at a normal pace and in normal conditions.
III	*"Marked limitation of ordinary physical activity";* e.g. angina occurs walking 1–2 blocks on the level and climbing 1 flight of stairs at a normal pace and in normal conditions.
IV	*"Inability to carry on any physical activity without discomfort – angina syndrome may be present at rest"*

From: Campeau L. *Circulation* 1976; **54**: 522. (http://www.ccs.ca).

Angina pectoris

Typically described as "choking", "tightening" or "heaviness". Levine's sign (hand clenched against the chest) may be present. Usually diffuse in nature, located to mid chest or xiphisternum with radiation to the left chest and arm, epigastrium, back or jaw. Typically lasting <10 min (duration >20 min may indicate acute coronary syndrome – infarction or unstable angina). Provoked by exertion, cold exposure, eating and emotional stress. May be worsened, or paradoxically relieved, by continuing exertion. Relieved by cessation of activity or nitrates. Typically graded using Canadian Cardiovascular Society (CCS) angina scale (Table 13.3).

Syncope

Transient loss or near loss (pre-syncope) of consciousness secondary to reduced cerebral blood flow – low CO or cerebral perfusion pressure. The patient may describe "drop attacks", a "funny turn", dizziness or tinnitus. The presence of associated symptoms, such as a premonitory aura, palpitation or chest pain should be actively sought. The differential diagnosis includes postural hypotension, neurologic disorders and cardiac disease.

Postural hypotension may be drug-induced (e.g. β-blockers, vasodilators), vasovagal (e.g. micturitional), orthostatic (>20 mmHg fall in systolic BP on standing) or secondary to aortocaval compression when supine in pregnancy. Diabetes mellitus and Parkinson's disease may cause autonomic dysfunction.

A witnessed seizure may indicate epilepsy as the cause, whereas pre-syncope associated with transient dysphasia, blindness (amaurosis fugax) or paresis suggests a thromboembolic or vasculopathic cause.

Stokes–Adams attacks

Causes of Stokes–Adams attacks include sinus arrest, heart block and VT.

Exertional syncope

Exertional syncope may suggest AS, coronary artery disease, pulmonary hypertension (PHT) or a congenital anomaly of coronary artery anatomy. A family history of syncope may indicate hypertrophic obstructive cardiomyopathy, takotsubo cardiomyopathy or an inherited cardiac conduction defect (long QT syndrome, Wolff–Parkinson–White syndrome).

Edema

"Anasarca", the accumulation of interstitial fluid in dependent areas such as the lower limbs and sacral area. Sodium and water retention may occur in cardiac failure, renal failure and malnutrition. Facial edema may suggest myxedema or SVC obstruction.

Palpitations

Awareness of heartbeat. "Thumping" sensation in chest, neck or back; "missed", "jumping" or "extra" beats; or "racing" of the heart. A common symptom in the absence of cardiac disease. May indicate significant dysrhythmia or abnormal cardiac function. Any relationship to exertion or ingestion of alcohol, caffeine or nicotine should be sought, as should symptoms suggestive of thyrotoxicosis.

Fatigue

A distinction should be made between lethargy or general malaise, and effort tolerance limited by chest pain, dyspnea, claudication or leg weakness. As static measures of cardiac (ventricular) performance often give no indication of functional reserve, it is essential to obtain a measure of maximal functional capacity and the rapidity of any decline. A simplified version of the Duke Activity Status Index (DASI) is shown in Table 75.5.

Miscellaneous

These include nausea, anorexia, dry mouth (disopyramide), nocturia and polyuria (diuretics), cough (ACE inhibitors), xanthopsia (digoxin toxicity), tinnitus and vertigo (chinchonism), headache (nitrates), photosensitivity (amiodarone), nightmares (propranolol), abdominal swelling/pain (ascites/hepatomegally).

Physical signs

Physical examination is conducted with the patient supine and reclining at 45°. The patient may be required to turn to the left, sit forward, stand or perform isometric exercise.

Observation (inspection)

General appearance

Conscious level, nutritional status, diaphoresis, xanthelasmata, systolic head nodding (de Musset's sign – AR) and signs of conditions associated with cardiac disease (Marfan's, Cushing's, and Downs syndromes, acromegally, system lupus erythematosus, rheumatoid arthritis, ankylosing spondylitis, muscular dystrophy).

Skin

Cyanosis, orange fingers (tobacco use), anemia, jaundice (hepatic congestion), malar flush, erythema (pressure sores, cardioversion burns), hemorrhagic palmar/plantar lesions (Janeway lesions – endocarditis), bruising and phlebitis (venepuncture, IV therapy and drug abuse).

Surgical scars

These include sternotomy (cardiac surgery), thoracotomy (mitral valvotomy, repair of coartation or patent ductus arteriosus – PDA), subclavian (pacemaker or cardiodefibrillator insertion), cervical (carotid endarterectomy), antecubital (coronary angiography), abdominal (aortic aneurysm repair).

Nail beds

Clubbing, cyanosis, splinter hemorrhages, arterial pulsation (Quinke's sign – AR), Osler's nodes (tender finger-tip nodules – endocarditis).

Cyanosis

Cyanosis is blue skin discoloration. May be peripheral (hypovolemia, low CO) or central (mucous membranes). The latter indicates a deoxygenated Hb concentration >5 g dl^{-1}. May not be manifest in severe anemia.

Respiratory rate

Tachypnea may indicate anxiety or underlying dyspnea. Episodic (Cheyne–Stokes) breathing is suggestive of severe cardiac failure.

Neck

Goitre, carotid abrupt carotid distension and collapse (Corrigan's sign – AR), and jugular veins.

Jugular veins

Pressure level and waveform. Level rarely 2 cm above sternal angle when patient reclined at 45° and falls on inspiration. Inspiratory rise suggests pericardial constriction (Kussmaul's sign). Elevated by anxiety, pregnancy, anemia, exercise, right heart failure and SVC obstruction (non-pulsatile). Giant a-wave (TS, PS, RVH, RA myxoma), cannon a-wave (complete heart block, VT, junctional rhythm, pacing anomaly), systolic cv-wave (TR), slow y-descent (TS), sharp/short y-descent (pericardial constriction), increased x-descent (RV volume overload, tamponade).

Mouth

Fetor oris, mucous membrane dryness, state of dentition, palate, systolic uvular pulsation (Müller's sign – AR).

Fundi

Hypertensive and diabetic changes, Roth spots (endocarditis).

Palpation
Skin
- Temperature, capillary refill, pitting edema.

Pulse
- Rate, rhythm, character/volume (bounding, anacrotic, collapsing, thready, irregular), respiratory variation, condition of vessel, radio-femoral delay.
- Pulsus alternans: amplitude varies on alternate beats – indicative of severe LV dysfunction.
- Pulsus bisferiens: combined anacrotic and collapsing pulse.
- Irregular pulse may indicate AF, sinus arrhythmia, multiple atrial or ventricular premature beats or SVT with variable A-V block.
- "Waterhammer" pulse of AR detected by palpating radial artery as arm is elevated – more easily appreciated in calf muscles when elevating leg.
- An arteriovenous fistula (dialysis, severe Paget's bone disease, PDA) may also produce a collapsing pulse.
- Delayed/absent femoral pulses (coarctation, dissection, AAA).

Neck
- Tracheal deviation, carotid thrill, radiated cardiac thrill.
- Suprasternal/manubrial pulsation (coarctation).

Precordium
- Apex beat is impulse of ventricular systole normally felt in fifth intercostal space (ICS) in midclavicular line. S$_4$ may be palpable in LVH.
- Thrills in MR, VSD, AS, PS, MS and PDA.
- Left parasternal (RV) heave in PS, PHT, MS.

Lung fields
- Vocal fremitus.

Abdomen
- Hepatic enlargement/pulsation, splenomegaly (endocarditis), ascites.

Percussion
Precordium

A crude estimate of cardiac size. Area of dullness increased by pericardial effusion and decreased by emphysema.

Lung fields

Pleural effusion, lobar collapse and pneumothorax.

Abdomen

Hepatomegaly and ascites.

Auscultation

Listen all over. Bell best for low frequencies, rigid diaphragm best for high frequencies. Murmurs

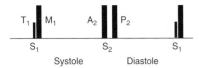

Figure 13.1 Normal heart sounds. First sound (S_1) = closure of TV and MV (loudest). Loudness of M_1 increased with sinus tachycardia, inotropes, thyroxine and delayed MV closure (reduce P-R interval and early MS). Splitting not usually audible – may indicate AV opening sound or myocardial injury (e.g. acute MI). Second sound (S_2) = closure of AV followed by PV. Splitting increased on inspiration as PV closure delayed. Inspiratory splitting increased with pulmonary hypertension, pulmonary stenosis and RBBB. Splitting reduced on expiration, and with LBBB, aging, early PHT and AS. Fixed splitting in ASD, VSD, massive PE. Paradoxical splitting (increases on expiration) by delayed AV closure – AS, LBBB, hypertension.

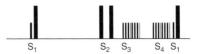

Figure 13.2 Third and fourth heart sounds. Third sound (S_3) = rapid early diastolic filling (protodiastolic gallop). May be normal in the young, otherwise pathological. Present in LV/RV failure, MR, TR, pregnancy, left → right shunts and anemia. Shorter and earlier in diastole in constrictive pericarditis. Fourth sound (S_4) = late diastolic filling (atrial systole). May be present in some tall athletes; otherwise pathological. May indicate reduced LV compliance (LVH, amyloid, ischemia). Precludes AF and severe MS. Summation gallop (S_3+S_4 superimposed) may occur in tachycardia.

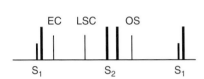

Figure 13.3 Clicks and snaps. Ejection click (EC): AS, PS and pulmonary hypertension (reduced on inspiration). Late systolic click (LSC): MV prolapse. Opening snap (OS): MS. Audible over whole precordium Indicates mobile MV leaflets, louder on expiration. Interval between A_2 and OS falls as LA pressure increases and rise with increased aortic pressure. Pneumothorax may produce systolic "clicking".

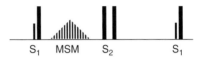

Figure 13.4 Mid ("ejection") systolic murmur (MSM). Follows AV/PV opening (crescendo-decrescendo). May be innocent (Grade ≤ III) or due to AV sclerosis, increased pulmonary flow (ASD, TAPVD), AS (harsh MSM in aortic area, soft A_2, split S_2) or PS (soft P_2, opening click, louder on inspiration).

exaggerated by inspiration (right heart origin), expiration (left heart origin), posture (left lateral, sitting forward), squatting, standing, and isometric exercise (MR in MV prolapse). Classic anatomic areas for auscultation of individual valves unreliable.

Peripheral vessels

- *Brachial arteries*: blood pressure measurement (by sphygmomanometer), estimation of respiratory paradox.
- *Carotid arteries*: bruit, radiated murmurs.
- *Abdominal arteries*: murmurs normal in 50% of young patients and 5% of over 50 years old. Renal or celiac and artery stenosis, splenic artery compression (tumor) or aneurysm.
- *Femoral arteries*: Traube's sign (booming systolic and diastolic "pistol shot" sounds over the artery in AR), Duroziez's sign (diastolic flow murmur heard in AR when artery partially compressed by stethoscope diaphragm).

Lungs

- Vesicular (normal) breath sounds.
- Bronchial breath sounds, crackles (crepitations) and wheeze (rales, rhonchi).
- Whispering pectoriloqy, broncophony and egeophony.

Precordium – heart sounds

Low-pitched sounds of short duration believed to be created by closing valve leaflets, opening valve leaflets and when structures "shudder" under sudden tension. Amplitude reduced by obesity, emphysema, pericardial effusion, AS, PS, low cardiac output and dextrocardia; increased by hyperdynamic circulation and in arterial hypertension/PHT; and varies in AF and CHB (Figures 13.1–3).

Precordium – cardiac murmurs

Vibrations caused by turbulent blood flow – more likely with high-velocity blood flow, low blood viscosity and an abrupt change in vessel/chamber diameter. Characterized by relationship to cardiac and respiratory cycles, location, radiation, acoustic quality and intensity (Table 13.4, Figures 13.4–11).

Table 13.4 Grading of cardiac murmurs

Grade	Characteristics
1/6	Only just audible, even under good auscultatory conditions
2/6	Soft
3/6	Moderately loud
4/6	Loud
5/6	Very loud
6/6	Audible with stethoscope lifted from chest wall

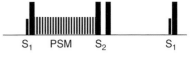

Figure 13.5 Pan (holo) systolic murmur (PSM). High-pitched apical PSM radiating to axilla with soft S_1 and S_3 in MR. Mid or late systolic click suggests MV prolapse. "Musical" PSM, louder on inspiration, at left lower sternal edge (LLSE) in TR. Harsh PSM at LLSE with thrill (~90%) suggests VSD.

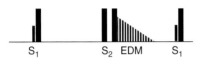

Figure 13.6 Early (immediate) diastolic murmur (EDM). *AR* – "blowing" decrescendo murmur at LLSE ± superimposed S_3. Murmur of functional MS (Austin Flint) may be present. *PR* – decrescendo murmur at left upper sternal edge (LUSE), louder on inspiration. Graham Steell (PR) murmur associated with MS and PHT.

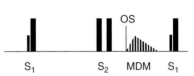

Figure 13.7 Mid diastolic murmur (MDM) following opening snap (OS). *MS* – rumbling apical MDM radiating to axilla, louder on expiration, loud P_2. Duration proportional to severity. In severe MS the OS occurs earlier ($\leq$70 mS after P_2) and is softer/inaudible and duration of MDM increases. *TS* – louder on inspiration. MDM may be caused by MV/TV thickening in rheumatic endocarditis (Carey Coombs) or by increased flow in VSD, PDA (MV) or ASD, TAPVD (TV).

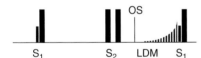

Figure 13.8 Late diastolic murmur (LDM) or presystolic accentuation. *MS* – MV flow in late diastole + atrial systole (S_4). OS typically $\geq$100 mS after P_2 in mild MS. S_4 precluded by AF.

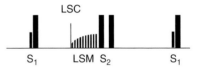

Figure 13.9 Late systolic murmur (LSM). MR/MV prolapse. May only be apparent after exercise.

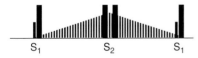

Figure 13.10 Continuous murmur. PDA ("machinery" murmur at LUSE with loud P_2), pulmonary arteriovenous fistula or surgical conduit (e.g. Blalock-Taussig, Waterston, Fontan).

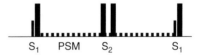

Figure 13.11 Venous hum. Partial obstruction of neck veins (especially in children). Obliterated by digital compression of veins. Important to differentiate from PDA.

Other sounds

Venous hum, friction rub and cardiorespiratory.

Further reading

Constant J. *Essentials of Bedside Cardiology*, 2nd edition. Totowa, NJ: Humana Press, 2002.

Non-invasive diagnostic tests

J. M. Tom Pierce and Sarah Marstin

Non-invasive diagnostic tests (Table 14.1) are undertaken to support the clinical impression of and to quantify the extent of cardiac disease. The investigations may be repeated over time to follow the progress of disease. Information may be supplemented with invasive investigations such as angiography when coronary artery disease is suspected.

Electrocardiography

The ECG represents the sum of myocardial voltage changes throughout the cardiac cycle along the vector of each of the leads recorded. It may be recorded from the skin surface, from the endocardium in the catheter laboratory or from the epicardium during certain open procedures requiring cardiac mapping. The simplicity of acquisition of the surface ECG makes it one of the most frequent tests performed.

The following processes affect the sum of myocardial voltage changes (Table 14.2):

- the frequency of atrial and ventricular systole
- the mass of the chambers undergoing depolarization

Table 14.1 Classification of non-invasive diagnostic techniques

Electrocardiography	Ionizing radiation	Non-ionizing imaging
Resting 12-lead ECG	CXR	Echocardiography
Exercise stress test	CT	MRI
Ambulatory ECG monitoring	Nuclear scintigraphy	
Intraoperative ECG monitoring		
Intraoperative ST segment analysis		

- the route by which depolarization occurs
- myocardial perfusion
- metabolic influences.

The ECG, in conjunction with markers of myocardial necrosis (e.g. troponin I), helps to establish the diagnosis of STEMI or NSTEMI.

Exercise ECG

Myocardial oxygen extraction is maximal at rest, so an exercise-induced increase in metabolic demand can only be met by increase in coronary blood flow. It follows therefore that coronary flow limitation in the setting of coronary artery stenosis has a far greater effect during exercise than at rest, thereby increasing the sensitivity of the ECG to detect ischemia.

Exercise ECG (ExECG) testing, using a treadmill or static cycle ergometer, is to investigate "cardiac-type" chest pain or exertional breathlessness. Both treadmill and cycle-based testing are limited to patients with the ability to exercise. In the Bruce protocol both the speed and gradient of the treadmill are increased at each stage, whereas in the modified Bruce protocol the treadmill speed remains constant during the first three stages. In the Naughton protocol, however, only the treadmill gradient is altered. Heart rate and blood pressure are recorded at each increase in workload and the ECG examined for evidence of ST segment depression. Myocardial ischemia is suggested by the development of chest pain, ST segment changes, failure to increase blood pressure or arrhythmias. Results are defined as positive, negative, equivocal and uninterpretable.

ExECG testing is relatively cheap and can be performed in the outpatient setting. It has low specificity

Core Topics in Cardiac Anesthesia, Second Edition, ed. Jonathan H. Mackay and Joseph E. Arrowsmith. Published by Cambridge University Press. © Cambridge University Press 2012.

Table 14.2 Overview of ECG abnormalities

	Abnormality	Description	Comments
Atrioventricular conduction	First-degree block	PR interval >200 ms One P wave per QRS	Seen in coronary artery disease, acute rheumatic fever, digoxin toxicity and electrolyte disturbance
	Second-degree block	Mobitz type I Progressive lengthening of PR interval Mobitz type II PR interval constant, occasional non-conducted beats 2:1 block: 2 P waves per QRS complex, normal P wave rate	Also known as Wenkebach Usually benign May herald complete heart block May herald complete heart block
	Third-degree block	Normal atrial depolarization, no conducted beats, usually wide QRS with ventricular rate <50/min	Ventricles excited by slow "escape" mechanism. Myocardial infarction, chronic fibrosis around bundle of His and in right bundle branch block. Consider pacing
Intra-ventricular conduction	Left bundle branch block	QRS >120 ms, late R-waves in I, aVL and V_{5-6}, no septal Q waves, deep S in V_1, tall R in V_6, associated with T wave inversion in lateral leads	Best seen in V_6 Always pathological, prevents further interpretation of ECG
	Left anterior hemi-block	QRS 100 ms, marked left-axis deviation, deep S in II, III, q in I ±aVL	
	Left posterior hemi-block	QRS 100 ms, right-axis deviation	
	Right bundle branch block	QRS >120 ms, RSR in V_{1-2}, dominant R and inverted T in V_1, usually normal axis	Best seen in V_1 May indicate RV problems, may be normal variant Bifasicular block: RBBB with left anterior hemiblock
Ischemia		ST depression >2 mm	
Infarction		Raised ST segments, +/−Q waves (>3 mm, >30 ms), normalization of ST segments, T wave inversion	
Hypertrophy	RA	Peaked P wave	
	LA	Bifid P wave	
	RV	RAD, tall R in V_1, T wave inversion V_{1-2}, deep S V_6, ± RBBB	
	LV	R in V_5/V_6 >25 mm or R in $V_5/6$ + S in $V_1/2$ >35 mm	

and sensitivity (65–70%) for coronary artery disease, although simultaneous transthoracic echocardiographic detection of regional wall motion abnormalities (RWMA) improves specificity. Low-grade stenoses (<50%) are difficult to detect, as are fixed stenoses with collateral blood flow. Contraindications to exECG include acute coronary syndromes, severe congestive cardiac failure and severe aortic stenosis. It may also be unsuitable for patients with physical disability, respiratory disease, peripheral vascular disease, left bundle branch block or A-V conduction abnormalities.

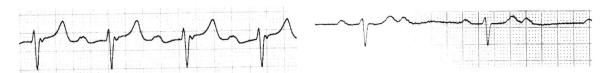

Figure 14.1 First-degree heart block (left) and 2:1 heart block (Mobitz II) (right).

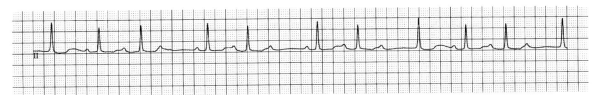

Figure 14.2 Wenckebach phenomenon (Mobitz I). The P-R interval gradually increases.

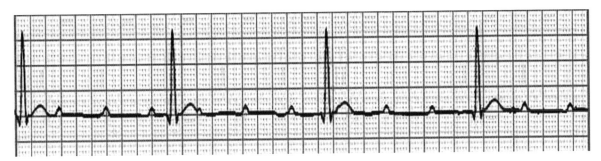

Figure 14.3 Third-degree (complete) heart block.

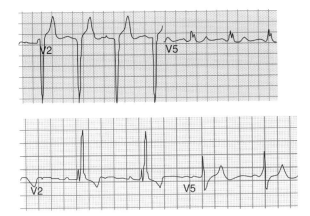

Figure 14.4 Left bundle branch block (upper) and right bundle branch block (lower).

Table 14.3 Limitations to the resting surface ECG

Temporal changes in the ST segment may be missed with a single recording

Small non-Q wave infarcts may fail to meet diagnostic criteria

Large transmural infarcts may obscure additional electrocardiographic events

The sensitivity to detect ischemia is limited by the position of the exploring electrode

Posterior cardiac events are often missed

Resting ECG may be normal even in the setting of three-vessel coronary artery disease

May fail to reflect the effect of exercise on myocardial perfusion

ECG changes lag behind changes in diastolic and systolic dysfunction with ischemia

Prone to skeletal muscle myopotentials obscuring changes

Table 14.4 The Bruce treadmill protocol and an example of one of the many modifications described. The target heart rate for the test is 220 minus patient age. For example, the test would be halted (regardless of ECG changes) for a patient aged 50 when a heart rate of 170 had been achieved

Bruce protocol			Modified protocol		
Stage	Speed (mph)	Grade (%)	Speed (mph)	Grade (%)	Duration (min)
1	1.7	10	1.7	0	3
2	2.5	12	1.7	5	3
3	3.4	14	1.7	10	3
4	4.2	16	2.5	12	3
5	5.0	18	3.4	14	3
6	5.5	20	4.2	16	3
7	6.0	22	5.0	18	3
8			5.5	20	3
9			6.0	22	3
10			6.5	24	3

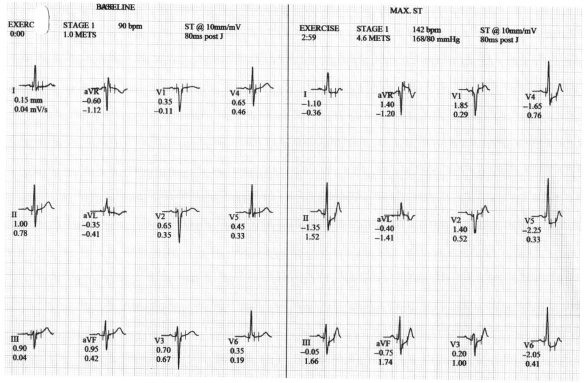

Figure 14.5 Exercise ECG summary print out from a patient undergoing low workload with significant ST segment changes. The depression of the ST segment is measured 80 ms after the J point. The maximum ST segment depression was 2.25 mm in lead V_5.

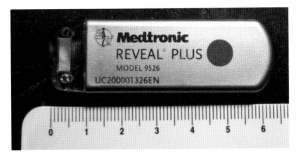

Figure 14.6 The Medtronic Reveal® implantable ECG recorder. The recording electrodes are on the left.

Ambulatory ECG

Ambulatory ECG monitoring, also known as Holter or continuous 24 hour recording, is a method used to aid the diagnosis of chest pain, palpitations or syncope that occur intermittently during normal daily activities. The ECG electrodes are applied to the chest and attached to a recording device which is carried by the patient for a period of 24–48 hours. Some devices comprise a patient-activated event monitor. Patients are required to complete a log of events to aid analysis and correlate physical activities with contemporaneous ECG changes. The recorder is interrogated to produce a printout or computer analysis of events.

Longer-term (up to 6–12 months) implantable ECG recorders are used to increase event detection rate. They may record data continuously or intermittently. Integral electrodes are placed subcutaneously in the left subclavian position. The Reveal® device is an example of a patient-activated intermittent loop recorder (Figure 14.6). When activated, data acquired in the minute before activation (the prodrome) and during symptoms are stored. The digital storage of data is limited to 45 min. The device may be interrogated transcutaneously and therefore may be left *in situ* if required. Both insertion and removal of the recorder can be conducted under local anesthesia.

Transthoracic echocardiography

Transthoracic echocardiography (TTE) is relatively quick and straightforward to perform, and provides qualitative and quantitative assessment of cardiac structure and function.

Although TTE is an extremely useful tool, it does have several limitations. Certain patient factors reduce echogenicity and therefore make image quality poor or unobtainable. These include obesity, pulmonary

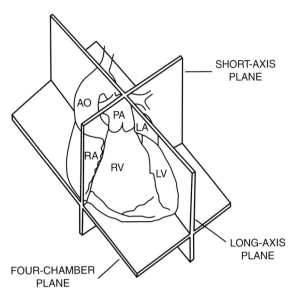

Figure 14.7 The thee basic image planes used in transthoracic echocardiography. The long axis extends from the LV apex through the A-V plane. The short axis lies perpendicular to the long axis. The four-chamber view lies perpendicular to both the long and short axis planes, and includes the LV apex, RV, LA and RA.

emphysema, interference from the ribs, an inability to lie in the lateral position, and the presence of surgical drains and anterior chest wall dressings. Findings are relatively operator-dependent and technical difficulties may limit both the quality and completeness of an examination. Spatial resolution is restricted to one wavelength (0.3 mm at 5 MHz) and depth resolution to 200 wavelengths (60 mm at 5 MHz). TTE is poor at imaging posterior structures and Doppler can only be used to estimate flow accurately if the angle of incident ultrasound is $<20°$. (See Figure 24.2.)

Stress echocardiography

Echocardiography can be combined with exercise testing or dobutamine-induced (40–60 µg kg^{-1} min^{-1}) stress in patients unable to exercise to allow qualitative assessment of ventricular performance with increase in heart rate. Occasionally, pacing or atropine is required to obtain an adequate HR response. Imaging dynamic changes in LV outflow obstruction in hypertrophic obstructive cardiomyopathy (HOCM) is also possible. Stress echocardiography is more sensitive than stress ECG at detecting ischemia. The value of the test rests in the visualization of functional changes with increased myocardial demand.

85

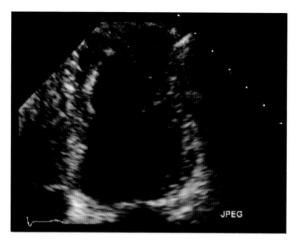 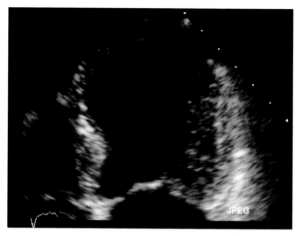

Figure 14.8 Still echo images taken at rest (left) and during dobutamine-induced stress (right) demonstrating significant ventricular dilatation. The patient had significant LAD stenosis.

Contrast echocardiography

Contrast agents can be employed to improve image quality by delineating the border between endocardium and ventricular cavity. Sonographic contrast agents are suspensions of microspheres filled with perfluorocarbon gas which enhance image resolution by acting as intravascular tracers. The insonated gas bubbles pulsate, with compression occurring at the peak of the ultrasound wave and expansion at the nadir. SonoVue® is a stabilized aqueous suspension of sulfur hexafluoride (2.5 μm microbubbles) within a shell of polyethylene glycol (macrogel 4000). After peripheral intravenous injection of 0.2–0.4 ml, the microbubbles traverse the pulmonary vascular bed to opacify the ventricular cavity. Further refinements allow quantification of coronary microcirculation by assessment of subendocardial opacification. This is particularly powerful during stress echocardiography

as a reduction in opacification is often easier to appreciate than a new RWMA. Allergic reactions to contrast agents have occurred and therefore, contrast is contraindicated in patients with recent unstable cardiac symptoms, a recent (<7 days) coronary intervention, class III and IV heart failure or serious arrhythmias.

Further reading

Chung EK, Tighe D. *Pocket Guide to Stress Testing*. London: Wiley Blackwell; 1997.

Garcia MJ. *Non-Invasive Cardiovascular Imaging: A Multimodality Approach*. London: Lippincott Williams and Wilkins; 2009.

Leeson P, Mitchell ARJ, Becher H. *Echocardiography (Oxford Specialist Handbooks in Cardiology)*. Oxford: Oxford University Press: 2007.

Otto CM. *Textbook of Clinical Echocardiography*, 4th edition. Philadelphia: Saunders; 2009.

15

Cardiac radiological imaging

Catherine V. Koffel and Maximilien J. Gourdin

Over the years, new cardiac radiological imaging modalities have been developed to assess the beating heart. A comprehensive non-invasive cardiac examination is now possible. The anesthesiologist must be aware of the indications and limits of each technique.

Chest radiography

A posteroanterior and lateral CXR provides information about the heart, the lungs, the great vessels and the thoracic skeleton (Table 15.1). The normal orientation of the cardiac valves in relation to the thoracic skeleton is shown in Figure 15.1. A plain preoperative CXR provides a baseline against which to judge postoperative images.

Table 15.1 Assessment of the preoperative chest radiograph before cardiac surgery

Cardiac silhouette

Cardiothoracic ratio ("normal" ≤50%)
LA enlargement
Calcification – LV wall, valvular, pericardial
Prostheses/pacing wires

Mediastinal silhouette

Calcification – aortic arch
Mediastinal widening
Tracheal deviation

Hila

Pulmonary arteries and veins
Lympadenopathy and other masses

Lung fields

Upper lobe blood diversion

Interlobular septal (Kerley B) lines
Perihilar ("bat's wing") consolidation

Diaphragm

Pleural effusion

Skeleton

Sternal wires – previous surgery
Rib notching
Retrosternal space – in redo-surgery

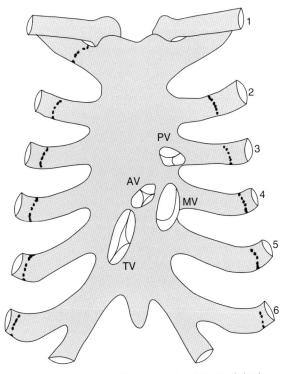

Figure 15.1 Orientation of heart valves in relation to skeletal structures visible on a plain posteroanterior CXR.

Core Topics in Cardiac Anesthesia, Second Edition, ed. Jonathan H. Mackay and Joseph E. Arrowsmith. Published by Cambridge University Press. © Cambridge University Press 2012.

Nuclear cardiology

Scintigraphy, positron emission tomography (PET) and single photon emission computed tomography (SPECT) detect gamma rays emitted by a radionuclide tracer administered to the patient. In contrast to scintigraphy imaging (planar 2D), PET and SPECT can provide information in three dimensions. The radionuclide tracers thallium (^{201}Tl), technetium-sestamibi (^{99m}Tc-sestamibi) and ^{99m}Tc-tetrofosmin are routinely used for SPECT and scintigraphy. Due to its shorter half-life (^{99m}Tc, 6 h versus ^{201}Tl, 72 h), a higher dose of ^{99m}Tc can be administered. Superior image quality at a lower radiation dose makes ^{99m}Tc the preferred tracer. The radionuclide tracers rubidium (^{82}Rb) and N-ammonia (^{13}N-ammonia) are used for PET.

Nuclear cardiac imaging techniques allow assessment of myocardial blood flow, myocardial viability and, when ECG-gated imaging is used, global and regional ventricular function. The main limitations of these techniques are relatively poor spatial resolution, soft-tissue attenuation artifacts and delivery of a significant dose of ionizing radiation.

Stress imaging

Myocardial imaging at rest and during exercise (stress) permits the assessment of myocardial perfusion (Table 15.2). Pharmacological stress, induced using a vasodilator (adenosine or dipyridamole) or an inotrope (dobutamine), can be used in patients unable to exercise. Multiple or severe inducible ischemic defects represent significant scintigraphic findings. ECG-gated acquisition gives improved diagnostic accuracy by allowing better distinction between true perfusion abnormalities and artifacts. It also allows evaluation of ventricular function.

Furthermore, viable myocardium can be identified either by perfusion (^{201}Tl or ^{99m}Tc-sestamibi; assessment of cellular membrane integrity) or by metabolic (fluorodeoxyglucose, ^{18}FDG) tracers. Myocardial viability is an important determinant of the likely benefits of revascularization therapy. The indications and effectiveness of myocardial perfusion imaging are summarized in Tables 15.3 and 15.4.

Computed tomography

High temporal and spatial resolution is required to visualize small and moving coronary arteries. This has been made possible by the development of

Table 15.2 Clinical significance of radionuclide tracer uptake during myocardial perfusion

Tracer uptake	Significance
Homogeneous	Normal myocardial perfusion (except when severe three-vessel disease: homogeneous uptake associated with poor LV function) Low risk of cardiac event (0.6% per year)
Reversible defect	Defect on stress study only Indicates reversible ischemia/viable myocardium High risk of cardiac event (~7–13% per year) Indication of revascularization therapy
Fixed defect	Defect on rest and stress study Indicates myocardial infarction

Table 15.3 Indications for myocardial perfusion imaging

Preoperative evaluation

Myocardial viability assessment

Risk stratification

Evaluation after PCI or coronary artery grafting

Medical therapy monitoring

PCI, percutaneous coronary intervention.

multidetector row CT (MDCT) – scanners with fast X-ray tube rotation speed and multiple detector rows. The use of first generation four-slice MDCT was limited by the need for slow heart rates (to reduce motion artifacts) and a long breath-hold time (up to 40 s – difficult for breathless patients). The latest generation of 64-slice, ECG-gated MDCT systems can acquire images of the cardiac anatomy, the coronary vessels and any stenoses in <10 s. Due to the high spatial resolution of 64-slice MDCT (~0.4 mm), >90% of coronary segments are evaluable with high sensitivity and good specificity. The presence of severe coronary calcification (Agatston score >400–600 units) reduces the sensitivity of the modality and makes it difficult to assess intraluminal narrowing. The clinical utility of coronary CT angiography (CTA) is summarized in Table 15.5.

Table 15.4 Assessment of coronary artery disease (CAD) by non-invasive radiological imaging methods

	Computed tomography	Magnetic resonance	PET/SPECT
Anatomical evaluation			
Non-invasive coronary angiography	Routine application Limited by coronary calcifications (pre-test Ca-scoring), temporal resolution (heart rate) Sensitivity 91%, specificity 80% High negative predictive value of 95%–98% Limited reliability for treatment decision	Research protocols and specialized centers Sensitivity 93% Specificity 58%	
Functional evaluation			
Rest and stress perfusion imaging	More experimental Limited by the increasing dose of radiation Underestimate the extent of ischemia	Routine application Enhancement of perfused tissue during first pass Gd-ceMRI Detection of CAD with sensitivity 91%, specificity 81%	Gold standard Detection of CAD with sensitivity and specificity > 90%
LV function	More experimental	Gold standard Assessment of biventricular ejection fraction, stroke volume, ventricular mass Prognostic value	Gated PET/SPECT Limited by low resolution
Myocardial viability	More experimental	Myocardial scar detection by late Gd-ceMRI Prognostic value	Gold standard Prognostic value

Gd-ceMRI, gadolinium contrast-enhanced magnetic resonance imaging.

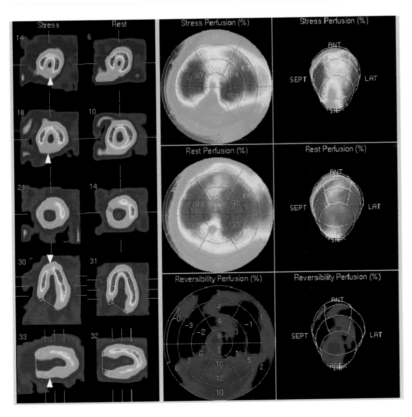

Figure 15.2 99mTc-sestamibi myocardial perfusion scintigraphy. Example of a patient with reversible apical and inferobasal perfusion defects (white arrowheads). Analysis of tracer uptake allows quantification and localization (20 myocardial segments) of the lesions.

The radiation dose administered during cardiac MDCT is high (~15–21 mSv) and associated with an increased lifetime risk of cancer. The risk is greater for women (breast cancer), young patients and combined cardiac and aortic scans.

Electron-beam CT (EBCT) and dual-source CT (DSCT) have been developed to overcome the temporal limitations of MDCT. However, EBCT offers lower spatial resolution and further clinical studies are required to evaluate the potential of DSCT.

Table 15.5 Clinical indications of coronary CT angiography

Detection of coronary artery stenosis

Low PPV (60–70%), selected patient (intermediate risk patient), high NPV

Coronary artery anomalies

Origin and course of aberrant coronary arteries, 3-D evaluation, high accuracy

Coronary stent imaging

Possible to rule out in-stent stenosis, affected by metal artifacts, low PPV

Coronary artery bypass grafts

Visualization of grafts with high accuracy (especially large venous grafts), limited by difficult assessment of native coronary artery, grafts occlusion or stenosis diagnosed with high PPV (>92%)

PPV, positive predictive value; NPV, negative predictive value.

Coronary artery disease

The presence of coronary arterial calcium is a marker of coronary atherosclerosis. Coronary calcium scoring by non-contrast enhanced EBCT and by MDCT is used for risk stratification in patients with coronary artery disease (CAD). The greater the amount of calcium, the greater is the likelihood of occlusive CAD. The presence or absence of coronary calcification does not, however, allow reliable distinction between stable and unstable plaques. Furthermore, the presence of calcification does not always correlate with coronary stenosis. Thus calcium scoring has low predictive positive value (PPV).

Since the introduction of 64-slice MDCT in 2004, non-invasive coronary CTA has become an alternative to invasive imaging techniques in many centers. Contrast-enhanced coronary CTA can be performed within 10 min and fast reconstruction makes the study immediately available for final interpretation. With the exception of distal segments and left circumflex coronary artery, evaluation of significant (>50%) coronary stenosis is possible with a high sensitivity and specificity (Table 15.4).

Coronary CTA is particularly useful for ruling out significant CAD. Due to its high negative predictive value (NPV), a normal coronary CTA reliably excludes significant coronary stenosis. The main limitations of MDCT are the inability to assess coronary artery stenoses in the presence of dense calcification

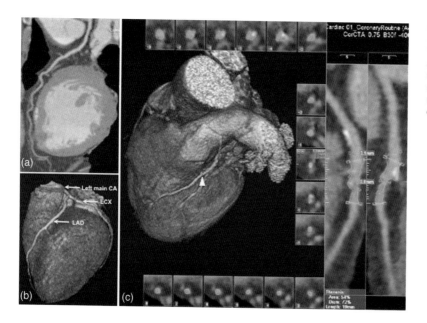

Figure 15.3 Coronary CT angiography. (a) Curved multiplanar reconstruction image of a normal LAD. Proximal, mid and distal segments are visualized. (b) 3-D volume-rendered image of normal coronary arteries. (c) 3-D and multiplanar reformatted images of coronary stenosis (arrow).

and the detection of coronary atherosclerotic lesions that are not flow-limiting. Hybrid systems, linking high-resolution anatomic CT imaging with the functional capability of PET/SPECT, have been developed to overcome the limitations of each technique.

Aortic disease

MDCT with advanced post-processing techniques or MRI can be used to evaluate the entire spectrum of the aortic disease. These two reference techniques provide crucial information about the aorta and surrounding structures, helping to display critical anatomical relationships to interventionists and surgeons. CTA remains the preferred technique for evaluation of suspected aortic rupture because of its availability, speed and very high sensitivity and specificity for this complication.

Pericardial disease

Motion-free MDCT imaging allows better visualization of the pericardium and is an additional technique for the diagnosis of pericardial disorders. The main advantage of CT is its high sensitivity for identifying pericardial calcification, making it the best modality for the diagnosis of constrictive pericarditis.

Valvular disease

Information regarding valvular anatomy and function derived from MDCT is described in Table 15.6.

Magnetic resonance imaging

Magnetic resonance imaging (MRI) uses the magnetic properties of atomic nuclei. Hydrogen nuclei (protons) in the body generate local and randomly oriented magnetic fields. The MR magnet provides a powerful static magnetic field to align the nuclei. Radiofrequency fields are then applied to alter the alignment and then removed. The energy released

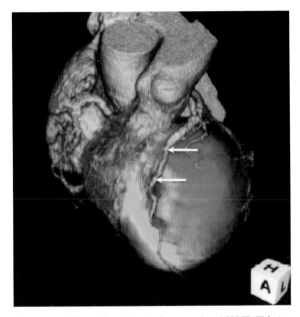

Figure 15.4 Three-dimensional volume-rendered SPECT/CT fusion image of clinical significant calcified LAD stenosis. The green area shows the corresponding perfusion defect.

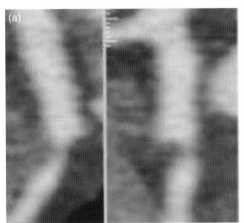
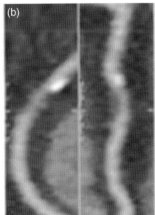
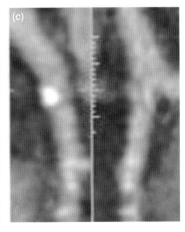

Figure 15.5 Coronary CT angiography. Non-invasive assessment of atherosclerotic plaque. (a) Non-stenotic lipid plaque (low density ~50 Hounsfield units; HU). These plaques are more often associated with acute coronary syndromes. (b) Fibrocalcified plaque. (c) Calcified plaque (>130 HU).

Table 15.6 Valve assessment with MRI and MDCT

	Cine MDCT	SSFP Cine MRI
Morphology	Excellent for leaflets, chordae and papillary muscle visualization (high spatial resolution) Accurate quantification of valve calcifications	Moderate Limited for chordae and papillary muscles
Function	Qualitative and quantitative assessment (planimetry) of valve stenosis and regurgitation Good correlation with transthoracic (TTE) and TEE Accurate evaluation of valve motion and mechanism of valve disease (cusps prolapse, restrictive cusps motion)	

SSFP, steady-state free precession.

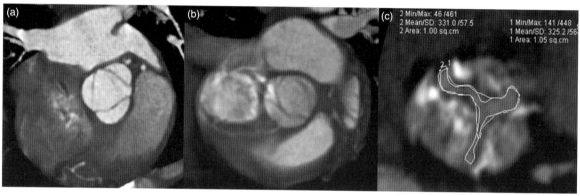

Figure 15.6 64-slice MDCT axial view of aortic valves. (a) Normal valve. (b) Bicuspid valve. (c) Measurement of AV orifice area by planimetry in a stenotic calcified valve.

as the nuclei return to their initial position is detected and used to produce the magnetic resonance image. With this technique, both two- and three-dimensional imaging is possible. A comprehensive MRI examination – static morphological images, cine MRI sequences, stress and rest perfusion MRI and ceMRI – can be time-consuming (~30 min depending on the sequence and protocol used).

The use of a 1.5 or 3.0 tesla magnet with a MR sequence called *steady-state free precession* (SSFP) imaging offers excellent signal-to-noise and contrast-to-noise ratios with fast image acquisition and superior image quality.

Injection of the contrast agent gadolinium diethylenetriaminepentaacetic acid (Gd-DTPA) improves the sensitivity of MRI. Gadolinium is less nephrotoxic than conventional radiocontrast agents, making contrast-enhanced MRI (ceMRI) an option for patients with renal impairment. Perfused tissue appears brighter during the first pass of Gd-DTPA (enhanced signal in spin-lattice relaxation time/T_1-weighted images).

MRI is now established as the non-invasive imaging modality of choice for the evaluation of the structure and function of the heart and blood vessels (Table 15.7).

Coronary artery disease

MRI can be used to detect CAD by both direct (i.e. angiographic) and indirect (i.e. perfusion) methods (Table 15.4). Low spatial resolution, poor reproducibility and a large percentage of non-assessable segments limit the use of coronary MR angiography.

The most important use of perfusion MRI is the assessment of myocardial viability (late Gd-ceMRI). The high PPV of perfusion MRI has been validated in several clinical studies. The presence of normal perfusion is predictive of a 99% chance of 3 year event-free survival.

MRI also provides accurate quantification of cardiac chamber volume and function as well as myocardial mass and is considered the gold standard for these measurements.

Table 15.7 Characteristics and common functional and morphological MRI indications

Indications

Myocardial ischemia and viability
Cardiac mass and inflammatory disease
Pericardial disease
Aorta disease
Congenital heart disease (morphology, shunt evaluation)
Arrhythmogenic RV dysplasia (ARVD)
Heart valve disease

Advantages

No ionizing radiation
No iodinated contrast material
Excellent soft-tissue contrast

Contraindications (~20% of patients)

Ferromagnetic foreign body
Aneurysm clip
Intraorbital metal
Non-MR-compatible implant
Claustrophobia

Aortic disease

MRI is particularly useful in patients with thoracoabdominal aortic aneurysm (oblique sagittal MRI images) and has the advantage of not exposing patients who require regular follow up to repeated doses of ionizing radiation (Table 15.7).

Valvular disease

Both MDCT and MRI allow accurate evaluation of heart valve function (Table 15.6). MRI planimetric (cine MRI) or continuity equation-based (phase contrast MRI) measurements of AV orifice area correlate strongly with TEE and TTE findings, and thus can be an alternative tool for the diagnosis of aortic stenosis and regurgitation.

Pericardial disease and cardiac masses

High soft-tissue contrast and the ability to acquire multiplanar and SSFP cine images make MRI the reference method for the evaluation of pericardial diseases and cardiac masses. The pericardium is seen on both T_1 and T_2-weighted (spin-spin relaxation time) MRI images as a thin band of low signal intensity. MRI can detect small or loculated effusions and acute pericarditis and is useful for the

Table 15.8 Comparison of cardiac radiological imaging methods for the diagnosis of cardiovascular diseases

	Chest X-ray (CXR)	Nuclear studies PET/ SPECT	MRI	MDCT
CAD				
Angiography	−	−	+	++ (Congenital coronary artery anomalies +++)
Perfusion images	−	+++	+++	+
Viability	−	++	+++	+
LV function	+	++	+++	+
Aorta				
Aneurysm	+	−	+++	+++
Dissection	−	−	+++	+++
Rupture	+	−	++	+++
Pericardial diseases	+	−	+++ (Constrictive pericarditis ++)	++ (Constrictive pericarditis +++)
Cardiac masses	+	−	+++	++
Heart valve	−	−	++	++
Aortic valve			++	++
Mitral valve			+	+
Congenital disease	+	−	+++	++

differentiation of constrictive pericarditis from restrictive cardiomyopathy.

Summary

Technical progress in cardiac radiological imaging has radically altered the diagnosis and management of cardiac and vascular disease. Many of these noninvasive tests, validated by large clinical trials, are now considered to be gold standards (Table 15.8).

Key points

- Myocardial perfusion imaging may identify ischemic myocardium that would benefit from revascularization.

93

- Contrast-enhanced MRI allows assessment of myocardial viability with a greater accuracy than FDG-PET/SPECT.
- Negative 64-slice MDCT coronary angiography reliably excludes significant coronary disease.
- The development of hybrid PET-SPECT/CT imaging enables the simultaneous assessment of the anatomic extent and functional consequences of coronary artery disease.
- MDCT and MRI are alternative modalities for valvular imaging with good correlation with echocardiography.

Further reading

Kaufmann PA. Cardiac hybrid imaging: state-of-the-art. *Ann Nucl Med* 2009; **23**(4): 325–31.

Pouleur AC, le Polain de Waroux JB, Pasquet A, Vanoverschelde JL, Gerber BL. Aortic valve area assessment: multidetector CT compared with cine MR imaging and transthoracic and transesophageal echocardiography. *Radiology* 2007; **244**(3): 745–54.

Vogel-Claussen J, Pannu H, Spevak PJ, Fishman EK, Bluemke DA. Cardiac valve assessment with MR imaging and 64-section multi-detector row CT. *Radiographics* 2006; **26**(6): 1769–84.

Invasive diagnosis techniques

16

Herve Schlotterbeck and Stephane Noble

Cardiac catheterization

Cardiac catheterization was originally developed as a means to measure pressures within the heart chambers and great vessels (Table 16.1). The introduction of radio-opaque contrast media led to the development of ventriculography and coronary angiography. These invasive procedures involve exposure to contrast media and ionizing radiation, and may be accompanied by both minor and life-threatening complications. Despite the development of new, non-invasive techniques (e.g. radionucleotide perfusion imaging and MRI), cardiac catheterization remains the most widely used method for assessing the severity and distribution of coronary artery disease. In addition to diagnostic information, cardiac catheterization permits therapeutic intervention (e.g. angioplasty, valvuloplasty) as well as assessing prognosis and aiding surgical planning.

Right heart

Right heart catheterization (RHC) is mainly indicated for patients with a history of unexplained dyspnea, valvular (particularly mitral) disease or intracardiac shunt. It is used in combination with left heart catheterization in only 10% of patients – arguably too infrequently given the relatively high incidence of pulmonary hypertension (PHT) in cardiac disease.

A radio-opaque catheter is inserted under local anesthesia via a large vein (e.g. femoral, internal jugular) and advanced through the RA and RV to the PA.

Table 16.1 Measurements obtained during left and right heart catheterization, and normal values

	Parameter	Measurement	Normal values	Units
LEFT	Arterial/aortic pressure	S/D (M)	<140/90 (105)	mmHg
	LV pressure	S/D_E	<140/12	mmHg
RIGHT	RA pressure	(M)	(<6)	mmHg
	RV pressure	S/D_E	<25/5	mmHg
	PA pressure	S/D (M)	25/12 (22)	mmHg
	PAWP	(M)	(12)	mmHg
	Cardiac index		2.5–4.2	$l\ min^{-1}\ m^{-2}$
	D_E volume index		< 100	$ml\ m^{-2}$
	$DavO_2$		< 5.0	$ml\ dl^{-1}$
	PVR		~100	$dyne\ s\ cm^{-5}$
	SVR		800–1200	$dyne\ s\ cm^{-5}$

S/D (M), systolic/diastolic (mean); D_E, end-diastolic. $DavO_2$, arteriovenous oxygen content difference.

Core Topics in Cardiac Anesthesia, Second Edition, ed. Jonathan H. Mackay and Joseph E. Arrowsmith. Published by Cambridge University Press. © Cambridge University Press 2012.

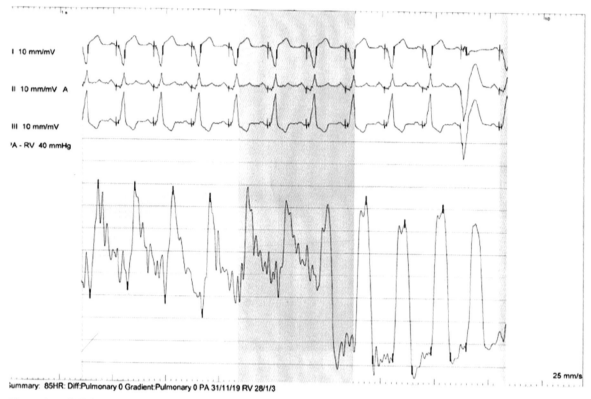

Summary: 85HR: Diff:Pulmonary 0 Gradient:Pulmonary 0 PA 31/11/19 RV 28/1/3

Figure 16.1 RHC showing a pull back from the PA to the right ventricle (RV). The mean PA pressure is in the normal range (19 mmHg).

Plain catheters may be deployed via the femoral vein, while insertion via the jugular or subclavian approach may be aided by the use of a balloon-tipped catheter. Each cavity has a characteristic pressure waveform profile (Figure 16.1). Pulmonary capillary wedge (occlusion) pressure, which can be obtained by wedging a plain catheter in a distal PA or by inflating the balloon, reflects LA and LV filling pressures.

The cardiac output can be measured using either thermodilution or the Fick method (requiring hemoglobin concentration and oximetric measurements in both PA and systemic arterial blood). (See Chapter 23.)

The anatomic location and hemodynamic significance of left-to-right shunts (i.e. ASD, VSD) can be assessed using oximetry at different vascular and cardiac levels (e.g. SVC, IVC, RA, RV and PA). Abnormally high SO_2 or a step increase in SO_2 will be found where a left-to-right shunt exists. The ratio of pulmonary to systemic blood flow (the shunt fraction; Qp/Qs) can be calculated using the shunt equation. (See Chapter 51.)

In patients with PHT, the wedge pressure and transpulmonary gradient (i.e. mean PA pressure – mean wedge) help to determine the origin of PA elevation (pre- vs. post-capillary). The rate of distal run-off following balloon occlusion, a technique known as PVR partitioning, may be particularly useful in the management of chronic thromboembolic PHT. In pre-capillary PHT, vasoreactivity testing using nitric oxide can be performed to identify patients who may benefit from long-term therapy with Ca^{2+} channel blockers. Pulmonary vascular resistance and PHT reversibility are routinely assessed in prospective heart transplant recipients as these parameters affect post-transplant outcome. RHC is undertaken after cardiac transplantation to assess graft function and to obtain endomyocardial biopsies.

The LA and LV can be instrumented via transeptal puncture, typically at the site of the fossa ovalis. This permits both the acquisition of diagnostic information (e.g. mitral stenosis) and therapeutic intervention (e.g. ASD/PFO closure, mitral valvuloplasty) (Figure 16.3).

The major complications of RHC include dysrhythmias, thrombosis, hemorrhage and PA rupture.

Table 16.2 Left heart catheterization procedures

Technique	Procedure	Information obtained
Manometry	Pressure measurements are made with the catheter in aortic root and LV cavity	AV gradient LVEDP
Angiography	The ostia or the coronary arteries, vein grafts or internal mammary artery are selectively cannulated and contrast-injected	Coronary anatomy, left or right dominance, location and severity of stenotic lesions, presence of collateral circulation, patency of bypass grafts
Ventriculogram	A pigtail catheter is advanced across AV into LV 35–45 ml contrast is rapidly injected	Ventricular size and function LV ejection fraction LV aneurysm Severity of MR
Aortogram	A catheter is placed in the aortic root. Contrast is injected manually	Severity of AR

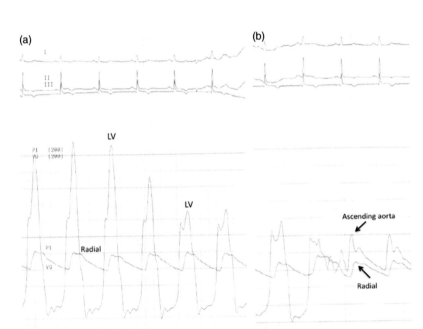

(a) (b)

Figure 16.2 (a) LHC with simultaneous recording of LV and radial artery (from the side port of the radial sheath) pressures during pull back inside the LV. This tracing shows an important intra-LV pressure gradient in a patient suffering from a mid-ventricular obstructive hypertrophic cardiomyopathy. (b) Pull back from the LV to the ascending aorta. The pressure curve in the ascending aorta shows the typical pointed-finger aspect described in cases of obstructive hypertrophic cardiomyopathy.

Left heart

A comprehensive left heart catheterization complete examination includes manometry, coronary angiography, left ventriculography and aortography (Table 16.2).

Coronary angiography

Fifty years after the procedure was first serendipitously performed by F. Mason Sones, selective coronary angiography remains the method most widely used to define coronary arterial anatomy. In addition,

it provides important information regarding coronary dominance (determined by the origin of the posterior descending artery), congenital anomalies, collateral blood supply and the presence of calcification.

In adults a 4–6 Fr (1.3–2 mm diameter) sheath is placed in a peripheral (femoral, brachial or radial) artery under local anesthesia. A series of long catheters (Figure 16.4) are then advanced through the sheath into the proximal aorta and LV cavity. Selective cannulation of the coronary ostia and subsequent injection of radio-opaque contrast allows

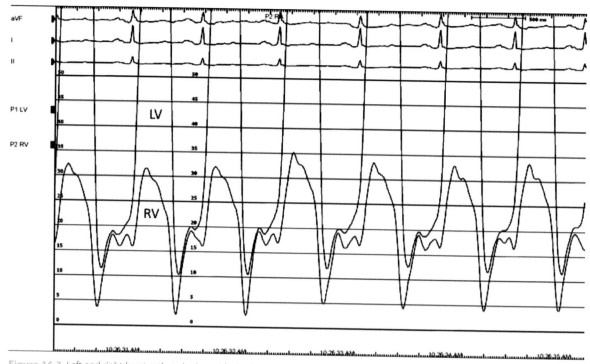

Figure 16.3 Left and right heart catheterization with simultaneous recording of LV and RV pressures in a patient with constrictive pericarditis (LVEDP = RVEDP and RV systolic pressure/RV end-diastolic pressure <3 mmHg).

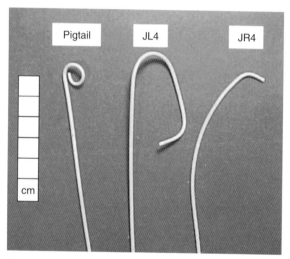

Figure 16.4 Commonly used adult (6Fr) cardiac catheters. Pigtail – for ventriculography. Judkins "left" (JL4) – left coronary artery. Judkins "right" (JR4) – right coronary artery.

demonstration of the coronary arterial anatomy. A reduction in luminal diameter >75% (>50% in left main stem) is considered significant (Figure 16.5).

The technique exposes patients to iodinated contrast media and ionizing radiation, both of which may be associated with complications. Although percutaneous coronary intervention (PCI) during LHC carries greater risk, major complications (e.g. death, stroke, myocardial infarction and dysrhythmia) occur in less than 0.1% of diagnostic procedures. Local vascular and hemorrhagic complications (e.g. hematoma, false aneurysm, distal ischemia) are the most common adverse events (2–8%) particularly when the femoral approach is used. Because of reduced hemorrhagic complications, use of the radial arterial approach is increasing. Rarer complications include allergic reactions to contrast media, contrast-induced nephropathy and late radiodermitis (Table 16.3).

Conventional coronary angiography has several limitations:

- as coronary angiography produces 2-D images, stenoses may be incorrectly evaluated in tortuous and angulated vessels. Moreover, stenoses are often evaluated in comparison with a seemingly normal reference segment that may actually be diseased;
- misinterpretations due to suboptimal contrast media injection, an inadequate number of orthogonal projections or catheter-induced coronary spasm;
- inter- and intra-observer variability in diagnosis and reporting.

Table 16.3 Complications of left heart catheterization

Site	Examples
Access site	Bleeding, hematoma, pseudoaneurysm Vascular injury – distal limb ischemia Infection
Vascular	Aortic dissection Renal, mesenteric, cerebral embolization
Cardiac	Coronary dissection/occlusion Myocardial infarction Dysrhythmia – including VF
General	Vasovagal syncope Contrast-induced nephrotoxicity Allergic reactions to contrast Radiodermatitis

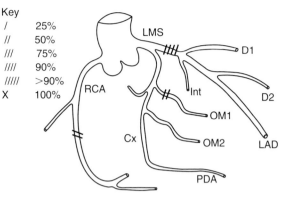

Key

/	25%
//	50%
///	75%
////	90%
/////	>90%
X	100%

Figure 16.5 An example of a coronary angiogram report showing left dominance, severe proximal LAD disease and mild disease in the mid right coronary artery (RCA) and the first obtuse marginal branch (OM1) of the circumflex artery (Cx).

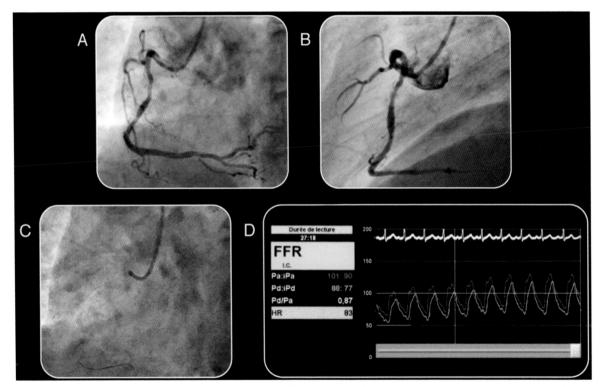

Figure 16.6 Functional coronary flow reserve (FFR) Panels a and b: two orthogonal views showing an intermediate lesion in the right coronary artery (RCA). Panel c: pressure wire advanced distally to the stenosis of interest (pressure measured at the transition between radio-opaque and transparent portions of the wire). Panel d: pressure tracings and results (in this case MAP=101.90 and mean distal RCA pressure = 88.77 gives FFR=0.87. FFR >0.8 is considered normal).

Some of these limitations can be overcome by assessing fractional flow reserve (FFR), which provides an index of the physiological significance of a coronary stenosis. A pressure-sensitive guidewire is advanced past the stenosis of interest (Figure 16.6) and FFR is calculated by dividing mean distal coronary pressure by the mean aortic pressure (measured simultaneously) at maximal hyperemia – typically induced by

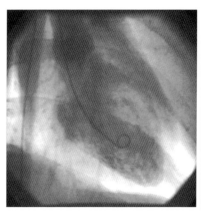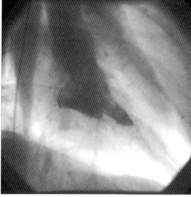

Figure 16.7 Normal diastolic and systolic left ventriculograms (right anterior oblique views).

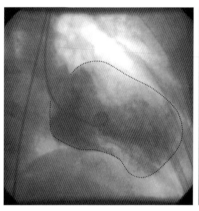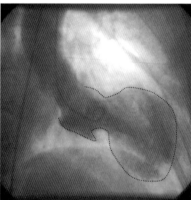

Figure 16.8 Diastolic and systolic left ventriculograms (right anterior oblique views) demonstrating LV cavity enlargement and a large apical aneurysm.

intravenous or intracoronary adenosine. FFR measurement is useful for the assessment of the hemodynamic impact of intermediate coronary artery lesions. Recent evidence suggests that FFR-guided PCI reduces the rate of stent implantation and decreases the incidence of myocardial infarction and death at 1 year.

Ventriculography and aortography

A high-volume contrast injection (35–45 ml) via a 6 Fr pigtail catheter positioned in the LV cavity provides information on LV ejection fraction, regional LV wall function and mitral regurgitation (semi-quantitative) (Figures 16.7 and 16.8). When the pigtail catheter is positioned in the aortic root, the aortic diameter and the presence of aortic regurgitation can be assessed with 45–55 ml contrast injection.

Intravascular ultrasound

Intravascular ultrasound (IVUS) is an intracoronary imaging technique that uses miniaturized ultrasound transducers to provide high-resolution, cross-sectional images, not only of the coronary artery lumen, but also of the vessel wall (Figure 16.9). In clinical practice, IVUS is used during interventional procedures, to assess angiographically ambiguous lesions and to provide additional information on left main stem disease.

In contrast to IVUS, coronary angiography provides a silhouette image of the vessel lumen – a *luminogram* – which may be confounded by the phenomenon of coronary remodeling. In stenosis of <40%, plaque accumulation is accompanied by an increase in arterial size, resulting in a stable lumen area. IVUS allows assessment of the extent of vessel

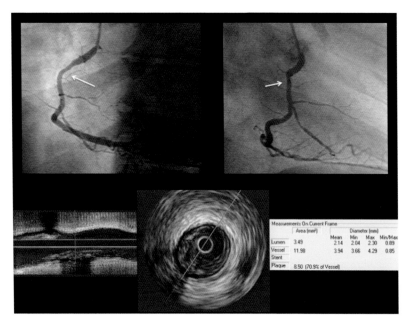

Figure 16.9 Intravascular ultrasound (IVUS). The arrows (top left and top right) show an intermediate angiographic lesion of the RCA investigated by IVUS. Longitudinal (bottom left) and cross-sectional (bottom center) IVUS images are shown. IVUS allows measurement of vessel, plaque and lumen diameter as well as lumen cross-sectional area.

wall disease that may not be detected by angiography. IVUS is not yet well suited to the detection of morphological features of atherosclerotic plaques; the resolution (100–150 μm) is too low to detect features such as thin fibrous cap (50–75 μm). Virtual histology, an additional IVUS imaging tool, applies spectral analysis of radiofrequency ultrasound signals to characterize plaque composition (fibrous, fibro-fatty, dense calcific, necrotic) in real time on the basis of tissue characteristics. Although this technique seems promising, its clinical usefulness remains to be confirmed.

Key points

- Cardiac catheterization remains the gold standard for imaging the coronary arteries.
- Serious complications are rare but may be life-threatening.
- FFR is useful for the hemodynamic assessment of intermediate coronary artery lesions.
- Right heart catheterization is an underused investigation.

Further reading

Baim DS. *Cardiac Catheterization, Angiography, and Intervention.* Philadelphia: Lippincott Williams and Wilkins; 2006.

Galiè N, Hoeper MM, Humbert M, *et al.* Guidelines for the diagnosis and treatment of pulmonary hypertension. *Eur Heart J* 2009; **30**(20): 2493–537.

Noble S, Heinonen T, Tardif JC. Imaging biomarkers of atherosclerosis. *Biomark Med* 2008; **2**(6): 555–65.

Tobis J, Azarbal B, Slavin L. Assessment of intermediate severity coronary lesions in the catheterization laboratory. *J Am Coll Cardiol* 2007; **49**(8): 839–48.

Chapter

17

Patient selection and risk stratification

Samer A. M. Nashef

It is questionable (and politically very incorrect!) whether doctors should at all "select" patients for procedures. What actually happens is that doctors decide they would be prepared to offer a procedure to a patient who then decides whether to go ahead or not. Both of these steps involve a similar thought process, the basis for which is outlined in this chapter.

For any medical treatment to be any use, it should provide one of two things: it should make the patient either feel better (improve the symptoms) or live longer (improve the prognosis). This applies to all medical intervention, from the prescription of a paracetamol (acetaminophen) tablet to open heart surgery. If you devise a treatment that improves neither symptoms nor prognosis, it is as useful as an ashtray on a motorbike and you may cheerfully consign it to the dustbin. The decision to proceed with a cardiac operation is therefore based on weighing the advantages (as indicated on symptomatic or prognostic grounds or both) against the main disadvantage, which is the risk of the operation. If the doctor thinks it is worthwhile on this basis, the operation is offered. If the patient thinks it worthwhile, the operation is accepted. Both need information to make a decision. This information is set out below.

Symptomatic indications

These are easy. As most patients prefer to take a tablet than have a hairy-armed surgeon cut them up with a knife, the symptomatic indication is always the same whatever the surgery: *failure of medical treatment* adequately to control the symptoms.

Prognostic indications

These are a little more complicated and differ between the various cardiac conditions. Some lesions have such an obvious impact on prognosis that the surgical option is virtually mandatory unless the risk is truly prohibitive. An example would be acute aortic dissection involving the ascending aorta. This carries a cumulative mortality of 1% for every hour of conservative treatment, so that by two days nearly half the patients would have expired. Luckily, most cardiac conditions are not like that, and the risk of conservative management needs to be assessed carefully and weighed against the risk of surgery. In some areas that information is still poorly defined, but in others there are clear guidelines based on quite good evidence. Some of these are outlined below.

Ischemic heart disease

The evidence for this comes from two aging but still valid studies carried out first in America and then in Europe. The American Coronary Artery Surgery Study (CASS) and a similar European study randomized patients with angina to either medical treatment (keep taking the tablets) or surgical treatment with CABG surgery. Patients who refused randomization were followed up on a register. With passing time, those treated surgically began to show a survival advantage. This was particularly marked in these groups (Table 17.1, listed in descending order of greater prognostic importance).

The presence of impaired LV function increases the prognostic advantage of surgery over medical treatment in all categories.

It can be seen from the above that coronary angiography is essential to assess the prognostic implications of IHD, and makes decision-making relatively straightforward. On prognostic grounds alone, a young otherwise fit patient with a 90% left main stem stenosis should be offered surgery, whereas an old,

Core Topics in Cardiac Anesthesia, Second Edition, ed. Jonathan H. Mackay and Joseph E. Arrowsmith. Published by Cambridge University Press. © Cambridge University Press 2012.

Table 17.1 Prognostic impact of CABG surgery

Survival benefit	Indication
+++	>50% stenosis of the main stem of the left coronary artery
++	Proximal stenosis of the three major coronary arteries: LAD, circumflex and right coronary arteries
+	>50% stenosis of two major coronary arteries including high-grade stenosis of the proximal LAD

unfit diabetic arteriopath with single vessel disease affecting only a branch of the circumflex coronary artery should not.

Aortic valve disease

The symptomatic indication is the same as everywhere else: failure of medical treatment adequately to control the symptoms. The prognostic indication depends on the lesion.

Stenosis

Strangely enough, prognosis here is directly related to symptoms! Patients are usually deemed to have significant AS when the gradient across the valve reaches 40 mmHg. Most patients with significant stenosis will continue to be asymptomatic for years. Sudden death or decompensation in asymptomatic patients with AS is as rare as hens' teeth. Indeed, it has been stated that the commonest cause of death in asymptomatic AS is AV replacement! When symptoms begin, however, the picture changes quite dramatically, with death or decompensation becoming a distinct possibility within a matter of months from the onset of symptoms (angina, dyspnea or exertional syncope). It therefore follows that the best time to operate is the day before symptoms appear. The impossibility of such a practice without a crystal ball means that most surgeons will treat the onset of symptoms as an indication for relatively urgent surgery.

Regurgitation

Here too, many patients are asymptomatic. The trouble with AR is that some hearts will tolerate a substantial amount of regurgitation for life, whereas others will dilate and fail. It can be difficult to predict

which will do what in future. Most surgeons and cardiologists will therefore look at a combination of three factors to determine the prognostic indication: the severity of the regurgitation, echocardiographic evidence of LV dilatation and evidence that the LV is "struggling" (strain pattern on the ECG).

Mitral valve disease

The symptomatic indication is the same as everywhere else: failure of medical treatment adequately to control the symptoms. The prognostic indication depends on the lesion.

The traditional teaching about MV disease is that it becomes hemodynamically important when the symptoms become bad, so that there is rarely an indication to offer mitral surgery to the asymptomatic patient. The improved results obtained with MV repair in particular and with mitral surgery in general have led many surgeons to challenge this accepted wisdom. The prognostic sequelae of untreated MS and MR are different: stenosis causes pulmonary hypertension (PHT) and regurgitation results in a LV dilatation and dysfunction. In both cases, delaying surgery until these complications are established means that the result of the operation and the long-term prognosis are not good. Current thinking is that mitral lesions should be treated on prognostic grounds if there is evidence of early development of PHT or early LV dysfunction (as shown by dilatation on echocardiography) even if symptoms are well controlled on medical treatment. Fortunately, in most patients, these developments tend to go in tandem with symptomatic deterioration, thus making decisions relatively easy.

Risk assessment

Now that we know the symptomatic and prognostic indications for the common cardiac conditions and thus the likely benefits of cardiac surgery, we need to find a method of determining the likely risk of operation, so that risk can be weighed against benefit. Fortunately, cardiac surgery is one field where risk is no longer calculated by guesswork but is almost an exact science, thanks to statistics, registers and the work of many individuals in the field. The late Michael Crichton (of ER and Jurassic Park fame) began his 1969 novel A Case of Need with the immortal words "all heart surgeons are bastards" and went on to describe the surgeon in the novel an "eight-percenter", meaning his operative mortality was 8% (in 1969, this was good). The message is that the mortality of cardiac surgery has for over 40 years been measured and incorporated into decisions about clinical care. Crude mortality, however, is not enough and even journalists understand that the risk profile of the patient has as much to do with outcome as the quality of surgical care that is given.

In the late 1980s, Victor Parsonnet [3], a New Jersey surgeon, published a landmark paper on a method of assessing risk of death in adult cardiac surgery by looking for certain risk factors and giving them points or weights, for example: diabetes, 3 points; hypertension, 3 points; aortic valve replacement 5 points and so on. After counting all the points, they are added to produce a number which is the predicted mortality of the proposed operation in that patient. The Parsonnet system found immediate favor in many cardiac surgical establishments throughout the world and is still used in some hospitals today, although many consider it to be of purely historic interest as it has been superseded by better models. Your author is particularly (and understandably) biased toward the European System for Cardiac Operative Risk Evaluation, or EuroSCORE. Apart from its rather snazzy acronym, the system is more powerfully discriminatory than Parsonnet and has been validated worldwide. The original model was an additive system (add up the points to get the percent predicted mortality – see Table 17.2).

Additive systems tend to underscore very high-risk patients who are better served by using the full logistic equation. This is a complex calculation which cannot be done at the bedside on the back of an envelope, but the EuroSCORE project group offer an online (www.euroscore.org) and downloadable calculator to calculate the logistic EuroSCORE and this is probably the model most widely used in the world currently.

The Society of Thoracic Surgeons (STS) in North America has for years offered an excellent risk model which is updated at regular intervals through its massive cardiac surgical database. The STS model is used extensively in North America but less so elsewhere and this may be due to its complexity. The most recent version (http://www.sts.org/sections/stsnationaldatabase/riskcalculator/) is in fact several risk models for various types of operation and some 40 questions must be answered to calculate the risk of CABG alone.

Most surgeons therefore use EuroSCORE, but as it was developed more than 10 years ago, it is now out of date. Several institutions and whole nations now outperform EuroSCORE predictions: for example, current UK cardiac surgical mortality is approximately 0.5 of EuroSCORE prediction. A formal renewal of EuroSCORE has just been completed and a new model (EuroSCORE II) is about to be published. At the time of writing, the paper has not yet completed peer review so it would be premature to incorporate its findings, but early indications are that it is well received and likely to become the international standard. EuroSCORE II is broadly similar to the original model, with a few notable exceptions: it incorporates insulin-dependent diabetes, has several levels of renal dysfunction, ignores ventricular septal rupture and pays more attention to urgency, NYHA class and the "weight" of the intervention. Unfortunately, there is no additive model, so you cannot calculate the risk on the back of an envelope, but there are on-line and downloadable "app" calculators already available for trial use.

Regardless of which model is used, it is important to adjust this to the performance of the unit in question before predicting the risk for the patient. If your unit's mortality is double or half what EuroSCORE predicts, you should adjust what you quote to the patient accordingly, for example:

$$\text{Predicted mortality} = \frac{\text{Patient EuroSCORE} \times \text{Hospital mortality}}{\text{Hospital logistic EuroSCORE}}$$

in other words, in Hospital X, where actual mortality is, say, 0.7 of predicted, the patient's logistic Euro-SCORE is multiplied by 0.7, reflecting the hospital's performance.

Conclusion

Determining the indication for cardiac surgery is now a piece of cake. It is so simple, even a cardiac surgeon can do it.

1. Work out the likely benefit (symptomatic and prognostic).
2. Work out the likely risk (use logistic EuroSCORE, or, when ready, EuroSCORE II corrected for your unit's performance).
3. Weigh the risk against the benefit.
4. Help the patient to make a decision.

105

Table 17.2 The additive European System for Cardiac Operative Risk Evaluation (EuroSCORE, 1999)

Factors	Comments	Points
General factors		
Age	Per 5 years or part thereof over 60	1
Sex	Female	1
Chronic pulmonary disease	Long-term use of bronchodilators or steroids for lung disease	1
Extracardiac arteriopathy	Any one or more of the following: claudication, carotid occlusion or >50% stenosis, previous or planned intervention on the abdominal aorta, limb arteries or carotids	2
Neurologic dysfunction	Severely affecting ambulation or day-to-day functioning	2
Previous cardiac surgery	Requiring opening of the pericardium	3
Serum creatinine	>200 μmol l^{-1} (2.3 mg dl^{-1}) preoperatively	2
Active endocarditis	Patient still under antibiotic treatment for endocarditis at the time of surgery	3
Critical preoperative state	Any one or more of the following: VT or VF or aborted sudden death, preoperative cardiac massage, preoperative ventilation before arrival in the anesthetic room, preoperative inotropic support, IABP or preoperative ARF (anuria or oliguria <10 ml h^{-1})	3
Cardiac factors		
Unstable angina	Rest angina requiring IV nitrates until arrival in the anesthetic room	2
LV dysfunction	Moderate (LVEF 30–50%)	2
	Poor (LVEF <30%)	1
Recent infarct	Within 90 days	2
Pulmonary hypertension	Systolic PA pressure >60 mmHg	2
Operative factors		
Emergency	Carried out on referral before the beginning of the next working day	2
Other than isolated CABG	Major cardiac procedure other than or in addition to CABG	2
Surgery on thoracic aorta	For disorder of ascending, arch or descending aorta	3
Postinfarct septal rupture		4

Key points

- Surgery is indicated on symptomatic grounds when symptoms are not adequately controlled by maximal medical therapy.
- Surgery is indicated on prognostic grounds in situations such as severe mitral regurgitation and left main stem coronary disease, regardless of the severity of symptoms.
- The use of validated risk models, such as EuroSCORE, allows rapid risk assessment at the point of care.

Further reading

CASS principal investigators and their associates. Myocardial infarction and mortality in the coronary artery surgery randomized trial. *N Engl J Med* 1984; **310**(12): 750–8.

Nashef SA, Roques F, Michel P, Gauducheau E, Lemeshow S, Salamon R. European system for cardiac operative risk evaluation (EuroSCORE). *Eur J Cardiothorac Surg* 1999; **16**(1): 9–13.

Parsonnet V, Dean D, Bernstein AD. A method of uniform stratification of risk for evaluating the results of surgery in acquired adult heart disease. *Circulation* 1989; **79**(Suppl 1): 3–12.

Roques F, Michel P, Goldstone AR, Nashef SA. The logistic EuroSCORE. *Eur Heart J* 2003; **24**(9): 882–3.

Basic principles of cardiac surgery

Samer A. M. Nashef

Despite the romantic notions attached to it, the heart is a muscular pump. When it "goes wrong", the cause is usually a faulty valve or a blocked pipe. Although it seems obvious that the management of plumbing or mechanical faults should be surgical, patients with these problems remained almost exclusively under the care of physicians during the first half of the twentieth century.

Early obstacles

Knowledge of the obstacles that delayed the development of heart surgery is useful. First, surgeons took some time to appreciate that lungs cannot breathe by themselves without an intact chest. Early attempts at thoracic surgery on spontaneously breathing patients anesthetized with chloroform and ether were doomed to failure.

The development of endotracheal intubation (1910s), muscle relaxants and positive-pressure ventilation (1940s) allowed some operations to be undertaken on the beating heart. Closed mitral valvotomy was carried out "blind", by inserting a finger or an instrument into the LA or LV to stretch, cut or tear open the fused rheumatic, stenotic valve. Closure of ASDs was undertaken by clamping the venae cavae (inflow occlusion), which rendered the heart bloodless and motionless for a short period of time. The RA was then quickly opened, the lesion repaired with indecent haste and the atrium closed with obscene rapidity. Prayers were then said for the heart to resume beating and for the brain to be intact. This approach resulted in some interesting complications, such as unintentional closure of the IVC orifice, the coronary sinus or worse: the tricuspid valve. It also explains why the first generation of cardiac surgeons became legends of surgical bravado. The reputation

still lingers, but in fact the specialty and its practitioners are now as worthy (and as dull) as accountants.

Breakthroughs

In the 1950s, two important developments took place. The first was the realization of the concept of an artificial heart (and lungs) to support the patient while the heart was being operated. The second was the exploration of systemic cooling to allow longer periods of cardiac standstill. Both had the same aim, that is to prolong the time available to fix a heart problem, and both had limited success. Cooling gave the surgeon some time to maneuver but was tedious and messy – the patient being lowered into an ice bath or sprinkled with ice-cold water. The early heart–lung machine was complicated, unreliable and needed some 20 units of blood to prime it and, although effective as an oxygenator, produced considerable aeroembolism and defibrination. As neither on its own was particularly user-friendly or safe, early cardiac surgery employed both techniques, with topical cooling providing a margin of safety in the likely event of pump failure. Nowadays, heart–lung machines are so reliable and perfusionists so obsessional that pump malfunction is extremely rare. Surgeons who still use active systemic cooling in routine cardiac surgery do so out of nostalgia and force of habit.

Cardiopulmonary bypass

Myocardial protection

Most cardiac operations rely on the heart–lung machine, which protects the patient while the heart is being operated (see Chapter 55). During CPB, the heart beats empty, but the coronary arteries are still

Core Topics in Cardiac Anesthesia, Second Edition, ed. Jonathan H. Mackay and Joseph E. Arrowsmith. Published by Cambridge University Press. © Cambridge University Press 2012.

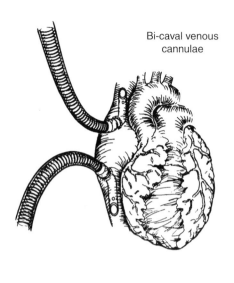

Bi-caval venous
cannulae

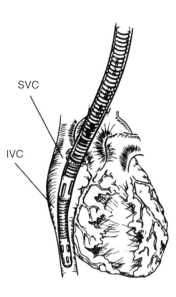

SVC

IVC

Figure 18.1 Techniques of venous cannulation. Bicaval (left) using simple armoured cannulae, and unicaval (right) using an armored two-stage cannula. Courtesy of Medtronic Ltd and reproduced with permission.

perfused from the aorta, which itself is perfused by the heart–lung machine. Opening the coronary arteries or the aorta results in a gush of blood, making surgery impossible. Clamping the aorta between the site of insertion of the aortic cannula and the origin of the coronary arteries produces a bloodless field, and makes intricate surgery possible. Clamping the aorta would cause the heart to become globally ischemic unless steps are taken to protect the heart itself (see Chapter 19).

Setting up

Most operations proceed along a pre-ordained path, so that cardiac surgery, if performed well, should be as predictable and boring as possible. After induction of anesthesia, skin preparation and draping, a median sternotomy is performed. Traditionally, the anesthesiologist deflates the lungs before the sternal saw divides the sternum, to reduce the risk of opening the pleura (if it is opened, it is not a big deal). Where needed, conduits for coronary bypass are harvested from the leg, arm or chest. The patient is then fully heparinized and the ACT used to confirm the adequacy of anticoagulation. Most cardiac units have rigid protocols for administering heparin. Purse-string sutures are inserted into the aorta to secure the cannula, which will deliver oxygenated blood from the heart–lung machine (the wise anesthesiologist stands well back during aortic cannulation and decannulation). Further purse-string sutures are inserted into the RA to secure the cannula or

cannulae, which drain venous blood into the heart–lung machine. There may be one atriocaval cannula or two separate caval cannulae (Figure 18.1).

Once everybody is happy with the ACT and the conduits are ready, the patient is "put on bypass". This is done by unclamping the "venous" or RA cannula and allowing it to drain RA blood into the oxygenator by simple gravity or siphonage. Oxygenated blood is then pumped into the aorta and the ventilator is switched off. During the first few minutes of CPB, the surgeon may make preparations for the operation, such as inspecting and preparing the coronary graft targets, inserting vents into the LV, LA, PA or aorta (to drain any residual intracardiac blood), or carrying out preliminary dissection and mobilization to achieve better exposure.

The juicy bits

The surgeon begins the central component of the operation by cross-clamping the aorta. This marks the beginning of the "cross-clamp" time. The heart is now ischemic and time is of the essence: at this point, the operation acquires a quantum leap in purposefulness, with palpable increase in efficiency and a decrease in idle chatter. Appropriate myocardial protection (Chapter 19) is achieved, usually by cardioplegia administration via the aortic root (this segment of aorta is now blocked by the clamp distally and the AV proximally so the solution can only flow down the coronaries). The heart stops and the "cardiac" part of the operation begins.

109

Coronary surgery

In a coronary operation, the target coronary artery is opened longitudinally with a sharp fine blade, distal to any stenosis. The arteriotomy is extended with fine scissors, and the distal coronary anastomosis or "bottom end" is constructed with fine continuous sutures joining the end of the conduit (saphenous vein, radial artery or mammary artery) to the coronary arteriotomy. This is an "end-to-side" anastomosis. If the same conduit is then used to graft another vessel, a sequential "side-to-side" anastomosis is performed. Additional cardioplegia may be given into the aortic root or via the grafts or both as the case proceeds. The left internal mammary anastomosis, usually to the LAD, is constructed last.

Aortic valve surgery

In AV surgery, the aorta is opened above the sinuses of Valsalva. If the patient has AR, antegrade cardioplegia must be administered directly into the coronary ostia, which are visible through the open aortotomy. Direct administration via the aortic root would simply distend the LV. AVR is carried out by removing the diseased valve, inserting interrupted sutures first into the annulus then into the sewing ring of the prosthesis, sliding the prosthesis on the sutures down into the annulus and tying the sutures. The aorta is then closed with a continuous suture.

Mitral valve surgery

MV surgery needs an incision in the LA, just medial to the right-sided pulmonary veins, and involves quite a bit of retraction of the atrium to gain access. This tends to deform the overlying RA, and is the main reason for using two caval cannulae rather than one atrial cannula for the bypass circuit. Mitral repair involves a number of different maneuvers, such as leaflet resection, annular plication or annuloplasty. Most units carrying out mitral repair rely heavily on TEE to analyze the nature of the mitral lesion and to confirm the success of the repair. MVR follows the same pattern as AVR. Once the mitral repair or replacement is completed, the left atriotomy is closed with a continuous suture.

De-airing

If a main heart chamber (atrium, aorta, PA or ventricle) has been opened as part of the procedure, it is important to evacuate air from the heart, especially the left side, before the heart is put back into the circulation and the air escapes to the brain. The many de-airing methods essentially rely on washing the air out with blood and saline. This may involve a fair amount of vigorous physical activity by the surgeon while the heart and sometimes the entire patient are shaken, stirred and repositioned to optimize the process. This, together with a request for restarting ventilation briefly to expel air from the pulmonary veins, is usually sufficient to rouse the sleepiest anesthesiologist from deepest torpor. It is also a reliable signal that the end, though not quite close enough, is now at least in sight.

Clamp-off

The aortic cross-clamp is then removed, allowing perfusion of the coronary arteries and the heart then begins to come to life. If myocardial protection has been optimal, the heart reverts to a normal sinus rhythm. If not, VF is the commonest dysrhythmia seen and internal cardioversion is carried out. Any proximal anastomoses (top ends) of coronary grafts are then carried out using a partially occluding or "side-biting" aortic clamp. The patient is then prepared for "coming off bypass". The lungs are ventilated and the perfusionist gradually occludes the RA cannula, thus allowing more blood to return to the heart and be pumped. The arterial pressure line begins to show pulsation as the heart gradually takes over the circulation. The heart–lung machine is then stopped and the atrial or caval cannulae removed.

. . . and finally

Heparin is reversed using its antidote, protamine, which often produces hypotension. This can be treated by transfusing blood from the pump into the patient via the aortic cannula. Hemostasis is secured (what a long and tedious process these three simple words describe!) and the chest is closed over the appropriate number of drains and epicardial pacing wires. The patient is then transferred to a critical care area for postoperative monitoring.

Off-pump surgery

In an effort to avoid the potential adverse effects of the heart–lung machine, many surgeons now perform coronary surgery without it, using clever contraptions to steady the bit of heart they are working on. Early reports suggest that it is feasible in some, if not most, coronary patients, and may reduce complications in high-risk patients. There is no cannulation, extracorporeal circulation or cross-clamping of the aorta. The absence of CPB means that these operations are more demanding of the anesthesiologist, who will need to work constantly on optimizing hemodynamics as the heart is mobilized, retracted and stabilized while continuing to support the circulation (see Chapter 30).

New developments

Efforts to reduce the invasiveness of cardiac surgery continue apace. Minimally invasive coronary surgery (MICS) can allow the left internal mammary artery to be grafted to the LAD through a small anterior thoracotomy without CPB. Percutaneous CPB with endoscopic surgery allows some operations to be carried out without dividing the sternum. Occasionally during MICS, conventional CPB, which necessitates a rapid sternotomy, is required. Most cardiac anesthesiologist classify this as "maximally invasive" cardiac surgery.

Equipment has been developed which replaces the surgeon's hands within the chest with small, robotic "hands" controlled by the surgeon from outside, another room or even another continent! The reader may wish to speculate on the motivation for all these developments at a time when cardiac surgery is phenomenally successful and has an enviable safety record. Are we motivated by a true desire to help the patients by reducing the invasiveness of our procedure, a desperate attempt to claw back from the cardiologists the large number of patients now treated by percutaneous intervention or do surgeons, like little boys, get bored with their predictable old "toys" and want new ones?

Key points

- Most routine cardiac surgical procedures follow a predictable and well-defined path.
- The principal aims of the surgeon are to complete the surgical procedure with the shortest ischemic time possible and secure hemostasis following CPB.
- Time invested in thorough de-airing and coronary reperfusion is generally rewarded with interest.

Traditional English operating room intermission

Crossword prize

Please fax answers and your contact details to +44 1480 364936 (01480 364936 from UK) to enter prize draw.

Prize draw will take place in August 2012 at Papworth Hospital.

First Prize – One free copy of Core Topics in Cardiac Anesthesia.

Second Prize – Two free copies of Core Topics in Cardiac Anesthesia!

Solution will be available at http://www.papworth-anaesthesia.org from September 2012.

Across

6 Warning signal in the style of the marines (5)

7 Man prone to be minister (8)

10 A form of line art seen in toilet (7)

11 More even praise (7)

12 Serious audience at home (7)

13 Slim and profligate, a pound for a penny (7)

14 The 4,17 watching the 4, 6dn, 27, 4, 26, by the 4,5 (numbers game) (11)

19 4,5 loch? He saw it happen (7)

21 Bush, removed from office, returned (7)

23 Nice kit in motion (7)

25 Keen to start building a chair in the city (7)

26 Killed racehorse backed by journalist (8)

27 Living creature (5)

Down

1 Care a bit about bugs (8)

2 I swing both ways, live and drink (6)

3 Model sits nicest for no artists (10)

4/5 Ted may be simple (4,6)

6 Not 17, please! (6)

8 Articles from dodgy dealers (7)

9 Sounds like real caviar in Cornwall (5)

13 Fish jokes, boys and girls (10)

15 Prevented state 4,5 (7)

16 An empty air, elegant and wild (8)

17 Conscious of a slipstream (5)

18 Sport is King! (6)

20 Some put on guest language (6)

22 Idols after heart beats (6)

24 Port stopper (4)

Chapter

19

Myocardial protection

Betsy Evans and David P. Jenkins

Most cardiac surgical procedures require temporary, intentional interruption of coronary blood flow by application of an aortic cross-clamp (AXC). The rationale behind this is to produce a bloodless surgical field and a flaccid heart, thereby ensuring a technically perfect procedure. Myocardial protection is the term used to describe the component of the operation primarily applied to reduce the obvious major disadvantage of aortic cross-clamping – that of myocardial ischemia. The aim of myocardial protection is therefore to preserve myocardial function by delaying the onset of ischemic injury. Myocardial ischemic injury has been traditionally subdivided into reversible (temporarily "stunned", but no cell necrosis) and irreversible (myocardial infarction, with myocyte necrosis). More recently, apoptosis (programmed cell death, without destruction of cell membranes) has been added as a third type of myocyte injury. To ensure that myocardial protection is best achieved, the specific agent must be delivered safely, reliably and uniformly to the myocardium. Attention to detail during cardiac surgery produces optimal outcomes; this is especially pertinent in the current era of operating on high-risk patients with impaired myocardial function.

Historical perspectives

In the early days of cardiac surgery, procedures were performed without consideration being paid to myocardial ischemia or necrosis. It was only with the advent of CABG surgery, in the 1970s, that the notion of intraoperative myocardial protection was considered. Abolition of myocardial injury is impossible to achieve since ischemia will occur as soon as the AXC is applied. Myocardial protection is a delaying strategy to enable sufficient time to perform the procedure before the onset of irreversible myocardial injury.

Bigelow's original report described unmodified ischemic arrest by decreasing myocardial oxygen demand (lowered metabolic rate) as a consequence of hypothermia. This method of protection had a definite temporal relationship with morbidity and mortality. Specific chemical solutions (cardioplegia) were subsequently devised to modify the course of ischemia. Melrose described the use of rapid, potassium-induced electromechanical diastolic cardiac arrest, which permitted cardiac surgery to be performed on a non-beating flaccid heart. The combination of hypothermia and cardioplegia became the "cornerstone" of myocardial protection, reducing myocardial edema and necrosis, and improving clinical outcome. The different components of cardioplegic solutions were systematically tested in isolated rat heart models at St Thomas' hospital by Hearse in the early 1970s and later applied to clinical practice by Braimbridge; an early example of bench to bedside research: hence the name St Thomas solution for crystalloid cardioplegia still used today. Bretschneider developed a low sodium solution in Europe at a similar time.

Contemporary practice

The majority of cardiac surgeons use some form of cardioplegia for myocardial protection. Recent modifications in myocardial protection strategies have concentrated on reducing reperfusion injury by adjusting the type and route of administration of cardioplegia. Blood-based solutions are now used by most surgeons, in preference to crystalloid solutions, because of their additional substrates, oxygen-carrying capacity and buffering potential.

Core Topics in Cardiac Anesthesia, Second Edition, ed. Jonathan H. Mackay and Joseph E. Arrowsmith. Published by Cambridge University Press. © Cambridge University Press 2012.

Table 19.1 Composition of commonly used cardioplegic solutions (concentrations in mmol.l^{-1}). Recipes for blood cardioplegia include: 4 parts blood to 1 part crystalloid (Ringer's 500 ml + STS2 25–50 ml); blood 500 ml + STS2 10 ml; blood 250 ml + Birmingham 50 ml

	St Thomas' 2 (STS2)	Plegivex® (STS1)	Ringer's	Birmingham
Na$^+$	110	147	147	
K$^+$	16	20	4	80
Ca^{2+}	1.2	2	2.25	
Mg^{2+}	16	16		20
Cl$^-$	160	204	155.5	
NaHCO$_3$	10			
Procaine HCl		1		

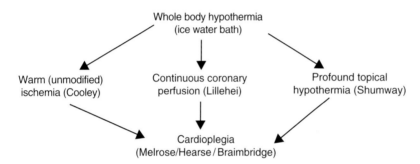

Figure 19.1 The evolution of myocardial management techniques. Whole body hypothermia was used to induce circulatory arrest (rather than protect the myocardium) before the advent of CPB systems. Variability in the degree of cooling and rewarming limited the efficacy of topical hypothermia.

There are numerous options for myocardial protection. The absence of conclusive prospective trials proving the superiority of any particular strategy means that surgeon preference still plays a role. Essential to all methods of myocardial protection is attention to detail and careful observation of the heart throughout surgery. It is important to realize that the ability of one surgeon to obtain good results with a particular myocardial protection technique does not necessarily mean that another surgeon or institution can achieve similar results. Specific groups of patients, however, present a challenge when considering myocardial protection:

- severely impaired LV or RV function
- LVH resulting from AS or hypertension together with severe coronary artery disease
- repeat (redo) revascularization procedures in the setting of partially occluded grafts or graft-dependent circulation.

Myocardial protection with cardioplegia

Rationale for cardioplegic arrest

Cardioplegia induces rapid diastolic arrest in the unperfused (ischemic) heart, preventing wasteful energy consumption and reducing metabolite accumulation. It provides a predictable and "safe" period of cardiac flaccidity and a bloodless field. It is frequently used during coronary revascularization and remains the preferred protection method for longer intracardiac procedures.

The constituents of modern cardioplegia solutions vary (Table 19.1), although most use K$^+$ as the arresting agent with varying concentrations of Ca^{2+}, glucose, buffers and Mg^{2+}. Cardioplegia has been proven in many experimental preparations and in clinical studies to give good myocardial protection. As the myocardium continues to receive a limited amount of non-coronary (bronchial and pericardial) collateral blood flow, cardioplegic solution is gradually washed out over 20–30 min after which further cardioplegia is required.

Following the institution of CPB and application of AXC, cardioplegia is usually administered through the coronary arteries (antegrade) via an aortic root cannula, directly into the coronary ostia or via a partially fashioned bypass graft (Figures 19.2 and 19.3). Typically 1000 ml is given over 3 min at a pressure of 70–80 mmHg. In the presence of AR, root

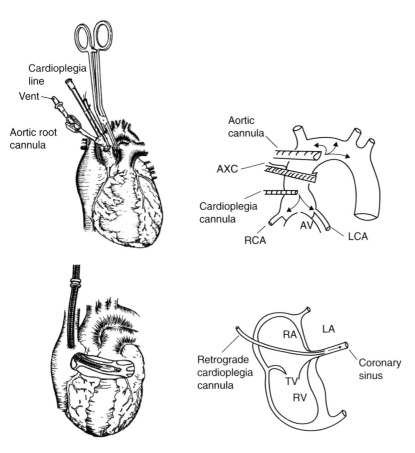

Cardioplegia line

Vent

Aortic root cannula

Aortic cannula

AXC

Cardioplegia cannula

RCA

AV

LCA

RA

LA

Retrograde cardioplegia cannula

TV

RV

Coronary sinus

Figure 19.2 Antegrade (top) and retrograde (bottom) administration of cardioplegia. A competent AV is required for effective cardioplegia administration via an aortic root cannula. Coronary sinus catheters usually have an inflatable cuff.

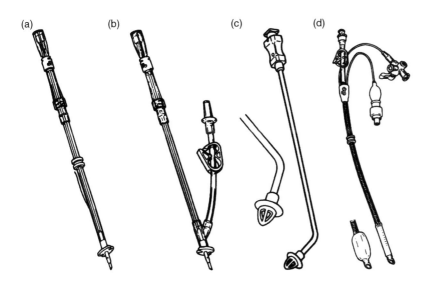

(a)   (b)   (c)   (d)

Figure 19.3 Examples of cardioplegia administration cannulae. (a) Aortic root cannula. (b) Combined aortic root cannula and vent. (c) Ostial cannula for direct coronary administration (with close-up of tip). (d) Elongated balloon-tipped retrograde cardioplegia cannula (with balloon deflated and inflated).

delivery of cardioplegia is contraindicated due to the risk of LV distension and reduced delivery to the coronary arteries.

Cold versus warm

Cold (4–10°C) cardioplegia is frequently supplemented by direct cardiac cooling with ice slush, cold saline or a cold jacket. The observation that hyperkalemic arrest alone is responsible for most of the reduction in myocyte metabolic demand achieved by cardioplegia has raised doubts about the need for topical cardiac cooling.

Infusing warm blood cardioplegia before and after cold cardioplegic arrest has been shown to preserve myocardial ATP levels. Similarly, cardioplegia enriched with Kreb's cycle substrates (glutamate or aspartate) also improves ATP preservation and restores energy stores more quickly than unmodified cold solutions. Warm blood cardioplegia induction or a terminal infusion of warm blood before cross-clamp release (a "hot shot") is advocated by some surgeons.

In 1991 Lichtenstein suggested that the heart could be maintained at a temperature of 37°C and myocardial metabolic function preserved throughout the ischemic period by maintaining continuous coronary perfusion. The randomized, prospective Warm Heart Trial (1994) compared normothermic with hypothermic cardioplegia in 2000 patients undergoing CABG surgery. The trial concluded that normothermic cardioplegia was associated with a reduced incidence of postoperative low CO syndrome. Hayashida reported a randomized study comparing the effects of cold (9°C), tepid (29°C) and warm (37°C) blood cardioplegia in 42 patients undergoing CABG surgery. Myocardial O_2 consumption (MVO_2) and lactate release were greatest with warm, intermediate with tepid and least with cold cardioplegia. Early postoperative LV function was best preserved after tepid cardioplegia with a lower incidence of post-surgery ventricular dysrhythmias and reduced blood loss. Although cold crystalloid cardioplegia is associated with excellent clinical outcomes in elective surgery, normothermic blood cardioplegia techniques seem to offer superior cardioprotection in high-risk situations.

Adjustments and additives to cardioplegia solutions

Beta-blockade is proven to reduce myocardial injury during ischemia and reperfusion, by lowering MVO_2

and sympathetic tone in addition to cell membrane stabilization.

Glucose-insulin-potassium solutions have been used commonly to treat ischemic myocardium in a variety of medical and surgical situations. However, the recent Insulin Cardioplegia Trial (2002) failed to demonstrate a significant benefit of insulin-cardioplegic solution in the setting of high-risk patients undergoing isolated myocardial revascularization.

Anti-inflammatory agents: cardioplegic solutions now include antioxidants such as reduced glutathione to combat free radicals generated during ischemia and to act as scavengers during initial reperfusion.

Blocking neutrophil adhesion to the endothelium and subsequent diapedesis in theory would lead to less post-bypass inflammation. Monoclonal antibodies to Mac-1, ICAM-1 and L- and P-selectin have all been shown experimentally to reduce post-ischemic reperfusion injury, but none of these agents have been put into clinical use.

Complement inhibitors have been shown in animal models to decrease neutrophil migration into ischemic myocardium. In 1999 Fitch reported a significant drop in postoperative myocardial injury, blood loss and cognitive impairment following the preoperative administration of recombinant monoclonal antibody for human C_5 in patients undergoing surgery with cardiopulmonary bypass. However, subsequently the larger multicenter PRIMO-CABG trial reported in 2004 that the use of pexelizumab (a C_5 complement inhibitor) had no significant effect on primary composite end-point (death or acute myocardial infarction within 30 days after surgery).

Na^+/H^+ *exchange inhibition:* protons accumulating during ischemia as a result of lactate accumulation are exchanged during reperfusion for sodium ions. The Na^+/K^+ pump is rendered inefficient due to ischemia-induced shortage of ATP, therefore intracellular sodium increases. The Na^+/Ca^{2+} exchanger removes the sodium, leading to intracellular calcium loading, which is responsible for the ischemia/reperfusion tissue injury. Inhibition of the Na^+/H^+ exchanger with cariporide has the effect of decreasing myocardial infarct size and improving post-ischemic functional recovery in experimental animal studies. However, the large prospective randomized GUARDIAN trial – designed to assess the potential protective effect of cariopride in patients with unstable angina, non ST-elevation myocardial infarction or undergoing high-risk percutaneous or surgical revascularization – failed to demonstrate any clinical benefit except in the surgical group.

Nitric oxide/L-arginine: nitric oxide is an endogenous endothelial product which is known to reduce myocardial ischemia/reperfusion damage in experimental animal models. It also has anti-apoptotic effects which further protect myocyte function. Experimental animal model data show that L-arginine-enriched blood cardioplegia increases nitric oxide release and improves myocardial protection with improved ventricular function recovery.

Cardioplegia delivery techniques

Normothermic cardioplegia strategies necessitated the development of novel delivery systems that enabled continuous coronary perfusion. Retrograde perfusion, via the coronary sinus, allows uninterrupted cardioplegia delivery and, in addition, better subendocardial distribution in areas supplied by stenosed coronary vessels or bypass grafts. The concept of retrograde cardioplegia is simple; it does, however, require correct catheter placement and monitoring of perfusion pressure (30–40 mmHg) to prevent perivascular hemorrhage and edema (Figure 19.2). Limitations of this technique result from shunting of blood directly into the atrial and ventricular cavities. This occurs because of the presence of thebesian channels and arterio-sinusoidal vessels (especially in the right coronary artery territory), which necessitate compensatory delivery flow rates greater than 100 ml min^{-1}.

The combination of antegrade and retrograde cardioplegia has been proposed to improve overall myocardial protection. This was confirmed in the CABG Patch trial (2000), which enrolled high-risk patients with reduced LV function. Blood cardioplegia was found to be superior to crystalloid cardioplegia, and combined cardioplegia better than antegrade cardioplegia alone. Although these benefits translated into reduced postoperative morbidity there was no significant difference in mortality.

Intermittent ischemia and reperfusion (cross-clamp/fibrillation)

This strategy, which has been used since the 1970s, does not involve the use of a myocardial protective agent. It is based, instead, on the fact that the heart can tolerate repeated periods of ischemia, of up to 15 min in duration, provided that there are brief periods of intervening reperfusion. The mechanism for myocardial protection is believed to be endogenous ischemic preconditioning (see Chapter 20). This method of myocardial management is now only used in a minority of centers; however, cardiac outcomes are not different from those seen using cardioplegic techniques. This technique is simple and particularly suited to CABG surgery where distal and proximal anastomoses can be fashioned alternately, thus enabling sequential revascularization of each coronary as the operation progresses. It is important, however, that the heart is not permitted to distend. Repeated application and removal of an AXC increases the risk of atheroembolism and stroke in patients with atheromatous disease.

Off-pump CABG surgery (OPCAB)

The technique of "off-pump" revascularization avoids the need for CPB. The principles of myocardial management are similar to cross-clamp/fibrillation. In OPCAB surgery the target vessel is stabilized with a mechanical device and then temporarily occluded with a snare to enable the distal anastomosis to be fashioned. This way only a single region of myocardium is rendered ischemic at any one time; the remainder of the heart beats to sustain the circulation. Many surgeons now utilize an intracoronary shunt to minimize localized ischemia.

Although perioperative myocardial ischemia, defined by cardiac enzyme release, is reduced in OPCAB surgery, this has yet to be translated into clinical benefits. A recent multicenter randomized trial comparing off-pump and on-pump revascularization in low-risk patients showed that the quantity and quality of revascularization were superior in the on-pump group.

Consequences of inadequate protection

The success of myocardial protection strategies used is often difficult to quantify. In some patients it may be obvious: difficulty weaning from CPB, the need for intra-aortic balloon pump or inotropic support, ECG changes and elevation of cardiac-specific enzymes and proteins. In others, signs can be more subtle: dysrhythmias, low CO due to myocardial stunning, and in the longer term myocardial fibrosis leading to lower ejection fraction and chronic heart failure.

117

Key points

- No single method of myocardial management has been shown to be superior under all conditions.
- The active (arresting) ingredient of most cardioplegia solutions is potassium.
- Ventricular distension should be avoided at all costs.
- Retrograde cardioplegia infusion may incompletely protect the RV.
- Inadequate myocardial protection may have life-threatening consequences in both the immediate and the long term.

Further reading

Cordell AR. Milestones in the development of cardioplegia. *Ann Thorac Surg* 1995; **60**(3): 793–6.

Jacob S, Kallikourdis A, Sellke F, Dunning J. Is blood cardioplegia superior to crystalloid cardioplegia? *Interact Cardiovasc Thorac Surg* 2008; **7**(3): 491–8.

Mentzer RM Jr, Jahania M, Lasley RD. Myocardial Protection. In: Cohn LH (Ed). *Cardiac Surgery in the Adult*. New York: McGraw-Hill, 2008. pp. 443–64. www.cardiacsurgery.ctsnetbooks.org/.

Walsh SR, Tang TY, Kullar P, Jenkins DP, Dutka DP, Gaunt ME. Ischaemic preconditioning during cardiac surgery: systematic review and meta-analysis of perioperative outcomes in randomised clinical trials. *Eur J Cardiothorac Surg* 2008; **34**(5): 985–94.

Chapter

20

Myocardial stunning, hibernation and preconditioning

Stefan G. De Hert

Interruption of coronary blood flow results in myocardial ischemia, which, if prolonged and unresolved, ultimately leads to cardiomyocyte death. While early restoration of blood flow is necessary to prevent myocardial cell death, reperfusion may itself result in tissue dysfunction. Reperfusion injury may cause arrhythmias, reversible contractile dysfunction (myocardial stunning) and endothelial dysfunction. Paradoxically, reperfusion may be lethal, causing cell death by necrosis and apoptosis. In contrast, chronic myocardial hypoperfusion causes contractile dysfunction by a mechanism known as hibernation (Table 20.1).

Myocardial stunning

Myocardial stunning refers to the occurrence of transient contractile dysfunction despite restoration of blood flow to previously ischemic myocardium. In most instances, the duration of dysfunction greatly exceeds the period of preceding ischemia. The pathogenesis of reperfusion injury is not fully understood, but several mechanisms appear to be involved (Figure 20.1). The major consistent metabolic abnormality in stunned myocardium is a reduction in intracellular adenosine triphosphate (ATP) concentration. Because this resolves with a time course that is roughly parallel to functional recovery, emphasis was initially placed on a potential role of high-energy phosphate stores in the development of myocardial stunning. However, more recently it has become obvious that ATP depletion has no major causal role in the development of reperfusion injury; instead reactive oxygen species and the disruption of the normal intracellular Ca^{2+} homeostasis have emerged as the major mechanisms. In addition, the susceptibility of "reoxygenated" cardiomyocytes to

Table 20.1 Terminology in myocardial ischemia

Stunning

- Transient systolic and diastolic dysfunction persisting after reperfusion
- Duration of stunning $>>>$ duration of ischemia
- Ameliorated by pretreatment and reversed by inotropes

Hibernation

- Regional wall motion abnormalities caused by chronic hypoperfusion
- Cardiomyocyte dedifferentiation and interstitial fibrosis
- Mechanism: adaptive versus apoptotic?
- Recovery rate/extent α severity of cardiomyocyte alteration and fibrosis

Preconditioning

- Exposure to a brief stimulus reduces subsequent injury from a sustained period of lethal ischemia
- Characterized by early and delayed windows of protection
- May be triggered by physical and pharmacological factors

display potentially injurious hypercontraction at an otherwise normal cytosolic Ca^{2+} concentration seems to be increased after a prolonged period of hypoxia. The resulting cytoskeleton fragility means that myocytes are no longer able to sustain normal contractile forces.

The crucial role of mitochondrial dysfunction in the pathogenesis of ischemia-reperfusion injury (IRI) has become increasingly evident in recent years. The key component in the development of IRI is the opening of nonspecific mitochondrial permeability transition pores (mPTP) located in the inner

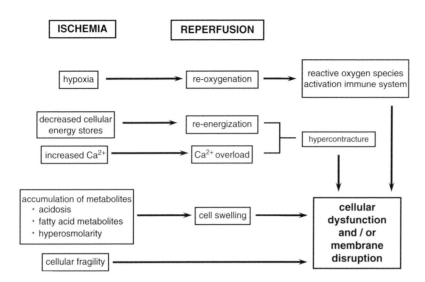

Figure 20.1 Events occurring in the course of ischemia-reperfusion injury.

mitochondrial membrane. Normally closed, mPTPs open in conditions of stress, such as IRI, causing metabolic uncoupling and loss of ATP generating capacity. Unrestrained, this leads to the loss of ionic homeostasis and, ultimately, necrotic cell death. In addition to their role in cell necrosis, brief mPTP opening leads to the release of cytochrome *c* and other molecules that initiate the apoptotic cascade. Apoptosis is a controlled cellular response to moderate cell injury. In contrast to necrotic cell death, which is the consequence of severe structural cell damage, cells that have entered the apoptotic process initially retain physical sarcolemmal integrity. The point where the process becomes irreversible is the activation of endonucleases that target genomic DNA. The contractile dysfunction from myocardial stunning can, however, be reversed with inotropes without potentiating further myocyte damage.

Myocardial hibernation

Myocardial hibernation refers to the clinical situation where chronic wall motion abnormalities are present in patients with ischemic heart disease without infarction. This entity represents the response of the heart to chronic hypoperfusion, where reduced myocardial contractility and regional myocardial oxygen consumption allow the cardiac myocytes to remain viable despite compromised oxygen supply.

The diagnosis of myocardial hibernation requires the presence of the following elements: reduced

coronary perfusion, regional contractile dysfunction in the presence of viable cardiomyocytes with intact cell membranes and ongoing metabolism. From a clinical perspective it is essential to distinguish viable, hibernating myocardium from non-viable, infarcted tissue. Cardiac function in patients with viable myocardium may improve after revascularization. In contrast, patients without viable myocardium are unlikely to benefit from revascularization. Dobutamine stress echocardiography and ^{18}fluorodeoxyglucose positron emission tomography appear to have the highest positive predictive value for segmental recovery after revascularization. (See Chapter 14.) Currently available techniques are less precise, however, in predicting recovery of global LV function.

Myocardial preconditioning

Myocardial preconditioning describes the phenomenon whereby exposure to a brief stimulus can reduce the subsequent injury from a sustained period of otherwise lethal ischemia. Like many organs, the heart possesses the remarkable ability to protect itself against the consequences of ischemia. In 1986, Murry and colleagues reported for the first time that short episodes of ischemia and reperfusion before a sustained ischemic event – early ischemic preconditioning – reduced infarct size (Figure 20.2).

Preconditioning represents a potent and consistently reproducible method of protection against ischemia. It decreases infarct size, post-ischemic cardiac dysfunction and arrhythmias. A prerequisite of

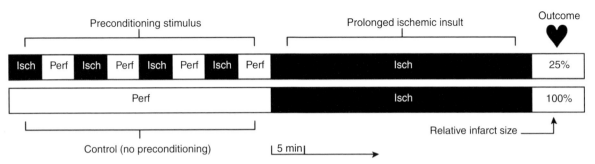

Figure 20.2 Canine model of early myocardial preconditioning described by Murry *et al.* (*Circulation* 1986; 74: 1124–36). Four 5-min periods of circumflex artery occlusion, each separated by 5 min reperfusion, reduced infarct area by 75% following a subsequent 40-min occlusion. Despite 50% more ischemia, infarct size was significantly reduced in preconditioned animals. Preconditioning could not attenuate damage after 180 min of ischemia, indicating that the time course of myocyte death could be delayed but not prevented.

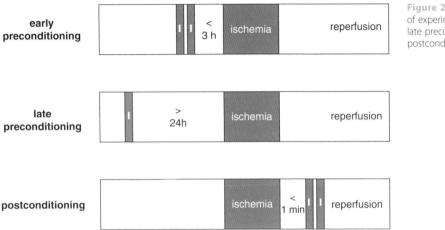

Figure 20.3 Schematic representation of experimental examples of early and late preconditioning and postconditioning.

the phenomenon is a delay (washout period) between the preconditioning trigger and the onset of ischemia. Ischemic preconditioning typically consists of two windows of cardioprotection: an early phase that occurs immediately and produces strong protection of limited duration (~2 h), and a late phase which occurs about 24 h after the initial stimulus and induces longer-lasting (3 days) but less pronounced protection (Figure 20.3).

Although the mechanisms involved in myocardial preconditioning remain to be fully elucidated, several steps have been identified (Figure 20.4). The signaling pathways mainly involve post-translational modification of proteins (translocation and phosphorylation). Protein kinase C (PKC) plays a central role as intracellular mediator, although tyrosine kinase and mitogen-activated protein kinases (MAPK) are also involved. During the early phase of preconditioning,

"cellular memory" is believed to result from translocation of PKC from cytosol to cellular membranes and more rapid activation of PKC during the prolonged ischemic period. The majority of experimental evidence indicates that mitochondrial K_{ATP} channel activation (opening) is of pivotal importance in the preservation of mitochondrial function during ischemia. Prevention of both mPTP opening and activation of necrotic and apoptotic pathways during reperfusion plays a key role in the protection conferred by the preconditioning stimulus. During the late phase of preconditioning, cellular memory is believed to result from the synthesis or activation of cytoprotective proteins, such as anti-oxidant enzymes and heat-shock proteins that stabilize the cytoskeleton.

A number of ischemic preconditioning protocols have been examined in the setting of cardiological

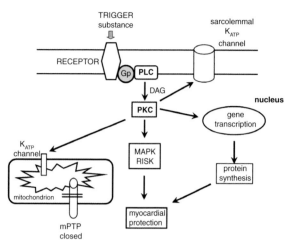

Figure 20.4 Schematic representations of some of the proposed mechanisms involved in early and late preconditioning and postconditioning. Receptor activation results in PLC activation. PKC is activated by DAG and myocardial protection is mediated by the MAPK and RISK pathways. At the level of the mitochondrion pre- and post-conditioning prevents mPTP opening upon reperfusion. Late preconditioning involves the synthesis of cytoprotective proteins. Gp, G protein coupled receptor binding; PLC, phospholipase C; DAG, diacylglycerol; PKC, protein kinase C; MAPK, mitogen-activated protein kinase; RISK, reperfusion injury salvage kinase; mPTP, mitochondrial permeability transition pore.

intervention and CABG surgery with varying results. Although the clinical application of an ischemic preconditioning protocol might reduce the consequences of myocardial IRI, it should be borne in mid that exposing an already diseased heart to ischemia, albeit transient, risks further jeopardizing myocardial function and cell survival.

In addition to the classic stimulus of short-term ischemia, physical stimuli (e.g. rapid pacing and hyperthermia) and several pharmacological agents have been shown to induce preconditioning. Furthermore, it has been demonstrated that pharmacological agents that either block or stimulate specific steps in the intracellular cascade of events can modify ischemic preconditioning. Unfortunately, many of the currently available pharmacological preconditioning agents have serious side effects: hypotension (adenosine), arrhythmias (adenosine, K_{ATP} channel openers) or possible carcinogenesis (protein kinase activators).

The observation that volatile anesthetics and opioids exhibit a preconditioning effect has led to the term *anesthetic preconditioning*. In contrast to the experimental setting, where anesthetic preconditioning consistently provides protective action against post-ischemic myocardial dysfunction and damage,

the results of clinical studies using a preconditioning protocol are less convincing. A major obstacle to the translation of experimental data to the clinical setting is the need for a predictable and well-defined period of myocardial ischemia. Fortunately, cardiac surgery provides a suitable experimental paradigm. While some cardiac surgical studies revealed biochemical or functional evidence of myocardial protection, others failed to demonstrate cardioprotection. A possible reason for this variability is the choice of preconditioning protocol. It has been recently demonstrated that protection using a *preconditioning* protocol (manifest as lower postoperative troponin release or better-preserved myocardial function) only occurs following intermittent, rather than continuous, anesthetic drug administration. However, clinically relevant cardioprotection in cardiac surgery has been described using a volatile anesthetic administered throughout the entire period of surgery, i.e. the period before ischemia (preconditioning), during ischemia and during reperfusion (postconditioning). In these studies, where sevoflurane was compared to propofol, the former was associated with a consistent reduction in postoperative troponin release and better preservation of myocardial function. In addition, recent data seem to indicate a lower incidence of perioperative myocardial infarction, in-hospital mortality and even 1-year mortality in patients receiving a volatile anesthetic. These observations were primarily obtained in CABG surgery patients. Outside this setting, data are less convincing; volatile anesthetics have been shown to exhibit protective properties in AV surgery but not in MV surgery. Also during percutaneous coronary interventions no protective effects have been observed.

Organ protection can also be achieved by inducing ischemia in tissues distant from the organ at risk, a phenomenon known as *remote preconditioning*. Several cardiac surgical studies have indicated that transient occlusion of blood flow to a limb is associated with reduced myocardial damage.

Myocardial postconditioning

In 2003, Zhao and colleagues introduced the concept of *ischemic postconditioning* – very brief periods of ischemia in the earliest stages of reperfusion (Figure 20.3). As with preconditioning, a well-defined interval between the ischemic insult and the postconditioning trigger is a prerequisite for protection. Postconditioning involves pathways similar to those involved in preconditioning, including activation of the phosphatidylinositol-3-kinase and MAPK pathways, although it remains to be seen which mechanism exerts the protective effect. Ultimately, postconditioning probably mediates cardioprotection through delayed or transient mPTP opening.

Postconditioning has been demonstrated in human myocardium and its potential clinical applications are obvious. In contrast to preconditioning, where the stimulus must be applied at a critical time point *before* the ischemic episode to be effective, postconditioning can be planned during and applied *after* the insult (e.g. during myocardial revascularization). Pharmacological postconditioning is preferable to the application of further ischemic insults to reperfused myocardium. Volatile anesthetic agents have been shown to confer cardioprotection through postconditioning effects.

Key points

- The use of inotropes to improve the performance of stunned myocardium does not induce cardiomyocyte damage.
- Identification of hibernating myocardium is the key to achieving functional improvement with myocardial revascularization.
- Ischemic preconditioning has been demonstrated in all species and all tissues.
- Pre-infarction angina may result in a smaller infarct as a result of ischemic preconditioning.
- Pharmacological preconditioning can be induced with volatile anesthetic agents and opioids.

Further reading

Crisostomo PR, Wairiuko GM, Wang M, Tsai BM, Morrell ED, Meldrum DR. Preconditioning versus postconditioning: mechanisms and therapeutic potentials. *J Am Coll Surg* 2006; **202**: 797–812.

De Hert S. Myocardial protection from ischemia and reperfusion injury. In Mebazaa A, Gheorgiade M, Zannad FM, Parrillo JE (Eds.), *Acute Heart Failure.* London: Springer-Verlag; 2008.

De Hert S, Vlasselaers D, Barbé R, Ory JP, Dekegel D, Donnadonni R, Demeers JL, Mulier J, Wouters P. A comparison of volatile and non volatile agents for cardioprotection during on-pump coronary surgery. *Anaesthesia* 2009; **64**: 953–60.

Fräßdorf J, De Hert S, Schlack W. Anaesthesia and myocardial ischaemia/reperfusion injury. *Br J Anaesth* 2009; **103**: 89–98.

Halestrap AP, Clarke SJ, Javadov SA. Mitochondrial permeability transition pore opening during myocardial reperfusion – a target for cardioprotection. *Cardiovasc Res* 2004; **61**: 372–85.

Pagel PS. Postconditioning by volatile anesthetics: salvaging ischemic myocardium at reperfusion by activation of prosurvival signalling. *J Cardiothor Vasc Anesth* 2008; **22**: 753–65.

Schinkel AFL, Bax JJ, Poldermans D, Elhendy A, Ferrari R, Rahimtoola SH. Hibernating myocardium: diagnosis and patient outcomes. *Curr Probl Cardiol* 2007; **32**: 375–410.

Zaugg M, Lucchinetti E, Garcia C, Pasch T, Spahn DR, Schaub MC. Anaesthetics and cardiac preconditioning. Part 1: signalling and cytoprotective mechanisms. *Br J Anaesth* 2003; **91**: 551–65.

Prosthetic heart valves

Yasir Abu-Omar and John J. Dunning

Since the first successful heart valve implantation by Dr Dwight Harken (Boston, USA) in 1960 in a patient with AS, there has been significant progress in both the design and durability of prosthetic valve substitutes. This, coupled with improved surgical expertise and perioperative management, has led to a continuing improvement in outcomes of patients undergoing valve replacement and repair procedures. Currently over 200 000 valve replacement and repair procedures are being performed annually worldwide.

Several valve substitutes are available – mechanical and biological prostheses. The decision to use a specific prosthesis or surgical technique is largely dictated by both patient factors (e.g. age, lifestyle, comorbidities, preference) and surgical factors. The use of minimally invasive transcatheter valve implantation in patients with a prohibitive surgical risk is discussed in Chapter 42. The following account will focus on the advantages, limitations and potential complications of currently available valves.

Mechanical valves

Mechanical heart valves have been available since the 1960s. They have evolved from the original caged-ball and tilting-disc designs, to the bileaflet prostheses which currently dominate the market.

Caged ball

The Starr-Edwards caged-ball valve was the first commercially available heart valve and was first implanted in 1960. It consists of a small ball held in place by a closed or semi-closed metal cage (Figure 21.1). It has been modified over the years and is a very durable valve with minimal risk of mechanical failure. Due to its suboptimal hemodynamics and increased risk of hemolysis and thrombogenicity, it has been largely replaced by more modern prostheses, but is still available and is used in the Third World due to cost considerations.

Table 21.1 Classification of implantable heart valves

Mechanical	Caged ball
	Caged disc
	Single-leaflet tilting disc
	Twin leaflet
Bioprosthetic[a]	Porcine heterograft (xenograft)
	Bovine pericardial
Homograft	Human homograft (allograft)
	Pulmonary autograft

[a] Bioprosthetic valves incorporate both biological and synthetic materials.

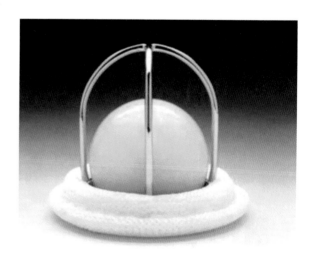

Figure 21.1 Starr–Edwards™ silastic ball valve. Still available and occasionally used. Smallest orifice for given annulus size. Cage fractures cause ball embolism and fulminant regurgitation.

Core Topics in Cardiac Anesthesia, Second Edition, ed. Jonathan H. Mackay and Joseph E. Arrowsmith. Published by Cambridge University Press. © Cambridge University Press 2012.

(a)

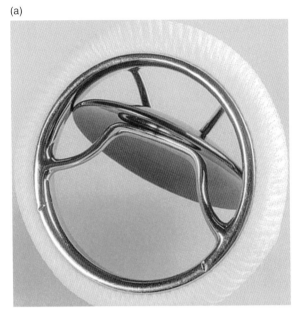

(b)

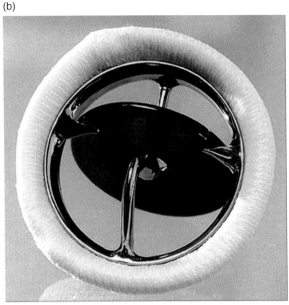

Figure 21.2 Tilting disc valves. (a) Bjork-Shiley: early models were reliable and extensively used. A design improvement enabling the disc to open at 70° caused an increase in strut failure rate in larger valve sizes. All models were subsequently withdrawn from the market. (b) Medtronic Hall™: most common valve of this type in use today. Extremely durable. Very low failure rate. Central hole in disc through which passes gooseneck-shaped central strut.

Tilting disc

The Bjork-Shiley tilting-disc valve was developed in the mid 1960s. The disc or single leaflet rotates on a single central strut with an opening angle of 75–85°. It offered better hemodynamic function than caged-ball valves. Strut fracture was reported with the Bjork-Shiley convexo-concave disc and led to its withdrawal. The Medtronic Hall tilting-disc valve is the contemporarily available representative of this type of prosthesis (Figure 21.2).

Bileaflet

These prostheses were developed in the late 1970s. Contemporary models are made of tungsten-impregnated graphite and mounted onto a sewing ring or cuff (Figure 21.3). The leaflets rotate on pivots and open to 75–80°. Modifications include alteration of the convexity of the leaflets, the opening angle, the hinge design, the height of the prosthesis and the size of the sewing ring or cuff. The latter modification was aimed at increasing the effective valve orifice area, thereby reducing the pressure gradient across the valve. Bileaflet valves are considered by many to be the "gold standard" and are the most frequently implanted mechanical prostheses.

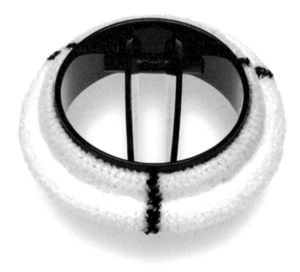

Figure 21.3 ATS Medical Inc. bileaflet mechanical valve. Another commonly used example is the St Jude Medical bileaflet valve (not shown). On TEE examination, this design is associated with one central and two peripheral regurgitant washing jets. The ATS version is said to be quieter and less thrombogenic than the St Jude. Both can be rotated within the sewing ring.

125

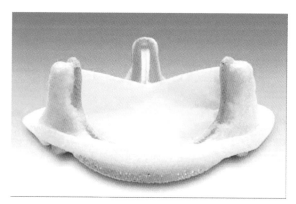

Figure 21.4 Carpentier–Edwards Perimount™ stented pericardial bioprosthesis. Tissue treatment eliminates up to 98% of pericardial phospholipids – a major calcium binding site. The stent is composed of Elgiloy® – an alloy of cobalt, chromium, nickel and molybdenum.

Biological valves

These can be divided into autografts, homografts and xenografts. Alternatively, they can be classified as stented or stentless.

Stented

These valves consist of porcine valve leaflets, or bovine or equine pericardium (Figure 21.4). The heterograft valve tissue is preserved in glutaraldehyde to significantly reduce antigenicity and susceptibility to calcification. The valves are mounted on a cobalt-chromium alloy stent and a cloth-covered sewing ring – the former providing structural support, the latter simplifying surgical implantation. Increased structural support is achieved at the expense of reduced effective valve orifice area.

Stentless

Stentless valves are implanted directly onto the native valve annulus without use of a rigid sewing cuff. They are implanted using two suture lines: one proximal to the annulus and one more distal. Accurate spatial distribution of the three commissures that support the leaflets is essential to ensure optimal valve function. The implantation technique is complex and technically more demanding than that for stented valves. Stentless AV prostheses can be used for aortic root replacement with re-implantation of the coronary arteries.

Stentless valves include autografts (from the same individual, e.g. pulmonary valve used to replace aortic valve), homografts (from a different individual, e.g. a

(a)

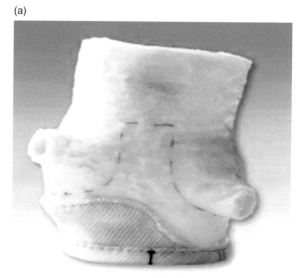

(b)

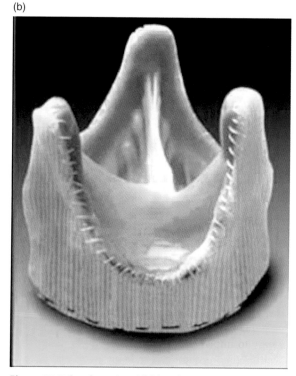

Figure 21.5 Stentless valves. (a) Edwards porcine Prima Plus™ stentless aortic bioprosthesis. (b) St Jude Medical Toronto SPV®. Removal of phospholipids reduces post-implantation calcium uptake.

cadaver) and hetero- or xenografts (from a different species, e.g. porcine, bovine; Figure 21.5). Theoretical advantages of stentless valves include minimal use of non-biological material, increased effective orifice area – reduced transvalvular gradient, and a closer reproduction of normal valve anatomy and hemodynamic performance.

In autograft valve replacement – the so-called Ross procedure – the excised AV is replaced by the native PV, which in turn is replaced by a homograft. It is usually reserved for younger adults and children as the autograft is thought to grow with the recipient. The procedure is technically very demanding and associated with greater potential for perioperative mortality and morbidity (see Chapter 52).

Surgical considerations
Hemodynamic performance

The goals of valve replacement are minimal transvalvular gradient and optimal hemodynamic function. In the aortic position, this is essential for postoperative normalization of LV mass and function (so-called reverse remodeling). An abnormally high postoperative gradient is the inevitable consequence of implanting a small prosthetic valve. The magnitude of *prosthesis-patient mismatch* is quantified by dividing the effective valve orifice area by body surface area. Mild degrees of mismatch are usually unimportant and may be seen following implantation of a mechanical or stented bioprosthesis. Severe forms, however, may be associated with reduced survival. Several techniques are available aiming at enlarging the aortic root or LVOT using an autograft or heterograft pericardium – which allows the implantation of a larger prosthesis. These procedures are technically demanding and associated with significant risk.

Choice of valve

The ideal valve prosthesis has the following characteristics:

- easy to implant
- inert
- possesses long-term durability
- has little or no transvalvular gradient
- not thrombogenic.

No valve currently available fulfils all these criteria.

In many cases the choice of valve is relatively straightforward; for example, use of a bioprosthesis in an elderly patient with AS. Other cases are less clear-cut, requiring a detailed discussion of the advantages and disadvantages of available valve types. In equipoise, the final decision may be simply a matter of personal preference. In recent years there has been a trend toward greater use of bioprostheses. This may in part be due to improved design and tissue preservation (increased durability, reduced reoperation rate) and increased recognition of the complications of long-term anticoagulation.

While pulmonary autografts and homografts provide the closest match to native valve function their use is limited by availability and the requirement for a higher level of technical expertise.

Excellent hemodynamic profiles and durability make mechanical prostheses the mainstay for valve replacement in younger patients. The risks of thromboembolic events and lifelong, mandatory anticoagulation (1–1.5% per year) have to be balanced against the risk of one or more reoperations. When implanted in a young recipient, the cumulative risks may compare unfavorably with the risk of reoperation after 10–15 years.

Although biological valves have a definite lifespan, patients do not typically require anticoagulation. They are therefore the valve of choice in patients where anticoagulation is contraindicated. They may also be used when anticoagulation monitoring is difficult or not available. Bioprostheses are also the valve of choice in the older patients who are unlikely to outlive the implanted valve. This is particularly true as the rate of structural deterioration is lower in elderly patients. In addition, patients with comorbidities that reduce long-term survival may be better served with a bioprosthesis.

In MV disease, valve repair is the operation of choice when possible as the results are superior to valve replacement. Structural deterioration of a mitral bioprosthesis is often more rapid than an aortic bioprosthesis. Another important consideration in the decision-making process regarding mitral valve replacement is that a large proportion of patients have chronic AF and may already be anticoagulated.

Renal failure

Patients with end-stage renal failure present a particular challenge. While it would appear sensible to avoid the risks of anticoagulation, bioprosthetic valves are known to undergo accelerated calcification in these patients. While several studies have reported no difference in outcome between tissue and mechanical

Table 21.2 Veterans Affairs Cooperative Study on Valvular Heart Disease. Causes of death (% of all deaths) 15 years after randomization, according to type and location of replacement valve

	Aortic valve replacement		Mitral valve replacement	
	Mechanical	Bioprosthetic	Mechanical	Bioprosthetic
Prosthesis-related	37%	41%	44%	57%
Cardiac – not prosthesis-related	17%	21%	31%	19%
Non-cardiac	36%	26%	18%	9%
Undetermined	10%	12%	7%	15%

From Hammermeister et al., 2000.

prostheses, the choice of prosthesis in renal patients remains unresolved.

Women of childbearing age

The choice of valve prosthesis in women of childbearing age is controversial. The principal areas of concern are the teratogenic and hemorrhagic effects of coumarins, and the hypercoagulable state of pregnancy. Of secondary importance are the potential effects of changes in cardiovascular physiology on prosthetic valve integrity. An autograft or heterograft may be a reasonable choice for patients who prefer a tissue valve. In isolated mitral regurgitation, valve repair is preferable to valve replacement. MS that becomes symptomatic during pregnancy may be temporized by valvotomy and treated definitively 6–8 weeks after delivery.

Complications
Valve-related mortality

The risk of early death after valve replacement is determined by a number of factors (see Chapter 17). Long-term survival is dependent on freedom from valve-related events such as thrombosis, thromboembolism, valve degeneration and infection, and anticoagulation events such as intracranial or GI hemorrhage. All patients face a small but finite risk of lethal valve-related complications.

Valve-related morbidity
Structural valve deterioration

Modern mechanical valves are resistant to structural dysfunction. Structural deterioration with bioprosthetic valves is related to both time since implantation

and patient age. The risk of valve failure requiring reoperation within 10 years of implantation is 40% in patients <40 years of age compared with 10% in those >70 years of age. The reasons for this observation are unclear but may be related to lower hemodynamic stresses in elderly patients.

In the Veterans Affairs Cooperative Study on Valvular Heart Disease, patients undergoing valve replacement were followed for 15 years. Primary valve failure was detected in 23% of patients following AVR and in 44% following MVR. Almost all of the primary valve failures occurred in those under 65 years of age.

In general terms, structural MV prosthesis deterioration is greater and starts earlier – deterioration starts at 5 years after MVR and 8 years following AVR. As outlined above, the most important patient factor is age; the younger the patient at the time of implantation, the greater the rate of structural valve deterioration.

Thromboembolism

This is one of the most important and serious complications. (Table 21.3) The embolic manifestations can be divided into peripheral (i.e. non-cerebral) or cerebral: transient ischemic attack, reversible ischemic neurologic deficit and stroke.

Valve thrombosis is rare (<0.2% per year), but potentially devastating and carries a high mortality. Hemodynamically stable patients with minimal thrombus (<5 mm thickness) can be treated with either IV heparin or a thrombolytic. Thrombolysis is associated with a high risk of thromboembolism. This strategy is more successful in patients with bileaflet aortic valves who have had symptoms <2 weeks. Unstable patients and those with extensive thrombosis are more likely to require surgical intervention.

Table 21.3 Veterans Affairs Cooperative Study on Valvular Heart Disease. Probability of death due to any cause, any valve-related complication, and individual valve related complications 15 years after randomization, according to type and location of replacement valve

	Aortic valve replacement		Mitral valve replacement	
	Mechanical ($n = 198$)	Bioprosthetic ($n = 196$)	Mechanical ($n = 88$)	Bioprosthetic ($n = 93$)
Death from any cause	0.66	0.76	0.81	0.79
Any valve-related complication	0.65	0.66	0.73	0.81
Systemic embolism	0.18	0.18	0.18	0.22
Bleeding	0.51[a]	0.30	0.53[a]	0.31
Endocarditis	0.07	0.15	0.11	0.17
Valve thrombosis	0.02	0.01	0.01	0.01
Perivalvular regurgitation	0.08[b]	0.02	0.17[b]	0.07
Reoperation	0.10	0.29	0.25	0.50
Primary valve failure	0.00	0.23[c]	0.05	0.44[c]

From Hammermeister et al., 2000.
[a] Risk of bleeding significantly higher with mechanical valve.
[b] Risk of perivavular regurgitation significantly higher with mechanical valve.
[c] Risk of structural failure significantly higher with bioprosthetic valve.

Anticoagulation is essential following heart valve implantation. Suggested therapeutic targets for the international normalized ratio (INR) vary from country to country. Recommendations for the UK and North America are shown in Tables 21.4 and 21.5 respectively. The key difference is that that American patients treated with warfarin also tend to receive aspirin.

Bleeding

Anticoagulation increases the risk of bleeding. This is compounded by concomitant administration of antiplatelet agents. The risks and benefits should be addressed preoperatively in every case and appropriate treatment guided by the recommendations above. The risk of a bleeding event in patients on warfarin ranges from 1.5 to 2.0% per patient-year and increases with age.

Prosthetic valve endocarditis

Infective endocarditis is a multi-organ system disease. There tends to be a relationship between the time since surgery and the causative organism (Table 21.7). Early infections are due to intraoperative contamination and skin flora (i.e. direct) whereas

Table 21.4 Therapeutic targets for anticoagulation after mitral and aortic valve replacement

	Aortic	Mitral
Bioprosthetic	Short term (<3 months): Long term (>3 months):	Warfarin (INR 2.0–3.0) Warfarin (INR 2.0–3.0) if patient in AF Aspirin if in sinus rhythm
Mechanical	Warfarin (INR 2.0–3.0) indefinitely	Warfarin (INR 2.5–3.5) indefinitely

later infections are commonly due to bacteremia from dental infections and non-cardiac operative sites (indirect).

It may be difficult to make the diagnosis of prosthetic valve endocarditis, and a high index of suspicion is required. Both pathological and clinical criteria are used. Pathological criteria include culture of microorganisms from an intracardiac abscess or an embolized vegetation. A histological diagnosis may be made from a vegetation or intracardiac abscess. The

129

Table 21.5 Level of evidence supporting recommendations for antithrombotic therapy in patients with prosthetic heart valves. ACC/AHA 2006 Guidelines (updated 2008)

	Aspirin (75–100 mg)	Warfarin (INR 2.0–3.0)	Warfarin (INR 2.5–3.5)	No warfarin
Mechanical valves				
AVR (low risk) <3 months	Class I	Class I	Class IIa	
AVR (low risk) >3 months	Class I	Class I		
AVR (high risk)	Class I		Class I	
MVR	Class I		Class I	
Biological valves				
AVR (low risk) <3 months	Class I	Class IIa		Class IIb
AVR (low risk) >3 months	Class I			Class IIa
AVR (high risk)	Class I	Class I		
MVR (low risk) <3 months	Class I	Class IIa		
MVR (low risk) >3 months	Class I			Class IIa
MVR (high risk)	Class I	Class I		

Antithrombotic therapy must be individualized. In patients receiving warfarin, aspirin is recommended in virtually all situations. Additional risk factors include: AF, LV dysfunction, previous thromboembolism, and hypercoagulable states. The international normalized ratio (INR) should be maintained between 2.5 and 3.5 for aortic disc valves and Starr-Edwards valves. *Circulation* 2008; 118(15): e523–661.

Table 21.6 Bleeding complications after cardiac valve replacement. Data from the Edinburgh Heart Valve Trial

	Follow-up	
	10 years	**20 years**
Bleeding: all episodes		
Mechanical	15.3%	55.6%
Bioprosthesis	7.5%	43.6%
Bleeding: major[a]		
Mechanical	11.7%	40.7%
Bioprosthesis	4.9%	27.9%

[a] Bleeding necessitating hospitalization or blood transfusion

Table 21.7 Causative organisms implicated in infectious endocarditis following valve surgery

Early (<60 days)

Staphylococcus epidermidis and *eureus*

Gram-negative organisms, diphtheroids

Fungi, mycobacteria, *Legionella*

Late (>60 days)

Streptococci

Staphylococcus epidermidis

presence of major and minor clinical criteria permits a clinical diagnosis of definite endocarditis to be made. The prevention, diagnosis and treatment of endocarditis are discussed in Chapter 71.

Paravalvular leak/hemolysis

Paravalvular leak may arise from a technical error during implantation or as a result of endocarditis. A severe paravalvular leak may require surgical correction particularly when it is associated with hemodynamic disturbance or hemolysis. The diagnosis is confirmed by the finding of a regurgitant jet that lies outside the valve sewing ring on angiography or echocardiography.

With modern mechanical and bioprosthetic valves hemolysis is uncommon. It can be subclinical or manifest as anemia and mild jaundice. Markers of hemolysis include anemia, reduced haptoglobin a reticulocytosis and elevated serum lactate dehydrogenase. Structural valvular dysfunction may cause significant hemolysis and warrants reoperation.

Key points

- Careful counseling prior to valve procedures is essential to ensure a satisfactory outcome.
- Mechanical valves are commonly used for AV replacement in young patients because their durability outweighs the risks associated with anticoagulation.
- Whenever possible, mechanical valves should be avoided in women of childbearing age.
- Bioprosthetic valves are indicated in elderly patients where the risks of anticoagulation are more important than device durability.
- The ideal and as yet unavailable valve prosthesis is durable, has an excellent hemodynamic profile and requires no anticoagulation.

Further reading

Bonow RO, Carabello BA, Chatterjee K, *et al.* 2008 Focused update incorporated into the ACC/AHA 2006 guidelines for the management of patients with valvular heart disease: a report of the American College of Cardiology/American Heart Association Task Force on Practice Guidelines. *Circulation* 2008; **118**(15): e523–661.

Hammermeister K, Sethi GK, Henderson WG, Grover FL, Oprian C, Rahimtoola SH. Outcomes 15 years after valve replacement with a mechanical versus a bioprosthetic valve: final report of the Veterans Affairs randomized trial. *J Am Coll Cardiol* 2000; **36**(4): 1152–8.

Oxenham H, Bloomfield P, Wheatley DJ, *et al.* Twenty year comparison of a Bjork-Shiley mechanical heart valve with porcine bioprostheses. *Heart* 2003; **89**(7): 715–21.

Routine clinical monitoring

Jörn Karhausen and Jonathan B. Mark

Clinical examination

The complexity of conditions encountered during cardiac surgery combined with relatively restricted patient access mandates the use of reliable, objective monitoring. Decision-making should always incorporate whatever clinical observations are available, but these rarely suffice during cardiac operations. While the anesthesiologists typically only has access to the head and neck, physical examination of these areas may be of critical importance. For example, unilateral facial blanching may indicate arterial (aortic) cannula malposition whereas chemosis and facial edema and flushing may indicate SVC obstruction.

Electrocardiography

Initially used exclusively for detection of arrhythmia, ECG monitoring has undergone technological advances that have substantially expanded the information that can be derived. However, there are a number of unique challenges to ECG monitoring in the intraoperative setting that require a detailed knowledge of its technical principles and pitfalls in order to assure reliable and effective use. The goals of intraoperative ECG monitoring are summarized in Table 22.1.

Table 22.1 Goals of intraoperative ECG monitoring

Heart rate monitoring

Detection of arrhythmia and conduction abnormalities

Detection of myocardial ischemia

Recognition of pacemaker malfunction

Indication of electrolyte disturbances

General considerations

The electrical potential generated by the heart is very weak, amounting to only 0.2–2 mV at the skin surface. Accordingly, electrodes should be placed with special care, with some sort of mildly abrasive skin preparation being used to ensure good electrode contact. This may prevent electrode malfunction or displacement; for example during rewarming, when there may be considerable diaphoresis.

Detection of myocardial ischemia

No gold standard exists for the clinical diagnosis of myocardial ischemia. Although the sensitivity of 12-lead ECG monitoring during exercise testing is 68%, the sensitivity of the ECG at rest is poor. Two patterns of ischemia may be distinguished by their ECG characteristics.

Subendocardial ischemia is most common in the perioperative setting and occurs when myocardial oxygen demand exceeds supply (so-called demand ischemia; Figure 22.1).

Contrary to common belief, the ECG distribution of changes in subendocardial ischemia does not localize coronary perfusion abnormalities. Furthermore, their magnitude does not indicate severity of ischemia but rather the probability that myocardial ischemia is present.

Transmural ischemia results from inadequate blood flow (so called supply ischemia; Figure 22.2). Unlike ST-segment depression in subendocardial ischemia, the leads displaying the ST-segment elevation indicate the anatomic location of the underlying ischemia and help to identify the culprit coronary artery.

Core Topics in Cardiac Anesthesia, Second Edition, ed. Jonathan H. Mackay and Joseph E. Arrowsmith. Published by Cambridge University Press. © Cambridge University Press 2012.

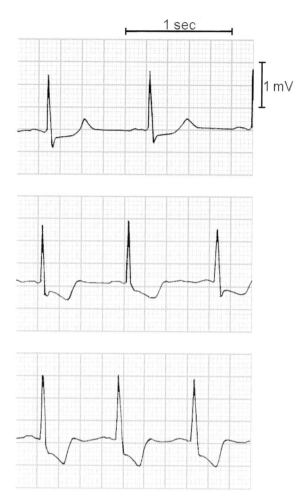

Figure 22.1 Subendocardial ischemia. ECG changes are characterized by horizontal or down-sloping ST-segment depression of 1 mm (0.1 mV) or greater in magnitude measured 60 ms after the J point lasting 1 min or longer. Adapted from Mark JB *Atlas of Cardiovascular Monitoring*. New York: Churchill Livingstone; 1998.

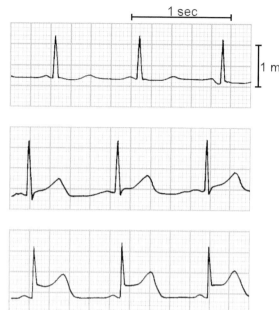

Figure 22.2 Transmural ischemia. ECG changes are characterized by ST-segment elevation (measured at the J point) of 1 mm or greater in magnitude in two or more limb leads or 2 mm or greater in two or more contiguous precordial leads. Adapted from Mark JB. *Atlas of Cardiovascular Monitoring*. New York: Churchill Livingstone; 1998.

Intraoperative ECG detection of myocardial ischemia is confounded by a number of factors commonly present in the operating room environment, including baseline ECG abnormalities, drug effects, hypothermia, LVH, patient positioning and intraoperative displacement of the heart (Figure 22.3).

In all cases, the ECG diagnosis of myocardial ischemia requires a complete appreciation of the patient's history and the clinical circumstances at the time of the observed changes. For the ECG to be an efficient and effective monitor for perioperative ischemia, attention must be paid to the following crucial details: selection and placement of leads, selection of appropriate bandwidth filter and adjustment of gain.

Lead selection

During cardiac procedures, ECG lead placement must not obscure the surgical field. Optimal lead selection depends in part on whether a three-lead or a five-lead system is used (Figure 22.4).

The five-lead ECG system allows true precordial lead monitoring, and hence improved sensitivity for the detection of myocardial ischemia, particularly when two or more leads are monitored (Table 22.2).

In the three-electrode system, leads are typically placed on the right shoulder, left shoulder and left leg. Standard bipolar limb lead selection allows monitoring of the inferior wall (II, III and aVF) and the lateral wall (I, aVL) but overall is less sensitive for detecting intraoperative ischemia. Various modifications have been developed to better reproduce precordial lead monitoring. For example, by placing the right arm lead in the right subclavicular region, the left arm lead in the V_5 position, and displaying lead I on the monitor; a modified bipolar lead (CS_5) is derived, which has a sensitivity comparable to lead V_5.

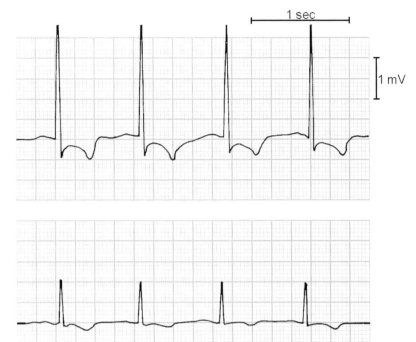

Figure 22.3 Effect of surgical chest retraction on ECG tracing. At baseline (top), lead V₅ shows a 27 mm R wave and 2 mm ST-segment depression. Following placement of the sternal retractor (bottom), the same lead displays a 10 mm R wave and a marked decrease in the magnitude of the ST-segment depression. Adapted from Mark JB. *Atlas of Cardiovascular Monitoring*. New York: Churchill Livingstone; 1998.

Filters and gain

Standard ECG gain is 10 mm/mV, and descriptions of ST-segment depression or elevation must be referenced to this standard (Figure 22.5).

The ECG potentials must be amplified and filtered before display. Whenever accurate ST-segment monitoring is needed, a *diagnostic mode* bandpass filter (0.05–100 Hz) should be used. Additional filtering, provided by the *monitor mode* bandpass filter (0.5–40 Hz) will attenuate baseline noise and high-frequency electrical interference (Figure 22.6). However, this additional filtering may hide pacing spikes or interfere with QRS and J-point recognition and deform ST-segment depression (Figure 22.7).

Computer-aided ST-segment monitoring

Automated ST trend analysis has become an important tool to overcome the unreliability of the human observer in detecting ST-segment changes over lengthy time periods (Figure 22.8).

Both the sensitivity and specificity of such devices have been disputed; there are no accuracy standards and manufacturers use differing means to test the performance of their algorithms. Consequently, a number of studies have demonstrated that automated ST analysis is vulnerable to computing errors. It is therefore imperative to verify computer-aided ST-segment analysis by comparing baseline with current ECG traces.

Arrhythmias and pacemaker function

The very-low-amplitude potentials produced by bipolar pacing leads make visualization of pacemaker spikes difficult. For this reason, most bedside monitors incorporate pacemaker spike enhancement to facilitate recognition of small high-frequency potentials (typically 5–500 mV with 0.5–2 ms pulse duration). These pacemaker spike enhancement algorithms can lead to artifacts if there is high-frequency noise within the lead system. Atrial and epicardial ventricular ECG tracings can be helpful for diagnosing complex conduction abnormalities and dysrhythmias during the postoperative period. Tracings are obtained from epicardial wires that are placed to allow temporary perioperative pacing. When the ECG is recorded from atrial leads, the atrial

Table 22.2 Sensitivity of individual ECG leads and their combination in the detection of ischemic episodes

Lead	Sensitivity
II	33%
V_4	61%
V_5	75%
II/V_5	80%
II/V_4	82%
V_4/V_5	90%
V_3/V_4/V_5	94%
II/V_4/V_5	96%
II/V_2–V_5	100%

From London *et al.* Anesthesiology 1988; 69: 232–41.

electrical activity is amplified compared to atrial signals seen on standard surface lead recordings.

Non-invasive blood pressure monitoring

Non-invasive blood pressure measurement is generally insufficient for monitoring the dynamic changes seen in cardiac surgical patients. In addition, because these techniques depend on pulsatile flow, they will not function during CPB or in patients with LV assist devices. However, non-invasive monitoring can be helpful as a back-up monitor or until invasive monitoring is established. Most automated systems are based on the oscillotonometric measurement method, which detects oscillations in cuff-pressure during gradual cuff deflation. The MAP is

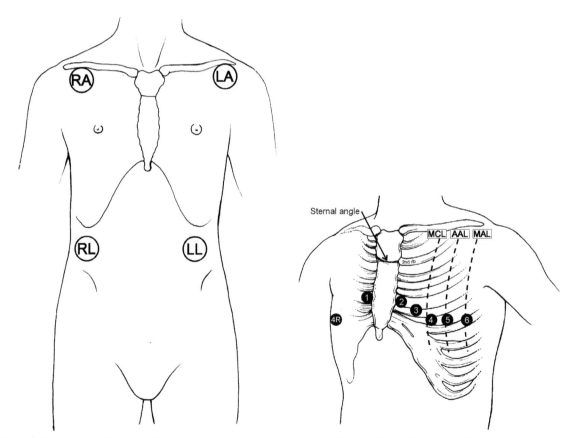

Figure 22.4 Five-lead ECG. One lead is placed on each extremity or near the shoulders and hips, and one lead is placed on the precordium in a standard position, generally V_5. This allows recording of the six standard frontal limb leads. With all limb electrodes acting as ground, a unipolar precordial lead can be recorded, generally V_5. Some authors have suggested that V_5 may be less sensitive at detecting ischemia compared to more medially located precordial leads V_4 or V_3. However, owing to the required sterile field during cardiac operations performed via median sternotomy, lead V_5 is the best choice. If RV ischemia is suspected, lead V_4R (*right* mid-clavicular line, 5th intercostal space) should be monitored. RA, right arm; RL, right leg; LA, left arm; LL, left leg; MCL, mid-clavicular line; AAL, anterior axillary line; MAL, mid-axillary line. Adapted from Mark JB. *Atlas of Cardiovascular Monitoring*. New York: Churchill Livingstone; 1998.

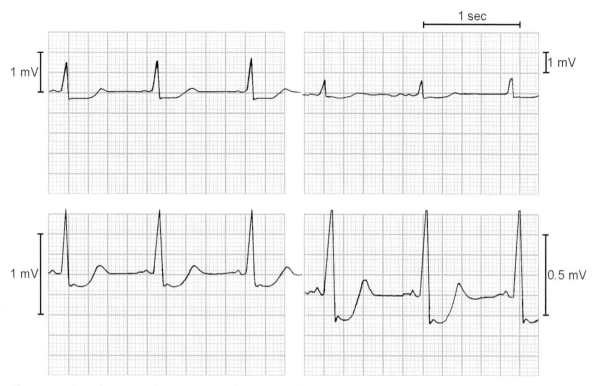

Figure 22.5 Gain adjustments. Adjusting gain can aid in wave visualization, but simultaneously exaggerates or minimizes ST-segment shifts. Adapted from Mark JB. *Atlas of Cardiovascular Monitoring.* New York: Churchill Livingstone; 1998.

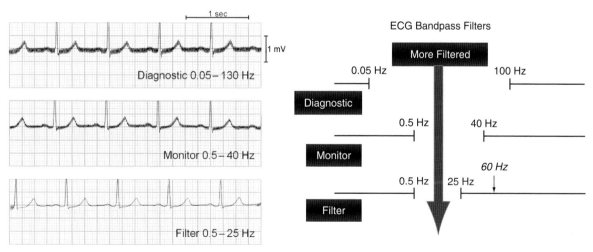

Figure 22.6 Filter settings and their effect on ECG tracing. High-frequency filters will reduce 60-Hz (US) or 50-Hz (Europe, South America) wall power source noise. Adapted from Mark JB. *Atlas of Cardiovascular Monitoring.* New York: Churchill Livingstone; 1998.

measured at the point of maximal oscillation, while systolic and diastolic readings are derived according to more empiric algorithms, such as oscillation onset for systolic pressure and oscillation disappearance for diastolic pressure. Therefore in acute care settings, such as the operating room and intensive care unit, MAP should be considered the most reliable value.

137

Oximetry

Despite the fact that a recent Cochrane review found no evidence that pulse oximetry influences the outcome of anesthesia, this technique is widely accepted as a standard of care for the rapid detection of hypoxemia. Measurements are based on the differences in absorption spectra of oxyhemoglobin and reduced hemoglobin exposed to red (660 nm) and infrared (940 nm) light sources. From this, a percentage of oxygenated hemoglobin (SpO_2) is derived through a pulse oximeter algorithm (Figure 22.9).

Interference from other tissues that absorb red and infrared light do not contaminate this

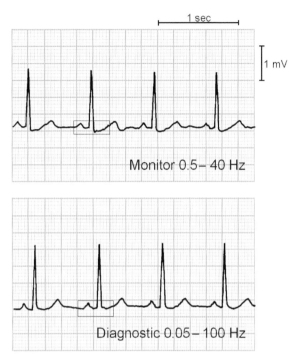

Figure 22.7 Filter settings and ST-segment abnormalities. Because the ST-segment and T wave reside in the low-frequency spectrum, low-frequency filtering may distort the ECG ST-segment and exaggerate the magnitude of ST-segment depression or elevation. Adapted from Mark JB. *Atlas of Cardiovascular Monitoring*. New York: Churchill Livingstone; 1998.

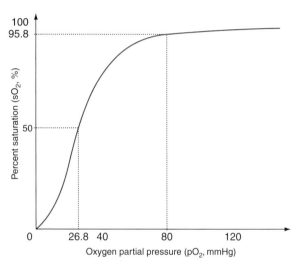

Figure 22.9 Pulse oximetry measures hemoglobin saturation, not PaO_2. Based on the shape of the normal hemoglobin dissociation curve, large increases in PaO_2 above 100 mmHg (7.6 kPa) will have little influence on SpO_2, while small decreases in PaO_2 below 60 mmHg (4.6 kPa) will cause large changes in hemoglobin saturation.

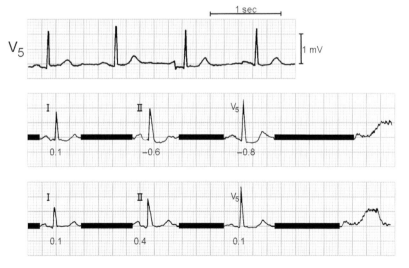

Figure 22.8 Computer aided ST-segment monitoring. After a baseline sampling interval, a digital QRS template is obtained and baseline reference points are established mathematically. These fiducial points are generally an isoelectric baseline point in the PR segment and the ST measurement point, 60 or 80 ms after the J point. Small changes in the ST segment position are measured relative to the isoelectric baseline and quantified to the nearest 0.1 mm (0.01 mV). The top panel shows a baseline ECG recording. The middle panel shows small ST-segment shifts and a trend line at the right edge shows the cumulative ST-segment shifts in all three leads. The bottom panel shows resolution of the ST-segment shifts. Adapted from Mark JB. *Atlas of Cardiovascular Monitoring*. New York: Churchill Livingstone; 1998.

measurement because absorption differences are derived from only the pulsatile (arterial) component. However, the accuracy of pulse oximetry may be altered by diminished tissue perfusion (limb ischemia, hypothermia, vasoconstriction), ambient light, intravenous dyes (e.g. methylene blue), carboxyhemoglobin, methemoglobin, decreased pulse pressure, nonpulsatile blood flow (decreased pulsatile signal strength versus the continuous absorption of the tissue) and electrocautery. For these reasons, pulse oximetry may be unreliable in the setting of cardiac surgery.

The pulse oximeter provides useful data beyond the hemoglobin oxygen saturation. Inasmuch as the oximeter plethysmograph resembles the peripheral arterial pressure waveform, the pulse oximeter is useful as a continuous pulse rate monitor. Additional applications of plethysmographic monitoring have focused on identifying respiratory variation during mechanical ventilation and assessing intravascular volume status and fluid responsiveness.

Temperature monitoring

Deliberate hypothermia is commonly used during CPB to provide organ protection, particularly of the brain, through a reduction in metabolic rate and attenuation of excitotoxic neurotransmitter release. Because persistent hypothermia has various adverse effects (e.g. coagulopathy, cardiac dysrhythmias), rewarming is essential prior to separation from bypass. During rewarming, the brain is most vulnerable to hyperthermia, and it is important to monitor temperature at a site that most accurately reflects cerebral temperature. There is debate regarding the optimal site for temperature measurement, since no single technique reliably reflects brain temperature, especially when changes occur rapidly. Because the clinical focus differs during cooling (core temperature) and rewarming (cerebral temperature), at least two temperature probes are generally used simultaneously.

- Nasopharyngeal or tympanic membrane temperature is recorded to estimate brain temperature.
- Esophageal temperature monitoring reflects the temperature of mediastinal structures. When cold fluids are used for direct cardiac cooling and myocardial protection, esophageal temperature will not reflect true core temperature.

- Pulmonary artery blood temperature, a measure of core temperature, can be monitored when a pulmonary artery catheter is in place.
- Bladder temperature reflects core temperature, but is highly dependent on urine flow and responds slowly to temperature changes during CPB.
- Rectal temperature measurements are slow to react to temperature changes and can be affected by stool.
- Skin temperature monitoring gives no indication of core temperature, but may be useful for assessing the core-peripheral temperature gradient.

Rewarming at the end of CPB should be instituted slowly as rapid rewarming may lead to unintended cerebral hyperthermia and increase the risk of neuronal injury. In addition, a difference between aortic inflow blood temperature and core temperature alters the solubility of gases dissolved in blood and, when $>10°C$, may lead to bubble formation. Rapid rewarming may also lead to a large temperature gradient between the core and periphery, which causes "afterdrop" core hypothermia as thermal energy redistributes postoperatively. (See Chapter 60.)

Further reading

Gainrossi R, Detrano R, Mulvihill D, et al. Exercise-induced ST depression in the diagnosis of coronary artery disease. A meta-analysis. *Circulation* 1989; **80**: 87–98.

Grigore AM, Murray CF, Ramakrishna H, et al. A core review of temperature regimens and neuroprotection during cardiopulmonary bypass: does rewarming rate matter? *Anesth Analg* 2009; **109**: 1741–51.

Li D, Yong L, Yong AC, Kilpatrick D. Source of electrocardiographic ST changes in subendocardial ischemia. *Circ Res* 1998; **82**: 957–70.

Mark JB. *Atlas of Cardiovascular Monitoring.* New York: Churchill Livingstone; 1998.

Mirvis DM, Berson AS, Goldberger AL, et al. Instrumentation and practice standards for electrocardiographic monitoring in special care units. A report for health professionals by a Task Force of the Council on Clinical Cardiology, American Heart Association. *Circulation* 1989; **79**: 464–71.

Pedersen T, Møller AM, Hovhannisyan K. Pulse oximetry for perioperative monitoring. *Cochrane Database of Systematic Reviews* 2009; **4**: CD002013.

Stone JG, Young WL, Smith CR, et al. Do standard monitoring sites reflect true brain temperature when

139

profound hypothermia is rapidly induced and reversed? *Anesthesiology* 1995; **82**: 344.

Thygesen K, Alpert JS, White HD, *et al.* Universal definition of myocardial infarction. *Circulation* 2007; **116**: 2634–53.

Wagner GS. Ischemia due to increased myocardial demand. In Wagner GS (Ed.), *Marriott's Practical Electrocardiography*, 9th edition. Baltimore: Williams and Wilkins; 1994. pp. 121–35.

Wagner GS, Macfarlane P, Wellens H, *et al.* AHA/ACCF/HRS recommendations for the standardization and interpretation of the electrocardiogram: part VI: acute ischemia/infarction: a scientific statement from the American Heart Association Electrocardiography and Arrhythmias Committee, Council on Clinical Cardiology; the American College of Cardiology Foundation; and the Heart Rhythm Society: endorsed by the International Society for Computerized Electrocardiology. *Circulation* 2009; **119**: e262–70.

Chapter

23

Invasive hemodynamic monitoring

Matthew E. Atkins and Jonathan B. Mark

Arterial blood pressure monitoring

Direct arterial pressure monitoring is ideal for beat-to-beat monitoring when rapid detection of hemodynamic changes is imperative. Although the direct technique requires additional expertise, equipment and expense, it is considered the gold standard for blood pressure monitoring and required during all major cardiac surgical procedures. In general terms, indications for arterial cannulation include anticipated major hemodynamic fluctuations or blood loss, presence of severe underlying cardiovascular disease, inability to obtain indirect measurements, and the need for frequent blood sampling. While the radial artery is the most frequently used site, other commonly used arterial cannulation sites include femoral and brachial. The axillary and dorsalis pedis arteries are used less frequently. Complications of arterial cannulation include: hemorrhage, thrombosis, vasospasm, distal ischemia, dissection, infection, inadvertent drug administration, pseudoaneurysm, and arteriovenous fistula formation. Vigilant monitoring of distal perfusion must be maintained and continued for several hours after decannulation to improve the detection of complications.

The MAP is nearly constant throughout the arterial tree and provides the most accurate single measure of the pressure driving blood flow to organs. In contrast, the values for systolic and diastolic blood pressure vary throughout the arterial tree. As the monitoring site moves more distally, the arterial pressure waveform changes – sharper systolic upstroke, higher systolic peak, delayed and less distinct dicrotic notch, more prominent diastolic wave and lower end-diastolic pressure (Figure 23.1). As a result, peripherally recorded arterial pressure waveforms have a wider pulse pressure than central aortic pressure. In addition, peripheral

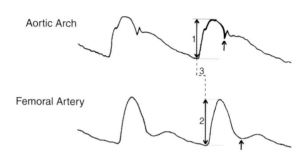

Figure 23.1 Although the mean pressure remains unchanged, the systolic and pulse pressure are both amplified as the monitoring site moves peripherally in the arterial tree.

pressure waveforms are often distorted by high-frequency artifacts and are subject to measurement system operating characteristics, notably the natural frequency and damping coefficient (see below).

In contrast to the normal distal pulse pressure amplification seen in peripheral arterial pressure traces, pressure waveforms recorded following hypothermic CPB often underestimate both systolic and mean central aortic pressure. These pressure waveform changes usually resolve within minutes to hours after discontinuation of CPB.

The radial artery is the preferred cannulation site because of its convenience and superficial location. The patient should be positioned with the wrist supinated and slightly extended. A "wrist roll" placed under the wrist facilitates extension. The puncture site should be prepared in a sterile fashion, and standard sterile barrier precautions should be utilized during the procedure. The operator's fingertips are used to palpate the pulse, and a small skin wheal with 1% lidocaine is made at the intended puncture site. A large skin wheal may make subsequent palpation of the pulse more difficult. Typically a 20 G cannula with integral stylette is advanced at an angle of 30–45°

Core Topics in Cardiac Anesthesia, Second Edition, ed. Jonathan H. Mackay and Joseph E. Arrowsmith. Published by Cambridge University Press. © Cambridge University Press 2012.

directly towards the pulse. When a flash of arterial blood is observed in the clear stylette hub, the cannula angle is decreased. If flow continues, the cannula and stylette are advanced another 1–2 mm to ensure intraluminal placement of the cannula tip. The cannula is then gently "pushed" off the stylette into the artery lumen. Some arterial catheterization kits have a wire that is passed into the lumen first, and then the cannula is threaded over the guidewire using a modified Seldinger technique. Proximal pressure is applied to the artery while the transducer tubing is attached to the cannula.

After the transducer and fluid-filled manometer tubing have been attached to the cannula, the system is levelled and zeroed. For monitoring the patient undergoing cardiac surgery, the system should be referenced to the level of the heart, i.e. the mid-axillary level. However, a position 5 cm posterior to the sternum at the level of the 4th intercostal space is preferable, as this mitigates the confounding effects of the hydrostatic pressure within the heart chambers. The high quality of modern disposable transducers obviates the need for gain calibration. During monitoring, the reference level should be checked frequently to exclude "zero drift". Patient or bed movement without adjustment of transducer height yields inaccurate pressure values.

The natural frequency and damping coefficient characterize the dynamic response of the monitoring system and influence the fidelity of the transduced waveform. The damping coefficient describes the forces acting on the monitoring system that determine how rapidly the system comes to rest (steady state) following a pressure change. A damping coefficient of 0.6–0.8 is optimal for most systems. Damping attenuates resonance within the pressure monitoring system, which occurs when a pressure wave strikes an elastic arterial wall and causes it to oscillate. The lowest frequency of these oscillations is called the fundamental frequency and corresponds to the patient's heart rate. The subsequent reverberations are multiples (harmonics) of the fundamental frequency. An *underdamped* system can lead to pressure measurement artifacts, including falsely wide pulse pressure, increased systolic blood pressure and exaggerated dicrotic notch. Conversely, an *overdamped* system may cause a slurred arterial upstroke, narrowed pulse pressure and waveform flattening. To optimize the dynamic response of the system, the natural frequency of the system should be at

least 8–10 times the fundamental frequency, roughly 15–20 Hz. This can be achieved by using short lengths of stiff extension tubing without extraneous ports, stopcocks, air bubbles or blood clots. These measures will improve the dynamic response of the system by increasing its natural frequency and avoiding excessive damping.

The natural frequency and damping coefficient of a pressure monitoring system can be determined by a square-wave flush test, performed by momentarily activating the fast flush valve and observing the resulting pressure waveform. By recording a strip of this flush test, one can determine the natural frequency by dividing the paper speed (25 mm s^{-1}) by the length of one cycle, measured between two adjacent pressure peaks or troughs on the strip. For example, if the distance between two peaks on the strip is 1 mm, and the paper speed is 25 mm s^{-1}, this yields a natural frequency of 25 Hz, and should accurately reproduce a waveform tracing with a fundamental frequency of 3 Hz (i.e. a heart rate of up to 180 beats per minute). The damping coefficient is derived by measuring the ratio of the amplitude of two adjacent pressure peaks and then referring to a lookup table or chart (Figure 23.2).

Central venous pressure monitoring

Central venous pressure (CVP), an estimate of RA pressure (RAP), is dependent upon intravascular volume, RV function and venous tone. Indications for central venous cannulation include anticipated large volume shifts, administration of drugs that cause venous irritation, total parenteral nutrition, frequent blood sampling, temporary venous pacing, fluid therapy in patients with inadequate peripheral access and (rarely) aspiration of venous air emboli.

Common sites for central venous cannulation include the internal jugular (IJV), subclavian and femoral veins. Complications include bleeding, hematoma, arterial puncture, arrhythmias, infection, pneumothorax, thrombosis, airway compromise, air embolism and nerve injury. Use of a subclavian vein is associated with the lowest infection rate and is preferred for long-term use. However, it is not compressible and its use is relatively contraindicated in coagulopathic patients. Use of the more compressible femoral veins is associated with a greater infection risk. The IJVs are relatively easy to cannulate, but lie in close proximity to the carotids, pleura and trachea.

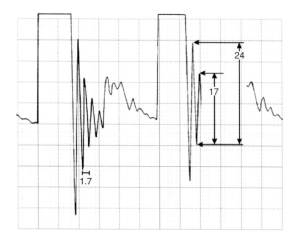
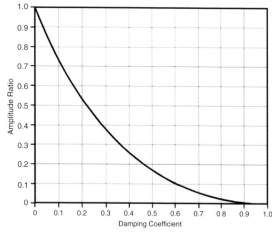

Figure 23.2 Calculation of natural frequency and damping coefficient. If the amplitudes of two adjacent peaks are 24 and 17, the ratio is 17/24 or 0.7, which yields a damping coefficient of 0.12.

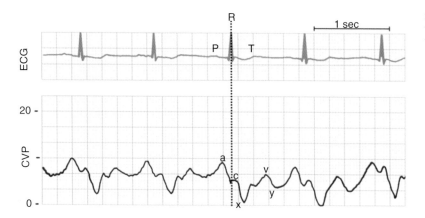

Figure 23.3 Normal CVP tracing. Note the timing of the waves in relation to the R wave on the ECG.

Multiple clinical studies and meta-analyses have shown that the use of ultrasound decreases both the rate of failed cannulation and the incidence of complications.

Although the CVP is often used as a surrogate for intravascular volume, an isolated CVP value, except when extremely high or low, is a poor indicator of volume status. CVP is affected by patient positioning, positive-pressure ventilation, TV integrity, RV dysfunction and pulmonary and pericardial disease. Consequently, trends in CVP provide a better guide.

Analysis of the RAP or CVP waveform reveals three systolic components (c-wave, x-descent, v-wave), and two diastolic components (y-descent, a-wave) (Figure 23.3). The a-wave represents atrial contraction, and the c wave closure of the TV at the beginning of systole. During the ensuing x-descent, rapid atrial

filling begins as the ventricle contracts and ejects, resulting in the v-wave at the end of systole. As the TV opens during diastole, CVP falls as blood rapidly flows into the RV during the y-descent. Blood flow from the vena cavae into the RA is maximal during the x and y pressure descents.

Several diagnostic clues to cardiac rhythm abnormalities can be gleaned from careful observation of the CVP waveform. In AF, absence of synchronized atrial contraction eliminates the a-wave. Atrial flutter may produce saw-tooth waves on the pressure tracing, known as f-waves. Junctional rhythm, complete heart block and ventricular tachycardia are all forms of atrioventricular (A-V) dissociation in which cannon a-waves may be evident. These result from atrial contraction against a closed TV during ventricular systole. Loss of A-V synchrony often causes sudden hypotension from a reduction in cardiac filling and CO.

Normal CVP (RAP) ranges between 0 and 8 mmHg. A number of pathological conditions can increase the CVP and alter the waveform. If TR is present, an elevated mean RAP is caused by a tall regurgitant *cv*-wave. A prominent *a*-wave combined with systemic hypotension may suggest RV diastolic dysfunction secondary to ischemia. CVP may approximate the PA wedge (occlusion) pressure (PAWP) in cardiac tamponade, with diastolic right and left heart pressure equalization being a characteristic hemodynamic finding.

Pulmonary artery catheterization

The pulmonary artery flotation catheter (PAFC) has been used to manage cardiac and critically ill patients since the 1970s. To date, however, no randomized trial or meta-analysis has been able to definitively demonstrate improved patient outcome. Some studies even suggest that PAFC use increases complications, length of stay and hospital costs. The PAFC allows direct measurement of RA, PA and PA wedge pressures. Additionally, mixed-venous oxygen saturation and RV cardiac output can be measured.

Complications of PAFC use include catheter knotting, pulmonary infarction and PA rupture as well as those associated with central venous cannulation (see above). Although rare (reported incidence 0.1–1%), PA rupture carries a mortality approaching 50%. To reduce the risk of this complication, the PAFC should never be left in the wedged position, nor should the balloon remain inflated for prolonged periods of time, as this may cause pulmonary ischemia and infarction. Any attempt to inflate the balloon while the catheter is "wedged" can result in PA rupture. In addition, the PAFC should be withdrawn a few centimeters following PAWP measurement, because the catheter may subsequently migrate distally. Likewise, the balloon must always be deflated when withdrawing the catheter to minimize risk of damaging the PV and TV.

PAFC placement is achieved by "flotation" through the right heart chambers, facilitated by a small (1.5 ml) balloon located at the catheter tip. The right IJV is the preferred site for PAFC insertion because it offers a direct route to the RV. From this site, the RAP tracing is typically acquired at a depth of 20–25 cm, the RV at a depth of 25–35 cm, and the PA at a depth of 35–45 cm. The PAWP is usually acquired at a depth of 50–60 cm. By keeping these

average distances in mind when advancing the catheter, one may reduce the risk of catheter knotting or kinking the catheter inside the heart. Alternative access sites for PAFC insertion include the subclavian and femoral veins, although successful placement can be more challenging. Maneuvers that aid PAC placement include head-down tilt (RA → RV), head-up and right lateral tilt (RV → PA) and transiently increasing CO (e.g. bolus ephedrine 10 mg IV).

Observation of the pressure waveforms (Figure 23.4) is essential to ensure correct PAFC placement. After wedging the PAFC in a distal PA, a *static* column of blood connects the catheter tip and LV during diastole (Figure 23.5). This is the physiological basis for using PAWP as an estimate of LVEDP. PAWP is also an indirect measure of LA pressure. It should be borne in mind that the LA pressure waveform will be delayed and damped by transmission through the pulmonary vasculature. The PAWP waveform closely resembles that of the RA, although it is delayed in relation to the ECG tracing.

The PAFC tip has a thermistor that allows CO measurement using the thermodilution technique. A fixed volume (usually 10 ml saline at room temperature) is injected into the RA, and temperature changes are recorded by the thermistor at the PAFC tip. The area under the temperature-time curve is inversely proportional to CO, which is calculated using the Stewart-Hamilton equation. Although the equation (Figure 23.6) appears complex, CO can simply be considered as the quotient of *thermal input energy* and the *area under the PA temperature curve*.

Knowledge of CO, CVP and MAP allows calculation of the systemic vascular resistance (SVR):

$$SVR = \frac{MAP - CVP}{CO}$$

Multiplying by 80 converts traditional Wood units to dynes s cm^{-5}.

Data derived from the PAFC may also help diagnose causes of shock (Table 23.1) and distinguish RV failure from LV failure. In both cases, the CO will be low and SVR high. In LV failure, filling pressures (i.e. RAP, PAWP) are elevated. By contrast, in RV failure, RAP is high, but PAWP low.

Dynamic markers of volume status

Dynamic markers appear to be much better at predicting which patients will respond to fluid therapy. During negative-pressure (spontaneous) ventilation,

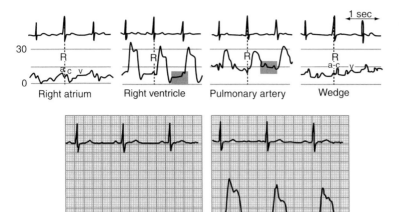

Figure 23.4 Characteristic pressure waveforms observed during PAFC insertion. Note the "diastolic step-up" between the RV and PA. The RV waveform lacks a dicrotic notch, and pressure *increases* steadily during diastole. In contrast, the PA waveform has a notch and the pressure *decreases* during diastole.

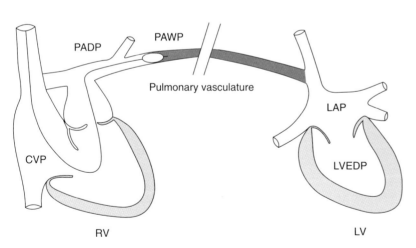

Figure 23.5 Estimating cardiac filling with the PAFC. The schematic shows the PAFC wedging in a proximal PA to measure indirectly downstream left heart filling pressures. The PA diastolic pressure provides an estimate of LA pressure and LV filling pressure (LVEDP), as pressure in the PA at the end of diastole usually equilibrates with downstream pressure in the LA. In critically ill patients, when the right and left ventricles may have different diastolic pressure–volume curves, the PA diastolic pressure offers a more accurate estimate of LV preload than the CVP. PAWP is measured closest to the LA, and therefore is subject to the least interference and error. Whenever "upstream" pressures are used to estimate LV filling, confounding factors may invalidate the estimate. Although LV compliance, HR, MV disease, PVR and alveolar pressure are key factors, RV compliance and TV and PV disease may also play a role. PAWP overestimates LVEDP when alveolar pressure exceeds intravascular pressure, in MS, in pulmonary hypertension and in the presence of tachycardia. In AR LV filling is underestimated, because all PAFC measurements are isolated from the continued retrograde inflow into the LV following MV closure.

Table 23.1 Hemodynamic parameters aid in determining the etiology of shock. Distributive shock, as in sepsis, neurogenic causes or anaphylaxis, is distinguished by an inappropriately low SVR

Shock	RAP	CO	SVR
Cardiogenic	High	Low	High
Hypovolemic	Low	Low	High
Distributive	Low	High	Low

$$Q = \frac{V_i \cdot (T_b - T_i)}{\int_0^\infty \Delta T_b(t) \cdot dt} \times \frac{S_i \cdot C_i}{S_b \cdot C_b} \times k$$

Figure 23.6 The Stewart-Hamilton equation. Q, cardiac output; V_i, injectate volume (ml); T_b, blood temperature; T_i, injectate temperature; S_i, injectate specific gravity (kg l^{-1}); S_b, blood specific gravity; C_i, injectate specific heat capacity (J kg^{-1} °C^{-1}); C_b, blood specific heat capacity; and the integral function that of blood temperature versus time (°C min).

Pulse Pressure Variation (PPV)

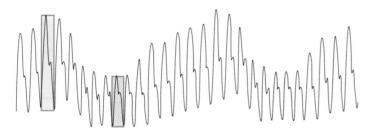

Figure 23.7 Pulse pressure variation (PPV) with positive-pressure mechanical ventilation. PPV >13% effectively identifies patients who will respond to volume administration with an increase in SV, CO and MAP.

$PP_{Max} = 150 - 70 = 80$

$PP_{Min} = 120 - 60 = 60$

$PPV = (PP_{Max} - PP_{Min})/([PP_{Max} + PP_{Min}]/2)$

$PPV = 80-60/([80+60]/2) = 29\%$

decreases in intrathoracic pressure may cause variation in CVP. A fall in CVP >1 mmHg during inspiration has been shown to predict response to volume. During positive-pressure (mechanical) ventilation, however, increases in intrathoracic pressure cause variation in both systolic and pulse pressures. Variations of greater than 10–15% have been shown to predict response to volume administration.

Key points

- The pressure waveforms *and* ECG should be continuously displayed to validate absolute values and examine the timing of cardiac events.
- Respiratory variation in CVP and arterial pulse pressure may be used to determine fluid responsiveness.
- During diastole, RV pressure increases and PA pressure decreases.

- If used during cardiac surgery, the PAFC should be withdrawn 5–10 cm prior to the onset of CPB to reduce the risk of catheter migration, pulmonary infarction and pulmonary artery rupture.

Further reading

Gelman S. Venous function and central venous pressure: A physiologic story. *Anesthesiology* 2008; **108**(*4*): 735–48.

Michard F, Boussat S, Chemla D, *et al.* Relation between respiratory changes in arterial pulse pressure and fluid responsiveness in septic patients with acute circulatory failure. *Am J Respir Crit Care Med* 2000; **162**(*1*): 134–8.

Michard F, Teboul J. Predicting fluid responsiveness in ICU patients: a critical analysis of the evidence. *Chest* 2002; **121**(*6*): 2000–8.

Schroeder RA, Barbeito A, Bar-Yosef S, Mark JB. Cardiovascular Monitoring. In: Miller RD (Ed.), *Miller's Anesthesia*, 7th edition. Philadelphia: Churchill Livingstone Elsevier; 2010.

Transesophageal echocardiography

Roger M. O. Hall

The growth in use of perioperative TEE over the last decade has been such that TEE is now considered to be a core component of modern cardiac anesthesia and intensive care. Its value as a monitor is complementary to traditional invasive pressure measurement and in some aspects is superior to them. This chapter will cover the physics of ultrasound, the principles of Doppler ultrasound, imaging modes, the format of a basic TEE examination and indications for TEE. The perioperative assessment of cardiac function using TEE is discussed in the next chapter.

Ultrasound physics

Ultrasound is sound whose frequency is above the audible range. Humans can hear sound with a frequency that is between 20 and 20 000 Hz, hence ultrasound is any sound with a frequency of greater than 20 kHz. Medically useful ultrasound, however, is usually in the range 1 to 10 MHz.

The "wave like" properties of ultrasound can be described in terms of frequency, wavelength, velocity and amplitude. Ultrasound causes alternating rarification and compression in tissues that are propagated through the tissue at the speed of sound for that tissue (Table 24.1).

The ultrasound wavelength in blood is 0.3 mm for a 5 MHz probe and 0.6 mm for a 2.5 MHz probe. The two-point discrimination (spatial resolution) of ultrasound is dependent upon wavelength, as the minimum distance that can be resolved between two objects is one wavelength.

A 1 MHz probe will be unable to distinguish between two structures less than 1.5 mm apart, whereas a 5 MHz probe can resolve structures 0.3 mm apart. Thus, as ultrasound wavelength shortens, image detail (resolution) increases (Figure 24.1).

Table 24.1 Sound velocity in lung, blood and bone

Tissue	Sound velocity (m s^{-1})
Lung (air)	300
Blood	1540
Bone	4000

Velocity (C) = Frequency (f) $\times$ Wavelength (λ)

As with radio waves – where short-wave (VHF) broadcasts have a smaller range than long-wave – ultrasound tissue penetration decreases as frequency increases. In clinical practice the maximum tissue penetration (attenuation) depth is equivalent to 200 wavelengths. The practical implication is that TEE is better at imaging structures that are closely related to the esophagus such as the LA and MV. Although anterior structures, such as the LV apex, are poorly imaged from the esophagus, they are accessible with transthoracic echocardiography.

Modern medical ultrasound equipment employs a series of piezo-electric crystals to alternately emit and receive ultrasound waves. A small number (~1%) of emitted waves are reflected back at interfaces between tissues of varying acoustic density. Given that ultrasound travels 1 cm in 13 μs, knowledge of the time interval between emission and reception allows the distance to the reflective interface can be calculated. Ultrasound waves reflected from interfaces at varying depths will be received at different times, which can be displayed as points a line. The strength (amplitude) of the reflected wave is represented by the size of the point. This is the basis of B mode echo.

Current imaging techniques are based on B mode imaging. In M mode a single B mode "line" is

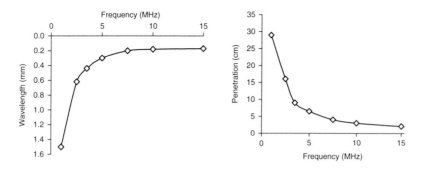

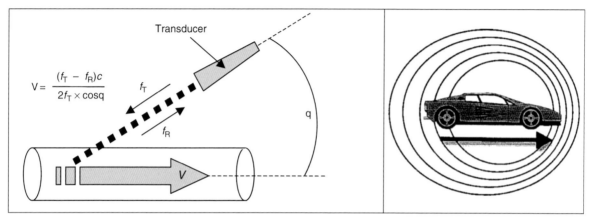

Figure 24.1 The inverse relationship between frequency and wavelength (spatial resolution) (left), and frequency and tissue penetration (right).

Figure 24.2 The Doppler principle. (Left) The mathematical relationship between blood flow velocity, change in frequency of reflected ultrasound, and angle between blood flow and ultrasound vectors. V, blood flow velocity; f_T, frequency of transmitted ultrasound; f_R, frequency of reflected ultrasound; θ, angle between blood flow and ultrasound beam. (Right) In the direction of motion the sequence of sound waves will be compressed, resulting in a higher sound frequency heard as the car approaches an observer and lower sound frequency as the car moves away. Reproduced with permission from Erb J. Basic principles of physics in echocardiographic imaging and Doppler techniques. In: Feneck R, Kneeshaw J, Ranucci M (Eds) *Core Topics in Transoesophageal Echocardiography*. Cambridge: Cambridge University Press; 2010.

sampled at a very high frequency (1000 s^{-1}) and the information is then displayed with depth information on the y-axis and time on the x-axis. Whilst this still only looks at one discrete anatomical line, motion of the region examined can be seen.

The classic echo display is 2D echo, which displays anatomic information in near real time with an easily understood two-dimensional format. This sector scan is actually made up of multiple B mode lines. Because the equipment is bound to the speed of sound, the speed at which the image can be updated (the *frame rate*) is inversely proportional to the scan depth and angle.

Factors increasing strength of returning signal are greater transmitted amplitude and an angle of incidence ~90°.

Modern TEE probes resemble a flexible gastroscope and contain arrays of piezo-electric crystals that can emit ultrasound at varying frequencies.

Doppler ultrasound

When sound waves are reflected from a moving target the wavelength of the reflected sound is altered in proportion to the velocity of the target. The resulting change in frequency, first described by Doppler and known as the *Doppler shift*, forms the basis of the vehicle "speed traps". The same principle can be employed by using ultrasound to measure the velocity of blood within the heart.

When the direction of blood flow is not parallel to the ultrasound beam, the velocity will be underestimated by a factor equal to the cosine of the incident angle. (Figure 24.2) In clinical practice an angle <20° (where the cosine = 0.94) produces acceptably accurate measurements.

Information about blood flow velocity obtained using Doppler ultrasound can be displayed in a number of ways. In *pulse wave Doppler* (PWD), the

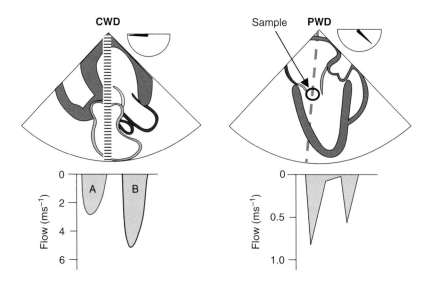

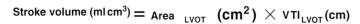

Figure 24.3 Measurement of blood flow velocity. (Left) Continuous-wave Doppler is used to measure high velocity flow across the AV in aortic stenosis. A, mild (peak gradient; 36 mmHg). B, severe (peak gradient; 100 mmHg). (Right) Pulsed-wave Doppler is used to measure diastolic transmitral blood flow velocity at the MV leaflet coaptation point. Note that PWD measures much lower velocities than the CWD.

Stroke volume (ml cm^3) = Area $_{LVOT}$ (cm^2) $\times$ VTI$_{LVOT}$ (cm)

Figure 24.4 Calculation of stroke volume and cardiac output using the velocity time integral. The clear center of the PWD pattern indicates laminar LVOT flow. If heart rate = 80 bpm, cardiac output = stroke volume (3.14 × 20) × 80 ≈ 5000 ml min^{-1}.

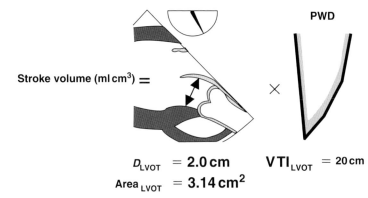

Stroke volume (ml cm^3) =

D_{LVOT} = 2.0 cm VTI$_{LVOT}$ = 20 cm

Area $_{LVOT}$ = 3.14 cm^2

velocity of blood flow is measured at a precise distance from the ultrasound probe. In *continuous wave Doppler* (CWD), the velocities of blood flow are measured at all points along the ultrasound beam without localization. In *color flow Doppler*, PWD is used to construct a map of blood flow velocities that is superimposed on the corresponding 2D image.

Once velocity is known it is then possible to estimate pressure gradients using a simplified form of the Bernoulli equation that describes the relationship between instantaneous pressure gradient and velocity.

$$\text{Pressure gradient} \approx 4 \times \text{Velocity}^2$$

A pressure gradient can be estimated in any part of the heart where a velocity can be measured. For example; if peak AV flow (using CWD) is 5 m s^{-1}

(Figure 24.3) then the estimated peak instantaneous pressure gradient is 100 mmHg (i.e. 4×5^2). This information can be combined with a pressure measurement to estimate the pressure in a second site. RV systolic pressure can be estimated from peak TV regurgitant velocity and RA pressure.

$$\text{Peak RV systolic pressure} = 4 \times (V_{TR})^2 + \text{RAP}$$

Flow can be measured in the great vessels to estimate cardiac output or across a regurgitant valve to assess the severity of the valve pathology. Stroke volume can be estimated by multiplying the distance blood travels in a cardiac cycle (*stroke distance*) by the cross-sectional area of the vessel at the *same* point.

As distance is the integral of velocity, the stroke distance can be obtained by integrating the velocity

149

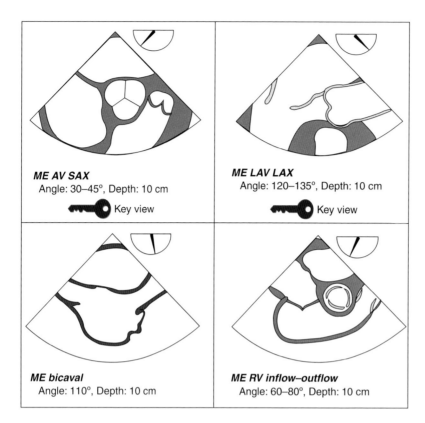

ME AV SAX
Angle: 30–45°, Depth: 10 cm
Key view

ME LAV LAX
Angle: 120–135°, Depth: 10 cm
Key view

ME bicaval
Angle: 110°, Depth: 10 cm

ME RV inflow–outflow
Angle: 60–80°, Depth: 10 cm

Figure 24.5 ME views at AV level.
(a) SAX: angle 30–45°; depth 10 cm.
(b) LAX: angle 120–135°; depth 10 cm.
(c) Bicaval: angle 110°; depth 10 cm.
(d) RV inflow-outflow: angle 60–80°;
depth 12 cm.

profile with respect to time. The result is known as the *velocity time integral* (VTI). (Figure 24.4)

Basic examination

A complete TEE examination requires some 20 views and includes the heart, the great vessels and the descending aorta. In practice, however, a satisfactory examination of the heart can be achieved rapidly using only 12 views – four each at the mid-esophageal AV level (Figure 24.5), mid-esophageal MV level (Figure 24.6) and transgastric level (Figure 24.7).

For teaching purposes at Papworth, we have found that trainees grasp the principles of TEE more quickly if the examination is initially limited to just six "key" views using the mid-esophageal short axis (30°) view of the AV – the so-called "*Mercedes Benz*" view – as a starting point. Once this very basic approach has been mastered, the examination is quickly expanded to 12 views. Only when the trainee has demonstrated competence at this level is the examination expanded to all 20 views. It is essential that the TEE examination be performed in a systematic manner; regardless of the order in which the standard views are obtained.

Although a complete TEE examination should include the confirmation and quantification of known pathological conditions, it is important not to miss undiagnosed lesions. Furthermore, the physiological impact of general anesthesia should be taken into account when estimating the severity of valvular lesions. Unexpected findings must be reported to the surgical team as they may significantly influence the conduct of the operation.

Limitations of TEE

The principal limitation of TEE is that it cannot be used to detect myocardial ischemia during the critical periods of induction of anesthesia, laryngoscopy, and tracheal intubation and extubation. The utility of TEE is also reduced by imaging artifacts and pitfalls. Two-dimensional TEE artifacts include acoustic shadowing, reverberations and side lobes. Doppler imaging artifacts include those caused by inappropriate intercept angle, aliasing and radiofrequency interference.

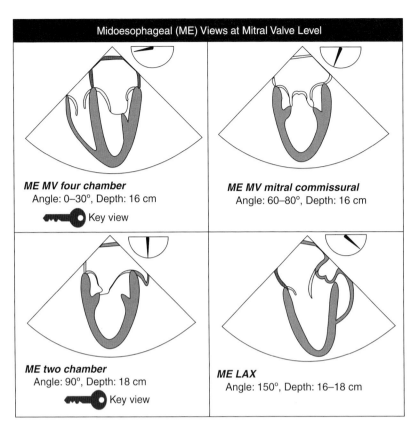

Figure 24.6 ME views at ME level.
(a) Four chamber: angle 0–30°; depth 16 cm.
(b) Mitral commissural: angle 60–80°; depth 16 cm.
(c) Two chamber: angle 90°; depth 18 cm.
(d) Long axis: angle 150°; depth 16–18 cm.

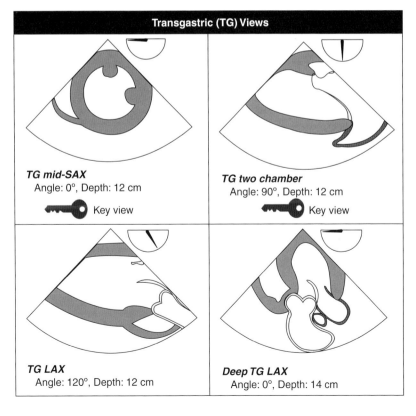

Figure 24.7 Transgastric views.
(a) Mid-SAX: angle 0°; depth 12 cm.
(b) Two chamber: angle 90°; depth 12 cm.
(c) LAX: angle 120°; depth 12 cm.
(d) Deep TG LAX: angle 0°; depth 14 cm.

Table 24.2 The impact of perioperative TEE on clinical decision-making

Undiagnosed ASD/PFO

Undiagnosed valvular pathology in coronary patients

Undiagnosed "second valve" pathology in valve patients

New regional wall motion abnormalities following revascularization

Assessment of adequacy of reparative surgical procedures

Congenital cardiac disease

ASD, atrial septal defect; PFO, patent foramen ovale.

Table 24.3 ASE/SCA 1996 Classification of indications for the use of perioperative TEE

Category	Examples
I	Evaluation of life-threatening instability in theater or the ICU that are not resolved using standard therapies Valve repair surgery Repair of congenital cardiac lesions Assessment of unstable aortic dissection or aortic aneurysms Surgery for HOCM and endocarditis
II	Assessment of prosthetic valve replacement Checking adequacy of de-airing Perioperative use for patients at increased risk of myocardial ischemia or hemodynamic instability
III	Intraoperative monitoring for emboli during orthopedic surgery Monitoring for placement of PACs, balloon pumps or defibrillators

Definition of categories: I – supported by the strongest evidence or expert opinion. TEE is frequently useful in improving clinical outcomes; II – supported by weaker evidence or opinion, evidence suggests it may be useful clinically; III – little current scientific or expert support, infrequently useful.
ASE, American Society of Echocardiography; SCA, Society of Cardiovascular Anesthesiologists; PAC, pulmonary artery catheter.

Indications

The putative benefits of perioperative TEE are largely based on consensus or "expert" opinion, rather than prospective, randomized controlled trials. Although the evidence that TEE improves outcome is weak, there is accumulating evidence that TEE alters cardiac surgical management.

Table 24.4 ASA/SCA 2010 indications for the use of perioperative TEE

Cardiac and thoracic aortic procedures

- Cardiac and thoracic aortic surgery
  For adult patients without contraindications, TEE should be used in all open heart (e.g. valvular procedures) and thoracic aortic surgical procedures and should *be considered in CABG surgeries* as well
  – to confirm and refine the preoperative diagnosis
  – to detect new or unsuspected pathology
  – to adjust the anesthetic and surgical plan accordingly, and
  – to assess the results of the surgical intervention
  In small children, the use of TEE should be considered on a case-by-case basis because of risks unique to these patients (e.g. bronchial obstruction)
- Catheter-based intracardiac procedures
  For patients undergoing transcatheter intracardiac procedures, TEE may be used.

Noncardiac surgery

- TEE may be used when the nature of the planned surgery or the patient's known or suspected cardiovascular pathology might result in severe hemodynamic, pulmonary or neurologic compromise
- If equipment and expertise are available, TEE should be used when unexplained life-threatening circulatory instability persists despite corrective therapy

Critical care

- For critical care patients, TEE should be used when diagnostic information that is expected to alter management cannot be obtained by transthoracic echocardiography or other modalities in a timely manner

ASA, American Society of Anesthesiologists; SCA, Society of Cardiovascular Anesthesiologists.

Recently published, the new North American practice guidelines for the use of perioperative TEE make a number of important changes to the previous (1996) guidelines. The key change is that "for adult patients without contraindications, TEE should be used in all open heart (e.g. valvular procedures) and thoracic aortic surgical procedures and should be considered in CABG surgeries as well" (Table 24.4). In some countries widening the indications to include routine AVR and CABG with preserved LV function has significant resource implications. Inclusion of this latter indication is particularly controversial.

Contraindications

The 2010 ASA/SCA guidelines suggest that TEE may be used for patients with oral, esophageal or gastric disease, if the expected benefit outweighs the potential risk, provided the appropriate precautions are applied. These precautions may include: considering other imaging modalities (e.g. epicardial echocardiography), obtaining a gastroenterology consultation, using a smaller probe, limiting the examination, avoiding unnecessary probe manipulation and using the most experienced operator.

Practice standards

The use of TEE is not without risk and may be contraindicated in the presence of esophageal pathology. Because the inexperienced echocardiographer may inappropriately interpolate suboptimal or missing information, the most common complication is misdiagnosis. Frequent sources of error include artifacts (e.g. side lobe and reverberation) that mimic intracardiac structures.

Key points

- Knowledge of the basic physical principles underlying medical ultrasound is essential for the effective use of perioperative TEE.

- Every TEE examination should be comprehensive, recorded for later inspection and formally interpreted in a report.
- Considerable time is required to develop competency in perioperative TEE.
- There are few contraindications to the use of TEE. Physical complications are rare but may be lethal.

Further reading

Feneck RO, Kneeshaw J, Ranucci M (Eds.). *Core Topics in Transesophageal Echocardiography*. Cambridge: Cambridge University Press; 2010.

Practice guidelines for perioperative TEE. A report by the ASA and SCA Task Force on TEE. *Anesthesiology* 1996; **84**: 986–1006.

Shanewise JS, Cheung AT, Aronson S, *et al.* ASE/SCA Guidelines for performing a comprehensive intraoperative multiplane TEE examination: recommendations of the ASE Council for Intraoperative Echocardiography and the SCA Task Force for Certification in Perioperative TEE. *Anesth Analg* 1999; **89**: 870–84.

Thys DM, Abel MD, Brooker RF, *et al.* Practice guidelines for perioperative transesophageal echocardiography. An updated report by the American Society of Anesthesiologists and the Society of Cardiovascular Anesthesiologists Task Force on Transesophageal Echocardiography. *Anesthesiology* 2010; **112**(5): 1–13.

Intraoperative assessment of ventricular function

Yeewei W. Teo and Andrew Roscoe

The assessment of LV and RV function is important for the intraoperative hemodynamic management. Because measurement of CO has long been used as a measure of ventricular function, the PAFC, which uses thermodilution to measure CO, has been considered the "gold standard". There are, however, significant risks associated with PAFC use, and PAWP is recognized as being a poor indicator of preload in patients with LV diastolic dysfunction. Less invasive technologies include esophageal Doppler (EDM), pulse contour analysis (PCA) and TEE. The EDM measures blood flow velocity in the descending thoracic aorta. CO is calculated by multiplying the integral of velocity with respect to time (i.e. VTI; the stroke distance), the estimated aortic cross-sectional area and HR. Errors in estimating the aortic radius are squared when calculating CO, magnifying any inaccuracy. A 10% error in radius will result in a 21% error in SV. Some studies have shown reasonable agreement with the PAC in hemodynamically stable patients. PCA devices are based on the principle that the systolic component of the arterial pressure waveform is proportional to SV. Limitations occur with rapid changes in vascular tone, dysrrhythmias and the use of the intra-aortic balloon pump. TEE is now established as the "gold standard" intraoperative cardiac monitor.

Left ventricle

Global systolic function

TEE allows direct visualization of cardiac performance. The standard transgastric (TG), mid-papillary short axis (SAX) view (Figure 25.1) is commonly "eyeballed" by the experienced sonographer to provide an estimate of preload and contractility.

Quantitative indices of global LV function include:

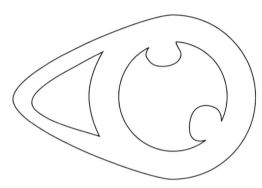

Figure 25.1 Transgastric mid-papillary short-axis view of the left ventricle.

(a)

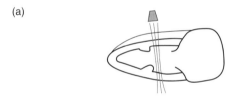

(b)

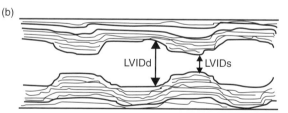

Figure 25.2 (a) Transgastric long-axis view of the LV with an M-mode beam passing just above the papillary muscles. (b) M-mode image of LV motion, showing internal diameter (LVID) in diastole and systole, used to calculate the fractional shortening.

Fractional shortening (FS): classically M mode is used in the TG long axis view (LAX) of LV (Figure 25.2). The internal diameter (ID) of the LV is measured in systole (s) and diastole (d), and the FS calculated. A normal value for FS is 25–42%.

Core Topics in Cardiac Anesthesia, Second Edition, ed. Jonathan H. Mackay and Joseph E. Arrowsmith. Published by Cambridge University Press. © Cambridge University Press 2012.

(a)

(b)

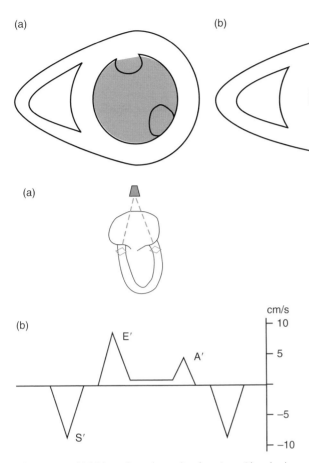

(a)

(b)

E′

A′

S′

cm/s
10
5
−5
−10

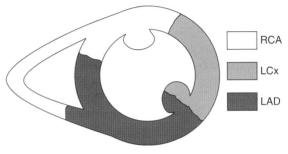

RCA
LCx
LAD

$$FS = [(LVIDd - LVIDs)/LVIDd] \times 100$$

An ejection fraction is predicted from this calculation using the Teichholz formula ($V = [7.0/2.4 + D] \times D^3$, where V is the volume and D is the echocardiographically measured internal dimension).

Fractional area change (FAC): using the TG mid-SAX view, the internal area (A) of the LV is traced in end-systole (ES) and end-diastole (ED) (Figure 25.3), and the FAC is calculated. A normal value for FAC is 50–65%.

$$FAC = [(LVEDA - LVESA)/LVEDA] \times 100$$

Stroke volume (SV): volumes can be calculated by measuring areas in two perpendicular planes (typically mid-esophageal 4-chamber and 2-chamber views) and then using Simpson's method (sum of a series of discs) to determine LV end-systolic and end-diastolic volumes:

$$SV = LVEDV - LVESV$$

SV may also be calculated by measuring the LV outflow tract (LVOT) diameter and by tracing the LVOT VTI in systole. The cardiac output is then determined by multiplying SV by HR

$$SV = VTI_{LVOT} \times AREA_{LVOT}$$

Ejection fraction (EF): This can be calculated from SV and LVEDV. The normal range for EF is 50–70%.

$$EF = (SV/LVEDV) \times 100$$

Pulsed-wave (PW) tissue Doppler imaging (TDI) of the basal myocardium can provide a quick method to estimate LV contractile function (Figure 25.4). An S' value greater than 8 cm s^{-1} is associated with an ejection fraction above 50%.

Regional systolic function

Following coronary artery occlusion systolic wall thickening and endocardial inward motion are reduced within five cardiac cycles. These signs precede ECG changes and increases in PAWP, making TEE a more sensitive indicator of myocardial ischemia. The regional wall motion abnormality (RWMA) is determined by the coronary artery involved. The

Table 25.1 Classification and scoring of regional wall motion abnormalities (RWMAs)

Class	Score	Myocardial thickening	Wall excursion
Normal	1	> 50%	Inward > 30%
Hypokinesia	2	10–50%	Inward 0–30%
Akinesia	3	< 10%	None
Dyskinesia	4	None/thinning	Outward
Aneurysmal	5	Thinning/aneurysmal	None/outward

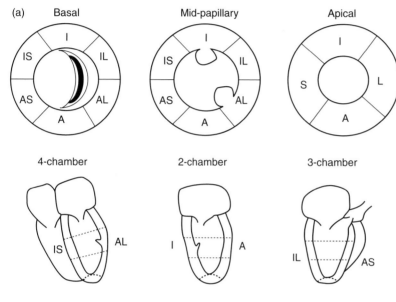

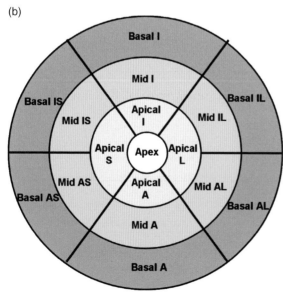

Figure 25.6 The LV segments: (a) mid-esophageal and TG views at basal, mid-papillary and apical levels, with anterior (A), antero-septal (AS), infero-septal (IS), inferior (I), infero-lateral (IL) and antero-lateral (AL) walls. (b) Seventeen-segment model.

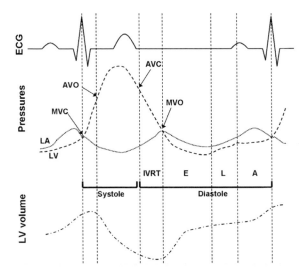

Figure 25.7 The four phases of ventricular diastole: isovolumic relaxation time (IVRT), early rapid filling (E), late filling (L) and atrial contraction (A). The pressure curves of the LA and LV show the timing of the opening (O) and closing (C) of the AV and MV.

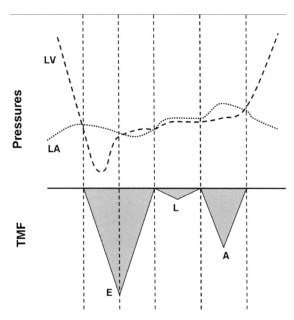

Figure 25.8 A normal transmitral flow pattern, consisting of early (E), late (L) and atrial contraction (A) waves.

TG mid-SAX view displays myocardium supplied by all three major coronary arteries (Figure 25.5).

For the purposes of RWMA evaluation, the LV myocardium is now divided into a 17-segment model. At basal and mid-papillary levels there are six segments; at the apical level there are four segments; the 17th segment is the true apex of the LV (Figure 25.6) – rarely visualized with TEE. Each segment is scored according to degree of dysfunction (Table 25.1). The sum for all the segments is divided by the number of segments visualized to produce a *wall motion index score*.

Diastolic function

Normal diastolic function allows for adequate LV filling with low LVEDP. Diastole extends from AV closure to MV closure. The phases of diastole include isovolumic relaxation time (IVRT), early rapid filling, late filling (diastasis) and atrial systole (Figure 25.7).

Indices of myocardial relaxation include:

Isovolumic relaxation time (IVRT): the initiation of myocardial relaxation occurs at the time of peak systolic pressure. When the pressure in the aorta exceeds that in the LV the AV closes and IVRT starts. When LV pressure falls below LA pressure the MV opens and IVRT ends. A normal IVRT is 70–90 ms. Impaired relaxation leads to an increase in IVRT >90 ms. With restrictive pathophysiology the IVRT decreases below 70 ms.

Transmitral flow (TMF): placing a PW Doppler sampling window at the tips of the MV leaflets as they open into the LV gives a typical TMF pattern. TMF starts as the MV opens and comprises three phases (Figure 25.8): rapid early filling (E wave), late filling (L wave) and atrial systole (A wave). LV filling is determined by the pressure gradient between the LA and LV when the MV opens, LV compliance, LV relaxation, atrial contraction and MV orifice area.

Diastolic dysfunction leads to changes in the ratio of the amplitude of the transmitral E and A waves (Figure 25.9). Initially E wave velocity decreases, but as dysfunction progresses, the E:A ratio reverts to that of a normal pattern (pseudo-normalization). When dysfunction becomes severe (restrictive pathology) the E wave velocity increases markedly.

Pulmonary venous flow (PVF): the use of PW Doppler in the left or right upper pulmonary veins gives a PVF pattern (Figure 25.10), consisting of two systolic waves (S_1 and S_2), a diastolic wave (D) and an atrial systole wave (A).

Diastolic dysfunction causes changes to the normal PVF pattern (Figure 25.11). As diastolic function worsens, the D wave initially decreases, then becomes greater than the S wave as restrictive pathophysiology predominates. The size and duration of the A wave increase as diastolic dysfunction progresses.

Normal function	Impaired relaxation	Pseudo-normal	Restrictive pathology

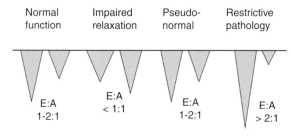

E:A 1-2:1   E:A < 1:1   E:A 1-2:1   E:A > 2:1

Figure 25.9 Changes in transmitral flow pattern with diastolic dysfunction.

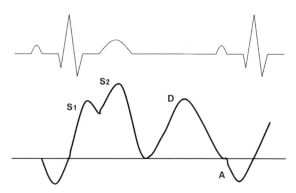

Figure 25.10 Normal pulmonary venous flow pattern. Systolic waves S_1 (atrial relaxation) and S_2 (mitral annular systolic excursion); diastolic wave (D) and atrial contraction (A) wave.

Tissue Doppler imaging (TDI): PW Doppler interrogation of the lateral mitral annulus reveals typical E' and A' waves. An E' wave less than 8 cm s^{-1} is associated with diastolic dysfunction.

Right ventricle

The RV is a complex structure – a triangular, crescent-shaped chamber containing muscle ridges (trabeculae carneae). This makes accurate measurement of volumes a difficult and time-consuming task in the intraoperative setting. Simpson's method can be used to determine RV volume, with the use of an ellipsoid or pyramidal model instead of a series of discs. Because RVEDV > LVEDV (50–100 ml m^{-2} versus 45–90 ml m^{-2}), normal RVEF is ∼10% less than the LVEF. RV stroke volume is dependent on preload and contractility and is very sensitive to changes in RV afterload. The mid-esophageal 4-chamber (Figure 25.12) and TG mid-SAX views are used to assess RV volume status and free-wall contractility.

Normal function	Impaired relaxation	Pseudo-normal	Restrictive pathology

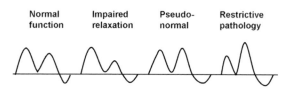

Figure 25.11 Changes in pulmonary venous flow pattern with diastolic dysfunction.

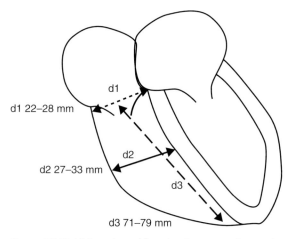

d1 22–28 mm

d2 27–33 mm

d3 71–79 mm

Figure 25.12 Mid-esophageal four-chamber view with normal values for RV dimensions.

RV hypertrophy is defined as RVED wall thickness >5 mm. RV systolic pressure can be estimated using continuous-wave Doppler interrogation of a TV regurgitation jet and applying the simplified Bernoulli equation ($P = 4V^2$).

Systolic function

RV systolic function may be assessed using:

Fractional area change (RVFAC): using the mid-esophageal 4-chamber view, RVEDA and RVESA are traced to give the RVFAC. A normal value is 30–60%.

Tricuspid annular plane systolic excursion (TAPSE): using M mode in the mid-esophageal 4-chamber view, the longitudinal motion of the lateral TV annulus is measured. A distance >15 mm indicates normal systolic function.

Tissue Doppler imaging (TDI): a systolic (S') wave velocity of the lateral TV annulus >12 cm s^{-1} is associated with normal RV contractility.

Diastolic function

Assessment of RV diastolic dysfunction is complex and still to be fully studied. It may be estimated by observing the RV filling pattern and hepatic vein flow profile.

Key points

- TEE provides a better estimate of preload than CVP or PCWP in ventricles with abnormal diastolic function.
- TEE is a sensitive indicator of myocardial ischemia.
- TEE allows direct visualization of LV and RV systolic and diastolic function.
- Although TEE can be used to measure CO, in practice the PAC is easier to use.

Further reading

Funk DJ, Moretti EW, Gan TJ. Minimally invasive cardiac output monitoring in the perioperative setting. *Anesth Analg* 2009; **108**(3): 887–97.

Haddad F, Couture P, Tousignant C, *et al.* The right ventricle in cardiac surgery, a perioperative perspective: I. Anatomy, physiology and assessment. *Anesth Analg* 2009; **108**(2): 407–21.

Lang RM, Bierig M, Devereux RB, *et al.* Recommendations for chamber quantification: a report from the American Society of Echocardiography Guidelines and Standards Committee and the Chamber Quantification Writing Group. *J Am Soc Echocardiogr* 2005; **18**(12): 1440–63.

Nagueh SF, Appleton CP, Gillebert TC, *et al.* Recommendations for the evaluation of left ventricular diastolic function by echocardiography. *J Am Soc Echocardiogr* 2009; **22**(2): 107–33.

Skubas N. Intraoperative Doppler tissue imaging is a valuable addition to cardiac anesthesiologists' armamentarium: a core review. *Anesth Analg* 2009; **108**(1): 48–66.

Weyman AE (Ed.). *Principles and Practice of Echocardiography*, 2nd edition. Philadelphia: Lea & Febiger; 1994.

Neurologic monitoring

Joseph E. Arrowsmith

Injury to the brain, spinal cord and peripheral nerves represents a significant cause of morbidity and disability after cardiac surgery. Although monitors of neurologic function have been available since the 1950s, their use remains uncommon and largely limited to enthusiasts and academic centers. The reason is undoubtedly the perception that neuromonitors are complex and costly devices that produce spurious results, and merely document neurologic injury – rather than allow prevention. Emerging evidence, however, suggests that modern neuromonitoring technologies – particularly when used together – can be used both to predict and to modify clinical outcome. Neurologic monitoring includes routine clinical observation, monitors of cerebral substrate (O_2, blood flow) and monitors of cerebral function (Table 26.1)

Clinical monitoring

The risk of neurologic injury is reduced by early detection of aortic cannula displacement and venous air entrainment, as well as the avoidance of hypoxia, hypoglycemia, acidosis, gross anemia, prolonged cerebral hypoperfusion and cerebral hyperthermia (Figure 26.1).

It should be borne in mind that cerebral perfusion pressure (CPP) is dependent upon MAP, intracranial pressure (ICP) and CVP. A marked elevation in CVP, even in the presence of a seemingly adequate MAP, may result in significant cerebral hypoperfusion. As continuous invasive hemodynamic monitoring is a mandatory component of cardiac anesthesia, the accuracy of the equipment used should be critically assessed at regular intervals.

Cerebral perfusion pressure $(\text{CPP}) = \text{MAP} - (\text{ICP} + \text{CVP})$

Table 26.1 Neurologic monitoring during cardiac surgery

Clinical	Arterial pressure
	Central venous pressure
	CPB pump flow rate
	Arterial oxygen saturation (SaO_2)
	Temperature
	Hemoglobin concentration
	Pupil size
	Arterial PCO_2
Substrate delivery	Transcranial Doppler (TCD) sonography
	Near infrared spectroscopy
	Jugular venous oxygen saturation
Cerebral activity	Electroencephalography (EEG)
	Somatosensory evoked potentials (SSEP)
	Auditory evoked potentials (AEP)
	Motor evoked potentials (MEP)
Other	Epiaortic ultrasound
	Transesophageal echocardiography

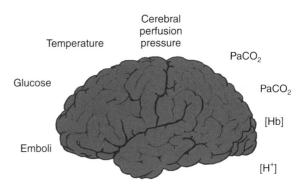

Figure 26.1 Factors affecting cerebral function during cardiac surgery. [Hb], hemoglobin concentration; [H⁺], hydrogen ion concentration.

Core Topics in Cardiac Anesthesia, Second Edition, ed. Jonathan H. Mackay and Joseph E. Arrowsmith. Published by Cambridge University Press. © Cambridge University Press 2012.

Table 26.2 Clinical applications of transcranial Doppler sonography

Detection of cerebral embolism during carotid endarterectomy and cardiac surgery

Detection of endoaortic balloon clamp migration during port access cardiac surgery

Diagnosis of circulatory arrest in raised ICP

Assessment of cerebral autoregulation

Assessment of CBFV in migraine

Detection and monitoring of post subarachnoid hemorrhage vasospasm

Hemodynamic assessment of vessels feeding arteriovenous malformations

Assessment of vertebrobasilar insufficiency

At temperatures >30°C cerebral autoregulation (flow-metabolism coupling) is essentially preserved so that cerebral blood flow (CBF) across a wide range of MAP is governed by $PaCO_2$. At $PaCO_2$ <23 mmHg (3.0 kPa) CBF may be reduced by more than half, leading to cerebral ischemia. Conversely, at $PaCO_2$ >68 mmHg (9 kPa) CBF may be more than doubled, resulting in the delivery of greater numbers of micro-emboli to the cerebral circulation. At lower temperatures, autoregulation is gradually lost and progressive cerebral "vasoparesis" renders CBF pressure-passive

Substrate delivery

Transcranial Doppler (TCD) sonography

Although the intact adult skull is impervious to the transmission of conventional ultrasound (5–10 MHz), insonation of the basal cerebral arteries is possible using low-frequency ultrasound (2 MHz) directed through regions of the skull where bone is thinnest (the temporal bones) or absent (the orbit and foramen magnum; Figure 26.2). Thus pulsed-wave TCD provides a non-invasive means of measuring cerebral artery blood flow velocity (CBFV) – an indirect measure of CBF (Figure 26.3).

CBFV can be calculated using the modified Doppler equation:

$$\text{CBFV} = \frac{c(F_S - F_T)}{2F_T \, \cos\theta}$$

where c = the speed of sound in human tissue ~1540 m s^{-1}, F_S = the frequency of reflected sound, F_T = the frequency of

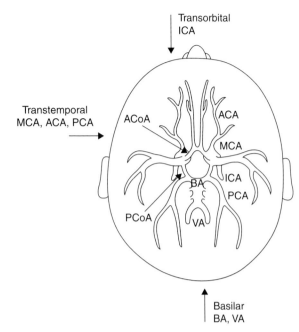

Figure 26.2 TCD ultrasound windows for examination of the basal cerebral arteries (the Circle of Willis) – submandibular approach not shown. ACA, anterior cerebral artery; ACoA, anterior communicating artery; MCA, middle cerebral artery; ICA, internal carotid artery; PCoA, posterior communicating artery; BA, basilar artery; PCA, posterior cerebral artery; VA, vertebral arteries.

transmitted sound – typically 2 MHz, and θ = the angle of incidence or insonation angle. In the absence of vasospasm or vessel stenosis, the pulsatility or Gosling Index is a reflection of cerebrovascular resistance.

$$\text{Gosling Index} = \frac{V_{SYS} - V_{DIAS}}{V_{MEAN}}$$

where V_{SYS} is systolic flow velocity, V_{DIAS} is diastolic flow velocity, and V_{MEAN} is weighted mean flow velocity.

Near infrared spectroscopy

Cerebral near infrared spectroscopy (NIRS) provides a non-invasive means of estimating regional cortical cerebral oxygenation. The physical principles underlying NIRS are summarized in Table 26.3.

Devices for clinical use typically employ self-adhesive sensors, applied to the skin on the sides of the forehead, away from the midline, and a remote processing and display unit. Between two and four wavelengths of infrared light are generated by photodiodes, and light emerging from the scalp is detected by optodes (Figure 26.4). NIRS algorithms typically assume that there is a fixed ratio of arterial:venous

Table 26.3 Physical principles underlying near infrared spectroscopy

Light in the visible spectrum (450–750 nm) penetrates biological tissues to a depth of only 10 mm, due to attenuation

By contrast, biological tissue is relatively translucent to infrared (650–1100 nm) radiation

Light traversing the brain is both scattered and absorbed

Absorption of light by colored substances ("chromophores") is concentration-dependent

Oxyhemoglobin (HbO_2) and deoxyhemoglobin (Hb) have different absorption spectra

The absorption of infrared light by HbO_2 and Hb is similar at 810 nm – the isobestic point

Hb has greater absorption at shorter wavelengths

HbO_2 has great absorption at longer wavelengths

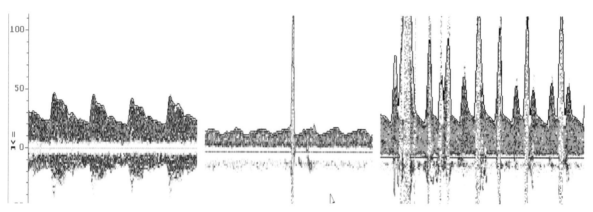

Figure 26.3 TCD examination of the MCA during CABG surgery; before (left), during (center), and immediately after (right) CPB. The high-amplitude signals (center and right) represent cerebral microemboli.

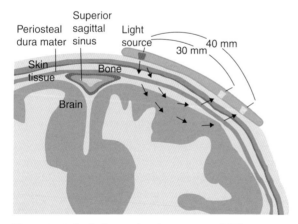

Figure 26.4 Cerebral near infrared spectroscopy (NIRS). (Courtesy of Somanetics Inc.)

blood (e.g. 1:3) in the sample volume; actual arterial: venous blood ratios are likely to be subject to both intra- and inter-individual variation. The use of more than one optode allows correction for the contribution made by blood in the scalp and skull, such that around 85% of the signal is from the brain. In contrast to conventional pulse oximetry, cerebral NIRS does not rely on the pulsatile component of the signal and can, therefore, be used during non-pulsatile CPB and deep hypothermic circulatory arrest (DHCA).

Cerebral NIRS has found a number of clinical applications in the setting of cardiac surgery: detection of cerebral ischemia; assessment of selective cerebral perfusion; and the prediction of perioperative neurologic injury, postoperative cognitive dysfunction, and duration of intensive care unit and hospital stay. In animal models, cerebral NIRS appears to provide a monitor of safe DHCA duration.

Jugular venous oximetry

Jugular venous oxygen saturation ($S_{JV}O_2$) is an invasive method of estimating the balance between global cerebral metabolism ($CMRO_2$) and cerebral oxygenation. The method is analogous to the use of mixed venous oximetry (S_VO_2) as a measure of whole body oxygen consumption and the adequacy of the systemic circulation.

$$CMRO_2 \approx CBF \times (S_aO_2 - S_{JV}O_2)$$

Using the Seldinger technique, a retrograde catheter is inserted into the internal jugular vein and advanced cephalad into the jugular bulb at the base of the skull. A lateral radiograph of the neck is required to confirm correct catheter placement. $S_{JV}O_2$ can be measured intermittently by drawing serial blood samples for blood gas analysis or continuously by using a fiberoptic catheter. The latter is prone to calibration drift. Normal values for $S_{JV}O_2$ are in the range 60–75%. Increased cerebral O_2 delivery or $\downarrow CMRO_2 \rightarrow$ $S_{JV}O_2$, whereas $\downarrow$ cerebral O_2 delivery or $CMRO_2 \rightarrow$ $S_{JV}O_2$.

In neurosurgical critical care, $S_{JV}O_2$ monitoring has been used to guide the management of raised ICP and cerebral hyperemia. In the setting of head injury $S_{JV}O_2$ <50% has been shown to be associated with a doubling of mortality.

In cardiac surgery, $S_{JV}O_2$ measurement may be particularly useful during CPB when systemic hypotension, cerebral hypoperfusion and anemia may have a significant impact on cerebral oxygenation. Excessive or rapid rewarming may produce cerebral hyperthermia and reduced $S_{JV}O_2$. The magnitude of

cerebral arterio-venous oxygen difference ($D_{AV}O_2$) during rewarming has been shown to correlate with cognitive dysfunction (Figure 26.6).

Cerebral function monitoring

Electroencephalography

The EEG is a representation of the spontaneous electrical activity of the cerebral cortex recorded through a series of scalp electrodes (Figure 26.7).

The potential differences (typically 20–200 μV) between pairs of electrodes or between each electrode and a common reference point are displayed continuously on up to 16 channels. The resulting output is

Table 26.4 Common causes of changes in cerebral oxygen delivery and consumption

	O₂ delivery	O₂ consumption
↑	Hypercapnia	Hyperthermia
	Hypertension	Pain
	Gross hypoxia	Light anesthesia
	Vasodilators (e.g. isoflurane)	Seizures
↓	Hypocapnia (<3.5 kPa)	Drugs
	Vasospasm	(e.g. thiopental)
	Hypotension	Stroke
	Low cardiac output	Coma
	Hypoxia	Hypothermia
	Anemia	Brainstem death

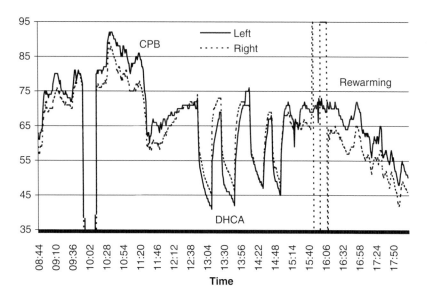

Figure 26.5 Near infrared spectroscopy monitoring during pulmonary thromboendarterectomy. Significant cerebral desaturation is seen at the onset of CPB, during four periods of hypothermic circulatory arrest (DHCA), and during rewarming.

163

Table 26.5 EEG waveforms

Waveform	Frequency (Hz)		Amplitude (μV)	Comments
Delta (δ)	1.5–3.5		>50	Normal during sleep and deep anesthesia, indication of neuronal dysfunction
Theta (θ)	3.6–7.5		20–50	Normal in children and elderly, normal adults during sleep, produced by hypothermia
Alpha (α)	7.6–12.5		20–50	Awake, relaxed, eyes open, mainly over occiput
Beta (β)	12.6–25		<20	Awake, alert, eyes open, mainly in parietal cortex, produced by barbiturates, benzodiazepines, phenytoin, alcohol
Gamma (γ)	25.1–50		<20	

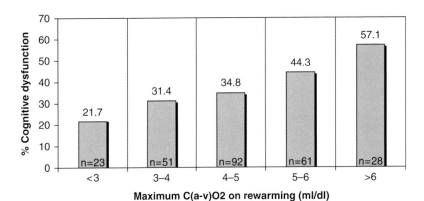

Figure 26.6 The frequency of cognitive dysfunction in relation to maximum cerebral arterial-venous oxygen content difference at normothermia in 96 patients with postoperative cognitive dysfunction. From Croughwell *et al. Ann Thorac Surg* 1994; 58(6): 1702–8. With permission.

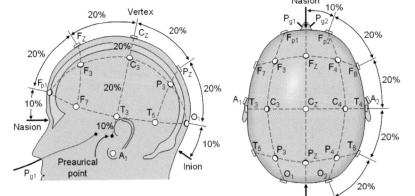

Figure 26.7 The internationally standardized 10–20 system of EEG electrode placement. F, frontal; Fp, frontal polar; C, central; O, occipital; P, parietal; T, temporal; A, ear lobe; Pg, nasopharyngeal. Right-sided placements are indicated by even numbers, left-sided placements by odd numbers and midline placements by Z. In addition, intermediate electrodes located at 10% positions may also be used. The location and nomenclature of these electrodes is standardized by the American Clinical Neurophysiology Society formerly the American Electroencephalographic Society. (Adapted with permission from Malmivuo J, Plonsey R. *Bioelectromagnetism – Principles and Applications of Bioelectric and Biomagnetic Fields*. New York: Oxford University Press; 1995.)

usually described in terms of location, amplitude and frequency. EEG frequency is conventionally grouped into one of four bands: δ, θ, α and β (Table 26.5). A normal awake adult has a posteriorly located, symmetrical EEG frequency of around 9 Hz (i.e. α rhythm).

Opioids and most anesthetic agents produce dose-dependent EEG slowing (↓ α and δ and θ) culminating

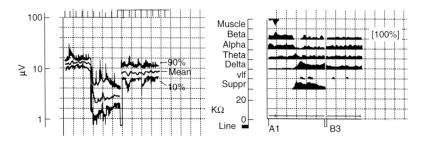

Figure 26.8 Typical CFAM tracing. The left trace displays the log-weighted-mean raw EEG amplitude distribution in μV, 10th and 90th centiles, and maximum and minimum amplitudes. The right trace displays; electromyography ("Muscle"), percentage α, β, θ, δ and very–low-frequency ("vlf" <1 Hz) activity, percentage of suppression ("Suppr.") < 1μV peak-to-peak, and electrode impedance in KΩ.

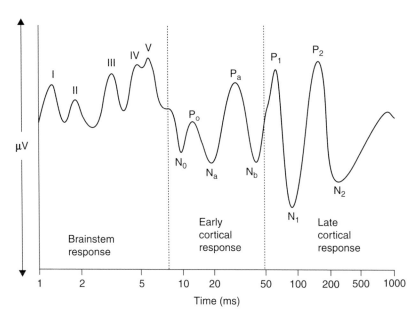

Figure 26.9 Auditory evoked potentials (AEPs). An auditory stimulus or "click" is repeated at regular intervals and signal averaging over several cycles is used to extract the AEP from background EEG activity. Short-latency (<10 ms) brainstem auditory evoked responses (BAERs) reflect neural activity between the cochlear nucleus (I) and the inferior colliculus (V). BAERs are unaffected by anesthesia but are temperature-sensitive, making them useful for monitoring the effects of cooling and rewarming. Mid-latency (10–100 ms) AEPs represent cortical processing – necessary for awareness and recall of auditory events. Analysis of early cortical AEPs forms the basis of "depth of anesthesia" monitors such as the bispectral index (BIS) monitor.

in periods of very low EEG amplitude – burst suppression. Nitrous oxide induces high-frequency frontal activity and decreased amplitude. Ketamine increases EEG amplitude at low doses, and slows the EEG at higher doses.

The EEG has long been regarded as the "gold standard" for the detection of cerebral ischemia. At constant temperature and depth of anesthesia, progressive ischemia produces a reduction in total power and slowing – decreased α and β power and increased δ and θ power. However, these changes typically only become apparent when CBF falls below half the normal value of 50 ml 100 g^{-1} min^{-1}. EEG amplitude attenuation of <50% or increased δ power is regarded as being indicative of mild ischemia, whereas >50% attenuation or a doubling in δ power is regarded as being indicative of severe ischemia. An isoelectric or "silent" EEG is seen when CBF falls below 7–15 ml 100 g^{-1} min^{-1}. While the EEG is sensitive to subtle changes in neuronal electrophysiology, it should be borne in mind that it is not specific for pathology.

Because the interpretation of continuous intraoperative multi-channel EEG monitoring is complex and time-consuming, a number of automated processed EEG systems have been developed. In the cerebral function monitor (CFM), the EEG signal is filtered to remove low-frequency activity and rectified to produce a single trace representing EEG power varying with both amplitude and frequency. The cerebral function analyzing monitor (CFAM) overcomes many of the shortcomings of CFM by displaying signal amplitude and frequency separately (Figure 26.8). A further method of EEG processing is power spectrum analysis.

165

Table 26.6 Multimodal neuromonitoring algorithm suggesting the cause of EEG slowing and suggested intervention

Time	Temp	MAP	CBFV	rCVOS	Problem – intervention
Any	NC	NC	NC	↑	Anesthesia-induced EEG depression. Dec depth anesthetic
PreCPB	NC	NC	↓ V_{SYS}	↓	Reposition aortic cannula
	NC	NC	↓ V_{DIAS}	↓	Reposition venous cannula
Onset CPB	NC	NC	NC	↓	Acute hemodilution – no intervention
On CPB	NC	NC	Emboli	↓	Neuroprotection protocol
	NC	↓	↓ V_{MEAN}	↓	Dysautoregulation – ↓ MAP
	↓	NC	↓ V_{MEAN}	NC	Normal flow-metabolism coupling
	↑	NC	NC	↓	Flow-metabolism uncoupling – increase depth of anesthesia
Post CPB	NC	NC	↓ V_{DIAS}	↓	Cerebral edema, obstructed cerebral microcirculation – Neuroprotection protocol

Adapted from Edmonds et al, J Cardiothorac Vasc Anesth 2001; 15: 241–50 and Austin et al, J Thorac Cardiovasc Surg 1997; 114: 707–15. A neuroprotection protocol may include administration of thiopental, phenytoin, corticosteroids or a free-radical scavenger. MAP, mean arterial pressure; CBFV, cerebral blood flow velocity; rCVOS, regional cerebral oxygen saturation; NC, no change.

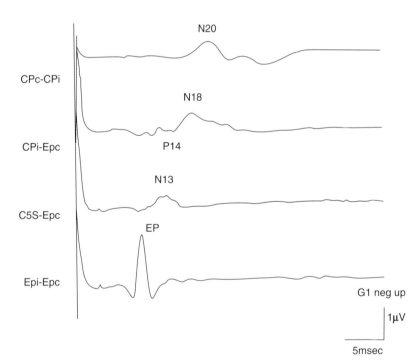

Figure 26.10 Normal median nerve SSEPs using minimum recommended montage. Electrode CPi denotes either CP3 or CP4, whichever is ipsilateral to the stimulated limb; CPc is the contralateral centroparietal scalp electrode. Epi and Epc refer to electrodes sited at Erb's point (brachial plexus) on the ipsilateral and contralateral sides, respectively. The C5S electrode is placed over the body of the fifth cervical vertebra.

Evoked potential monitoring

Sensory evoked potentials (SEP) are the electrical responses of the CNS to peripheral stimulation. Typically a stimulus is delivered at regular intervals and an averaged evoked response is extracted from background electrical activity. In clinical practice the stimulus may be visual (VEP), auditory (AEP; Figure 26.9) or somatosensory (SSEP; Figure 26.10). In contrast, motor evoked potential (MEP) monitoring employs transcutaneous transcranial electrical stimulation of the motor cortex and measurement of the evoked electromyography. Use of the MEP technique is precluded by complete neuromuscular blockade. Lower limb SSEPs and, more recently, MEPs have been be used in spinal and major vascular surgery to monitor spinal cord function and prevent postoperative paraplegia.

Multimodal monitoring

Although single-modality monitoring may produce useful information, it is possible that potentially adverse events may not be detected. Furthermore, observed changes may lead to a misinterpretation of events. By reducing the impact of the technical limitations and disadvantages of each individual monitor, multimodal monitoring offers improved detection of cerebral ischemia, permitting targeted intervention to reduce neurologic injury. A typical monitoring scheme will include both routine (i.e. MAP, CVP, temperature) and specialized (e.g. EEG, NIRS and TCD) measures.

With the exception of profound hypothermia, EEG slowing is the principal manifestation of cerebral ischemia. For this reason EEG slowing is considered a precondition for most intervention algorithms.

Key points

- The risk of neurologic injury is reduced by early detection and intervention.
- At normothermia, the EEG is a sensitive measure of cerebral ischemia.
- TCD measures cerebral blood flow velocity – not cerebral blood flow rate.
- NIRS monitoring during CABG surgery has been shown to be predictive of adverse outcome.
- Multimodal neuromonitoring has been shown to improve clinical outcome.

Further reading

Arrowsmith JE, Ganugapenta MSSR. Intraoperative brain monitoring in cardiac surgery. In Bonser R, Pagano D, Haverich A (Eds.), *Brain Protection in Cardiac Surgery*. London: Springer-Verlag; 2011.

Routine coronary heart surgery

Premedication, induction and maintenance

Paul H. M. Sadleir and Andrew I. Gardner

The aims of anesthesia for cardiac surgery are prevention of perioperative cardiac ischemia and arrhythmias, tight hemodynamic control, avoidance of non-cardiac complications and early tracheal extubation. The following description is only applicable to low-risk patients undergoing elective CABG surgery.

Preoperative assessment

For the majority of elective patients, preoperative assessment should take place several days before surgery in a pre-admission clinic. This allows an assessment of the patient's ability to withstand the intended surgical procedure, and provides an opportunity to explain anesthetic procedures and obtain consent for specific interventions. Having an interval between assessment and surgery permits the early identification of potential problems, allows additional investigations to be undertaken, and alerts support services, such as transfusion, pacing and critical care, of likely demand. This approach significantly reduces the likelihood of delays or cancellation on the day of surgery – particularly important for patients considered suitable for admission to hospital on the day of surgery.

The presence of previously documented symptoms and signs (see Chapter 13) should be verified, the results of preoperative investigations (in particular coronary angiography and echocardiography) reviewed, and any new or undiagnosed problems excluded. A more detailed discussion of the objective assessment of operative risk can be found in Chapter 17. The main determinants of perioperative risk are summarized in Table 17.2.

In addition to a routine systematic preoperative history and examination, specific areas of interest include:

- intended conduit harvest sites: may restrict placement of monitors and cannulae
- recent history of anticoagulant therapy (see below)
- permanent pacemaker/implantable defibrillator: may need reprogramming before induction of anesthesia
- esophageal pathology: may be a relative or absolute contraindication for TEE
- religious or cultural beliefs (e.g. Jehovah's Witness and blood product transfusion).

All regular anti-anginal, anti-hypertensive and anti-cardiac-failure medications should be continued in the preoperative period (Table 27.1).

The optimal timing of cessation of antiplatelet and anticoagulant therapy is determined by balancing the risk of perioperative bleeding against the risk of thrombotic complications.

- Thienopyridines should be discontinued at least 5 days before surgery.
- Aspirin withdrawal remains controversial: continuation of therapy during the 5 days before surgery may reduce early (in-hospital) mortality and improve graft patency without increasing the risks of re-operation for bleeding or transfusion. However, published evidence is inconclusive; in many centers concern about the risk of hemorrhagic complications still prompts aspirin cessation 7–10 days before surgery.
- Other antithrombotic agents used in secondary prevention, such as tirofiban or unfractionated heparin by infusion, are typically withdrawn 2–4 hours before surgery.

Table 27.1 A guide to which regular medications should be continued until the day of surgery

Continue	Controversial	Discontinue
Statins (decreases in-hospital mortality and need for RRT)	Aspirin ACE inhibitors	Thienopyridines (e.g. clopidogrel, prasugrel)
β-Blockers (reduced risk of post-CABG AF)	Angiotensin receptor blockers	GP IIb/IIIa inhibitors (e.g. tirofiban)
Nitrates		Diuretics
Calcium antagonists		NSAIDs
K$^+$channel openers		MAO inhibitors
Corticosteroids		Biguanides (metformin)[a]
Anti-dysrhythmics		
Bronchodilators		

[a] Hypoglycemic agents should be managed according to institutional protocols to maintain normoglycemia during the fasting period.
RRT, renal replacement therapy; ACE angiotensin converting enzyme; GP, glycoprotein; MAO, monoamine oxidase.

Table 27.2 Examples of premedicant drugs in cardiac anesthesia

Oral (90–120 min prior to induction of anesthesia):

> Lorazepam 2–4 mg
> Temazepam 10–20 mg
> Clonidine 100–150 μg
> Methadone 0.1–0.2 mg/kg

Intramuscular (45–60 min prior to induction of anesthesia):

> Morphine sulfate 0.2–0.3 mg/kg + hyoscine hydrobromide 200–400 μg

Patients are often given supplemental oxygen after the administration of sedative premedicants.

Premedication

Despite trends in other anesthetic subspecialties, sedative premedication remains common in cardiac anesthesia. The stated goals are minimization of the risk of cardiac ischemia secondary to anxiety, hypertension and tachycardia while at the same time avoiding respiratory depression. Although opioids, benzodiazepines and antihistamines are commonly prescribed, the final choice of drugs is subject to institutional variability (Table 27.2). Longer-acting amnestic drugs have the advantage of covering the early ICU period. As respiratory depression is a known sequel of sedative premedication, supplemental oxygen should be prescribed and administered until induction of anesthesia.

Preparation

As for all anesthetic procedures, the availability of drugs, equipment and staff (surgeon, nursing staff, perfusionist) should be checked prior to the patient's arrival in the operating suite. Drugs that should be immediately available include inotropes, anti-dysrhythmics, calcium, magnesium, heparin and protamine (Table 27.3).

Anesthetic/operating room

On arrival the identity of the patient should be verified and consent for surgery confirmed in accordance with the World Health Organization (WHO) "Safe Surgery" checklist. The availability of cross-matched blood should also be checked. The operative site should be clearly marked if appropriate (e.g. thoracotomy, radial artery harvest site). Non-invasive monitoring (ECG, NIBP and pulse oximetry) is then instituted prior to any anesthetic procedures.

Vascular access and invasive monitoring

Cannulae are sited under local anesthesia in a forearm vein (14 G) and the non-dominant radial artery (20 G). In the case of non-dominant radial artery harvest,

Table 27.3 Preparation for cardiac anesthesia

Equipment

- Anesthetic machine, laryngoscopes and intubation aids, suction apparatus
- Monitoring (standard anesthetic monitoring plus pressure transducers, depth of anesthesia monitoring, TEE, ABG, ACT)
- Infusion pumps and transfusion apparatus
- Arterial and venous cannulae
- Defibrillator and external pacemaker box
- Ultrasound for venous access

Drugs to be drawn up
Anesthetic

- Local anesthetic (lidocaine)
- Analgesic (e.g. fentanyl, sufentanil, remifentanil, alfentanil)
- Muscle relaxant (e.g. pancuronium, rocuronium)
- Induction agent (e.g. etomidate, propofol, midazolam)

Cardiovascular

- Vagolytic (atropine, glycopyrrolate)
- Vasopressor (metaraminol, phenylephrine)
- β-Blockers

Other

- Intravenous fluids
- Prophylactic antibiotics
- Anticoagulant (heparin)
- Antifibrinolytic agents (tranexamic acid, aminocaproic acid)

either the dominant radial artery or femoral artery may be cannulated. An intravenous infusion is then commenced, and arterial pressure transduced and monitored. Femoral arterial pressure monitoring is used when both radial arteries are required for conduits.

Insertion of central (i.e. internal jugular or subclavian) venous cannulae may then be undertaken; however, in many centers this is deferred until after induction of anesthesia. The use of ultrasound to guide internal jugular vein cannulation has been shown to reduce complications and the number of attempts required.

Inserting a PAFC in low-risk CABG surgery patients has little impact on clinical management or outcome, and routine use of the device is declining. A PAFC sheath may, however, be inserted for central vascular access, and has the advantage of

facilitating subsequent PAFC insertion if indicated after separation from CPB. Many cardiac anesthesiologists use a PAFC sheath in combined or complex procedures and in patients with poor LV function.

Depth-of-anesthesia monitoring by processed EEG devices may reduce the incidence of awareness in this population known to be at high risk. An additional advantage of using these devices is that it is possible to reduce the dose of anesthetic agents and consequently reduce drug-induced cardiovascular depression and cost.

Epidural

Thoracic and cervical epidural analgesia have been used for postoperative analgesia in cardiac surgery. This controversial aspect of cardiac anesthesia is discussed in Chapter 72.

Induction

In some centers, induction of anesthesia takes place in a separate anesthetic room. The benefits of a quiet environment, patient privacy and reduced "turnover" time have to be balanced against the risk of cardiovascular collapse requiring urgent CPB.

Many techniques have been described for the induction and maintenance of anesthesia for cardiac surgery. There is no ideal single agent and there is no place for a "mono-agent" technique. The characteristics of an ideal cardiac anesthetic agent include:

- unaltered hemodynamics
- lack of myocardial depression
- lack of coronary vasoconstriction or steal
- non-anesthetic cardioprotective effects
- residual analgesia
- rapid onset, offset and titration.

Following a period of preoxygenation, balanced anesthesia is induced with a combination of induction hypnotic, opioid and neuromuscular blocking drugs (Table 27.4). Moderate doses of opioid attenuate the response to laryngoscopy and intubation while causing minimal myocardial depression, and allow a reduction in the dose of hypnotic anesthetic agent required. Muscle relaxants provide ideal intubating conditions, prevent patient movement or shivering, and reduce oxygen consumption. Contrary to traditional teaching, many anesthesiologists

Table 27.4 Drugs for the induction of anesthesia

Induction agents

Etomodate 0.15–0.30 mg kg^{-1}
Propofol 1.0–1.5 mg kg^{-1}
Midazolam 0.05–0.10 mg kg^{-1}
Thiopental 3–4 mg kg^{-1}

Opioids

Fentanyl 5–10 μg kg^{-1}
Sufentanil 0.5–1.0 μg kg^{-1}
Remifentanil 0.5–2.5 μg kg^{-1} → 0.05–0.50 μg kg^{-1} min^{-1}
Alfentanil 50 μg kg^{-1} → 1 μg kg^{-1} min^{-1}

Neuromuscular blockers

Pancuronium 0.10–0.15 mg kg^{-1}
Rocuronium 0.5–0.9 mg kg^{-1}
Vecuronium 0.1 mg kg^{-1}
Atracurium 0.6 mg kg^{-1}

administer the muscle relaxant early to patients without obvious airway problems to prevent opioid-induced coughing or chest wall rigidity. Pancuronium is commonly used because of its long duration of action and sympathomimetic action which attenuates the bradycardia associated with high-dose opioid anesthesia and β-blockade. Rocuronium has the advantage of rapid onset (decreasing the risk of stomach insufflation which may result in degradation of TEE images), and the useful property that it can be reversed with a selective relaxant binding agent (sugammadex) if residual blockade is present at time of emergence.

Transfer to operating room

When an anesthetic room has been used for induction it is necessary to transfer the patient to the operating room. Although this procedure has the potential for complications (e.g. accidental avulsion of lines and tubes), observing simple precautions can minimize them.

On arrival in the operating room, the patient should first be re-connected to the ventilator, the capnograph, pulse oximeter and ECG. Pressure areas are checked and padded. A temperature probe should be inserted, and TEE probe if indicated. Pressure transducers are then re-connected and re-zeroed. Venous lines are checked for patency and access to three-way taps confirmed before the patient is

Table 27.5 Procedures following induction of anesthesia

Tracheal intubation	**Secure tube to side of mouth and exclude tongue compression**
Mechanical ventilation	Tidal volume 6–8 ml kg^{-1} to maintain normocapnea FiO$_2$ of 0.6 in air Although theoretically possible to use N$_2$O in early pre-CPB period, failure to switch to air could increase risk of air embolus. Most anesthesiologists now avoid N$_2$O
Maintain anesthesia	Volatile or intravenous agents
Secure additional vascular access	Central venous – if not undertaken prior to induction. Use short internal jugular lines (10–12 cm) or do not insert >12 cm from skin puncture
Urinary catheterization	A suprapubic catheter may be inserted at end of case and before transfer to ICU if transurethral catheterization is not possible
Antibiotic prophylaxis	Covering skin organisms to prevent surgical site infection (sternal wound infection and mediastinitis) and dictated by local protocols (usually β-lactam or glycopeptide antibiotics)
Temperature monitor	Nasopharyngeal/bladder
Patient protection	Eyes closed and taped. Heels padded. Knees slightly flexed Protect ulna and radial nerve pressure points
TEE probe	If indicated, it is easier to insert before the patient is prepared and draped for surgery
Gastric tube	Nasogastric/orogastric tube is used in some centers to reduce postoperative nausea and vomiting. May be used to vent stomach prior to insertion of TEE if it is suspected that the stomach has been insufflated during induction
Confirm patency of peripheral lines	Peripheral and central venous lines should run freely. Arterial line should aspirate easily
Depth of anesthesia monitoring	If not applied prior to induction

Table 27.6 Anesthetic check list prior to start of surgery

Ventilation

Zero monitoring lines

The Five "A"s   **A**ccess

                           Anesthesia

                           Arterial gas

                           ACT (baseline)

                           Antibiotics

Check cross-matched blood

Table 27.7 Degrees of anesthetic and surgical stimulation

High	Low
Laryngoscopy	Post intubation
Tracheal intubation	Preparing and draping
Skin incision	Surgical "delays"
Sternotomy	Mammary artery harvesting
Sternal retraction	
Sternal elevation	

prepared and draped for surgery. To avoid inadvertent intra-arterial drug administration, it is essential that arterial and venous injection ports are physically separated and clearly labeled.

Drug infusion lines should be checked and correct functioning of infusion pumps should be confirmed.

Maintenance

Both volatile agents (0.5–1 MAC) and propofol (3–4 mg kg^{-1} h^{-1} or target controlled infusion 1.5–3 µg ml^{-1}) are commonly used for the maintenance of anesthesia prior to the onset of CPB.

Volatile agents are known to confer a degree of cardioprotection by virtue of ischemic pre- and post-conditioning, although the clinical relevance is yet to be determined (see Chapter 20).

A supplemental dose of opioid is frequently administered a few minutes before sternotomy, and anesthetic requirements may vary according to surgical stimulation. When assessing volume status, the anesthesiologist should be aware that the harvest of bypass graft conduits may result in significant concealed hemorrhage.

The ECG, and TEE if present, should be monitored for evidence of myocardial ischemia. The use of surgical retractors and retrocardiac swabs may make ECG interpretation difficult. The surgeon should be alerted if there is doubt about the presence of ischemia. Attempts may be made to treat these changes pharmacologically with systemic administration of GTN or a β-blocker (e.g. esmolol). CPB should be instituted if ischemic changes persist or circulatory collapse ensues. Completion of conduit harvesting can then continue during "non-ischemic" CPB – i.e. prior to aortic cross-clamping.

Following pericardotomy, the anesthesiologist should observe the heart to gain an appreciation of its size, filling and contractility. Fluid administration is guided by MAP, CVP and TEE findings. There appears to be little to choose between crystalloid and colloid solutions, although glucose-containing solutions are best avoided.

Key points

- Although patients are extensively investigated from a surgical point of view, preoperative anesthetic assessment will often identify issues that require further attention.
- The goals of cardiac anesthesia are tight hemodynamic control and avoidance of perioperative cardiac ischemia.
- Supplemental oxygen should be administered to the patient when sedative premedication is given.
- Good communication between anesthesiologist, surgeon and perfusionist is vital for safe transition to CPB.

Further reading

Augoustides JG, Cheung AT. Pro: ultrasound should be the standard of care for central catheter insertion. *J Cardiothorac Vasc Anesth* 2009; **23**(5): 720–4.

Bybee KA, Powell BD, Valeti U, *et al.* Preoperative aspirin therapy is associated with improved postoperative outcomes in patients undergoing coronary artery bypass grafting. *Circulation* 2005; **112**(9 Suppl): I286–92.

Duncan AI, Koch CG, Xu M, *et al.* Recent metformin ingestion does not increase in-hospital morbidity or mortality after cardiac surgery. *Anesth Analg* 2007; **104**(1): 42–50.

Engelman R, Shahian D, Shemin R, *et al.* The Society of Thoracic Surgeons practice guideline series: Antibiotic prophylaxis in cardiac surgery, part II: Antibiotic choice. *Ann Thorac Surg* 2007; **83**(4): 1569–76.

Frässdorf J, De Hert S, Schlack W. Anaesthesia and myocardial ischaemia/reperfusion injury. *Br J Anaesth* 2009; **103**(1): 89–98.

Reich DL, Fischer GW. Perioperative interventions to modify risk of morbidity and mortality. *Semin Cardiothorac Vasc Anesth* 2007; **11**(3): 224–30.

World Health Organization. *WHO safe surgery checklist.* 2009. http://www.who.int/ patientsafety/safesurgery/en/ (accessed 23 November 2011).

Routine conduct of cardiopulmonary bypass

Barbora Parizkova and Stephen J. Gray

CABG surgery is the most common indication for CPB. While there is considerable diversity in the way CPB is practiced, one single requirement is universal – clear and unambiguous communication between the individuals that constitute the operating room team: surgeons, anesthesiologists, perfusionists and nurses.

Preparation

The CPB system is assembled, primed and tested before the patient is anesthetized. Disposable CPB systems are supplied "closed" (with arterial and venous lines in continuity) to preserve sterility and to allow circulation of prime before connection to the patient. While still closed, the prime is warmed (37°C) and filtered to remove bubbles and particulate matter. An adult CPB system typically requires around 1500 ml of prime, consisting of crystalloid, colloid or blood as well as heparin, calcium and mannitol. The precise "recipe" is institution-dependent.

It is essential for the perfusionist to document the patient's height, weight and hematocrit. This allows the calculation of "safe" pump flows (based on body surface area) and the likely requirement for packed red cells.

Communication

Preceding each case all team members must be aware of the intended sites of incision, cannulation technique, myocardial protection and temperature management strategy. The safe conduct of CPB requires all team members to be aware of the following key events:

- heparin administration
- commencement of CPB and announcement when "full flow" is reached

- lungs "off" after "full flow" achieved
- lungs "on" before attempting to wean from CPB
- termination of CPB
- protamine administration.

Anticoagulation

Adequate systemic anticoagulation, usually with unfractionated heparin, is an absolute requirement for CPB. Anticoagulation often precedes or accompanies cannulation of the aorta but the precise timing is subject to considerable variation. The advantages of early heparinization (salvage of blood lost during conduit harvesting and readiness for urgent CPB) have to be balanced against the disadvantages (increased hemorrhage from operative sites). A heparin dose of 300 units kg^{-1} (3 mg kg^{-1}) is usually sufficient. A point-of-care anticoagulation monitor is used to give an objective measure of the adequacy of anticoagulation. An ACT >300 s is required for cardiotomy suction and >400 s for the institution of CPB. Heparin resistance must be considered if a therapeutic ACT cannot be achieved despite additional doses of heparin. Antithrombin (AT) deficiency can be treated by giving blood products or AT-concentrate.

In many centers, a lysine analog (e.g. tranexamic acid or aminocaproic acid) is used to reduce blood loss and transfusion requirements. If used, it is recommended that lysine analogs be administered after heparinization to reduce the risk of thrombotic complications.

Cannulation

Arterial cannulation always precedes venous cannulation. The ascending aorta is the commonest site, although femoral and subclavian arteries are occasionally used. Excessive hypertension (e.g. MAP >80 mmHg) should be avoided at the time of arterial cannulation to reduce the risk of localized arterial dissection. The relatively narrow diameter of arterial cannulae increases resistance to blood flow, potentially leading to large pressure gradients, high-velocity jets and turbulence. This "jetting" effect increases the risk of arterial dissection and atheroembolism and flow. Correct positioning of the arterial cannula is confirmed by the presence of a pulsatile blood-prime interface in the arterial line and by monitoring arterial line pressure.

Venous cannulation for routine CABG surgery is carried out using a single large cannula inserted via RA appendage and directed towards the IVC. When combined with procedures requiring access to the RA or LA, cannulation of the cavae is typically required. Venous return to the CPB reservoir is passive (siphon- or gravity-dependent). This is influenced by the height of the operating table and tubing diameter. RA cannulation is often accompanied by hemodynamic instability, dysrhythmias, impaired venous return and hemorrhage. For this reason, and because of the ease of fluid administration via the arterial cannula, arterial cannulation invariably precedes venous cannulation.

Additional cannulae are placed for cardioplegia administration (aortic root, coronary sinus) and venting (superior pulmonary vein, main PA, LV apex). Venting refers to the removal of blood from the heart to prevent distension during diastolic arrest.

Initiating CPB

The perfusionist initiates CPB by releasing the arterial line clamp and slowly increasing pump flow. The venous clamp is then released, which allows blood to drain into the venous reservoir under gravity and decompresses the right heart. Transient hypotension, the result of a reduction in blood viscosity secondary to acute hemodilution, is common and usually responds to increasing pump flow or the judicious use of vasoconstrictors. The mnemonic "AVID" is a useful aide-memoire for the main issues upon initiation of CPB (Table 28.1).

Mechanical ventilation can be discontinued once full CPB flow has been established. It is customary to disable anesthesia machine alarms (e.g. apnea, hypotension, asystole) for the duration of CPB.

A sudden increase in arterial line pressure at the onset of CPB may indicate line occlusion, malposition of the arterial cannula or arterial dissection. A high CVP coupled with poor venous drainage indicates a poorly positioned venous cannula, an air-lock or kinking of the tubing.

In some centers the effects of acute hemodilution are to some extent mitigated by the use of a retrograde autologous prime technique immediately before the institution of CPB. The cardiotomy reservoir is primed to its minimal level and "topped up" to a safe level with ~400 ml heparinized arterial blood drained from the CPB arterial line.

Cardiovascular management during CPB

The ideal characteristics of optimal CPB have yet to be described. Current controversies in CPB management are discussed in Chapter 63. There is, however, wide agreement that prolonged periods of hypoxemia, hypotension and hypoperfusion are deleterious. Typical targets for CPB for CABG surgery are shown in Table 28.2.

Pump flow rate and arterial pressure

During normothermic CPB, a pump flow of 2.2–2.5 l min^{-1} m^{-2} is typically used to main vital organ perfusion. Nowadays most routine CABG surgery undertaken with CPB uses non-pulsatile or constant pump flow. Evidence of adequate tissue perfusion is gained by regularly monitoring MAP, urine output, arterial blood gases, SvO_2 and acid-base status. The factors that influence the minimum safe pump flow rate are summarized in Table 28.3.

Because O_2 consumption falls with decreasing temperature (~7%/°C), pump flow is usually reduced during hypothermic CPB. Very low pump flow rates are avoided because of the risk of inadequate organ perfusion.

In most centers, an arterial pressure of 50–60 mmHg is maintained during CPB. During hypothermic CPB, brief periods of hypotension (30–40 mmHg) are tolerated by most patients. Applying Ohm's law to the circulation (MAP = CO × SVR), hypotension can be treated by increasing pump flow rate, administering a vasoconstrictor or both.

Hematocrit

Dilutional anemia is an inevitable consequence of CPB. Severe anemia is associated with low pre-operative hematocrit, low body mass and large

Table 28.1 "AVID" – key considerations at the onset of CPB

A	**Arterial inflow**	
	Arterial blood oxygenated?	Color/oximetry
	Arterial cannula malposition?	Unilateral facial edema and anisocoria
		High arterial line pressure
	Evidence of aortic dissection?	High arterial line pressure
		↓ Reservoir level
		↓ or ↑ radial artery pressure
		Inability to arrest heart with antegrade cardioplegia
V	**Venous inflow**	
	Venous drainage good?	Reservoir levels maintained
		RA not distended and ↓ CVP
	Evidence of SVC obstruction?	Heart rotated about base for surgical access,
		↑ CVP, facial engorgement or conjunctival edema
I	**Incomplete bypass**	
	Evidence of incomplete CPB?	Pulsatile arterial and PA pressures
		↓ Venous drainage
		Aortic insufficiency
		Considerable bronchial venous flow
		Target pump flow not reached
D	**Drugs**	Reduce or discontinue vasoactive drug administration
		Discontinue ventilation

Table 28.2 Physiological considerations during CPB

MAP	50–70 mmHg
CVP	0 – 5 mmHg
Pump flow	2.2–2.5 l min^{-1} m^{-2} (at normothermia)
SvO2	>65%
Hematocrit	>0.20–0.25
Arterial blood gases	Alpha-stat preferred management during hypothermic CPB
Plasma glucose	90–162 mg dl^{-1} (5–9 mmol l^{-1})

Table 28.3 Factors determining minimal safe pump flow during CPB

Body surface area

Hematocrit

Temperature

Depth of anesthesia

Neuromuscular blockade

Systemic vascular resistance

Anesthesia

Adequate anesthesia must be maintained throughout CPB. The cardiac anesthesiologist needs to be aware of the impact that heparin administration, hemodilution, hypothermia and extracorporeal sequestration have on the efficacy of anesthetic drugs. These effects are summarized in Chapter 12. When a propofol infusion is used to maintain anesthesia during normothermic CPB, the rate of administration is usually left

priming volume. The beneficial effects of hemodilution (reduced viscosity, improved microvascular flow) have to be balanced against increased tissue edema (reduced oncotic pressure). A hematocrit of 22–25% appears to represent a reasonable trade-off between unacceptable anemia and excessive transfusion.

unaltered. By contrast, the onset of CPB removes the anesthesiologist's ability to administer a volatile anesthetic agent via the lungs. When used as the principal agent for maintenance after induction, failure to subsequently administer a volatile agent via the CPB oxygenator may result in awareness. This is possibly why intravenous anesthesia remains popular despite a lack of ischemic preconditioning properties.

Cardioplegia

Depending on institutional practice, either the perfusionist or the anesthesiologist may be responsible for the delivery of cardioplegic solutions. Crystalloid cardioplegia can be prepared before the onset of CPB. In contrast, blood cardioplegia cannot be prepared until after the onset of CPB because it requires the addition of heparinized blood to a crystalloid base solution. Cardioplegic solutions must be free of air and particulate matter. The administration of cardioplegia is usually associated with rise in serum K^+ and hypotension secondary to vasodilatation. The principles underlying cardioplegia are discussed in Chapter 19.

Rewarming

Restoration of normothermia is achieved by the heat-exchanger, which warms blood as it passes through the oxygenator. Rewarming should be a gradual process to avoid excessive thermal gradients, incomplete thermal equilibration and neurologic injury. Excessively rapid blood rewarming denatures plasma proteins and may induce bubble formation. Despite its accuracy, nasopharyngeal temperature monitoring may underestimate cerebral venous temperature by up to 3.4°C when rewarming is very rapid. As little as 0.5°C hyperthermia may exacerbate ischemic CNS injury. Conversely, inadequate rewarming combined with further heat loss during chest closure results in shivering, vasoconstriction, increased O_2 consumption and coagulopathy. In practice the difference between arterial inflow and nasopharyngeal temperature should be <4.0°C, and SvO_2 should be >65% during rewarming.

De-airing

Removal of intracardiac air following CABG surgery is usually only necessary when an open-heart procedure (e.g. LV aneurysmectomy or valve surgery) has been performed concurrently. Air is typically expelled via a ventriculotomy or proximal aortotomy. In both cases the lungs are ventilated, to expel air from the pulmonary circulation, and the patient is positioned to ensure that the venting site is superior. Transventricular deairing is performed in the Trendelenberg position, whereas deairing via the ascending aorta is performed in the supine position. Confirmation of the adequacy of deairing is greatly assisted by TEE.

Defibrillation

Occasionally, removal of the aortic cross-clamp (coronary reperfusion) may trigger VT or VF. Prolonged VF with LV distension must be avoided, as it significantly increases myocardial O_2 consumption and may cause subendocardial ischemia. Defibrillation is typically accomplished using a 5–10 J biphasic (10–20 J monophasic) shock delivered using internal paddles.

Pacing

Temporary pacing can be established via insulated steel wires sutured onto the epicardium. These are tunneled through the chest wall and connected to a pacemaker device. The small risks of myocardial damage during insertion and hemorrhage following removal have to be balanced against the potential therapeutic benefit. The perception of this balance is subject to considerable variation, with some surgeons using atrial and ventricular wires in all cases, and others reserving them for high-risk cases. Generally speaking, the placement of pacing wires may be omitted in low-risk cases (i.e. uncomplicated CABG with HR >70 that responds to atropine). Atrial wires may be considered redundant in patients with chronic AF.

In the operating theater environment, fixed-rate, dual-chamber pacing (i.e. "DOO", rate 80–100, AV delay 120–150 ms) is the mode of choice as it is insensitive to diathermy radiofrequency interference. The atrial and ventricular pacing voltages should be high enough to ensure reliable capture. An excessively high atrial pacing voltage may produce simultaneous ventricular activation and impede diastolic filling (*cv*-waves on CVP pressure trace and arterial hypotension). Similarly, incorrect connection of the pacing cable to the pacemaker may also have unexpected and

Table 28.4 The TRAVVEL checklist for termination of CPB

T Temperature	Nasopharyngeal 36–37°C
R Rate	Stable cardiac rate and rhythm. Fixed-rate epicardial pacing may be required
A Air	Techniques to remove intracardiac air. TEE may be used to confirm adequacy
V Venting	Venting lines either clamped or removed before coming of CPB
V Ventilation	Mechanical ventilation restarted. Left lower lobe expansion visually confirmed (if pleura open)
E Electrolytes	Normalize metabolic indices: base excess < -5 mmol l^{-1}, PO$_2$ >75 mmHg (10 kPa), PCO$_2 \approx 40$ mmHg (5 kPa), hematocrit >22%, K$^+$ >4.5 mmol l^{-1}
L Level	Operating table, re-zero pressure transducers

unwanted effects. The pacemaker should be changed to "DDD" mode before transfer to ICU.

Weaning from CPB

The mnemonic "TRAVVEL" (Table 28.4) provides a useful checklist prior to terminating CPB. After the anesthesiologist has restarted mechanical ventilation, the perfusionist gradually occludes the venous line, thereby increasing RV preload. The fall in venous drainage is matched by a gradual reduction in pump flow as the heart begins to eject. The venous line is clamped after termination of CPB, but the arterial line is used as a conduit for the transfusion of blood from the venous reservoir. At this point volatile anesthetic administration – if used – should revert to the anesthesiologist and all anesthesia machine alarms should be reactivated.

Decannulation

Following termination of CPB, the venous cannula and vents are removed. Before giving protamine, any residual pericardial and pleural blood is returned to the venous reservoir and cardiotomy suction discontinued thereafter. After alerting the perfusionist, a test-dose of protamine (10–20 mg) is then given and the patient observed for 1–2 minutes. If no major adverse hemodynamic instability occurs, the remainder of the dose (~1.0 mg for each 100 units of heparin given) is then administered over 2–5 min. Mild protamine-induced hypotension is common and generally responds to transfusing blood from the venous reservoir via the aortic cannula. Following removal of the aortic cannula, the anesthesiologist assumes sole responsibility for fluid administration. In some centers, where the aortic cannula is removed shortly after administration of the protamine test-dose,

the anesthesiologist must be prepared to respond rapidly to profound hypotension. In many centers any blood remaining in the CPB system is drained and returned to the patient. Both the anesthesiologist and surgeon must agree to this, as subsequent reinstitution of CPB is made more difficult.

Hemostasis

The adequacy of heparin reversal should be confirmed by ACT measurement. Further arterial blood analysis is undertaken to assess oxygenation, ventilation, hematocrit and K$^+$. Closure of the pericardium or sternum may be accompanied by hemodynamic instability. Chest reopening may be required if "tamponade" graft kinking occurs.

Preparing for transfer

As surgery draws to an end, preparations for transfer to the ICU should be made. The airway, vascular lines, pacing wires, catheters and surgical drains should be adequately secured and protected when moving the patient from the operating table. Because hypotension and dysrhythmias may occur, the patient should be monitored throughout transfer. Occasionally a coronary air embolus may induce severe hypotension or VF. Deferring transfer should be considered if the cardiac rhythm is unstable or when MAP <60 mmHg. An additional supply of oxygen, ventilation apparatus, intravenous fluids and emergency drugs should be immediately available.

Key points

- Clear and unambiguous communication between surgeon, anesthesiologist and perfusionist is essential to the safe conduct of CPB.

- Excessive hypertension should be avoided during aortic cannulation.
- Confirmation of adequate anticoagulation must be obtained before use of cardiotomy suction.
- Pump flows are based on patient body surface area and temperature.
- Mechanical ventilation should be restarted and all anesthesia alarms reactivated when terminating CPB.

Further reading

Ghosh S, Falter F, Cook D (Eds.). *Cardiopulmonary Bypass.* Cambridge: Cambridge University Press: 2009.

Gravlee GP, Davis RF, Stammers AH, Ungerleider RM (Eds.). *Cardiopulmonary Bypass: Principles and Practice*, 3rd edition. Philadelphia: Lippincott Williams and Wilkins; 2008.

Murphy GS, Hessel EAII, Groom RC. Optimal perfusion during cardiopulmonary bypass: An evidence-based approach. *Anesth Analg* 2009; **108**(5): 1394–417.

29

Routine early postoperative care

Maura Screaton

The high volume and repetitive nature of cardiothoracic surgical critical care has meant that in many centers nursing staff have taken over much of the routine postoperative care previously undertaken by medical staff. The use of critical care pathways and protocols allows senior nurses to manage uncomplicated cases relatively independently, with medical staff only being consulted when patient progress deviates from a clearly defined pathway. Because new members of the medical staff may not be accustomed to this style of patient care, it is essential that they read and understand the protocols, appreciate the indications for medical referral and be aware of management steps prior to referral. Medical staff without previous cardiothoracic ICU experience should be guided through several straightforward cases in order to understand the key principles.

ICU admission and handover

The ICU should ideally be located adjacent to and on the same floor level as the operating suite. Invasive monitoring should be continued throughout transfer to the ICU.

Priorities on arrival are:

Capnography	Confirmation of adequate ventilation
Invasive monitoring	Transducers leveled and re-zeroed
Oximetry	Confirmation of peripheral oxygenation
ECG	Rate and rhythm
Pacing	Switch from fixed-rate to demand mode

It is essential that all relevant patient, anesthetic and intraoperative details are clearly conveyed to the admitting nurse.

- Patient details
  - Name, age and preoperative risk factors
  - Allergies/drug sensitivities
- Surgical
  - Planned and actual surgical procedure performed
  - Complications and other significant events
  - Ease of weaning from CPB
  - Optimal cardiac filling pressures in operating room
  - Hemodynamic support – vasoactive drugs, pacing, IABP
- Anesthetic
  - Vascular line types and insertion sites
  - Laryngoscopy grade – particularly if tracheal intubation was difficult
  - Current drug infusions and administration rates
  - Blood products administered (and ordered for later administration)
  - Fluids administered, urine output and use of hemofiltration during CPB
  - Post-CPB blood gases, ACT, glucose, K^+ and hematocrit
  - Pending laboratory investigations
- Patient-specific ICU goals
  - Acceptable ranges for MAP, CVP, (LAP, PCWP, CO)
  - Expected duration of sedation and mechanical ventilation
- Investigations
  - A baseline CXR is routinely undertaken in some centers to check line and ETT positions.

Sedation and ventilation

Although it may be possible to wean patients from mechanical ventilation before leaving the operating room, most anesthesiologists consider that the risks of bleeding, hemodynamic instability and hypothermia outweigh any potential benefits. Simple volume controlled ventilation is adequate for the majority of patients using 10 breaths per minute, a tidal volume of 6–8 ml kg^{-1} and 60% oxygen. ABG analysis is used to guide changes in ventilator settings to maintain PO$_2$ >75 mmHg (>10 kPa) and PCO$_2$ 38 mmHg (~5 kPa). Sedation and mechanical ventilation are usually continued for 2–4 h in order to allow rewarming and exclude significant bleeding.

Criteria for patient extubation by nurse	
Airway	Ability to protect airway. Intubation not difficult.
Breathing	Adequate ventilation and oxygenation
Circulation	Hemodynamic stability
Metabolic	Base deficit <5 mmol l^{-1}
CNS	"Appropriate"

Analgesia

Median sternotomy is associated with moderate to severe postoperative pain. Effective postoperative analgesia reduces pain on movement and deep inspiration, facilitating early weaning from mechanical ventilation. In most centers intravenous morphine is the analgesic of choice. Although non-steroidal anti-inflammatory drugs are effective they should be used with caution in patients with a coagulopathy or impaired renal function. The use of epidural analgesia is discussed in Chapter 72.

Hemodynamic goals

The maintenance of adequate systemic perfusion is vital to the preservation of cerebral, myocardial and visceral function.

Common early postoperative hemodynamic problems include hypertension, hypotension, tachycardia and bradycardia.

Hypertension

Pain, hypoventilation and intolerance of the endotracheal tube may all cause hypertension. Treatment

HR	Usually 60–100
Rhythm	Preserve sinus rhythm
MAP	60–80 mmHg
CVP	6–10 mmHg (on IPPV)
Perfusion	Good peripheral perfusion
Urine output	>0.5 ml kg^{-1} h^{-1}

should be directed at the underlying cause. If hypertension persists despite good analgesia, adequate ventilation, resedation or tracheal extubation, a vasodilator (e.g. SNP or GTN) should be used.

Hypotension

Reduced preload, contractility and afterload may contribute to hypotension. Most commonly hypotension is caused by hypovolemia secondary to urinary loss, hemorrhage and peripheral vasodilatation. Hypotension that does not respond to a colloid challenge (200–400 ml) is an indication for additional support. Temporary pacing should be optimized before instituting inotropic therapy. If possible, hemodynamically unstable tachyarrhythmias should be converted pharmacologically or electrically. Further investigation with a CXR (to exclude concealed hemorrhage), a PAFC or TEE is indicated in patients with refractory hypotension.

Tachycardia

Possible causes include pain, hypovolemia, inotropic/chronotropic therapy and tamponade. The diagnosis of tamponade is discussed in more detail in Chapter 65.

Bradycardia

Epicardial pacing wires allow rapid treatment of bradycardias. In the absence of AF, atrial demand (AAI) pacing is preferable to ventricular demand (VVI) pacing because of the contribution of atrial systole to CO. Dual chamber (DDD) pacing is required if A-V conduction is impaired.

Communication with relatives

The day of surgery is understandably stressful for family and friends. It is good practice for either medical or nursing staff to contact relatives by telephone within the first hour of ICU admission to give a brief report. Relatives should be encouraged to telephone or visit thereafter.

Hemorrhage

Bleeding is an inevitable consequence of cardiac surgery. Excessive postoperative bleeding, however, is abnormal and associated with increased morbidity and mortality. Bleeding, which may be overt or covert, is frequently described as being "surgical" (i.e. from a blood vessel), "anesthetic" (i.e. coagulopathic) or both! Overt blood loss through mediastinal and pleural drains is relatively easy to diagnose, whereas the diagnosis of covert hemorrhage requires a high degree of clinical suspicion.

Time	Acceptable blood loss (ml kg^{-1} h^{-1})
1st hour	3
2nd–4th hours	2
5th–12th hours	1

In an effort to identify patients requiring surgical re-exploration earlier, some units use a blood loss nomogram (Figure 29.1). This method allows better visualization of bleeding trends and a comparison with other patients operated on at the same institution. Re-exploration must be considered if hemorrhage exceeds the 95th centile for two successive hours. The development of algorithms for the investigation and management of excessive postoperative bleeding can help decision-making. Early re-exploration of a bleeding patient is associated with improved outcome.

Fluid and electrolyte balance

Fluid intake (crystalloid and colloid), urine output and chest tube drainage are recorded hourly. Following CPB, most patients are in positive crystalloid balance. Total crystalloid intake (oral and intravenous) is restricted to 750 ml m^{-2} in the first 24 h, and 1000 ml m^{-2} day^{-1} thereafter. Colloid (e.g. hydroxyethyl starch, succinylated gelatin, blood) is given when the patient has low MAP with low CVP or oliguria.

The serum K$^+$ concentration should be maintained between 4.5 and 5.5 mmol l^{-1}. Hypokalemia is common for several reasons – preoperative diuretic therapy, hemodilution, the humoral response to

surgery, catecholamine use and significant post-CPB diuresis. Hypokalemia is associated with dysrhythmias and must be aggressively corrected. If the K$^+$ concentration is <4.5 mmol l^{-1}, KCl 10 mmol is given via the central venous line over 10 min, whereas if the K$^+$ concentration is <4.0 mmol l^{-1}, KCl 20 mmol is given over 20 min.

Hyperkalemia is less common in the early postoperative period. No action is usually required if the K$^+$ concentration is <6.5 mmol l^{-1}. In the absence of cardiac dysfunction a K$^+$ concentration of >6.5 mmol l^{-1} may be treated with a loop diuretic (e.g. furosemide 20 mg) or a dextrose (25 g) and insulin (15 units) infusion. Intravenous calcium salts (e.g. CaCl$_2$ 10 mmol) may be considered in the presence of cardiac dysfunction.

Oliguria

Oliguria is defined as a urine output <0.5 ml kg^{-1} h^{-1} for two consecutive hours and may have a prerenal, renal or post-renal cause. Anuria is unusual and may indicate a blocked urinary catheter. Before intervening, the patient's chart should be reviewed to establish the normal preoperative blood pressure and to exclude reduced renal perfusion pressure (i.e. MAP-CVP). An incorrectly positioned IABP may cause renal artery occlusion.

Fluid challenge
250 ml over 10 min
Repeated if rise in CVP not sustained after 30 min

Diuretic
e.g. furosemide 20 mg or mannitol 0.25 g kg^{-1}

Increase MAP/CO
Consider pacing
Inotrope e.g. dopamine 2–5 μg kg^{-1} min^{-1}

Metabolic acidosis

Mild metabolic acidosis is common following cardiac surgery. In the absence of significant renal impairment, a persistent acidosis may indicate inadequate CO and visceral ischemia. Because the base deficit is a useful "barometer" of the effectiveness of treatment, alkaline solutions (e.g. sodium bicarbonate) should not be administered unless there is evidence of end-organ dysfunction (i.e. myocardial depression).

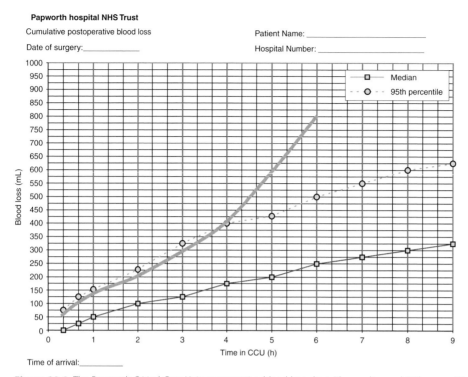

Figure 29.1 The Papworth Critical Care Unit postoperative blood loss chart. The median and 95th percentile ICU blood loss is plotted against time. In the example shown, an abrupt increase in the expected rate of bleeding for two consecutive hours should prompt surgical re-exploration. (Courtesy of C. Gerrard and A. Vuylsteke, ICU, Papworth Hospital.)

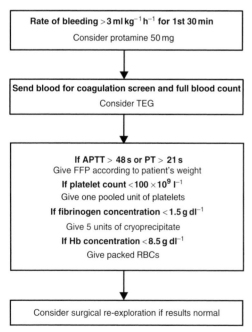

Figure 29.2 Simple algorithm for dealing with excessive hemorrhage after cardiac surgery. PT, prothrombin time.

Gastrointestinal problems

Abdominal distension with absent bowel sounds, nausea and vomiting is relatively common. Although nasogastric tubes are used routinely in some centers, their use may increase the risk of nosocomial respiratory tract infection. The presence of a gastric bubble on a CXR should prompt insertion of a nasogastric tube. Nausea and vomiting may be treated with phenothiazines (e.g. prochlorperazine) or serotonin antagonists (e.g. ondansetron).

Failed tracheal extubation

Failure to maintain adequate ventilation or gas exchange after tracheal extubation is rare. Reintubation and reinstitution of mechanical ventilation should be considered in the presence of significant bleeding, neurologic impairment or hemodynamic instability. Although a review of the anesthetic record may predict an easy reintubation, it should be remembered that vocal cord or glottic edema may make laryngoscopy and intubation more difficult. In most cases early, elective intervention is preferable to an emergency reintubation following cardiorespiratory collapse. The essential requirements for reintubation are:

- skilled assistance
- full hemodynamic monitoring
- laryngoscopes, endotracheal tubes
- intubation aids
- suction apparatus
- functioning capnograph
- induction agent and muscle relaxant
- vasopressor and other emergency drugs
- colloid solution
- sedative drug infusion(s).

First postoperative day

Timing of chest drain removal is a surgical decision. The drains are usually removed when there is no air leak and residual drainage is <25 ml h^{-1} for two consecutive hours.

The arterial line is removed before the patient is transferred to the surgical floor or ward, although it may be retained if the patient is being transferred to a stepdown or high-dependency area.

Epicardial pacing wires are usually left *in situ* even if the drains are taken out. They are normally removed on the fifth or sixth postoperative day.

The central venous line is retained and any lumen not in use should be flushed with heparinized saline and capped. It is usually removed on the third or fourth postoperative day. The pharmacological treatment of tachyarrhythmias (e.g. AF) is greatly facilitated if the line is not removed too early.

The urinary catheter is retained for at least 2 days. Accurate fluid balance is essential as oliguria frequently precedes postoperative complications.

Key points

- Problems in the early postoperative period are common – most can be effectively managed by the application of locally developed protocols.
- Demand (rather than fixed-rate) pacing should be used to reduce the risk of VF.
- Maintain a high index of suspicion for covert bleeding and tamponade.
- Good communication between anesthesiologists, intensivists, surgeons and nursing staff is fundamental.

Chapter

30

Off-pump coronary surgery

Jonathan H. Mackay and Joseph E. Arrowsmith

The term "off-pump" coronary artery bypass (OPCAB) encompasses a number of techniques during which myocardial revascularization is performed without employing extracorporeal circulation. Although the term "beating heart surgery" has been used interchangeably with OPCAB, it should be borne in mind that CABG surgery can be performed on a beating heart "on-pump".

History

Prior to the introduction of CPB in the 1950s, all cardiac surgery was performed on a moving heart in a bloody operative field. CPB and cardioplegic arrest

effectively relegated beating-heart surgery to centers unable to afford the costs associated with CPB. In time, the suspicion that many of the complications of cardiac surgery were secondary to CPB led to the "rediscovery" of beating-heart surgery. Re-evaluation of the technique and the development of cardiac stabilization devices, retractors and intracoronary shunts has facilitated widespread uptake of OPCAB. In essence cardiac surgical practice has come full circle (Figure 30.1).

Initially OPCAB was practiced only by enthusiasts and restricted to low-risk patients requiring one or two bypass grafts on the anterior cardiac surface. The demonstration that OPCAB is both safe and

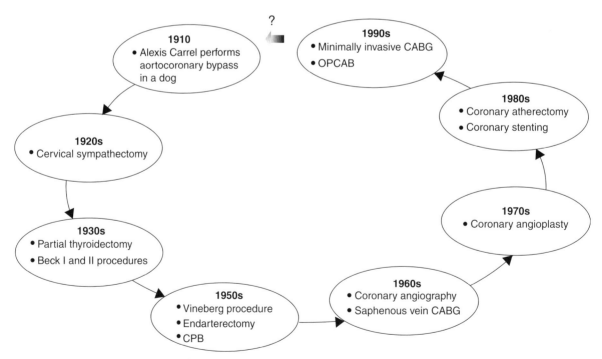

Figure 30.1 The surgical management of coronary artery disease – a century of evolution.

186 *Core Topics in Cardiac Anesthesia, Second Edition*, ed. Jonathan H. Mackay and Joseph E. Arrowsmith. Published by Cambridge University Press. © Cambridge University Press 2012.

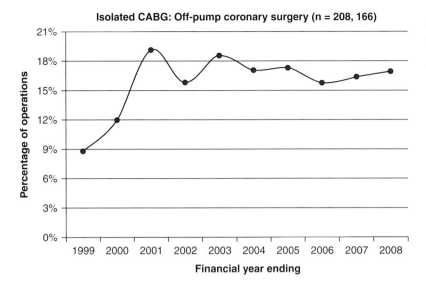

Isolated CABG: Off-pump coronary surgery (n = 208, 166)

Figure 30.2 Trends in OPCAB surgery in the UK 1999–2008. From: Society for Cardiothoracic Surgery in Great Britain & Ireland. *Sixth National Adult Cardiac Surgical Database Report 2008, Demonstrating quality* (http://www.scts.org).

efficacious in high-risk patients with multi-vessel disease led to a broadening of indications. The uptake of OPCAB surgery varies widely between centers and individual surgeons. Although in some centers >90% of isolated revascularization procedures are performed off-pump, the vast majority of US surgeons perform <5% of their cases without CPB. The same could probably be said for the UK, where the proportion of OPCAB procedures appears to have reached a plateau (Figure 30.2).

Rationale

Interest in OPCAB has been driven by a desire to avoid the perceived ill effects of CPB, develop less invasive surgical approaches and reduce costs. To some extent commercial pressures and the wide availability of information about OPCAB has contributed to both cardiologist and patient demand for the technique. Objective evidence that OPCAB has achieved these aspirations has been difficult to obtain.

Although no consensus exists, there are groups of patients for whom OPCAB is technically difficult. It may be unwise, therefore, to use the technique in patients with a deep intramuscular LAD or diffusely diseased coronaries or in those who require extensive endarterectomy. In addition, many surgeons consider active ischemia with hemodynamic compromise to be a contraindication.

Surgical approach

The majority of OPCAB procedures are performed through a conventional median sternotomy. Not only

does this approach provide excellent access to the heart and the internal mammary arteries, it facilitates the rapid institution of CPB, if required.

In the small number of patients with single vessel (LAD) disease who are not suitable for percutaneous intervention, a limited anterior short thoracotomy (LAST) may provide sufficient surgical access for minimally invasive direct coronary artery bypass (MIDCAB). Proponents of MIDCAB cite reductions in length of hospital stay, postoperative infection rates and postoperative analgesic requirements as reasons to pursue the technique. Those opposed to MIDCAB cite the not insignificant "conversion" rate, limited resuscitation access, *increased* postoperative analgesic requirements and the absence of long-term graft patency data as reasons *not* to pursue the technique.

Multivessel coronary revascularization via a median sternotomy will necessitate displacement of the heart from its natural position. The uptake of OPCAB has been greatly assisted by the introduction of single-use and reusable mechanical stabilization devices and double or triple limb intracoronary shunts. The Medtronic Octopus™ has the advantage of attaching to the surface of the heart via suction cups and reduces the degree of cardiac chamber compression caused by other devices. (Figure 30.3)

Anesthetic management

From the anesthetic view point, conventional CABG can be conveniently divided into three readily identifiable epochs: the period between induction of

187

Table 30.1 The rationale for OPCAB surgery – putative benefits and areas of controversy

	Advantages	Disadvantages
General	Avoids air and particulate emboli from extracorporeal circuit Avoids risk of cannulation site injury (i.e. aortic dissection) Avoids median sternotomy for single vessel disease	Labour-intensive anesthesia Technically challenging Cannot be extended to deal with incidental intracardiac pathology (e.g. MR) Anterior thoracotomy may be more painful than median sternotomy
Myocardial	No requirement for cardioplegia Transient interruption to normal coronary blood flow ↓ Release of markers of myocardial injury (i.e. troponins, creatine kinase) ↓ Incidence of perioperative infarction ↓ Myocardial reperfusion injury	Potential for incomplete revascularization Quality of coronary anastomoses uncertain Long-term graft patency uncertain Impact on postoperative AF unclear
Neurologic	No requirement for aortic cannulation ↓ Cerebral microemboli – ↓↓ if all aortic instrumentation avoided ↓ Incidence of delirium and stroke – in large retrospective studies	↓ Cognitive dysfunction unproven
Renal	↓ Risk of dialysis-dependent renal failure in patients with pre-existing renal dysfunction	↓↓ Cardiac output during posterior (e.g. circumflex) grafting
Pulmonary	Ventilation and pulmonary circulation maintained throughout procedure	No significant improvement in lung function despite ↓ inflammatory response
Gastrointestinal	Avoidance of embolic complications	No significant reduction in incidence of GI complications
Hematologic	Full heparinization may be avoided ↓ Hemorrhage and blood product requirements	Claims for significant ↓ transfusion requirements unblended and may be biased
Immunologic	↓ Systemic inflammatory response Avoids increases in vascular permeability and total body water associated with CPB	
Cost	↓ Duration of intensive care and length of hospital stay ↓ Disposable costs (i.e. CPB equipment) ↓ Use of blood and blood products	Perfusionist and CPB system required to be available on "stand-by"

anesthesia and the onset of CPB, the period of CPB itself, and the period between the termination of CPB and the end of surgery. During CPB pump flow rate (i.e. cardiac output), SVR and MAP are all amenable to manipulation. In contrast, during OPCAB the period of CPB is replaced by intermittent episodes of cardiac displacement and coronary occlusion, during which distal coronary anastomoses are fashioned. Myocardial ischemia, dysrhythmias, cardiac compression, A-V valve distortion and regurgitation, caval (inflow) occlusion and RV outflow obstruction all conspire to reduce both CO and MAP. This is,

therefore, a busy time for the anesthesiologist: providing the surgeon with adequate access to the lateral and posterior cardiac surfaces while minimizing the hemodynamic consequences.

General considerations

Patients scheduled for OPCAB surgery should undergo the same preoperative assessment and management as those scheduled for conventional CABG with CPB. Similarly, the goals of intraoperative anesthetic management – prevention of perioperative

Table 30.2 Anesthetic drugs for OPCAB surgery

Premedication	Short-acting benzodiazepines. Avoid lorazepam
Induction agents	Similar to "on-pump"
Opioids	Remifentanil use may expedite earlier extubation
Muscle relaxants	Pancuronium considered acceptable by many. Shorter-acting agents may be preferred by those aiming for early or "on-table" extubation
Maintenance	TIVA techniques using propofol are popular. Volatile techniques

Table 30.3 Causes of hemodynamic instability during OPCAB surgery

Reduction of venous return

RV and LV compression

Ventricular septal displacement secondary to chamber compression

Valve distortion and regurgitation (particularly the MV)

Partial aortic clamping (side-biting clamp for proximal anastamoses)

Conduction system ischemia leading to heart block (particularly during RCA grafting)

(a) 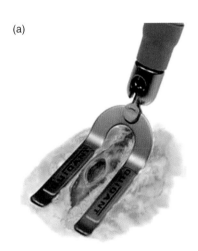 (b)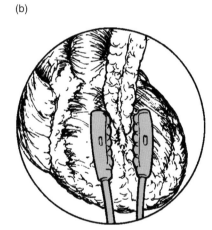

Figure 30.3 (a) The Guidant stabilization device (Courtesy of Guidant Corporation). (b) The Octopus™ suction stabilization device (Courtesy of Medtronic Inc.)

cardiac ischemia, tight hemodynamic control, minimizing cardiovascular depression and avoidance of non-cardiac complications while providing adequate depth of anesthesia – are identical. The requirement for a double-lumen endotracheal tube and lung isolation to improve surgical access via a LAST incision should be discussed with the surgeon before induction of anesthesia.

Because recovery following OPCAB is often more rapid than that following conventional surgery, anesthetic techniques have evolved to facilitate early extubation. As might be expected, no single anesthetic technique has been shown to be superior.

Monitoring

Surgical retraction, elevation and rotation of the heart may impede venous return and ventricular outflow. It follows that the hemodynamic impact is typically greatest when the heart is positioned for circumflex and posterior descending artery grafting, and that the rationale for advanced intraoperative monitoring is the early detection of a fall in CO.

Despite the theoretical advantage of truly continuous CO monitors (e.g. esophageal Doppler), there is little evidence to suggest that intermittent PAFC-based monitoring results in poorer clinical outcomes. In the setting of OPCAB, some anesthesiologists argue that arterial pressure monitoring and capnography provide a rapid and reliable means of detecting a fall in CO!

More subtle changes in regional ventricular wall function can only be effectively detected with TEE. As discussed in Chapter 25 (Teo and Roscoe), myocardial ischemia reduces systolic myocardial thickening and inward motion long before changes in the surface

189

Table 30.4 Intraoperative monitoring for OPCAB surgery

Basic monitoring

Multi-lead ECG with ST analysis
Hemodynamic – MAP, CVP
Airway – FiO_2, $FetCO_2$, SpO_2
Temperature, urine output, arterial blood gases, ACT

Advanced monitoring

Cardiac output measurement	PAFC (intermittent or continuous) Esophageal Doppler monitoring (EDM) Pulse-contour monitoring
Regional wall motion	Transesophageal echocardiography (TEE)
Neurologic	Transcranial Doppler (TCD) EEG Near infrared spectroscopy (NIRS)

ECG become apparent. During cardiac elevation, reliance must be placed on the mid-esophageal views, as the transgastric views may be unobtainable.

In a small number of centers, advanced neurologic monitoring is used to detect critical reductions in global and regional cerebral blood flow. As with all neurophysiological monitoring during surgery, the relationship between observed changes and clinical outcome is inconsistent and unreliable. At present there is no objective evidence that using TCD, near infrared cerebral spectroscopy (NIRS) or electroencephalography – either alone or in combination – has any impact on clinical outcome in the setting of OPCAB surgery.

Heat conservation

In anticipation of rapid recovery and early postoperative extubation, intraoperative heat loss should be minimized and active warming measures employed. Convective and radiant losses from prolonged exposure of thoracic contents present a considerable challenge and, unlike conventional CABG, there is no rewarming period. Various methods have been advocated to minimize the incidence and severity of hypothermia (Table 30.5).

Table 30.5 Heat conservation during OPCAB surgery

Maintenance of high ambient temperature (~25°C)

Use of heated mattress

Use of sterile lower body forced air blanket (after saphenous vein harvest)

Use of intravenous fluid warming device

Use of insulating material to reduce cranial heat loss

Hemodynamic management

The options to ameliorate the cardiovascular disturbances that may occur during OPCAB surgery are physical, pharmacological and electrical (Table 30.6). In the early days of beating-heart surgery, a pharmacologically induced bradycardia (<40 bpm) was favored by many surgeons. Improvements in cardiac stabilization, recognition of the importance of maintaining vital organ perfusion, and growing operator confidence have reduced the importance of heart rate control. To maintain CO and avoid the risks of ventricular distension, some surgeons prefer to operate on a heart paced at 80–90 bpm.

Table 30.6 Hemodynamic management during OPCAB surgery

Physical

Fluid administration – avoidance of hypovolemia (fluid requirements >> conventional CABG)
Maintenance of cerebral perfusion – avoidance of gross CVP elevation
Posture – use of Trendelenburg position and lateral tilt
Opening right pleural cavity to reduce the impact of cardiac rotation
IABP in high-risk cases

Pharmacological

↓ Heart rate – esmolol (intravenous diltiazem in USA)
↑ Contractility – inotrope
Vasoactive drugs – GTN, SNP, α_1-agonists
Antiarrhythmics – K^+, Mg^{2+}

Electrical

↑ Heart rate – fixed rate, epicardial atrial pacing (AOO)

Anticoagulation

Interruption of normal blood flow and manipulation of vascular endothelium necessitates some degree of

Table 30.7 The Veterans Affairs (VA) Randomized On/Off Bypass (ROOBY) Study

Methodology

Randomized, prospective study conducted at 18 VA medical centers (2002–2008)
2203 patients scheduled for urgent or elective CABG. Randomized to on-pump or off-pump
Primary short-term (30 day) end points: composite of death or complications
Primary long-term (1 year) end points: all-cause mortality; need for revascularization; nonfatal infarction
Secondary (1 year) end points: completeness of revascularization; graft patency; neuropsychological outcomes

Results (off-pump vs. on-pump)

No significant difference in primary short-term composite adverse outcomes (7.0% vs. 5.6%, $P = 0.19$)
Significant increase in primary long-term composite adverse outcomes (9.9% vs. 7.4%, $P = 0.04$)
Significantly more patients had fewer bypass grafts than planned (17.8% vs. 11.1%, $P < 0.001$)
Significantly reduced graft patency (82.6% vs. 87.8%, $P < 0.01$)

Comments

Many procedures performed by trainees under direct supervision
Levels of operator experience with OPCAB widely different
Rate of conversion to CPB in off-pump group (12.4%) was 5 times that reported in national STS database

From: Shroyer AL, et al. N Engl J Med 2009; 361(19): 1827–37.
STS, Society of Thoracic Surgeons.

anticoagulation. In the vast majority of cases the drug of choice is unfractionated heparin because of its predictable pharmacology. Opinion is divided as to the dose of heparin that should be used. While some surgeons favor full anticoagulation (i.e. 300 IU kg^{-1} and ACT >400 s), the majority prefer partial anticoagulation (i.e. 100–150 IU kg^{-1}). Full anticoagulation facilitates the rapid institution of CPB but may increase bleeding. Reversal of anticoagulation is also subject to considerable variation. Practices include complete reversal, partial reversal and no reversal.

Postoperative management

Although the goals of postoperative management are similar to "on-pump" CABG, it is important to appreciate subtle differences in analgesic requirements, fluid management and temperature control.

Postoperative analgesic requirements are dependent on the type of surgical incision, the type and dose of intraoperative analgesics and the use of local or regional anesthetic techniques. The pain associated with median sternotomy is largely unaltered by the use of CPB and it should be borne in mind that patients undergoing OPCAB may have received substantially less intraoperative analgesia. For patients with a LAST incision, intrapleural analgesia, intercostal blockade and paravertebral blockade can produce excellent analgesia, without the risk of a perispinal hematoma associated with central neuraxial techniques. Suboptimal analgesia should not, however, be the price paid by the patient for early extubation.

Patients undergoing OPCAB are not subjected to the considerable fluid load associated with CPB and administration of cardioplegic solutions. For this reason their intraoperative and postoperative fluid requirements are greater.

The use of adequate intraoperative measures to prevent heat loss and maintain body temperature should render the OPCAB patient relatively immune from the so-called "after-drop" phenomenon commonly seen after hypothermic CPB. While intraoperative measures should be continued into the early postoperative period, hyperthermia should be avoided.

Institution of CPB

In some cases conversion to "on-pump" surgery is required, although the indications and thresholds for conversion vary considerably. Indications for CPB include: inadequate surgical access, gross hemodynamic instability, refractory dysrhythmia and the diagnosis of new valvular pathology requiring surgical correction. Full anticoagulation is required for CPB.

191

Outcome and complications

The complications of OPCAB surgery are similar to those of conventional CABG surgery. Although the reported rates of complications following OPCAB are lower in many published series, it should be borne in mind that study populations may not be comparable. In most of the large, "off-pump" versus "on-pump" series reported to date, there was no randomization and patients in "off-pump" groups had fewer bypass grafts. This observation has led some to raise the issue of incomplete revascularization. The reality is that for a study to detect a postoperative mortality reduction from 3% to 2% with 80% power and a 5% type I error >8000 patients would have to be recruited.

The future

The uptake of OPCAB surgery will only increase if large randomized studies conclusively demonstrate lower complication rates and equivalent graft patency rates. Recognition of the importance of aortic atheroma in the genesis of neurologic injury has led to a reduction or avoidance of instrumentation of the proximal aorta. New devices, capable of forming a proximal anastomosis without aortic clamping, are increasingly becoming available.

Key points

- The use of OPCAB appears to have reached a plateau.
- In contrast to conventional CABG with CPB, OPCAB places additional demands on the anesthesiologist.
- Displacement of the heart from its natural position is frequently associated with hypotension and a reduced cardiac output.
- The assertion that OPCAB reduces the incidence and severity of major complications remains one of the greatest polarizing issues in cardiac surgery.

Further reading

Hoff SJ. Off-pump coronary artery bypass: techniques, pitfalls, and results. *Semin Thorac Cardiovasc Surg* 2009; **21**(3): 213–23.

Kuss O, von Salviati B, Börgermann J. Off-pump versus on-pump coronary artery bypass grafting: a systematic review and meta-analysis of propensity score analyses. *J Thorac Cardiovasc Surg* 2010; **140**(4): 829–35.

Shroyer AL, Grover FL, Hattler B, *et al.* On-pump versus off-pump coronary-artery bypass surgery. *N Engl J Med* 2009; **361**(19): 1827–37.

Chapter

31

Aortic valve disease

Jonathan H. Mackay and Joseph E. Arrowsmith

The AV is composed of three semilunar cusps, left (posterior), right (anterior) and non-coronary, which are related to the three sinuses of Valsalva (Figure 31.1). The main functions of the AV are to permit unimpeded LV systolic ejection and to prevent regurgitation of LV stroke volume during diastole. The normal adult AV orifice area is 2–4 cm^2.

Aortic stenosis

Aortic stenosis (AS) is defined as a fixed obstruction to systolic LV outflow.

Clinical features

Patients may be asymptomatic for many years, although normally present with one or more of the classic triad of symptoms: angina, syncope or breathlessness. Less fortunate patients may present with sudden death. Fifty percent survival rates from onset of symptoms are as shown in Table 31.1.

Pathology

In most cases, AS is an acquired disease. Degenerative calcification causes thickening and stiffness of the leaflets. It is associated with advanced age (>70 years) and is often associated with MV annular calcification. Chronic rheumatic AV disease causes commissural fusion and AR is more common.

Bicuspid AV, with a prevalence of 2%, is one of the commonest congenital heart lesions. Patients with a bicuspid AV have a shorter latency period to symptom onset due to earlier degeneration and calcification.

More rarely, AS may be at a supra- or sub-valvular level. Similar principles of anesthetic management apply.

Table 31.1 Survival rates from onset of symptoms in aortic stenosis

Presenting symptom	50% Survival rate
Angina	5 years
Syncope	3 years
Breathlessness	2 years

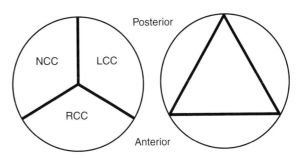

Figure 31.1 The aortic valve (as seen on TEE at ~30°) during diastole (left) and systole (right). NCC, non-coronary cusp; RCC, right coronary cusp; LCC, left coronary cusp.

Pathophysiology

The fixed obstruction to LV ejection causes chronic LV pressure overload and increased wall tension (Figure 31.2). This increase in wall tension is offset by the development of concentric LVH at the price of diastolic dysfunction secondary to impaired relaxation and reduced compliance, manifest as elevated LVEDP (Figure 31.3). LV end-diastolic dimensions are usually preserved in early AS.

Angina pectoris

An imbalance between myocardial O$_2$ supply (MDO$_2$) and demand (MVO$_2$) may occur even in the absence of

Core Topics in Cardiac Anesthesia, Second Edition, ed. Jonathan H. Mackay and Joseph E. Arrowsmith. Published by Cambridge University Press. © Cambridge University Press 2012.

significant coronary artery disease. The combination of LVH and wall tension increases systolic MVO$_2$, while a reduction in coronary perfusion pressure decreases MDO$_2$ (Figure 31.4).

Syncope

Syncope typically occurs on exertion. SV is limited in moderate or severe AS giving a "fixed" or "limited" CO. Inability to compensate for exercise-induced peripheral arterial vasodilatation is the most common explanation for syncope. Ventricular dysrhythmia is another potential cause.

Breathlessness

Breathlessness is the most sinister of the triad of symptoms and may herald the onset of LV decompensation/dilatation. Increased LVEDP necessitates higher left-sided filling pressures, which lead to pulmonary congestion (Figure 31.5). Decompensation arises when the LV wall tension can no longer be maintained by systolic wall thickening and the LV dilates. LV dilatation is associated with increased wall tension (Laplace's law).

Investigations

- *Electrocardiograph (ECG)*: increased R and S wave amplitude, T wave inversion (strain pattern) in anterior chest leads.
- *Two-dimensional echo*: AV anatomy and function, LV function, aortic root size. Typical features are:

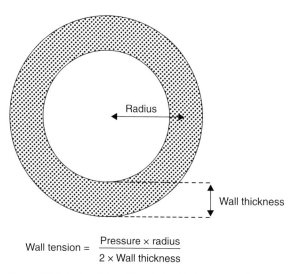

$$\text{Wall tension} = \frac{\text{Pressure} \times \text{radius}}{2 \times \text{Wall thickness}}$$

Figure 31.2 Laplace's Law. The relationship between wall tension (stress), intracavity pressure, radius of curvature and wall thickness.

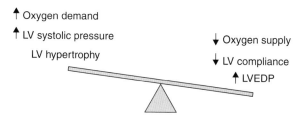

Figure 31.4 The imbalance between myocardial oxygen supply and demand in AS.

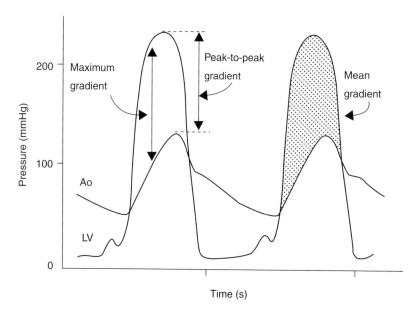

Figure 31.3 Pressure waveforms obtained simultaneously from the LV cavity and the aortic root in aortic stenosis. The *peak-to-peak* gradient is measured in the catheter laboratory and is the difference between the peak systolic pressures in the LV cavity and aortic root. Note that peak aortic root pressure is reached later than peak ventricular pressure. The maximum or *instantaneous* gradient is usually measured by continuous-wave Doppler ultrasound.

leaflet thickening, calcification, reduced opening. Planimetric measurement of AV orifice area (AVA) is unreliable in the presence of calcification.

- *Color-flow Doppler:* turbulence across valve. Does not permit assessment of severity. May demonstrate associated regurgitation.
- *Continuous-wave Doppler:* because alignment of the ultrasound beam with blood flow through the AV is easier, transthoracic echocardiography (TTE) provides a more accurate assessment of AV gradient than TEE using the deep transgastric view (Figure 24.7d). Peak AV gradient = 4 × peak velocity^2 (modified Bernoulli equation). AVA can be measured using the continuity equation (Figure 31.6).

- *Coronary angiography:* to exclude coronary disease. Mandatory in males >40 years or females >50 years.
- *Ventriculography:* LV function, peak-to-peak AV gradient (Figure 31.3).

Anesthetic goals

Sinus rhythm and the late diastolic "atrial kick" are very important in these poorly compliant hearts. Atrial contraction can account for 30–40% diastolic filling in these patients (cf. 15–20% in normal patients). AF and nodal rhythms result in failure to maintain preload and are poorly tolerated.

Table 31.2 ACC/AHA classification of severity of aortic stenosis in adults

	Mild	Moderate	Severe
Valve area (cm^2)	>1.5	1.0–1.5	<1.0
Valve area index (cm^2 m^{-2})	–	–	<0.6
Jet velocity (m s^{-1})	<3	3–4	>4
Peak gradient (mmHg)	36	36–64	>64
Mean gradient (mmHg)	<25	25–40	>40
Dimensionless severity index^a	–	0.25–0.50	<0.25

^{a} VTI$_{LVOT}$/VTI$_{AV}$.
ACC, American College of Cardiology; AHA, American Heart Association; VTI, velocity-time integral.

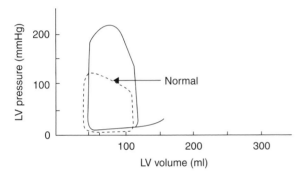

Figure 31.5 Left ventricular pressure–volume loop in aortic stenosis. Note elevated end-diastolic pressure, elevated systolic pressure and preservation of stroke volume.

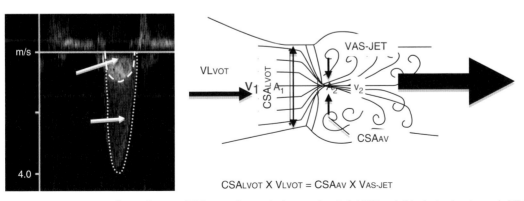

$$CSA_{LVOT} \times V_{LVOT} = CSA_{AV} \times V_{AS\text{-}JET}$$

Figure 31.6 Estimation of AV orifice area (AVA) using the continuity equation. Left: LVOT and AV velocity time integrals (VTIs) are calculated by tracing the LVOT and AV continuous-wave Doppler velocity envelopes, which in this case are superimposed. The VTI is the distance travelled by blood during systolic ejection. Right: the product of VTI and cross-sectional area (CSA) remain constant for LVOT and AV. Multiplying the VTI by the CSA of the structure through which the blood is flowing yields the stroke volume. AVA = (VTI$_{LVOT}$ × CSA$_{LVOT}$)/VTI$_{AS\text{-}JET}$, where VTI$_{LVOT}$ is the VTI of LVOT blood flow, CSA$_{LVOT}$ is the CSA of the LVOT and VTI$_{AS\text{-}JET}$ is VTI of the stenotic AV jet. **195**

TEE provides a better direct objective measure of LV filling (i.e. LV end-diastolic area) than the PAFC (i.e. PAWP), but the former is not available during the critical period of induction of anesthesia.

Tachycardia may cause myocardial ischemia by reducing diastolic coronary perfusion and should be avoided. Bradycardia should also be avoided due to the "limited" CO. Systolic function is usually well preserved in the early stages of AS. Maintaining contractility is usually only a problem in end-stage AS associated with LV decompensation. Attempts to improve SV by reducing afterload are misguided and dangerous in AS, as afterload is effectively fixed at the AV level. The anesthetic technique must, therefore, preserve SVR.

In the post-CPB period following AVR for stenosis (i.e. when the fixed obstruction to LV outflow has been removed) the anesthesiologist should anticipate significant rebound arterial hypertension. Untreated hypertension may increase bleeding and the risk of aortic dissection during decannulation. The conventional management of hypertension in this setting includes vasodilators, posture-induced preload reduction and volatile anesthetic agents. Deliberate "nodal" A-V pacing (i.e. A-V delay <15 ms) can be used in

Table 31.3 Anesthetic considerations in aortic stenosis

Preload	"Better full than empty"
HR	60–80 is ideal
Rhythm[a]	Preserve sinus rhythm
Contractility	Maintain (but most tolerate mild depression)
SVR	Maintain (or slight ↑) to maintain coronary perfusion pressure

[a] Following AVR the placement of ventricular pacing wires is considered mandatory because of the high incidence of A-V block.

extreme circumstances to effectively remove the contribution of late diastolic LV filling.

Treatment of hypotension

Hypotension is common following induction of anesthesia and must be anticipated. Initial treatment is usually IV fluid and a vasoconstrictor to maintain preload and afterload respectively. Early intervention is required to prevent an inexorable downward spiral of hypotension leading to myocardial ischemia and cardiac arrest. If cardiac arrest does occur, external cardiac massage is generally ineffective. Survival after prolonged arrest is unusual without the facility for rapid institution of CPB.

Aortic regurgitation

Aortic regurgitation (AR) is defined as diastolic leakage across AV which causes LV volume overload.

Clinical features

Presenting features are highly dependent on whether the etiology is acute or chronic.

- *Chronic AR*: compensatory LV changes allow many patients with chronic AR to be asymptomatic for >20 years. Symptoms, typically breathlessness on exertion, accompany LV decompensation. Angina is less common in AR than AS because the increase in MVO_2 with volume overload is smaller than that with pressure overload.
- *Acute AR*: typically presents with acute pulmonary edema, tachycardia and poor peripheral perfusion.

Pathology

AR may be secondary to dilatation of the aortic root, abnormalities of the valve leaflets or a combination of

Table 31.4 The etiology of aortic regurgitation

Aortic root dilatation	Congenital	Marfan's syndrome
	Acquired	Longstanding hypertension, aortic dissection, atheromatous aortic disease, syphilitic aortitis, connective tissue disorders
Leaflet abnormality or damage	Congenital	Bicuspid AV (frequently become incompetent after fourth decade and have well recognized association with coarctation of aorta)
	Acquired	Aortic dissection, chronic rheumatic heart disease, infective endocarditis, connective tissue disease (e.g. systemic lupus erythematosus, rheumatoid arthritis, ankylosing spondylitis), balloon valvuloplasty

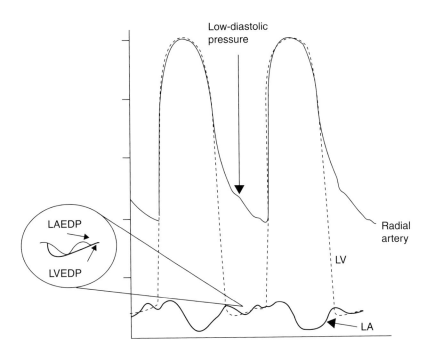

Low-diastolic pressure

Radial artery

LV

LA

LAEDP

LVEDP

Figure 31.7 Pressure waveforms for AR. A fall in diastolic pressure leads to a widening of pulse pressure.

both. Both aortic dissection (discussed in Chapter 36) and infectious endocarditis cause acute AR. Endocarditis causes leaflet perforation and vegetations may impede diastolic leaflet closure.

Pathophysiology

Factors affecting the severity of AR (Figure 31.7) include:

- size of orifice area
- diastolic pressure gradient across the AV
- length of diastole (inversely related to HR).

In both chronic and acute AR, the primary problem is LV volume overload. In chronic AR, the increase in diastolic filling volume induces adaptive changes in the LV. Muscle elongation results in an increased LV radius and eccentric LVH. Unlike MR, where the LV offloads into the LA during the early part of ejection, there is no reduction in LV pressure during systole. LV wall thickness increases to match the increased radius and reduce wall tension (Laplace's law). True compliance is changed only slightly but the ventricle operates much further to the right on the pressure–volume curve (Figure 31.8).

Hearts in chronic AR, so-called "bovine" hearts, can develop the largest LVEDV of all the valvular heart lesions. Systolic SV is increased (LVEDV increases by more than LVESV) in order to compensate for diastolic

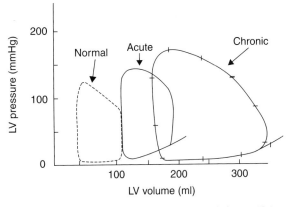

Figure 31.8 Pressure–volume loops for acute and chronic AR. In chronic AR, LVEDV and SV are greatly increased. In acute AR, where there has been no adaptive increase in LV compliance, the increases in LVEDV and SV are smaller.

regurgitant volume and maintain an "effective" SV. Although Starling mechanisms initially maintain LV systolic function, increasing LVEDV eventually leads to decompensation evidenced by a decrease in the slope of the end-systolic pressure–volume relationship. The rise in LVESV is accompanied by a fall in LV ejection fraction (LVEF).

Acute AR causes diastolic volume *and* pressure overload in a normal-sized, non-compliant LV. The acute rise in LVEDP reduces coronary perfusion

197

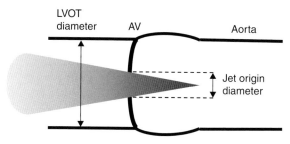

Figure 31.9 Color-flow Doppler echocardiographic assessment of the severity of AR using the ratio of jet origin diameter to LVOT diameter (<0.3 = mild, 0.3–0.6 = moderate, >0.6 = severe). Measurement of the *vena contracta* diameter (the narrowest part of the incompetent AV) and the proximal isovelocity surface area (PISA) are advanced color-flow Doppler methods used to estimate regurgitant orifice area – a measure of AR severity. A detailed description of these techniques can be found in any standard echocardiography textbook.

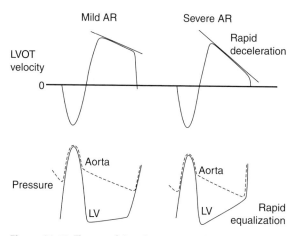

Figure 31.10 The use of diastolic regurgitant flow deceleration (pressure half-time method) to grade the severity of AR. Mild AR >400 ms, moderate AR 250–400 ms, severe AR <250 ms. The mathematical principles underlying the method are summarized in the next chapter – Figure 32.6.

pressure and causes early closure of the MV and the requirement for higher LA filling pressures.

Investigations

- *Two-dimensional echo:* AV leaflet pathology, aortic root dimensions, LV function. LV end-systolic dimension >5.5 cm and LVEF <50% are signs of systolic dysfunction and are indications for surgery.
- *Color-flow Doppler:* to assess width of regurgitant jet at origin in relationship to width of LVOT. Diastolic flow reversal in the descending aorta suggests severe AR. The presence and severity of any associated MR needs to be established.

Table 31.5 Anesthetic considerations in aortic regurgitation

	Acute AR	Chronic AR
Preload	Increase ++	Increase
HR	Fast	Medium to fast
Rhythm[a]	Sinus	Sinus
Contractility	Inotropic support	Maintain/support
SVR	Low – maintain	Low

[a] Following AVR the placement of ventricular pacing wires is considered mandatory because of the high incidence of A-V block.

- *Continuous-wave Doppler:* calculation of regurgitant valve orifice size using the pressure half-time method (Figure 31.10). Diastolic regurgitant blood flow velocity decreases more rapidly in severe AR.
- *Coronary angiography:* to exclude coronary disease.

Anesthetic goals

Preload needs to be greater in acute AR to overcome higher LVEDP. A modest tachycardia shortens diastole and reduces regurgitant flow. It also reduces the time for anterograde filling through the MV, which reduces LV distention, lowers LVEDP and improves coronary perfusion. In acute AR and the latter stages of chronic AR, sinus rhythm is particularly beneficial because it facilitates anterograde LV filling.

Contractility must be maintained, inotropic support is often required in acute AR.

Afterload reduction lowers the diastolic AV gradient and, therefore, the regurgitant volume. Vasodilator therapy is commonly used to delay the development of systolic dysfunction. Afterload reduction may not be tolerated in the presence of a low diastolic blood pressure, particularly in the emergency setting.

Treatment of hypotension

Strategies are based on inotropes and vasodilators. The IABP is contraindicated due to its tendency to worsen regurgitation and cause LV dilatation.

Key points

- AS produces both systolic and diastolic LV dysfunction.
- Tachycardia, *severe* bradycardia and vasodilatation are poorly tolerated in AS.

- Hypotension should be treated early in AS to prevent hemodynamic collapse.
- Deliberate "nodal" A-V pacing can be used in extreme circumstances to treat hypertension following AVR for AS.
- Volume overload in chronic AR results in the largest LVEDV of all the valvular heart lesions.
- A-V conduction abnormalities are common after AV replacement. Epicardial pacing and close

monitoring after ICU discharge are considered mandatory.

Further reading

Van Dyck MJ, Watremez C, Boodhwani M, Vanoverschelde JL, El Khoury G. Transesophageal echocardiographic evaluation during aortic valve repair surgery. *Anesth Analg* 2010; **111**(1): 59–70.

Zigelman CZ, Edelstein PM. Aortic valve stenosis. *Anesthesiol Clin* 2009; **27**(3): 519–32.

Chapter

32

Mitral valve disease

Jonathan H. Mackay and Francis C. Wells

In the first edition we wrote that "The recent trends towards repair, rather than replacement of the MV, together with increased use of perioperative TEE, have stimulated cardiac anesthesiologist to gain a greater understanding of MV anatomy". Now we have to say that it is *essential* for a cardiac anesthesiologist to be properly skilled in MV imaging. Indeed, in many institutions, three-dimensional TEE is becoming a standard adjunct to MV surgery.

The normal adult MV area is 4–6 cm^2. Unlike other heart valves, the MV consists of two asymmetric leaflets. The *aortic* (anterior) leaflet makes up 65% of the valve area but its base forms only 35% of the circumference. The *mural* (posterior) leaflet usually consists of three main scallops, although there may be up to five. The leaflets are joined at the anterolateral and posteromedial ends of the commissure (Figure 32.1). The aortic MV leaflet shares the same fibrous attachment as the non-coronary cusp of the AV.

The complete valve apparatus consists of the leaflets, which arise from the A-V junction, and the *chordae tendinae*, which connect the leaflets to the papillary muscles, which in turn are muscular projections from the non-compacted layer of the LV (Figure 32.2). There are two principal fibrous condensations that form the trigones; postero-superior and antero-inferior. They are placed approximately equidistant within the sector of the valve between the two lateral ends of the commissure. This fibrous condensation extends for up to a third of the circumference of the orifice. It is commonly misstated that there is a complete annulus of circumferential fibrous tissue.

- During diastole – MV leaflet opening should permit unimpeded flow from LA to LV.
- During systole – coaptation of the MV leaflets protects the pulmonary circulation from high LV pressures.

The tensor apparatus consisting of chordae tendinae and papillary muscles make significant contributions to LV function and ejection fraction.

MV surgery is still most often undertaken through a sternotomy though right thoracotomy may be used particularly for redo MV surgery. Minimal-access surgery, which entails peripheral cannulation and a mini right thoracotomy, is becoming more widespread. Its benefits await substantiation by a prospective randomized study (see Chapter 34).

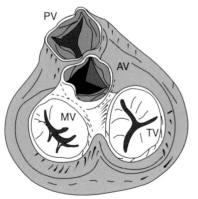

Figure 32.1 Anatomy of the cardiac valves (viewed from above).

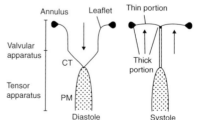

Figure 32.2 Mitral leaflet opening during diastole, and coaptation (central overlap) and apposition (relative height of leaflets) during systole. CT, chordae tendinae; PM, papillary muscle.

Core Topics in Cardiac Anesthesia, Second Edition, ed. Jonathan H. Mackay and Joseph E. Arrowsmith. Published by Cambridge University Press. © Cambridge University Press 2012.

Mitral stenosis

Mitral stenosis (MS) in adults is defined as area <2 cm^2 and classified as severe or critical when the valve area is <1 cm^2.

The vast majority of cases are secondary to rheumatic fever, though a history of an earlier acute febrile illness is often absent. Leaflet thickening and commissural fusion occur secondary to the inflammatory process. Other valve disease, particularly involving aortic and tricuspid valves, is common. Pure MS is less common than mixed stenosis and regurgitation, as a result of the fixed orifice.

Clinical features

Breathlessness on exertion is the commonest presentation and the onset is usually insidious. Other presentations include hemoptysis, AF or peripheral embolic events.

Pathophysiology

Fixed obstruction to blood flow between LA and LV creates a pressure gradient across the MV. Left atrial pressure (LAP) increases to maintain CO.

$$\textbf{Pressure gradient} = [\textbf{Flow rate}/(\textbf{K} \times \textbf{valve area})]^2$$

where K is the hydraulic constant. Elevated LAP and the presence of low LVEDP result in an increased MV gradient (Figure 32.3).

The consequences of elevated LAP include:

- LA hypertrophy and, later, dilatation
- atrial fibrillation
- reduced pulmonary compliance
- pulmonary hypertension and eventually RV "stress" and TR.

AF reduces LV filling particularly when associated with fast ventricular rates. Pulmonary hypertension is initially reversible but becomes irreversible following sustained chronic elevation of PVR.

The LV pressure–volume loop in MS is small and shifted to the left due to reduction in LV pressure and volume loading (Figure 32.4).

LV systolic function may be depressed due to myocardial fibrosis and chronic underloading. Figure 32.5 illustrates the effect of reducing valve area on the relationship between transmitral flow rate and pressure gradient. Decreasing MV area has a dramatic effect on the flow rate required to generate the

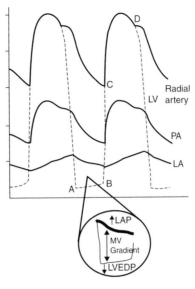

Figure 32.3
Pressure curves for MS.

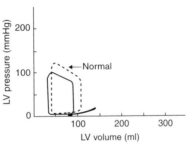

Figure 32.4
LV pressure–volume loop in MS.

diastolic pressure gradient at which pulmonary edema develops.

Investigations

Two-dimensional echo: leaflets thickened, possibly calcified, doming and reduced opening.

Pulsed-wave Doppler gradient (pressure half time; PH-T): MV inflow is quantified with pulsed or continuous-wave Doppler. The rate of fall of blood flow velocity of the E (early diastolic filling) wave is attenuated in MS. The PH-T method uses the slope of E wave deceleration to calculate MVA. Calculation of MVA by the PHT method is unreliable in the presence of an incompetent aortic valve. Aortic regurgitation contributes to LV diastolic filling, causing transmitral blood flow velocity to decline more rapidly. The net result is an underestimation of the severity of MS.

Color-flow Doppler: the proximal isovelocity surface area (PISA) method can be used to estimate valve orifice area.

$$\textbf{MV orifice area (cm}^2) = 220/\textbf{PH-T (ms)}$$

201

Anesthetic goals

High LAP is required to overcome the resistance to LV filling. Excessive preload may cause LA distension and AF. Control of heart rate is paramount. Tachycardia does not allow time to for LV filling and results in reduced LVEDV. Bradycardia is poorly tolerated due to relatively fixed SV. Loss of sinus rhythm can decrease CO by 20%. Consider synchronized direct current (DC) shock in acute onset AF – if no LA thrombus present.

SVR needs to be maintained particularly in patients with tight stenosis and an active sympathetic nervous system. LV contractility is rarely a problem in pure MS where greater emphasis should be placed on protecting the RV from increases in PVR and pulmonary hypertension.

Treatment of hypotension

Hypotension is usually associated with tachycardia. Consider DC cardioversion if tachycardia is due to acute-onset AF. Sinus tachycardia is generally best treated initially with volume and phenylephrine. Esmolol is useful if these measures fail to improve hemodynamics.

External CPR is unlikely to be successful in patients with severe MS. In the event of full-blown cardiac arrest, the emphasis should be on institution of internal cardiac massage and emergency CPB.

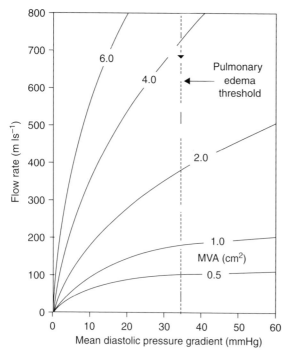

Figure 32.5 Rate of transmitral diastolic blood flow versus mean diastolic MV gradient for normal (4–6 cm^2) and stenotic MVs (0.5–2 cm^2). MVA, mitral valve area.

Table 32.1 Anesthetic considerations in mitral stenosis

Preload	High
HR	Avoid tachycardia
Rhythm	Sinus rhythm better than AF
SVR	Maintain
Contractility	Maintain
PVR	Avoid increase

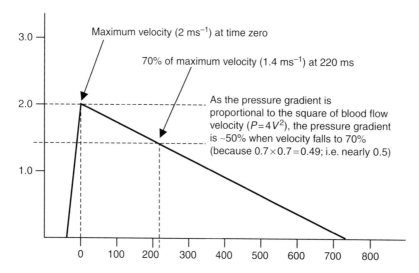

Figure 32.6 Estimation of mitral valve orifice area (MVA) using diastolic transmitral blood flow velocity to calculate the pressure half-time (PH-T). The pressure half-time is defined as the time required for the magnitude of the instantaneous transmitral pressure gradient to fall by half. From the modified Bernouilli equation P = 4 × V^2 (where P = pressure and V = velocity) it can be deduced that for pressure to halve, velocity must fall by 30%. In the example above, the PH-T is 220 ms, which gives a MVA = 220/220 = 1.0 cm^2.

Surgery

Percutaneous transeptal balloon valvotomy is an alternative to surgery in patients with favorable valve morphology (noncalcified, pliable leaflets and absence of commissural calcification) in the absence of significant MR or LA thrombus. Valvotomy is a palliative procedure and recurrence is common. Patients with valvular calcification, thickened fibrotic leaflets and subvalvular fusion have higher incidences of complications and recurrence, and fare better with open surgery.

Mitral regurgitation

Mild MR is a common finding in patients with ischemic heart disease undergoing cardiac surgery. Most of these patients do not require surgical intervention to the valve. Lesions typically amenable to repair include myxomatous degeneration, mural (posterior) leaflet prolapse and chordal rupture. Cardiac anesthesiologists can assist the surgical decision-making process using TEE by providing information on etiology, severity and likely natural history of the regurgitant lesion.

Pathology

Acute MR is usually due to rupture or ischemia of a papillary muscle or rupture of chordae tendinae. Posterior papillary muscle dysfunction is more common than anterior papillary dysfunction, because the former is supplied by a single coronary artery whereas the latter is supplied by two coronary arteries.

- *Myxomatous degeneration of valve leaflets* most commonly affects mural (posterior) > aortic (anterior) leaflet, chordae thin and prone to rupture. Leaflets appear redundant and thickened. Size disproportion between mitral leaflets and LV cavity causes prolapse.
- *Chronic rheumatic heart disease* leads to scarring and contraction of chordae and leaflets, which become thickened and often calcified.
- *Ischemic mitral regurgitation* leads to papillary muscle dysfunction with reduced contractility and consequent prolapse, mitral annular dilatation, papillary muscle rupture.
- *Endocarditis* leads to leaflet perforation, chordal rupture, vegetations, abscess formation or scarring may interfere with coaptation.

- *Congenital* cleft or fenestrated mitral leaflets, double orifice MV and endocardial cushion defects.

Clinical features

Breathlessness on exertion and easy fatigability are the commonest presentations for chronic MR. Symptoms frequently deteriorate with the onset of AF. Patients with acute MR do not have time to develop LA enlargement and may present with acute LV failure and pulmonary edema.

Pathophysiology

The effect of systolic ejection of blood into the low-pressure LA is largely dependent on whether the onset of MR is acute or chronic.

- *Acute MR* results in a sudden increase in LAP. The LA and LV are not accustomed to increased volume load. Increased LVEDP and increased LAP result in acute pulmonary edema. SVR increases to maintain blood pressure. The balance between myocardial O_2 supply and demand is adversely affected by reduced CO and increased HR. There is a particularly high risk of subendocardial ischemia when acute MR is secondary to ischemic papillary muscle dysfunction or rupture.
- *Chronic MR* results in LV volume overload, LV dilatation and a rightward shift of the LV pressure–volume loop (Figure 32.7). Increased LVEDV occurs without any increase in LVEDP early in the course of the disease process.

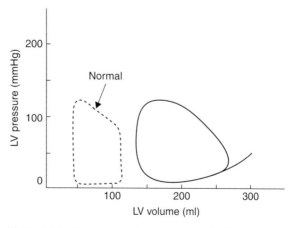

Figure 32.7. LV pressure–volume loop in chronic MR.

Anesthetic goals

Patients with chronic MR are frequently in AF. Sinus rhythm is useful, but less critical than for other valve lesions, as the blood entering the LV in late diastole is immediately returned to the LA in early systole.

Reduced afterload is generally desirable because of improved forward flow. Patients with non-ischemic MR tolerate a lower MAP than patients with AR because coronary perfusion pressure (i.e. aortic root pressure) is maintained during diastole.

Treatment of hypotension

The risk of downward spiraling hypotension, resistant to medical treatment, is less than in stenotic valvular lesions. *Hypotension therefore rarely interferes with the important and interesting task of acquiring good TEE images of the valve.* Nevertheless profound hypotension may occur, particularly in MR secondary to acute ischemia. Patients with a competent AV usually respond to small doses of phenylephrine, otherwise inotropes are first-line treatment.

Investigations

The LA provides an excellent acoustic window for examination of the mitral valve. TEE is superior to TTE for examining posterior cardiac structures. MV repair and endocarditis surgery are both high-level indications for intraoperative TEE.

Transesophageal echo

The surgeon needs information about the etiology and functional severity of MR.

Two-dimensional

A thorough 2-D examination using esophageal and transgastric views provides the cornerstone of MV evaluation. Figure 32.8 illustrates the scanning planes through the MV for mid-esophageal views at 0, 60, 90 and 150°.

The diagrammatic representation of Carpentier's classification of MR is shown Figure 32.9.

Color-flow Doppler

MR jets appear red or yellow on color flow Doppler as blood flow is towards the transducer. Doppler studies of MR are highly dependent on loading conditions.

Table 32.2 Anesthetic considerations in acute and chronic mitral regurgitation

	Acute MR	Chronic MR
Preload	Maintain	Maintain
HR	Maintain	Control ventricular rate
Rhythm	Sinus preferable	Generally in AF
SVR	Maintain coronary perfusion	Slight decrease normally tolerated
Contractility	Support	Maintain
PVR	Maintain	Maintain

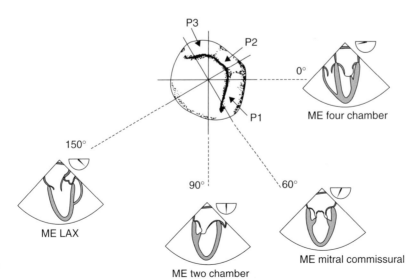

ME four chamber

150°

ME LAX

90°

ME two chamber

60°

ME mitral commissural

0°

P3

P2

P1

Figure 32.8 Mid-esophageal (ME) TEE scanning planes perpendicular to the MV demonstrating the effect of ultrasound plane rotation. P1, anterior scallop of mural (posterior) leaflet; P2, middle scallop of mural leaflet; P3, posterior scallop of mural leaflet. All three scallops of the mural leaflet can usually be visualized with the mid-esophageal 60° (commissural) and 150° views.

Table 32.3 Features of MR to look for on 2-D echocardiography

Leaflets	Structure: are the leaflets thin and pliable?
	Movement: do the leaflets open well?
	Coaptation: is the point where the leaflets meet below annulus?
	Apposition: are both leaflets at same height relative to annulus at the end of systole?
Annulus	Size: is the annulus dilated?
Subvalve	Structure: is there chordal lengthening, thickening or rupture?
LV	Structure: is there LV dilatation?
	Function: is a regional wall motion abnormality affecting papillary muscle function?

Table 32.4 Assessment of the severity of mitral regurgitation

Size of regurgitant jet is proportional to

- Size of orifice, pressure gradient, compliance of LA and LV

Classification of jets

- Orientation (central or eccentric), size of jet (volume of LA filled)

Assessment of severity of MR

- Color flow Doppler in several planes: measure proportion of LA filled by color
- Blunting or reversal of systolic pulmonary venous flow
- Calculation of regurgitant fraction (i.e. difference in forward flow through MV vs. second site such as AV. Note: the AV must be competent)
- Radius of proximal isovelocity surface area (PISA)
  The velocity of blood converging on the MV increases as it nears the regurgitant valve during ventricular systole.
  When the velocity exceeds the Nyquist limit, aliasing occurs
  Interface between aliasing velocities forms a semicircular line
  Radius of curvature of this line (distance between MV orifice and semicircular line) is proportional to the severity of MR

Pitfalls of color-flow Doppler

- Gain settings on echo machine, direction of regurgitant jet, influence of cardiac rhythm, atrial preload, afterload

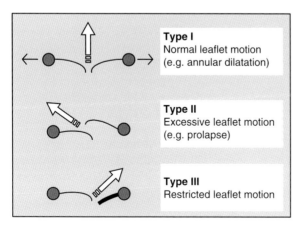

Type I
Normal leaflet motion
(e.g. annular dilatation)

Type II
Excessive leaflet motion
(e.g. prolapse)

Type III
Restricted leaflet motion

Figure 32.9 Diagrammatic representation of the Carpentier classification of MR. The direction of the regurgitant jet (open arrow) often aids determination of the etiology. A central jet is usually due to annular dilatation (type I, normal leaflet motion), whereas an eccentric jet may indicate leaflet prolapse (type II, excessive leaflet motion) or restriction (type III, restricted leaflet motion). The jet is directed "away" from a prolapsing leaflet and "towards" a restricted leaflet.

As the Doppler shift is a function of the cosine of the angle of incidence, the severity of MR may be underestimated in the presence of an eccentric regurgitant jet. For the same reason, if the jet is angled away from the ultrasound plane – the so-called *third-dimension effect* – measurements of the velocity of the regurgitant jet will be underestimated (Figure 24.2).

The apparent severity may be significantly influenced by the hemodynamic state of the anesthetized patient. Relative hypovolemia and reduced SVR may lead to an underestimation of severity. Pharmacological intervention may be required to reproduce near-normal resting conditions (Table 32.4). It is important not to confuse a hypercontractile LV in the setting of reduced afterload with good LV systolic function.

Table 32.5 Surgical solutions for mitral regurgitation

Carpentier type	Mechanism	Solution
Type I	Annular dilatation	Annuloplasty ring
	Leaflet perforation	Pericardial patch
Type II	Posterior leaflet prolapse (cord rupture/ elongation)	Quadrangular resection + simple/sliding annuloplasty
	Anterior leaflet prolapse	Posterior leaflet flip over; Gortex® cords; Edge to edge (Alfieri) apposition
	Commissural prolapse	Resection/plicaton; edge to edge; partial homograft
Type III	Restricted leaflet motion	Challenging – difficult to repair

Table 32.6 Mechanical complications of mitral valve repair

Problem	Mechanism	Discussion
Regurgitation	Leaflet distortion	Badly positioned or ill-sized annuloplasty ring
	Paravalvular leak	Gaps between the sutures or annuloplasty sutures cutting out through the annulus creating a hole between the ventricle and the LA
Stenosis	Severe reduction of MV orifice	May be trivial – all degrees possible
		Repeat surgery may be indicated
LVOT obstruction	Systolic anterior motion of anterior MV leaflet (SAM)	Anterior leaflet moves into LVOT during systole

Surgery

In comparison to MV replacement with complete valve excision, MV repair is associated with better preservation of LV function. There is less risk of bacterial endocarditis, reduced need for postoperative anticoagulation, lower operative mortality and better long-term survival with repair. Virtually all type I and the majority of type II lesions are amenable to satisfactory repair. Common problems and their solutions are shown in Table 32.5.

Emergency surgery in the setting of acute MR carries greater morbidity and mortality. LA enlargement, which typically accompanies chronic lesions and facilitates surgical access, is normally absent in MR of acute onset.

Surgical repair of rheumatic and ischemic (type III) lesions is challenging. Extensive rheumatic leaflet calcification often leaves little pliable leaflet tissue remaining. Partial or complete homograft replacement or the use of pericardial extension has yet to demonstrate long-term stability and durability.

Myocardial ischemia may result in type I (annular dilatation), type II (papillary muscle rupture) or type III (fibrosis of subvalvular apparatus) lesions. The mechanisms of MR are often complex – having more to do with LV function than a structural valve abnormality. Type III lesions caused by fibrotic distortion of the ventricular wall following infarction are particularly difficult to repair. Ischemic rupture of the head of a papillary muscle is best treated with valve replacement as reattachment of the papillary muscle head all too frequently breaks down. Patients with mild MR will often improve with coronary revascularization alone. More severe regurgitation may be better treated with valve replacement with preservation of the subvalvular apparatus.

The mechanical complications of mitral MV include persistent regurgitation, iatrogenic stenosis and LVOT obstruction (Table 32.6).

High-velocity regurgitant jets may produce severe hemolysis. Anemia and hematuria may necessitate repeat surgery. Obstruction of the LVOT secondary to SAM is a rare complication, ranging from severe (failure to wean from CPB) to mild/transient (exertional symptoms). The etiology of SAM is demonstrated in Table 32.7.

Postoperative management specific to the MV repair patient includes anticoagulation, treatment of dysrhythmias and prevention of secondary infection.

● Anticoagulation

Table 32.7 Etiology of systolic anterior motion of the aortic (anterior) mitral leaflet (SAM)

Etiology	Mechanism	Prevention/treatment
Excessive height of the posterior leaflet	Pushes anterior leaflet into LVOT in early systole. As systole progresses the leaflet is carried further and further into the LVOT producing potentially complete obstruction	Ensure that the posterior leaflet is not left too tall when being reconstructed
Small/rigid annuloplasty ring		Use of appropriate ring size
Septal hypertrophy	Reduces LVOT diameter	
LV cavity size	Reduces LVOT diameter	Avoidance of hypovolemia Cautious use of inotropes

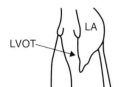

Figure 32.10 The mechanism of LVOT obstruction due to systolic anterior motion of the anterior mitral leaflet.

If in sinus rhythm after surgery:

- long-term anticoagulation not necessary
- evidence for use of anti-platelet therapy weak.

If in AF after surgery:

- Anti-coagulation indicated at the level determined by AF as the primary indication.
- Dysrhythmias
  - AF is the most common dysrhythmia – particularly in the elderly
  - onset often accompanied by hypokalemia/ hypomagnesemia
  - amiodarone has replaced digoxin as first-line therapy
  - amiodarone continued until at least first outpatient clinic visit.
- Infection

The risk of bacterial endocarditis is lower following MV repair than MV replacement.

Changes in international guidelines since the last edition mean that antibiotic prophylaxis is *no longer recommended* before dental, genitourinary and gastrointestinal surgery (see Chapter 63).

Consult local or national formulary for latest details.

Up to 50% of patients in AF before surgery will revert to sinus rhythm when the atrial stretching effect of MR has been corrected. The likelihood and durability of reversion to sinus rhythm are determined by the duration of AF prior to surgery.

Key points

- Mitral subvalvular apparatus is important for normal LV function.
- Tachycardia and *severe* bradycardia are poorly tolerated in MS.
- The assessment of LV function is difficult in severe MR.
- Relative hypovolemia and reduced SVR during anesthesia may lead to underestimation of severity of MR.

Further reading

Bonow RO, Carabello BA, Chatterjee K, *et al*. ACC/AHA 2008 guideline update on valvular heart disease: focused update on infective endocarditis. *J Am Coll Cardiol* 2008; **52**: 676–85.

Wilcox BR, Cook AC, Anderson RH. *Surgical anatomy of the heart*, 3rd edition. Cambridge: Cambridge University Press; 2004.

Tricuspid and pulmonary valve disease

Ving Yuen See Tho

The tricuspid valve

The TV apparatus consists of three membranous leaflets (anterior, septal and posterior), the annulus, papillary muscles, chordae tendinae and the RV. Normal TV area is 7–9 cm^2, making it the largest cardiac valve (Figure 32.1).

Tricuspid stenosis

Tricuspid stenosis (TS) is defined as a fixed obstruction to RV filling due to TV orifice narrowing. It is most commonly of rheumatic origin, often occurring in combination with regurgitation. Rheumatic TS is invariably associated with MV and, sometimes, AV disease. Non-rheumatic TS is rare; causes include congenital atresia or stenosis, right heart tumors (e.g. RA myxoma), endomyocardial fibroelastosis, carcinoid syndrome and prosthetic valve endocarditis.

Clinical features and pathophysiology

Patients present with features of systemic venous hypertension and RV failure – dyspnea, fatigue, peripheral edema, hepatomegaly and ascites. The JVP exhibits a dominant "a" wave and a slow "y" descent. The opening snap and high-pitched, mid-diastolic murmur are best heard at the left lower sternal edge. A pansystolic murmur heard at the same location may indicate concomitant TR (Figure 13.7).

Clinically significant TS develops when TV area <2 cm^2 and the transtricuspid gradient >2 mmHg. The relative changes in RA pressure and RVEDP mirror left heart pressure changes in MS (Figure 33.1).

Investigations

- ECG: tall peaked P waves in II, III and aVF indicate RA enlargement. AF or flutter may be present.

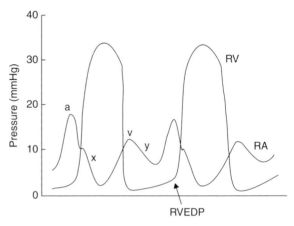

Figure 33.1 RA and RV pressure waveforms in TS. The RAP tracing shows the prominent "a" wave and a slow "y" descent. At end-diastole, there is a significant pressure gradient between the RA and RV due to the elevated RAP and drop in RVEDP.

- 2-D echo: TV leaflets appear thickened with restricted movement. Leaflet doming may be seen. Calcification uncommon. RA grossly enlarged in severe TS.
- Doppler: RV inflow velocity increased, giving rise to elevated pressure gradient.
- Right heart catheterization: determines pressure gradient, CO and valve area.

Anesthetic goals

These are broadly similar to those in MS (Table 32.1). The need for adequate preload – to maintain CO – has to be balanced against the risk of worsening venous congestion. AF and other supraventricular tachycardias may cause rapid cardiovascular collapse and should be treated promptly. Impaired RV coronary blood flow secondary to arterial hypotension should be avoided.

Core Topics in Cardiac Anesthesia, Second Edition, ed. Jonathan H. Mackay and Joseph E. Arrowsmith. Published by Cambridge University Press. © Cambridge University Press 2012.

Table 33.1 Echocardiographic classification of tricuspid stenosis

	Normal	Mild	Moderate	Severe
Mean pressure gradient (mmHg)	1	<2	2–6	>6
Valve area (cm²)	7–9	4–7	2–4	<2

Surgery

The need for surgery is determined by both the severity of symptoms and stenosis (Table 33.1). TV surgery is usually performed with other valve procedures. Surgical options include open commissurotomy and valve replacement. Percutaneous balloon valvotomy is relatively contraindicated in the presence of significant TR.

Triscupid regurgitation

Tricuspid regurgitation (TR) is defined as retrograde blood flow from RV into RA during systole.

Mild or "physiological" TR is present in as many as 70% of asymptomatic, normal individuals. Clinically significant TR is usually functional in origin – occurring secondary to RV enlargement and dilatation of the tricuspid annulus. Primary TR is rare; causes include Ebstein's anomaly, infective endocarditis, anorexogens (e.g. fenfluramine, phentermine), rheumatic heart disease and carcinoid syndrome.

Clinical features and pathophysiology

Isolated TR may be tolerated for many years without symptoms. Like TS, patients with significant TR present with fatigue, dyspnea, exercise intolerance and the features of systemic venous hypertension. The JVP is characterized by a prominent *cv*-wave, an absent *x*-descent, and a sharp *y*-descent (Figure 33.2).

Investigations

- ECG: nonspecific ST segment and T wave abnormalities in the right precordial leads suggest RV dysfunction. Q waves in the inferior or posterior leads may indicate RV infarction. Right axis deviation, tall R waves in V1 and V2, tall P waves and incomplete RBBB suggest pulmonary hypertension (PHT). AF may be seen.

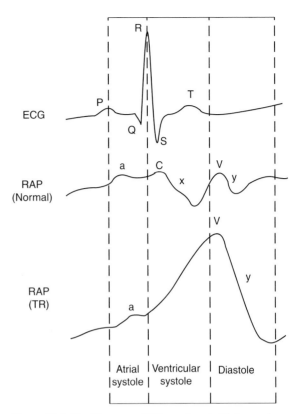

Figure 33.2 The RA pressure (RAP) waveform in TR shows a large *cv*-wave caused by the regurgitant jet, disappearance of the *x*-descent and a steep *y*-descent. The JVP may feel pulsatile with a systolic thrill in patients with severe TR, and may be confused with the carotid pulse.

- Chest radiograph: cardiomegaly due to RV enlargement which fills the retrosternal space on the lateral film. Prominent hilar vasculature.
- Two-dimensional echo: dilated hepatic veins. Diastolic interventricular septum (IVS) flattening in RV volume overload and systolic IVS flattening in RV pressure overload.
- Doppler: estimated PA systolic pressure = 4 × (peak TR jet velocity)² + RA pressure.

Anesthetic goals

As TR is usually secondary, the anesthetic management is dictated by the primary pathology. In general, the hemodynamic goals in patients with TR are similar to those for chronic MR (Table 32.2). Hypercarbia, hypoxia, acidosis and other factors that increase PVR should be avoided and consideration given to the use of pulmonary vasodilators. Airway pressures during

209

Table 33.2 Echocardiographic classification of tricuspid regurgitation

	Mild	Moderate	Severe
TR jet area (cm^2)	<5	5–10	>10
VC width (cm)	–	–	>0.7
PISA radius (cm)	<0.6	0.6–0.9	>0.9
Hepatic vein flow	Systolic dominance	Systolic blunting	Systolic reversal

VC, vena contacta; PISA, proximal isovelocity surface area.

mechanical ventilation should be minimized to avoid reduced RV filling.

Surgery

Patients with moderate to severe functional TR in the presence of a dilated annulus or PHT will require plication or annuloplasty during concomitant left-sided valvular surgery. In patients with primary TR, surgery is indicated when medical therapy fails to control symptoms. If valve replacement is necessary, bioprosthetic valves are preferred as they are associated with a lower risk of thromboembolic complications.

The pulmonary valve

The PV separates the RV outflow tract (RVOT) from the main PA. Its structure mimics that of the AV, comprising three cusps, each with its own sinus of Valsalva, and a sinotubular junction. The normal adult PV has an orifice area of 2 cm^2 and an annulus which has ventricular muscular attachments, making it susceptible to the effects of RV preload and afterload.

Pulmonary stenosis

Pulmonary stenosis (PS), defined as RVOT narrowing, may be subvalvular, valvular, supravalvular or proximal pulmonary arterial. In the majority of cases, PS is congenital and valvular in nature – characterized by commissural fusion, leaflet thickening and doming. PS secondary to leaflet dysplasia, a feature of Noonan's syndrome, is less common. Supravalvular stenosis may be found in congenital rubella and Williams syndromes, while subvalvular or infundibular stenosis is often associated with a VSD (e.g. tetralogy of Fallot,

double chamber RV). Physiological proximal arterial PS is frequently seen in neonates. Acquired PS is rare; causes include carcinoid syndrome and rheumatic heart disease. External compression by a tumor or sinus of Valsalva aneurysm may lead to PV narrowing.

Clinical features and pathophysiology

Patients with mild PS usually present with an asymptomatic systolic murmur detected during routine examination. Children with moderate to severe PS may develop exertional dyspnea, which should prompt early intervention. In contrast, adults often remain asymptomatic regardless of disease severity. The features of severe PS are those of systemic venous congestion and RV failure. A right → left shunt across a patent foramen ovale or ASD may produce cyanosis. A prominent venous a-wave, a precordial thrill and a parasternal heave indicate severe PS (see Figure 13.4).

As in AV stenosis, CO is maintained in the face of worsening PS and increased PV gradient by (right) ventricular hypertrophy. PS is said to be "critical" when CO is inadequate. Diastolic RV dysfunction – reduced RV compliance secondary to RVH, elevated RVEDP and prominent venous a-waves – occurs at an early stage. Analogous to end-stage AS, RV pressure overload causes RV systolic dysfunction – RV dilatation, TR and systemic venous congestion.

Investigations

- ECG: may show evidence of RVH and right axis deviation (RAD).
- Chest radiograph: often normal. In severe PS, the PA may be prominent with decreased pulmonary vascular markings in addition to an enlarged RA and RV.
- Two-dimensional echo: leaflets may be thickened, calcified or dysplastic depending on etiology. Other findings may include systolic doming, post-stenotic PA dilatation and RVH. Muscular subvalvular stenosis and an associated VSD should be excluded when adult PS is suspected.
- Doppler: used to determine the peak velocity and estimate the PV gradient (Figure 33.3).

Anesthetic goals

Patients with PS often have other structural cardiac abnormalities which need to be considered in the perioperative period. In general terms, the hemodynamic goals for patients with PS are similar to those for patients with AS. However, modest elevation of heart rate (80–100 bpm) is preferred to ensure forward flow through the stenotic PV as this occurs predominantly during systole (Table 31.3). Subendocardial blood flow falls as the RV hypertrophies. Aortic root pressure should be maintained to ensure adequate coronary perfusion and prevent RV subendocardial ischemia. In contrast to AS, there is no absolute requirement to maintain "post-stenotic" afterload – i.e. PVR.

Table 33.3 Echocardiographic classification of pulmonary stenosis

	Mild	Moderate	Severe
Peak velocity (m s^{-1})	<3	3–4	>4
Peak gradient (mmHg)	5–26	27–64	>64
Valve area (cm^2)	>1.0	0.5–1.0	<0.5

Pulmonary regurgitation

Pulmonary regurgitation (PR) is defined as retrograde blood flow from PA into RV during diastole. Like TR, mild "physiological" PR is a frequent echocardiographic finding in normal hearts. In adults, pathological PR is most commonly due to annular dilatation secondary to pulmonary hypertension. PR is also a common finding after surgical intervention for PS, and a frequent complication of surgery for tetralogy of Fallot. Consequently, a significant number of patients with severe PR presenting for valve replacement will have already undergone some form of cardiac surgery. Other causes include infective endocarditis, carcinoid syndrome, rheumatic heart disease, PA catheter trauma and connective tissue disorders (e.g. Marfan's syndrome). Congenital causes, such as absent pulmonary valve syndrome, are extremely rare.

Clinical features and pathophysiology

PR is well tolerated in both children and adults, with the majority of patients remaining asymptomatic for

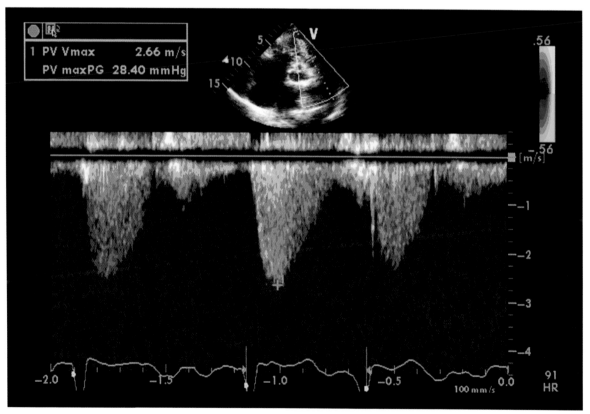

Figure 33.3 Continuous-wave Doppler applied across a stenotic PV. The peak velocity is 2.66 m s^{-1}, which corresponds to a peak gradient of 28.4 mmHg, indicating mild PS.

many years. As the disease progresses, exercise intolerance and clinical features of right heart failure may arise as a result of RV dilatation and failure. Patients presenting late often have irreversible RV dysfunction, which places them at an increased risk of ventricular arrhythmias and sudden cardiac death. Clinical examination may reveal a parasternal heave, a soft diastolic murmur at the left upper sternal edge, and a loud P_2. In the presence of PHT, a high-pitched early diastolic (Graham Steell) murmur may be audible (see Figure 13.6).

Analogous to AR, PR produces RV volume overload with subsequent dilatation and A-V valvular regurgitation. In addition, RV myocardial stretching impairs action potential conduction, leading to QRS complex prolongation and ventricular tachyarrhythmias.

Investigations

- ECG: may show evidence of RVH, RBBB, RAD and arrhythmias.
- Chest radiograph: normal in up to 50% of patients; may show dilatation of the pulmonary trunk and central pulmonary arteries.
- Two-dimensional echocardiography: flattening of IVS during diastole. Severity of PR can be determined by assessing jet width and extent of penetration into the RVOT on color flow Doppler (cf AR).
- Cardiac magnetic resonance: gold-standard imaging modality in the assessment and follow-up of patients with PR. RV function and severity of PR can be accurately assessed to aid timely intervention in patients with chronic PR.

Anesthetic goals

These are broadly similar to those for patients with chronic AR (Table 31.5). While reducing PVR reduces the regurgitant volume, there is no requirement to reduce SVR. As a consequence higher systemic arterial pressures are both desirable and well tolerated.

Carcinoid heart disease

Carcinoid refers to a neoplastic process in amine- and peptide-producing (amine precursor uptake decarboxylation – APUD) cells arising from primitive gut neuroectoderm. In a small proportion of cases, carcinoid may arise in a bronchus or gonad. Carcinoid

syndrome refers to a constellation of symptoms and signs caused when vasoactive substances (e.g. serotonin, prostaglandins, histamine) bypass hepatic and pulmonary inactivation and enter the systemic circulation. The syndrome is characterized by episodic bronchospasm, flushing, GI hypermotility and cardiovascular symptoms.

Clinical features and pathophysiology

Carcinoid heart disease is found in >50% of patients with carcinoid syndrome. Almost all patients with carcinoid heart disease have liver metastases. A gonadal carcinoid may drain directly into the IVC. A significant number of patients with symptoms of heart failure die within a year. One in five patients with carcinoid tumors present with symptoms and signs of right heart failure secondary to TV and PV disease. TR is found in practically all patients, followed by PR, and less commonly TS and PS. Left-sided valvular disease is uncommon and frequently associated with a shunt.

Characteristic pearly white fibrous plaques may be deposited anywhere on the endocardium and may cause restrictive diastolic dysfunction. Subvalvular involvement causes restriction and distortion of valve anatomy.

Investigations

- ECG: abnormalities are often nonspecific. QRS voltage may be reduced.
- Chest radiograph: findings are also usually nonspecific, and include cardiomegaly, prominence of the right heart chambers and pulmonary congestion. Pleural effusions and plaques may be seen late in the disease.
- Two-dimensional echocardiography: the TV and PV leaflets appear thickened, retracted and sometimes fixed in a semi-open position. Thickening and shortening of the subvalvular apparatus is commonly seen. Any right-sided valvular abnormality may be present, but TR is almost universal. Other findings include RA and RV dilatation with evidence of RV volume overload and reduced ejection fraction.
- Doppler: characteristic "dagger-shaped" signal on CWD (Figure 33.4).
- Biochemical screening: serotonin is the major vasoactive amine secreted by carcinoid tumours and is metabolized to 5-hydroxyindoleacetic acid

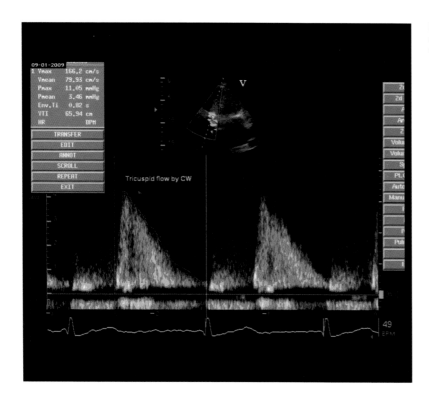

Figure 33.4 Dagger-shaped CWD signal characteristic of severe TR in a patient with carcinoid heart disease.

(5-HIAA), which is excreted in the urine; 24-hour urinary concentration of 5-HIAA is the key to establishing the diagnosis as well as assessing disease progression and response to treatment. Patients with carcinoid heart disease have characteristically much higher levels of urinary 5-HIAA and serum serotonin than those without cardiac involvement.

Surgery

Open valvular replacement is the treatment of choice for carcinoid heart disease and should be considered in symptomatic patients with worsening RV function. Despite recent case reports describing the use of bioprosthetic valves, most surgeons opt for mechanical valves on the grounds that they are more resistant to carcinoid plaque deposition. In patients with hepatic metastases who may require repeated embolization therapy, the use of bioprothetic valves largely removes the risks (i.e. bleeding and thromboembolism) associated with warfarin therapy. Cardiac and carcinoid symptoms should be stabilized on medical therapy prior to surgery. Somatostatin analogs, such as octreotide, which bind to somatostatin receptors have become the mainstay of medical therapy.

Anesthetic goals

These are largely dictated by the primary cardiac lesion and RV function. In addition, measures should be undertaken to prevent excessive release of the vasoactive substances and intractable hypotension – "carcinoid crisis".

Preventing carcinoid crisis

Factors which can precipitate a crisis include hypothermia, hypotension, hypercarbia, emotional stress and certain drugs (e.g. thiopental, atracurium, succinylcholine and morphine).

Benzodiazepines may be used as an induction agent and as an anxiolytic in the immediate preoperative period. Etomidate, steroidal muscle relaxants (e.g. vecuronium, rocuronium, pancuronium) and synthetic opioids (e.g. fentanyl and sufentanil) have all been shown to be safe.

An octreotide infusion should be started before induction of anesthesia and continued into the postoperative period. Additional doses may be given during as necessary. Serum glucose concentration should be monitored closely as octreotide suppresses insulin production and elevates blood glucose levels.

213

Treatment of hypotension

Hypotension may be caused by RV dysfunction, carcinoid crisis, blood loss and post-CPB vasodilatation. Intraoperative TEE, in addition to invasive CVP and PAP monitoring, can assist diagnosis. Hypovolemia should be treated with fluid replacement, and if a carcinoid crisis is suspected, a bolus of octreotide should be administered. Poor ventricular function can be managed safely with exogenous catecholamines, calcium and phenylephrine. Since the introduction of octreotide, previous concerns about catecholamine-induced carcinoid crisis have proven unfounded.

Key points

- TR is most commonly functional, occurring secondary to pulmonary hypertension, RV volume overload and tricuspid annular dilatation.

- Factors increasing PVR should be avoided intraoperatively.
- The main anesthetic challenges in carcinoid heart disease are intraoperative RV failure and carcinoid crisis.

Further reading

Castillo JG, Filsoufi F, Adams DH, Raikhelkar J, Zaku B, Fischer GW. Management of patients undergoing multivalvular surgery for carcinoid heart disease: the role of the anaesthetist. *Br J Anaesth* 2008; **101**(5): 618–26.

Chan KMJ, Zakkar M, Amirak E, Punjabi PP. Tricuspid valve disease: pathophysiology and optimal management. *Prog Cardiovasc Dis* 2009; **51**(6): 482–6.

Minimally invasive cardiac surgery

Andrew C. Knowles and Jose Coddens

In common with many other branches of surgery, there is increasing interest in the use of minimally invasive techniques to perform traditionally "open" cardiac operations. Many of these techniques incorporate incisions other than a full median sternotomy, one-lung ventilation, peripheral CPB, endoscopes and novel endovascular devices. As a consequence, so-called "minimally invasive cardiac surgery" (MICS) presents significant anesthetic challenges and is invariably heavily dependent on intraoperative TEE.

Preoperative assessment

The anesthesiologists should be involved at an early stage in the multidisciplinary assessment of the patient being considered for MICS. The particular points for MICS are:

Cardiovascular

- Define cardiac pathology, quantify ventricular performance and exclude other pathology (e.g. valvular incompetence and venous drainage anomalies).
- Exclude significant extracardiac (e.g. aortic) atheromatous disease.
- Adequacy of femoral vessels for CPB cannulation.

Respiratory

- Airway assessment and pulmonary function tests to ensure the suitability for one-lung ventilation.
- CXR: normal lung fields. Absence of pathology that may impede surgical access.

Gastrointestinal

- TEE is mandatory to guide safe positioning of CPB cannulae.

Table 34.1 Scope of minimally invasive cardiac surgery

Mitral valve repair/replacement

Tricuspid valve repair/replacement

Removal of atrial mass

Repair of atrial septal defect/patent foramen ovale

Redo surgery to avoid repeat sternotomy

- Contraindications to TEE (e.g. carcinoma, stricture, esophageal varices, previous radiotherapy or diverticuli) must be excluded.

Conduct of anesthesia

In addition to routine monitoring, bilateral radial artery pressure monitoring should be considered if an endo-aortic balloon clamp is to be used. Right radial pressure monitoring permits detection of distal balloon clamp migration and innominate artery occlusion. Transcranial Doppler sonography and cerebral oximetry may be used to monitor the cerebral circulation (Chapter 26).

A comprehensive TEE examination is required to confirm patient suitability for a MICS approach.

Either a double-lumen endotracheal tube or a single-lumen tube and bronchial blocker may be used to facilitate one-lung ventilation. Fiberoptic bronchoscopic confirmation of tube position is desirable, and the anesthesiologist should be prepared to deal with hypoxemia during one-lung ventilation. Because the use of internal defibrillation "paddles" may not be possible during MICS, external defibrillation pads should be placed on the patient's chest before surgery.

Core Topics in Cardiac Anesthesia, Second Edition, ed. Jonathan H. Mackay and Joseph E. Arrowsmith. Published by Cambridge University Press. © Cambridge University Press 2012.

Jugular vein cannulation

The right internal jugular vein is preferred. In addition to a standard central venous catheter, the jugular vein is cannulated with a large-bore venous cannula for CPB. In addition, a coronary sinus catheter or pulmonary artery vent may be required.

Ideally, jugular vein cannulation should be performed using ultrasound guidance and TEE confirmation of Seldinger wire passage into the RA. TEE is essential for the correct positioning of the venous CPB cannula and coronary sinus catheter. A small

Table 34.2 Transesophageal echocardiography in MICS

Confirm cardiac pathology

Assess function of cardiac valves

Evaluate chamber size and ventricular function

Inspect ventriculo-arterial and veno-atrial connections

Exclude intracardiac shunt

Exclude pericardial or pleural fluid

Ascending aorta	Diameter <4 cm if endo-aortic balloon clamp to be used Presence of atheroma/dissection

Aortic valve competence – to allow effective delivery of cardioplegia

MICS, minimally invasive cardiac surgery.

dose of heparin (i.e. up to 5000 IU) is often administered up to 5000 IU prior to insertion of the venous CPB cannula to prevent clot formation prior to full heparinization.

Femoral cannulation

In some centers a single venous CPB cannula is introduced via a femoral vein and advanced under TEE guidance across the RA into the SVC. Similarly TEE may be used to aid femoral arterial cannulation and endo-aortic balloon clamp positioning.

Conduct of surgery

Once one-lung ventilation is established, a small right lateral thoracotomy is performed. This provides a clear view of the pericardium, which is then opened to reveal the junction of RA and LA. CPB is then commenced. Any disparity between monitored radial or femoral arterial pressure should prompt immediate TEE examination of the thoracic aorta. Following inflation of the endo-aortic balloon clamp under TEE guidance (long axis ~120° view) cardioplegia can be delivered in to the aortic root.

One or more endosurgical ports are then inserted to allow the introduction of surgical instruments and an endoscopic camera (Figure 34.4). In addition, the surgical field is insufflated with carbon dioxide to hasten the absorption of gaseous emboli post CPB.

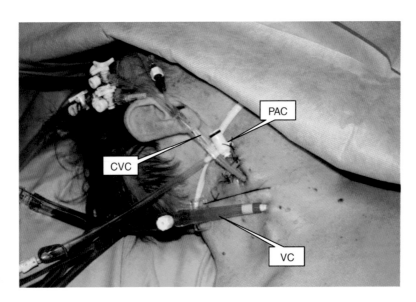

Figure 34.1 Jugular venous cannulation for minimally invasive cardiac surgery. A triple-lumen central venous catheter (CVC), venous CPB cannula (VC) and pulmonary artery catheter introducer sheath (PAC) have been inserted.

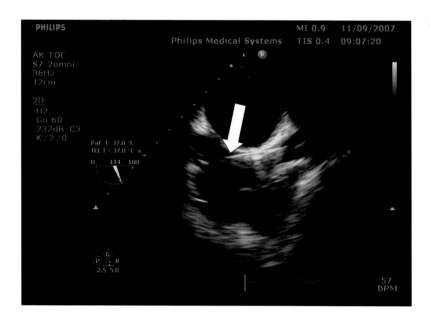

Figure 34.2 J wire in right atrium.

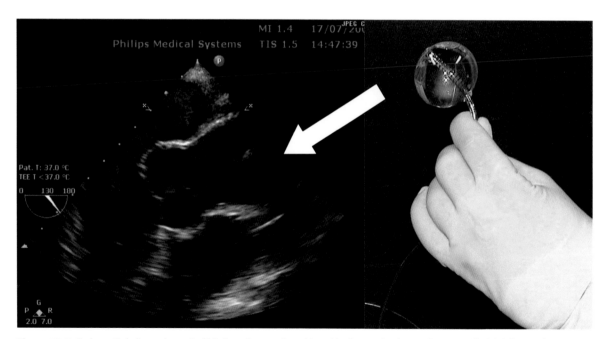

Figure 34.3 Endo-aortic balloon clamp. (Left) Balloon (arrowed) positioned in the proximal ascending aorta. (Right) Balloon inflated with saline.

Aortic clamping

Unique to MICS is the equipment used to replace the conventional aortic cross-clamp. Either an endo-aortic balloon clamp (inserted via femoral or sub-clavian artery) is inflated in the proximal ascending aorta or an external clamp is introduced via the right chest and the ascending aorta clamped externally. Whereas the latter method is used under direct vision, the former requires TEE guidance. Cardioplegia can be delivered either via the distal port of the

217

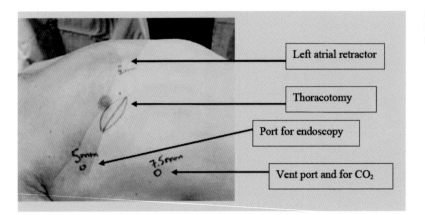

Figure 34.4 Location of thoracic incisions for minimally invasive cardiac surgery.

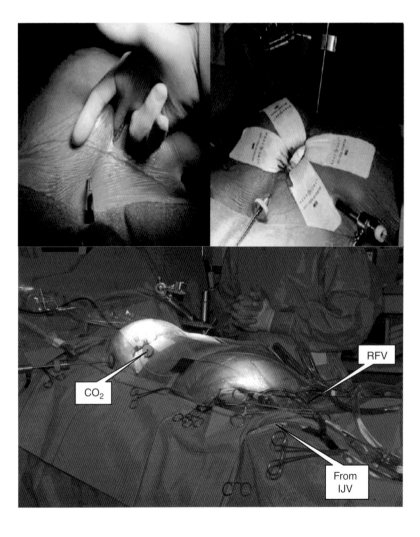

Figure 34.5 Sub-mammary incision with CO_2 insufflation line (CO_2) and camera port. Arterial cannula in right femoral artery. Cannula from right femoral vein (RFV) to line from right internal jugular vein (IJV) via "Y" connector.

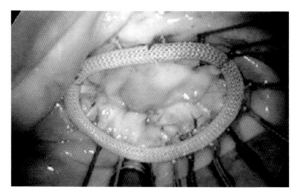

Figure 34.6 Surgeon's view of completed minimally invasive mitral valve repair.

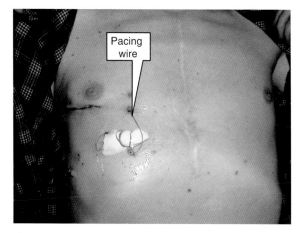

Figure 34.7 Minimally invasive mitral valve repair in a patient who has previously undergone conventional cardiac surgery. Note the healed sternotomy wound and use of temporary ventricular epicardial pacing wires.

endo-aortic balloon clamp or via a separate aortic root cannula. In addition, a coronary sinus catheter may be used to deliver retrograde cardioplegia.

Post cardiopulmonary bypass

Following completion of surgery the usual requirements for discontinuation of CPB apply. At this time one-lung ventilation may still be requested to facilitate thorough inspection of the heart to confirm hemostasis. Temporary expansion of the right lung prior to weaning from CPB increases PaO_2 and reduces hypoxic pulmonary vasoconstriction. This maneuver may improve hemodynamics in the presence of RV dysfunction. TEE is then used to assess the adequacy of any valvular repair, assess ventricular performance and exclude aortic dissection.

Before moving the patient to the ICU, the jugular venous CPB cannula is removed with the patient in

Table 34.3 Putative benefits of minimally invasive cardiac surgery

Patient satisfaction

Decreased length of hospital stay

Decreased wound burden/less trauma

Eliminate sternal wound complications

Improved surgical visualization

the reverse Trendelenburg position to reduce venous pressure. Care must be taken to avoid air entrainment during this procedure.

After oral and endobronchial suction, the double-lumen endobronchial tube (if used) is exchanged for a normal, single-lumen endotracheal tube.

Postoperative care

The path to tracheal extubation continues in a traditional fashion, with patients requiring a median of 24–48 h of ICU/high-dependency care. In most centers opioids are used as the main analgesic supplemented with local anesthetic wound infiltration, intercostal nerve blocks or paravertebral blocks. Although non-steroidal anti-inflammatory drugs are often very efficacious, their use is typically delayed until normal renal function is confirmed. Patients undergoing MICS appear to achieve full mobilization quickly, allowing the opportunity for early hospital discharge.

Key points
- MICS may be the option of choice for patients undergoing redo cardiac surgery.
- Anesthesiologists should be involved in multidisciplinary preoperative planning.
- The anesthesiologist plays a pivotal role in the provision of myocardial protection.

Further reading

Galloway AC, Schwartz CF, Ribakove GH, *et al.* A decade of minimally invasive mitral repair: long-term outcomes. *Ann Thorac Surg* 2009; **88**(4): 1180–4.

Lebon JS, Couture P, Rochon AG, *et al.* The endovascular coronary sinus catheter in minimally invasive mitral and tricuspid valve surgery: a case series. *J Cardiothorac Vasc Anesth* 2010; **24**(5): 746–51.

Modi P, Hassan A, Chitwood WR Jr. Minimally invasive mitral valve surgery: a systematic review and meta-analysis. *Eur J Cardiothorac Surg* 2008; **34**(5): 943–52.

35

Redo surgery

Jon Graham

Redo surgery has greater risk compared to first operations. The frequency of redo valve surgery continues to increase but there has been a reduction in reoperations for coronary artery disease. This decrease is probably due to percutaneous interventions and use of mammary and other arterial conduits in preference to saphenous vein grafts. Improvements in surgical, anesthetic and perfusion techniques have reduced morbidity and mortality.

↑**RISK**
- more complex surgery
- advanced patient age
- advanced cardiac disease
- advanced comorbidities

Anesthetic preparation

Redo surgery is often more complex and prolonged. It requires dissection of adhesions with increased likelihood of damage to the RV and existing conduits, blood loss and coagulopathy. It is essential for the anesthesiologist to be prepared for the increased likelihood of hemodynamic instability and hemorrhage in the pre-CPB period (Table 35.1).

Safe resternotomy

In redo cardiac surgery, the back of the sternum may be close to, or even attached to, the aorta, innominate vein, RA, RV and coronary bypass grafts. Injury to these structures during resternotomy may result in hemorrhage and cardiovascular instability. Damage to a patent arterial graft supplying the LAD territory may result in myocardial ischemia, dysrhythmia or cardiac arrest.

Table 35.1 Anesthetic priorities for redo surgery

Preoperative	Communication with surgeon and perfusionist Confirm strategies to reduce bleeding and transfusion Consideration of monitoring required (e.g. TEE, PAFC)
Before sternotomy	Substantial venous access Avoid conduit harvest sites (e.g. when radial artery grafts planned) Attach external defibrillation/pacing electrodes Draw up heparin Check immediate availability of blood CPB circuit primed and perfusionist in operating room Femoral vessels prepared, exposed or cannulated
During sternotomy	Consider "head up" (reverse Trendelenberg) position to reduce RV volume Consider GTN infusion Discuss discontinuation of mechanical ventilation with surgeon
Post CPB	Anticipate hemodynamic support required (e.g. inotropes, IABP) Anticipate difficulties with hemostasis

GTN, glyceryl trinitrate; IABP, intra aortic balloon pump.

An essential part of surgical planning is an assessment of the risk of damaging structures posterior to the sternum during resternotomy. In addition to reviewing the coronary angiogram and lateral CXR, chest CT or CT angiography may be required. In the event of massive hemorrhage or graft injury during

Core Topics in Cardiac Anesthesia, Second Edition, ed. Jonathan H. Mackay and Joseph E. Arrowsmith. Published by Cambridge University Press. © Cambridge University Press 2012.

Table 35.2 Surgical access for CPB following catastrophic hemorrhage

Stage of procedure	Cannulae *in situ*	Surgical strategies
Immediately following sternotomy	No femoral vessel cannulation	Cannulation of femoral artery Cardiotomy sucker → femoral artery CPB
	With femoral vessels cannulated	Femoro – femoral CPB
Later in dissection	No aortic or femoral artery cannulation	Cannulation of femoral artery Cardiotomy sucker → femoral artery CPB
		Cannulation of aorta Cardiotomy sucker → aorta CPB
		Cannulation of aorta and RA Conventional CPB
	With aortic or femoral artery cannulation	Cardiotomy sucker → aorta CPB, or Cardiotomy sucker → femoral artery CPB

resternotomy, immediate commencement of CPB is usually required. In these circumstances, adhesions and bleeding may make aortic and RA cannulation difficult. Pre-sternotomy precautions range from identifying and preparing the femoral vessels to femoral cannulation and institution of peripheral CPB. The latter approach allows graft injury or catastrophic hemorrhage to be managed with greater safety but requires sternal and mediastinal dissection to be performed in a heparinized patient.

Resternotomy is typically performed using a specialized oscillating saw. Dissection is then required to expose the aorta and RA for cannulation and CPB. In the event of major hemorrhage, direct pressure should be applied to the site of bleeding and heparin given. The route to CPB largely depends on preparations made prior to sternotomy (Table 35.2).

It should be borne in mind that redo surgery can be performed without median sternotomy. Mitral surgery may be performed via a right thoracotomy (Chapter 32); limited coronary bypass grafting via a left thoracotomy; and AV replacement via a mini-sternotomy or using transfemoral or transapical catheter techniques (Chapter 42).

Dysrthymia

Damage to the heart or existing bypass grafts during resternotomy and manipulation of the heart during subsequent dissection may cause hemodynamically significant dysrhythmias. Because exposure may be insufficient to allow use of internal defibrillator paddles, external defibrillator pads must be placed on the patient's lateral chest walls before induction of anesthesia.

Myocardial protection

Effective myocardial protection is more difficult in redo surgery in the presence of patent coronary artery bypass grafts. Retrograde cardioplegia, delivered via the coronary sinus, is commonly used in this situation because:

- anterograde cardioplegia is unlikely to reach myocardium supplied by a patent internal mammary artery graft;
- following application of an AXC, proximal vein grafts and a mammary artery graft will continue to supply oxygenated blood to the myocardium; temporary graft occlusion may be required to achieve adequate myocardial protection with retrograde cardioplegia;
- administration of anterograde cardioplegia through existing vein grafts may result in distal atheroembolism.

Because retrograde cardioplegia alone is unlikely to provide adequate RV protection, a combination of retrograde and anterograde cardioplegic techniques is used.

221

Table 35.3 Strategies to reduce bleeding and transfusion requirements in redo cardiac surgery

Preoperative	Consider erythropoietin, iron supplementation, Consider autologous blood donation Consider ceasing antiplatelet drugs Investigate and correct existing coagulopathy
Pre-sternotomy	Consider use of lysine analog Consider normovolemic hemodilution Establish cell salvage
Postoperative	Salvage of shed mediastinal blood Avoid hypertension

Managing hemorrhage

Strategies to reduce hemorrhage and transfusion requirements during redo cardiac surgery are summarized in Table 35.3 and discussed in more detail in Chapter 58.

Key points

- Redo cardiac surgery is associated with increased morbidity and mortality.
- Preoperative planning and effective risk management in the pre-CPB phase are essential.
- The presence of patent coronary artery bypass grafts has important implications for myocardial protection in redo cardiac surgery.

Further reading

Cohn LH (Ed). *Cardiac Surgery in the Adult*, 3rd edition. New York: McGraw-Hill; 2007.

Fazel S, Borger MA, Weisel RD, *et al.* Myocardial protection in reoperative coronary artery bypass grafting. *J Card Surg* 2004; **19**(4): 291–5.

Machiraju VR. How to avoid problems in redo coronary artery bypass surgery. *J Card Surg* 2004; **19**(4): 284–90.

Aortic dissection

Andrew C. Knowles and John D. Kneeshaw

Acute aortic dissection is one of the most common cardiothoracic surgical emergencies. An understanding of pathophysiology and aims of surgical management is essential.

Description

Aortic dissection is the separation of the intima and media of the aortic wall. It usually occurs as a result of a small tear in the intima (typically in the ascending aorta) where blood enters under pressure, separates the layers of the aortic wall and creates a false lumen. The dissection can involve part or the entire aortic circumference. Propagation of the dissection is dependent on absolute blood pressure, pulse pressure and the rate of systolic arterial pressure rise ($\delta P/\delta t$). Distal propagation is common and, as the dissection progresses, may occlude branches and compromise organ blood supply. Proximal extension is less common but may result in aortic valve disruption, coronary artery occlusion or rupture into the pericardium. A subsequent "re-entry" tear in the intima allows blood entering the false lumen to re-enter the true lumen. The causes of aortic dissection are listed in Table 36.1.

Anatomy

The aorta is divided into four main segments – the ascending, the arch, the descending (thoracic) and the abdominal aorta. The wall of the aorta comprises three layers. The inner layer of intima consists of endothelium supported by a basement membrane. The media, which is made up of smooth muscle, collagen and elastin, provides both structural integrity and elasticity. The outer adventitia contains the *vasa vasorum* that supply nutrients to the arterial wall.

Table 36.1 Causes of aortic dissection

Arterial hypertension	Advanced age, smoking, dyslipidemia, cocaine use
Connective tissue disorders	Marfan's syndrome, Ehlers-Danlos syndrome, Turner's syndrome, hereditary fibrillinopathies
Pregnancy	
Iatrogenic intimal injury	Aortic cannulation, IABP, cardiac catheterization
Hereditary vascular diseases	Bicuspid aortic valve, coarctation
Aortic aneurysm	

Classification

Aortic dissection is classified according to both duration of symptoms and anatomy. Aortic dissection is termed "acute" if the diagnosis is made within 2 weeks of the initial onset of symptoms – otherwise it is termed "chronic".

The Stanford classification is based on involvement of the ascending aorta (type A dissection involves the ascending aorta; whereas type B does not) and is useful because of the contrasting treatment options. The International Registry of Acute Aortic Dissection (IRAD) reports hospital mortality for patients with type A dissection of 27% if managed surgically and 56% if treated with medical therapy alone. Nearly 1 in 3 patients with type A dissection will die after admission to hospital. In contrast, type B dissection, which is predominantly managed without surgery, has an overall hospital mortality of 13%.

The DeBakey classification further subdivides dissection on an anatomic basis (see Figure 36.1). Of note, Michael DeBakey (1908–2008) suffered an

Core Topics in Cardiac Anesthesia, Second Edition, ed. Jonathan H. Mackay and Joseph E. Arrowsmith. Published by Cambridge University Press. © Cambridge University Press 2012.

aortic dissection aged 97. Despite initially refusing the operation, he became the oldest patient to undergo the surgery for which he was famous.

Subsequent studies have shown that intramural hemorrhage, intramural hematoma and luminal ulcers may be signs of evolving dissection or additional dissection subtypes. This has resulted in the etiological classification system (Table 36.2).

Clinical features

Acute aortic dissection can present with a diverse range of signs and symptoms (Table 36.3). As diagnosis may be difficult, a high index of suspicion is necessary. The high mortality associated with acute aortic dissection mandates early diagnosis and confirmation of anatomic distribution – critical in deciding whether surgery is indicated.

Diagnosis

Delay in establishing a diagnosis is associated with significant morbidity. It is important to determine the location of the initial tear, the extent of propagation and the severity of associated complications (aortic root dilatation, AR, MI and tamponade). Diagnostic tests include:

- *ECG*: mandatory in a patient with chest pain, but cannot differentiate between acute MI secondary to coronary artery disease from ostial coronary involvement in acute dissection.
- *CXR*: although the mediastinum may be widened, a normal CXR does not exclude dissection.
- *Specialized imaging*: contrast aortography provides unrivalled information about coronary artery involvement and was historically considered the gold standard; it is rarely used nowadays. Contrast spiral CT, MRI and TEE are now the key to both confirming the diagnosis and determining management strategy. Table 36.4 compares the diagnostic value of each of the imaging techniques.
  - *CT*: is rapid and non-invasive but requires the administration of nephrotoxic contrast media.
  - *TEE*: can be performed at the bedside but requires sedation or general anesthesia, and is highly operator-dependent. It is rarely

Table 36.2 Etiological classification of aortic dissection

Class 1	Classic aortic dissection with an intimal flap between true and false lumen
Class 2	Medial disruption with formation of intramural hematoma or hemorrhage
Class 3	Discrete or subtle dissection without hematoma, eccentric bulge at tear site
Class 4	Plaque rupture leading to aortic ulceration, penetrating aortic atherosclerotic ulcer with surrounding hematoma, usually sub-adventitial
Class 5	Iatrogenic and traumatic dissection

Reproduced with permission from Svennson *et al. Circulation* 1999; 99: 1331–6.

DeBakey ...	I	II	III
Stanford ...	A	A	B

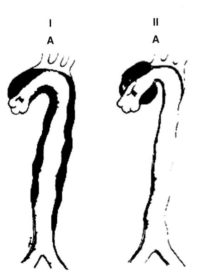 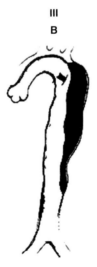

Figure 36.1 Classification of aortic dissection. In DeBakey type I, the intimal tear occurs in the ascending aorta with propagation of the dissection to the arch and distal thoracic aorta (DTA). In type II, a tear in the ascending aorta does not propagate beyond the innominate artery. In type III, the tear is beyond the origin of the left subclavian artery. The Stanford classification simply divides dissections into either type A or type B. Type A involves the ascending aorta regardless of the extent of the dissection. Type B lesions involve the DTA distal to the origin of the left subclavian artery.

Table 36.3 Symptoms and signs of acute aortic dissection

Pain	Sharp, tearing or ripping – maximal intensity at time of onset Retrosternal in proximal dissection Interscapular/ back in descending dissections Site of pain may move as dissection advances Abdominal pain may indicate mesenteric ischemia
Syncope	Severe pain, cardiac tamponade or obstruction of cerebral vessels Up to 20% have syncope without typical pain or neurologic findings
Dyspnea	Severe aortic regurgitation Extrinsic bronchial constriction MI secondary to coronary artery involvement
Other	*Hemoptysis:* bronchial compression/rupture *Hoarseness:* recurrent laryngeal nerve compression
Stroke	Carotid/subclavian (vertebral) artery involvement in dissection Altered conscious level
Shock	↑HR, ↓BP, diaphoresis, oliguria, cyanosis Anxiety and pain may cause ↑HR and ↑BP
Pulse deficits	Unequal upper limb blood pressures "White arm" – subclavian artery occlusion
Murmur	Aortic regurgitation – new early diastolic murmur Heart sounds may be soft in the presence of pericardial effusion

conducted outside cardiac surgical centers because tachycardia and hypertension during insertion of a TEE probe may worsen prognosis. In addition, isolated lesions in the distal ascending aorta and aortic arch may not be visible.

- *MRI:* provides high-resolution images but is time-consuming and is not universally available.
- *Biomarkers:* there is currently no readily available biomarker for acute aortic dissection. Damage to the aortic media in aortic dissection causes release of smooth muscle myosin heavy chains into the circulation. While a positive biomarker assay may raise the index of suspicion in a patient with an atypical presentation, it will not replace advanced imaging techniques.

Management

Type B dissection is usually managed conservatively (i.e. medically). The majority heal by fibrosis but ultimately a small number may require surgery. Surgery in the acute phase is only required in the presence of vital organ (e.g. renal, mesenteric) ischemia, aneurismal dilatation, aortic rupture or continuing pain. Endovascular stenting is increasingly being used as a less invasive alternative to surgery in patients with chronic type B dissection. Endovascular therapies may be particularly useful in the amelioration of malperfusion syndromes in both type A and type B aortic dissection.

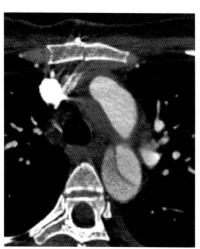
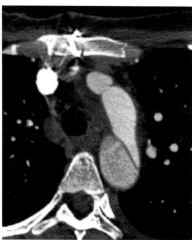

Figure 36.2 Contrast-enhanced CT of a patient after repair of an acute type A aortic dissection. The dissection flap can clearly be seen in the aortic arch and proximal descending aorta. An ascending aortic interposition graft is used to remove the risk of tamponade and dissection of the coronary artery ostial.

Table 36.4 Comparison of diagnostic value of imaging techniques in aortic dissection

	Spiral contrast CT	TOE	MRI
Sensitivity	>95%	Up to 99%	95–100%
Specificity	87–100%	89%	95–100%
Classify dissection	+++	++	+++
Differentiate true and false lumens	++	++	++
Localize intimal tear, flap and re-entry sites	+	+	++
Assess side branch involvement	+++	++	+++
Detect and assess AR	–	+++	++
Detect pericardium or pleural extravasation	+++	+++	+++
Coronary artery involvement	–	+	+

By contrast, type A dissection requires immediate surgery to prevent death by proximal extension (MI, tamponade or severe AR). Proximal extension is prevented by replacing a segment of the ascending aorta with a synthetic interposition graft. Additional procedures such as AV replacement or repair and CABG may also be required.

Initial management

Blood pressure control prior to surgery is paramount. This mandates invasive monitoring and the use of analgesics, anxiolytics and vasoactive drugs (e.g. vasodilator and β-blockers). Reducing the rate of aortic pressure change (i.e. dP/dt) reduces propagation driving force. A combination of drugs may be required to reduce myocardial contractility, HR and SVR (Table 36.5).

Patient transfer

Most patients with aortic dissection are admitted to hospitals without cardiac surgical facilities. Patients with type A dissection must be transferred to a specialist unit for further investigation and treatment. Effective medical therapy must be initiated prior to transfer. Substantial IV access and invasive arterial are mandatory. Central venous access may be desirable. Aggressive blood pressure control must continue during transfer. For this reason a medical escort with experience in advanced resuscitation and use of vasoactive drugs is essential. Ideally all medical notes, the results of any investigations and cross-matched blood should accompany the patient.

Table 36.5 Pharmacological blood pressure control in acute aortic dissection

β-Blockers	Esmolol: An ideal agent; high β_1 specificity, short duration of action, easily titratable Labetalol: combined α and β-blockade
Vasodilators	GTN: coronary artery dilatation desirable SNP: more potent and predictable action; reflex tachycardia may be troublesome
Analgesics	Opioids: pain control should not be overlooked Avoid NSAIDs

Anesthesia

Surgery should be expedited once the diagnosis is confirmed. Whenever possible a brief history should be taken and physical examination performed. At least six units of cross-matched blood must be available.

A rapid sequence induction should be considered in every case. The choice of anesthetic technique should take into account the need for hemodynamic stability – particularly during laryngoscopy. As the surgical approach is invariably via a sternotomy, a single-lumen ETT tube is used.

Monitoring

In addition to standard monitoring procedures, a left upper limb arterial line is preferred because of the risk of innominate artery involvement. If the arch vessels are to be isolated, a femoral arterial line is required.

A large-bore (8F) central venous cannula is often used for rapid transfusion. Repair of aortic dissection is a category I indication for TEE, and should be considered in every case (Chapter 24). Nasopharyngeal and bladder temperature monitoring should be used if deep hypothermic circulatory arrest (DHCA) is anticipated (Chapters 60 and 61).

Surgery

The patient is placed in a supine position with the groins exposed and prepared for possible femoral cannulation. Full anticoagulation and femoral artery cannulation are often undertaken prior to median sternotomy to allow sucker-CPB in the event of rupture or to facilitate arch replacement. Resistance to heparin is not uncommon. Where possible, conventional atrial-aortic CPB is then established. If DHCA is required to facilitate aortic arch repair, selective anterograde or retrograde cerebral perfusion may be considered. In many centers lysine analogs have replaced aprotinin as a means of reducing bleeding and transfusion requirements.

Postoperative care

The patient should remain sedated and mechanically ventilated for the initial postoperative period. Meticulous blood pressure control is essential to reduce stress on surgical suture lines and aortic wall. Due to the importance of maintaining CO, greater emphasis is placed on vasodilatation rather than reducing myocardial contractility. There is a high incidence of coagulopathy and postoperative hemorrhage. Bedside tests of coagulation (e.g. thromboelastography, platelet function analyzer) are useful in guiding blood component therapy. It is important to normalize core temperature, acid base status, hematology and biochemistry. Assessment of neurologic function should be performed prior to tracheal extubation.

Complications

- Myocardial dysfunction (dysrhythmia, impaired contractility)
- Embolic injury (thrombus, atheroma, air)
- Hemorrhage (coagulopathy, surgical)
- neurologic dysfunction (dissection, paraplegia, embolic stroke, hypoperfusion)
- Renal impairment (dissection, low cardiac output state)
- Respiratory impairment

Key points

- Acute aortic dissection can present with a diverse range of symptoms and signs. A high index of suspicion may be required to make the diagnosis.
- Type A dissection is a surgical emergency associated with high mortality.
- Mortality is due to aortic rupture, tamponade, myocardial infarction or massive stroke.
- Tight blood pressure control is mandatory in aortic dissection.

Further reading

Emrecan B, Tulukoğlu E. A current view of cerebral protection in aortic arch repair. *J Cardiothorac Vasc Anesth* 2009; **23**(3): 417–20.

Erbel R, Alfonso F, Boileau C, *et al.* Task Force on Aortic Dissection, European Society of Cardiology. Diagnosis and management of aortic dissection. *Eur Heart J* 2001; **22**(18): 1642–81.

Svensson LG, Kouchoukos NT, Miller DC, *et al.* Society of Thoracic Surgeons Endovascular Surgery Task Force. Expert consensus document on the treatment of descending thoracic aortic disease using endovascular stent-grafts. *Ann Thorac Surg* 2008; **85**(1 Suppl): S1–41.

Tsai TT, Nienaber CA, Eagle KA. Acute aortic syndromes. *Circulation* 2005; **112**(24): 3802–13.

Tsai T, Trimarchi S, Nienaber C. Acute aortic dissection: Perspectives from the International Registry of Acute Aortic Dissection (IRAD). *Eur J Vasc Endovasc Surg* 2009; **37**(2): 149–59.

Chapter

37

Aortic arch surgery

Andrew C. Knowles and Coralie Carle

The arch of the aorta is a continuation of the ascending aorta at the level of the sternal angle. It lies posterior to the manubrium sterni and anterior to the trachea. The arch therefore begins *proximal* to the brachiocephalic artery and ends *distal* to the left subclavian artery and ligamentum arteriosus. The three branches of the arch are the brachiocephalic, left common carotid and left subclavian arteries. The arch becomes continuous with the descending aorta at the lower border of the body of T_4. Conditions affecting the aortic arch include dissection, traumatic rupture and aneurysmal dilatation. Aortic dissection is discussed in Chapter 36.

Traumatic rupture

Indirect or blunt (deceleration) injury to the aorta is much more common than penetrating (e.g. gunshot or stabbing) injury. Road traffic accidents (RTA) and falls from significant heights account for the majority of non-penetrating injuries. In fact aortic injury is second only to head injury as the cause of death following RTA.

In 95% cases the site of aortic rupture is the isthmus – the site of insertion of the ligamentum arteriosum – where the relatively fixed arch joins the more mobile descending thoracic aorta (DTA). The condition carries considerable immediate mortality (85%), with the majority dying before they reach hospital. A patient will only survive until hospital admission when the rupture is contained by the aortic adventitia or surrounding structures. Surgical repair of a tear at the isthmus is undertaken via a left thoracotomy, involving the same principles and practice as those for surgery on the DTA. On rare occasions, delaying surgery may be necessary to avoid the risks of CPB in the presence of other injuries.

Aneurysm

An aortic aneurysm is a permanent, localized dilatation of the aorta with a diameter that is at least 50% greater than normal. The aneurysm can be described as fusiform (symmetrical dilatation of the whole circumference, resembling a narrow cylinder) or saccular (dilatation of a segment of the circumference, resembling a small sac). The incidence increases with age and has been reported as 6 per 100 000 person-years.

Pathogenesis

Aneurysms form in areas of weakness within the aortic wall and gradually increase in size until rupture. This occurs in accordance with Laplace's law (Chapter 31) applied to a cylinder where wall tension is proportional to transmural pressure and aortic radius. Aortic arch aneurysms, which represent 10% of thoracic aortic aneurysms, enlarge faster and rupture more frequently than other thoracic or abdominal aneurysms. The etiology of thoracic aortic aneurysms is shown in Table 37.1.

Clinical features

Aneurysms commonly present as an incidental finding during investigation for other conditions or at necropsy following sudden death. Symptoms are typically absent until enlargement encroaches on surrounding structures (Table 37.2). The sudden onset of severe retrosternal or interscapular pain radiating to the neck or jaw may indicate impending rupture. The presence of hemodynamic collapse and signs of hemothorax or hemopericardium suggest established rupture.

Core Topics in Cardiac Anesthesia, Second Edition, ed. Jonathan H. Mackay and Joseph E. Arrowsmith. Published by Cambridge University Press. © Cambridge University Press 2012.

Table 37.1 The etiology of thoracic aortic aneurysms

Atherosclerosis	The main cause of thoracic aortic aneurysms
	The principal co-factor is hypertension
	Aortic wall ischemia and decrease in medial nutrient supply occurs as a result of:
	  – gross intimal thickening with massive fibrosis and calcification
	  – an increase in the distance between endothelium and media
	  – adventitial fibrosis and *vasa vasorum* occlusion

Cystic medial degeneration	Fragmentation and loss of elastic tissue Loss of smooth muscle cells
Congenital	Marfan's and Ehlers-Danlos syndromes Presents in younger age group Defective synthesis of glycoprotein fibrillin, a component of the elastic tissue of the medial layer
Inflammatory	Polyarteritis Kawasaki's disease, Takayasu's aortitis, Behçet's arteritis Destroys the medial layer, leading to wall weakness
Infective	Bacterial, fungal, syphilis Destroys the medial layer, leading to wall weakness

Mechanical	Post (aortic) stenotic dilatation
	Turbulence distal to a bicuspid AV or aortic coarctation may result in aneurysmal dilatation
	Post-traumatic – blunt chest trauma (RTA)
	               – aortic cross-clamping
	               – post use of intra-aortic balloon pump

Table 37.2 The origins of symptoms associated with thoracic aortic aneurysm

Sympathetic efferents	Ascending: precordial pain Arch: jaw and neck pain Descending: interscapular pain
Mediastinum	Hemopericardium, hemothorax
Recurrent laryngeal nerve	Hoarseness
Trachea	Stridor
Esophagus	Dysphagia
SVC	Edema and engorgement
Aortic root dilatation	AR, congestive heart failure
Asymptomatic	Incidental finding

Diagnosis

Imaging techniques are used to confirm the location, size, rate of growth, impact on adjacent structures and operability of the aneurysm.

- *CXR* This is generally poor in detecting arch pathology and may appear "normal". It may be difficult to differentiate an aneurysm from other mediastinal masses. Enlargement of the aortic knuckle and tracheal deviation are suggestive of an aneurysm, whereas mediastinal widening suggests dissection or rupture.

- *Aortography* This was previously considered the gold standard for delineating the aortic arch and its branches. In view of the likely age of the patient, the potential benefits of concurrent coronary angiography must justify the risks associated with the use of contrast media.

- *CT* This is the most widely used non-invasive imaging technique. Image acquisition times with spiral CT are of the order of a few seconds. Contrast enhancement may be required to demonstrate rupture and extravasation.

- *MRI* This can provide clear images of the aorta and its branches without contrast media. Prolonged image acquisition sequences may not, however, be suitable for hemodynamically unstable patients.

229

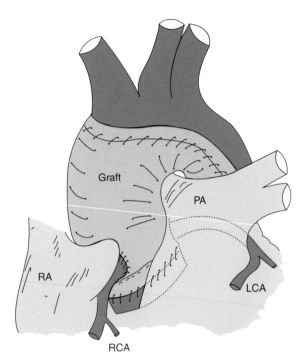

Figure 37.1 Example of a patch graft repair of the ascending aorta and aortic arch. The distal end of the graft is attached to the under surface of the arch. The right (RCA) and left (LCA) coronary arteries have been reimplanted into the proximal end of the graft.

- *TEE* This can be performed (under sedation) relatively rapidly at the bedside but incomplete imaging of the aortic arch limits its utility. Ventricular and valvular performance can be readily assessed.

Surgery

Surgical repair of the aortic arch is performed in the supine position via a median sternotomy. The procedure typically involves the replacement of either part or all of the arch with re-implantation of the arch vessels. In many cases an aortic (Carrel) patch is used to anastamose the arch vessels to an aortic graft (Figure 37.1). Surgical repair of the distal aortic arch and DTA are discussed in Chapter 36.

Anesthetic management

Patients presenting acutely with a ruptured aortic arch aneurysm should be managed using the approach outlined for Type A aortic dissection in Chapter 36.

Patients with a chronic aortic aneurysm require careful assessment to guide both the extent and timing of surgery. The rate of aneurysmal expansion is an exponent of aortic diameter. Even in the absence of symptoms, aortic diameter dictates prognosis and, therefore, the timing of intervention.

Preoperative assessment

The goal of preoperative assessment prior to elective surgery is the exclusion of concomitant cardiovascular, respiratory, renal and neurologic disease. These are very common in aortic surgery patients and the principal causes of perioperative morbidity and mortality.

Arterial hypertension should be well controlled before surgery to minimize the risks of perioperative hemodynamic instability and myocardial ischemia. Coronary artery disease is also common and concomitant surgical revascularization may be necessary.

Respiratory function should be formally assessed and optimized (smoking cessation, humidified oxygen, inhaled bronchodilators, physiotherapy and aggressive treatment of intercurrent infection).

Preoperative renal impairment, which is common in this typically elderly population, is an independent predictor of postoperative renal failure and, in turn, mortality.

Significant carotid artery stenosis (>80%) increases the already elevated risk of neurologic injury associated with aortic arch surgery. The extent of the planned surgery together with the methods of cerebral protection to be used must be discussed with the surgical team.

In the emergency situation, the time for preoperative evaluation is limited. In most cases the role of the anesthesiologist is to establish substantial venous access, initiate invasive monitoring and resuscitate the patient.

Monitoring

In addition to standard intraoperative monitoring and TEE, bladder or rectal temperature monitoring should be used if DHCA is anticipated. In practice femoral and bilateral radial arterial pressure monitoring is used if the arch vessels are to be isolated. The use of non-invasive cerebral monitoring (e.g. NIRS) may assist in detecting and limiting neurologic injury.

Induction

The maintenance of hemodynamic stability is paramount. A standard cardiac anesthetic technique is appropriate for most elective cases. A rapid sequence induction should be considered in emergency cases.

Cerebral protection

Aortic arch surgery requires the temporary interruption of anterograde cerebral blood flow. The primary method for providing protection against cerebral injury is DHCA. A period of circulatory arrest for up to 30–40 minutes at a body temperature of 15–18°C is tolerated by the majority of patients. More recently two techniques have been developed with the aim of reducing this cerebral morbidity on the basis that some flow is better than no flow. These are retrograde cerebral perfusion (RCP) and selective anterograde cerebral perfusion (SACP). The intention of these techniques is to ensure some oxygen delivery to the brain while normal (anterograde) flow is interrupted. The disadvantages of DHCA include a relatively short "safe period" and the harmful effects of profound hypothermia (Chapter 61).

Postoperative care

Postoperative care is essentially the same as that following repair of the ascending aorta (Chapter 36).

The key principles include: maintenance of normothermia, blood pressure control, maintaining hemodynamic stability and correction of coagulopathy.

Key points

- Traumatic or aneurysmal rupture of the aortic arch is a surgical emergency with a high mortality.
- Preoperative optimization is essential for patients undergoing elective aortic arch surgery.
- Surgery of the aortic arch is likely to involve circulatory arrest and may involve the use of selective cerebral perfusion techniques.

Further reading

Emrecan B, Tulukoğlu E. A current view of cerebral protection in aortic arch repair. *J Cardiothorac Vasc Anesth* 2009; **23**(3): 417–20.

Singh S, Hutton P. Anaesthesia for thoracic and thoraco-abdominal aortic disease – Part 2: Anaesthetic management and neuroprotection. *Curr Anaesth Crit Care* 2006; **17**(1–2): 109–17.

Descending thoracic aorta surgery

38

David Riddington and Harjot Singh

The descending thoracic aorta (DTA) extends from the distal aortic arch to the diaphragm. Conditions of the descending thoracic aorta (DTA) that present for surgery can be broadly classified into four main groups (Table 38.1).

The term "aortic syndrome" is often used to describe the spectrum of aneurysm, dissection, intramural hematoma and penetrating aortic ulcer. The focus of this chapter is anesthesia for elective DTA surgery.

Table 38.1 Conditions affecting the descending thoracic aorta

Aneurysm

Dissection

Rupture

Developmental anomalies (coarctation and vascular rings)

Aneurysm

The etiology of DTA aneurysm is multifactorial and is summarized in Table 37.1 (Chapter 37).

A contained rupture secondary to infection or trauma results in a false or pseudo aneurysm – a collection of thrombus and connective tissue lying outside the wall of the aorta.

The Crawford classification (type I–IV) depends on the extent of involvement of thoracoabdominal aorta (Figure 38.1).

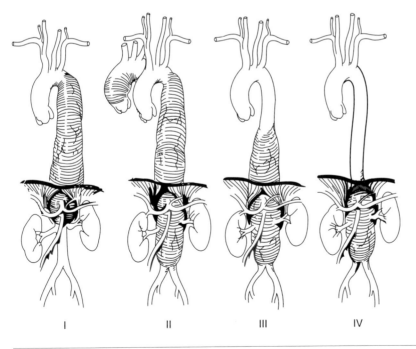

Figure 38.1 The Crawford classification of descending thoracic aortic aneurysms.

I   II   III   IV

Core Topics in Cardiac Anesthesia, Second Edition, ed. Jonathan H. Mackay and Joseph E. Arrowsmith. Published by Cambridge University Press. © Cambridge University Press 2012.

Clinical features

DTA aneurysms are commonly asymptomatic and an incidental finding on CXR or echocardiography. Nonspecific pain in the chest, back or abdomen suggests aneurysmal expansion, impending rupture or leakage. Other symptoms and signs include:

- dyspnea, wheeze, cough or recurrent pneumonia – bronchial compression
- hemoptysis – bronchial or pulmonary parenchymal erosion
- hoarseness – left recurrent laryngeal nerve compression
- dysphagia – esophageal compression
- Horner's syndrome – stellate ganglion compression
- acute hemodynamic compromise – rupture into pleura, pericardium or esophagus. Some compression symptoms may be postural.

Natural history

Aneurysmal growth rate is non-linear, increasing as the aneurysm grows in size. Patients with a DTA diameter ≥6 cm face a 14% annual risk of rupture or dissection. Surgery is recommended when the maximal diameter is 6.0–6.5 cm. Because aneurysmal growth in Marfan's syndrome is both accelerated and unpredictable, surgery may be considered at an earlier stage. Surgery may also be indicated for leaking or ruptured aneurysm, persistent pain or pseudoaneurysm formation.

Surgical approaches

Surgical access is typically achieved using a left thoracic postero-lateral incision in the fifth intercostal space with excision of the sixth rib to allow access to proximal DTA and distal aortic arch. Depending upon the extent of aneurysm, the incision may be extended into the abdomen. The diaphragm is taken down peripherally and the retroperitoneal space exposed. Management of the systemic circulation during surgery can be conveniently considered in three categories:

1. The "clamp and sew" or "clamp and run" technique (Figure 38.2).
2. Partial bypass:
   - application of cross-clamp with decompression of the proximal aorta and provision of distal aortic perfusion by a shunt (Figure 38.3)
   - left heart bypass (Figure 38.4)
   - partial femoral-femoral bypass (Figure 38.5).
3. Full CPB with DHCA (Figure 38.6).

Endovascular approaches

Endovascular techniques have emerged as an alternative to open surgery in those patients with suitable aortic anatomy, particularly those with significant comorbidities (Table 38.2).

Anesthetic management

The anesthetic management of these patients is extremely challenging for the following reasons:

- co-existing coronary artery disease is common and accounts for half of early deaths;

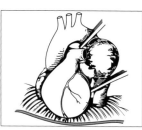

Advantages
Simplest method

Disadvantages
Very dependent on short cross–clamp time
Distal organ ischemia
Proximal arterial hypertension
Metabolic acidosis

Figure 38.2 DTA surgery with proximal and distal aortic cross–clamp.

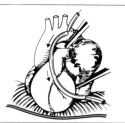

Advantages
Controls proximal hypertension primarily by
↓ LV afterload, ↓ myocardial wall stress
↑ splanchnic and renal perfusion
Prevention of metabolic acidosis
Heparin-coated conduit therefore systemic anticoagulation not required

Disadvantages
No facility for oxygenation or maintaining normothermia

Figure 38.3 DTA surgery with proximal and distal cross-clamps and simple shunt.

233

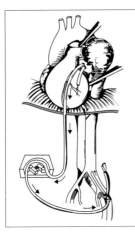

Advantages
Improved spinal cord / renal perfusion
Ability for rapid infusion of warm fluids
Supplementary extracorporeal oxygenation

Disadvantages
Requires full anticoagulation
Risk of vascular injury
Air / particulate embolism – stroke
Interference with the operative field
↑ operative time
↑ risk of major hemorrhage

Figure 38.4 DTA surgery with left heart (left atrial – femoral) bypass. In some centers the system incorporates a closed venous reservoir.

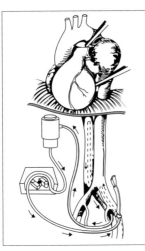

Advantages
No clutter of operative field
Supplementary oxygen is provided
Circuit can be used for full CPB if required
Distal perfusion cardiac output independent

Disadvantages
Systemic heparinization
Requires venous reservoir, oxygenator and roller pump

Figure 38.5 DTA surgery with femoral-femoral bypass.

	Advantages
Temp 15°C	Minimal aortic dissection
	No proximal AXC
	Bloodless surgical field
MAP < 20 mmHg	*Disadvantages*
	↑ Blood loss

Figure 38.6 DTA surgery with full CPB and deep hypothermic circulatory arrest.

- application of an aortic cross-clamp (AXC) induces significant; hemodynamic changes.
- the high risk of spinal cord, renal and mesenteric injury;
- the potential for coagulopathy and massive blood loss;
- the requirement for one-lung ventilation for left thoracotomy.

Vascular access

A multi-lumen central venous cannula and large-bore single-lumen venous cannulae are essential. An 8F central venous cannula and a large (14G or larger) peripheral venous cannula should be considered the minimum. A rapid infusion device capable of delivering warmed fluid at up to 500 ml min^{-1} is highly desirable.

Arterial cannulation proximal *and* distal to the aneurysm and proposed sites of aortic cross-clamp application is essential. Because the left subclavian artery may be obstructed during proximal aortic clamping the right radial artery is preferred for proximal pressure monitoring. Because the left femoral artery is commonly used for femoral bypass, the right femoral artery is preferred for distal pressure monitoring.

Table 38.2 Indication, contraindications, benefits and complications of endovascular approaches to DTA

Prerequisites

- Anatomical location of aneurysm
- Morphology of aneurysm
- Adequate distal vascular access
- 10–15 mm non-tapering aorta at proximal and distal end of aneurysm (so-called "neck length")
- Minimal abdominal and thoracic aortic tortuosity

Contraindications

- Inadequate vascular access
- Excessive aortic tortuosity
- Excessive aortic mural thrombus
- A neck length <10 mm distal to left subclavian artery or above celiac or mesenteric arteries

Putative benefits

- Applicable in patients unsuitable for open repair
- Obviates need for thoracotomy and major dissection
- Decreased incidence of paraplegia
- Decreased blood loss
- Decreased systemic inflammatory response
- Decreased ICU and hospital stay

Complications

- Renal failure, bowel ischemia, lower limb ischemia
- Stroke, paraplegia, myocardial infarction
- Aortic rupture
- Vascular access site complications
- Endoleak (graft ends, between graft segments or from segmental arteries)
- Graft migration and erosion
- Graft infection

Monitoring

Insertion of a silicone lumbar (L3–4 or L4–5) CSF drain 14–16G is considered to be both a therapeutic and a monitoring maneuver. Monitoring spinal cord function is discussed below.

The use of a PAFC is a matter for personal preference and institutional policy. If used, however, additional venous access will be required. It should be borne in mind that a PAFC catheter positioned in the left pulmonary artery may produce spurious PAWP values during one-lung ventilation.

Transesophageal echocardiography is frequently used to monitor cardiac function, check bypass cannula placement and detect malperfusion during femoral

bypass. Aneurysmal compression of the esophagus should be considered a relative contraindication to TEE.

One-lung ventilation

Isolation of the left lung and one-lung ventilation (OLV) facilitates surgical exposure and minimizes trauma to the non-dependent (i.e. left) lung. The anesthesiologist should be alert to the possibility of aneurysmal compression of the upper airways. Direct enquiry about postural respiratory symptoms, a review of radiological investigations and preoperative lung function testing (flow volume loop) may facilitate diagnosis and guide airway management strategy.

- Double-lumen tube (DLT): protects the dependent (i.e. right) lung from soiling from blood from left intrapulmonary hemorrhage caused by surgical retraction in a heparinized patient. Using a right-sided DLT has the advantage of avoiding instrumentation of the left main bronchus, but care must be taken to avoid occlusion of the right upper lobe bronchus. Using a left-sided DLT eliminates concern about right upper lobe ventilation; however, aneurysmal compression of the left main bronchus may hinder placement and risks aneurysm rupture. The DLT is usually replaced with a single-lumen endotracheal tube at the end of the procedure. In cases of difficult intubation or airway edema the tube may be withdrawn 2–3 cm and the bronchial cuff deflated.
- Bronchial blocker: may be used if lung isolation cannot be achieved with a DLT. The major drawbacks to this approach are less secure lung isolation and limited access for endobronchial suction. If bronchus blocker use is contemplated, the largest possible endotracheal tube (i.e. ≥8.0 mm) should be used to permit easy introduction of a fiberoptic bronchoscope and positioning of the blocker.

Implications of aortic cross-clamping

Most surgical approaches to DTA aneurysms involve application of an aortic cross-clamp (AXC). The proximal clamp is placed either distal to the left subclavian or between the left subclavian and left common carotid arteries. Clamping the proximal DTA produces a more marked increase in aortic arch pressure than clamping the abdominal aorta. The anesthesiologist must be aware of the other physiological consequences of both AXC application and AXC removal (Table 38.3).

Table 38.3 Physiological affects of aortic cross-clamp application and removal

Clamp application	Clamp removal
↑ SVR – sudden impedance to aortic outflow	↓ SVR – "declamping shock"/reactive hyperemia
↑ LVEDP (preload) – blood volume redistribution	Pulmonary hypertension
↑ Contractility and ↑ coronary blood flow	Sequestration of blood in capacitance vessels
↑ Catecholamines, renin and angiotensin	Ischemic metabolite actions
↑ Intraspinal (CSF) pressures	Alteration of liver, kidney and gut integrity

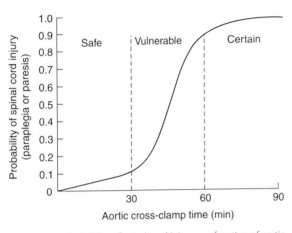

Figure 38.7 Probability of spinal cord injury as a function of aortic cross-clamp duration without distal perfusion. The likelihood of injury is <10% below 30 min, and >90% above 60 min. The risk of paraplegia is greatest following surgery for Crawford types I and II DTA.

Table 38.4 Spinal cord injury: patient and perioperative factors

Patient factors	Perioperative factors
Spinal cord blood supply	Duration of AXC
Patient age	Degree/duration of hypotension
Aortic dissection/rupture	Reperfusion injury
Aneurysm location and extent	CSF pressure
	Loss of intercostal/lumbar arteries
	Hyperglycemia

The net effects of AXC application are elevation of proximal aortic pressure, LVEDP, PAWP, PAP and CVP, and a reduction in distal aortic pressure, spinal cord perfusion pressure and renal blood flow. The magnitude of these effects is dependent upon AXC application site, the extent of collateral blood flow, LV function, diastolic filling pressures, vasodilator use and distal perfusion techniques. Hypertension proximal to the AXC may be managed with SNP, GTN, volatile agents, esmolol, phentolamine or diazoxide. Vasodilators should be discontinued in anticipation of AXC removal to prevent "declamping shock". Clear communication between surgeon, anesthesiologist and perfusionist allows time for preparation to deal with the hemodynamic and metabolic consequences of AXC removal. Typical measures include intravenous fluid, vasopressors, inotropes, sodium bicarbonate and increased minute ventilation. Slow or partial release of the AXC by the surgeon may be used to reduce the deleterious effects of abrupt AXC removal.

Spinal cord protection

Paraplegia secondary to spinal cord ischemia is the most feared and devastating complication after otherwise successful DTA surgery. The condition is unpredictable and affects up to 30% of patients (Figure 38.7). It most commonly manifests immediately after surgery, but the onset may be delayed by up to 3 weeks. Although many causes have been suggested it is difficult to predict which patients will develop paraplegia. Spinal cord ischemia is thought to occur as a result of both intraoperative factors, such as reduced perfusion pressure, spinal cord edema and increased CSF pressure following AXC application, and patient factors, such as vascular anatomy and the presence of collaterals (Table 38.4).

The gravity of this complication warrants some discussion of the vascular anatomy of the spinal cord. The arterial supply of the spinal cord is derived from the anterior and posterior spinal arteries (Figure 38.8). The anterior spinal artery is a midline structure formed from branches of each vertebral artery. It supplies the whole of the cord anterior to the posterior grey columns. The smaller posterior spinal arteries are derived from the inferior cerebellar arteries. In its rostral course, spinal branches of the

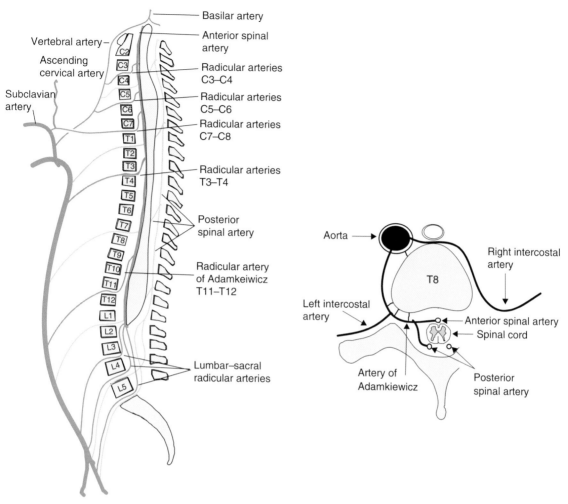

Figure 38.8 The arterial supply of the spinal cord. The largest of the anterior radicular arteries in the artery of Adamkiewicz has a variable origin between T5 and L1 (left). Ligation of intercostal arteries may cause bleeding and reversal of distal blood flow, resulting in spinal ischemia (right). Reproduced with permission from Sidhu VS. Anterior spinal artery syndrome following coronary artery bypass graft surgery. In: Arrowsmith JE, Simpson J (Eds). *Problems in Anesthesia: Cardiothoracic Surgery*. London: Martin Dunitz; 2002.

vertebral, deep cervical, intercostal, lumbar, iliolumbar and lateral sacral arteries support the spinal arteries. The anterior radicular arteries, which vary in size and number, tend to be larger in the T4–T9 region; the largest of these is known as the artery of Adamkiewicz. It has a characteristic hairpin bend that perfuses the spinal cord distal to its junction with the anterior spinal artery. It is this portion of the spinal cord, where collateral blood supply is minimal, that is at the greatest risk of ischemia from prolonged cross-clamping or sustained hypotension. Although the artery may arise anywhere from T5 to L1, the origin lies between T5 and T9 in 15% of patients, and between T9 and T12 in 60% of patients (i.e. above T12 in 75% of patients). The 25% of patients in whom

it arises below T12 are at increased risk of intraoperative spinal ischemia.

Strategies to reduce the incidence and severity of spinal cord injury include physical measures, neurophysiological monitoring and pharmacological neuroprotection (Table 38.5).

Current evidence suggests that CSF drainage reduces the incidence of paraplegia. A spinal drain is inserted in the lumbar region before the operation and CSF pressure is maintained at 10 mmHg, by free perioperative drainage (Figure 38.9). The drain should be clamped during patient movement and positioning and must be checked regularly to ensure patency. In the absence of neurologic deficit, the drain can be clamped 24 h after surgery and removed 48 h after surgery.

It is prudent to avoid removing the catheter while the patient is coagulopathic or if the CSF is heavily blood-stained. Lower motor neuron signs in the legs (flaccidity, weakness and areflexia) should prompt rapid

Table 38.5 Strategies to reduce the risk of spinal cord ischemia and paraplegia

Physical	Increased spinal cord perfusion pressure CSF drainage Distal perfusion techniques and reducing AXC time Reattachment of intercostal and lumbar arteries – Consider superior and inferior supply to the spinal cord by subclavian and internal iliac artery Hypothermia (systemic 32–33°C, epidural, intrathecal)
Monitoring	Distal arterial pressure monitoring – avoidance of hypotension *SSEP monitoring:* slow response time and provides no information about anterior horn cell function *MEP monitoring:* readings affected by volatile agents and neuromuscular blockade
Pharmacological unlicensed indications	*Systemic agents:* corticosteroids, barbiturates, naloxone, calcium antagonists, glutamate antagonists, free radical scavengers *Intrathecal agents:* papaverine, magnesium

intervention – maneuvers to further reduce CSF pressure and increase arterial blood pressure. The development of new neurologic signs one or more days after surgery should prompt consideration of epidural hematoma and infection, and requires urgent investigation (i.e. MRI and neurosurgical assessment).

The structural and functional integrity of the spinal cord can be monitored throughout surgery using evoked potential monitoring. Both motor evoked potentials (MEP) and somatosensory evoked potentials (SSEP) are established methods of spinal cord monitoring. MEPs, which assess descending pathways, are elicited by transcranial stimulation of the motor cortex. The evoked potentials are recorded either in epidural space or from a leg muscle. Multi-level SSEPs, which assess ascending pathways, are produced by stimulating a peripheral nerve (usually the posterior tibial nerve) and recording cervical or cortical responses. SSEPs are subject to the influence of hypothermia (↓ conduction velocity, ↓ amplitude, ↑ latency), anesthesia and electrical interference. MEP and SSEP monitoring have high sensitivity but relatively low specificity for spinal cord ischemia.

Patient positioning

Prolonged right lateral position demands scrupulous attention to pressure points, neurovascular bundles and eyes.

Postoperative analgesia

Surgery on the thoracoabdominal aorta is associated with considerable postoperative pain. The use of

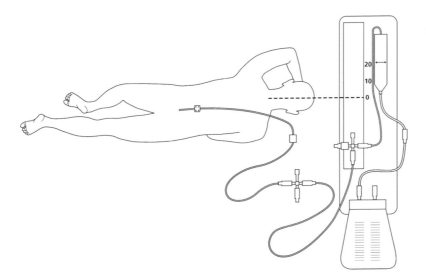

Figure 38.9 CSF drainage system. Serious side effects occur in less than 1%.

intraoperative epidural analgesia in the setting of systemic heparinization is discussed in Chapter 72. Hypotension and the difficulty of distinguishing between the neurologic effects of central neuraxial block and postoperative paraplegia dictate that solutions for epidural infusion should contain an opioid in combination with a relatively low concentration of local anesthetic. In some centers an epidural catheter is only sited when postoperative coagulopathy has been corrected and paraplegia excluded. Alternatives to epidural analgesia include continuous paravertebral blockade and intravenous opioids. The high risk of postoperative renal dysfunction and ARF precludes the routine use of NSAIDs.

Dissection

Dissection of the DTA is usually managed medically (Chapter 36). Indications for surgery in Stanford type B (DeBakey type III) dissection include rupture, ongoing pain, expansion and end-organ ischemia.

Transection

Aortic rupture may follow sudden deceleration, or blunt or penetrating injuries. The majority (80%) occur just distal to the origin of the left subclavian artery near the attachment of the ligamentum ateriosum – a point of aortic fixation where shearing forces are maximal. Regardless of cause, the prognosis is poor.

It is considered acute if free hemorrhage or peri-aortic hematoma is less than 8 days old. The diagnosis is based on a pressure differential between upper and lower extremity, loss of aortic arch contour, mediastinal widening and a high index of suspicion. Signs and symptoms of aortic rupture are nonspecific.

The diagnostic triad of increased upper extremity arterial pressure, decreased lower extremity arterial pressure, and mediastinal widening is present in more than 50% patients. Other symptoms and signs are given in Table 38.6.

The treatment is surgical – either by an open or an endovascular approach. Expectant (medical) management may be appropriate in a stable patient with other injuries (e.g. head injury). Open surgical repair involves excision with end-to-end anastomosis, patching or interposition grafting. In most cases, a "clamp and sew" technique is used, although shunting or partial CPB may be considered.

In a recently published review of over 7000 patients with traumatic aortic transection, mortality

Table 38.6 Symptoms, signs and radiological features of acute aortic transection

Symptoms	Dyspnoea Retrosternal/interscapular pain Hoarseness and dysphagia
Signs	Penetrating wound/rib or sternal fractures Upper extremity BP >> lower extremity BP Left pleural effusion Systolic flow murmur over precordium or medial to left scapula
Radiological features	Mediastinal widening Left-sided pleural collection Associated rib, clavicular or sternal fractures

was significantly lower in patients who underwent endovascular repair compared with open repair (9% vs. 19%). Spinal cord ischemia, end-stage renal disease and infective complications were also less common after endovascular repair.

Coarctation

Coarctation – narrowing of the aorta near the subclavian artery – may present in adulthood with upper extremity hypertension, radio-femoral delay and weak or absent pulse in the lower extremities (Figure 51.2). There may be proximal or distal aneurysmal enlargement and other cardiac abnormalities, notably bicuspid aortic valve. The CXR may demonstrate rib notching secondary to the development of large collaterals.

Traditionally, coarctation has been treated with open surgical repair via a left thoractomy. This may involve simple resection and end-to-end anastomosis, or more complex procedures such as prosthetic patch aortoplasty or subclavian flap aortoplasty. More recently, however, endovascular techniques have been employed in cases where contemporaneous procedures (e.g. aortic valve replacement) are not required.

Key points

- Surgery for DTA has substantial morbidity and mortality.
- A multidisciplinary discussion of surgical approach, distal perfusion and neuroprotective strategies is essential.

- Paraplegia following DTA surgery may occur despite all precautions.
- Endovascular approaches to DTA repair are associated with reduced morbidity and mortality.

Further reading

Arrowsmith JE, Ganugapenta MSSR. Intraoperative brain monitoring in cardiac surgery. In Bonser R, Pagano D, Haverich A (Eds.), *Brain Protection in Cardiac Surgery*. London: Springer-Verlag; 2011. pp. 83–111.

Cina CS, Abouzahr L, Arena GO, *et al.* Cerebrospinal fluid drainage to prevent paraplegia during thoracic and thoracoabdominal aortic aneurysm surgery: a systemic review and meta-analysis. *J Vasc Surg* 2004; **40**: 36–44.

Fedorow CA, Moon MC, Mutch WA, Grocott HP. Lumbar cerebrospinal fluid drainage for thoracoabdominal aortic surgery: rationale and practical considerations for management. *Anesth Analg* 2010; **111**(1): 46–58.

Murad MH, Rizvi AZ, Malgor R, *et al.* Comparative effectiveness of the treatments for thoracic aortic transaction. *J Vasc Surg* 2011; **53**(1):193–9.

Rousseau H, Bolduc JP, Dambrin C, *et al.* Stent-graft repair of thoracic aortic aneurysms. *Tech Vasc Interventional Rad* 2005; **8**: 61–72.

San Norberto García EM, González-Fajardo JA, *et al.* Open surgical repair and endovascular treatment in adult coarctation of the aorta. *Ann Vasc Surg* 2010; **24**(8): 1068–74.

Permanent pacemakers and implantable defibrillators

Maros Elsik and Simon P. Fynn

Widening indications for implantation have increased the prevalence of permanent pacemakers (PPMs) and implantable cardioverter defibrillators (ICDs). As these devices have become more complex, the potential for perioperative interference and reprogramming has grown. Patients treated with these devices are at increased risk of perioperative morbidity and mortality during cardiac surgery. The evidence base to guide perioperative management of patients with cardiac devices is derived predominantly from case series and expert opinion rather than prospective, randomized clinical trials.

Permanent pacemakers

In its most basic form, a PPM consists of a generator (incorporating electrical circuits and a battery) and a pacing lead, designed to sense cardiac electrical activity and, if necessary, deliver a cardiac stimulus to prevent bradycardia. Technological advances have resulted in increasing complexity of devices and leads, with complex algorithms regulating cardiac activity.

PPMs most commonly consist of an atrial and/or a RV lead. Leads must have the capacity to sense and pace the respective chamber, depending on device set-up and programming. Leads most commonly have single (unipolar) or dual (bipolar) electrodes, the latter separated by a few millimeters. In a unipolar lead setup the implanted generator serves as an electrode completing the electric circuit. Unipolar pacing produces noticeable pacing spikes on the standard ECG because of the large size of the electrical vector (representing the physical space between a unipolar cardiac lead and the pacemaker generator). For the same reason, unipolar sensing is more susceptible to interference, such as that caused by thoracic skeletal muscle contraction. A bipolar set-up is less prone to

interference though a pacing spike may not be easily seen on a standard filtered ECG.

Conditions for which there is evidence or general agreement that implantation is beneficial, useful and effective are summarized in Table 39.1.

Device classification provides a concise means of communicating chamber or chambers paced, chamber or chambers in which native depolarizations are sensed and how sensing affects pacing pattern. The original three-position code (1974) has evolved to the five-position North American Society of Pacing and Electrophysiology/British Pacing and Electrophysiology Group (NASPE/BPEG) generic pacemaker code (Table 39.2).

The original fixed-rate VOO ventricular pacemakers were superseded by VVI systems, which sense spontaneous ventricular depolarization and inhibit the delivery of unnecessary ventricular stimuli. VVI pacemakers have a ventricular escape interval, defined as the time after a paced or sensed beat that a pacemaker waits before delivering a pacing stimulus. VVI pacing is appropriate for chronic AF with slow ventricular rate. Most currently implanted PPMs are dual-chamber devices (DDD) capable of pacing and sensing both atrium and ventricle. These versatile devices are more hemodynamically efficient than ventricular pacing alone. Rate-adaptive DDDR devices, which enable HR and CO to increase during exercise, are more physiological. Additional programmable features of DDDR devices include maximal upper rate, minimal lower rate, activity threshold, rate response, and acceleration and deceleration times. Mechanisms of rate adaptation vary. Piezoelectric crystals can detect vibration and body movement. Other sensors detect acceleration, ECG events (e.g. QT interval), myocardial contractility, minute ventilation volume, central venous blood temperature or oxygen saturation

Core Topics in Cardiac Anesthesia, Second Edition, ed. Jonathan H. Mackay and Joseph E. Arrowsmith. Published by Cambridge University Press. © Cambridge University Press 2012.

Table 39.1 Indications for permanent pacemaker implantation

Acquired A-V block (in adults)	Third-degree A-V block with symptomatic bradycardia or documented asystole, neuromuscular disorders, following A-V node ablation
Chronic bifascicular and trifascicular block	Intermittent second-degree (Mobitz type II) A-V block, intermittent third-degree A-V block
AV block following acute MI	Persistent second-degree A-V block; transient third-degree A-V block; need not be symptomatic
Sinus node dysfunction	Documented symptomatic bradycardia; frequent sinus pauses
Prevention of tachycardia	Sustained, pause-dependent VT in which efficacy of pacing has been documented
Carotid sinus hypersensitivity	Recurrent syncope due to carotid sinus stimulation
Heart failure	Cardiac resynchronization therapy – symptomatic heart failure (NYHA class >2) with impaired ventricular function with widened QRS complex
Specific conditions	Hypertrophic cardiomyopathy; idiopathic dilated cardiomyopathy; cardiac transplantation – persistent bradycardia

ACC/AHA/HRS 2008 Guidelines for Device-Based Therapy of Cardiac Rhythm Abnormalities. Indications for pacing in children, adolescents and patients with congenital heart disease (not shown) are broadly similar.

Table 39.2 The NASPE/BPEG five-position generic pacemaker code

Position	I	II	III	IV	V
Category	Chamber(s) paced	Chamber(s) sensed	Response to sensing	Rate modulation	Antitachycardia functions
Code	O	O	O		O
letters	A	A	T	O	P
	V	V	I	R	S
	D	D	D		D

NASPE, North American Society of Pacing and Electrophysiology; BPEG, British Pacing and Electrophysiology Group. O, none; A, atrium; V, ventricle; D, dual (A+V); T, triggered; I, inhibited; R, rate modulation; P, anti-tachycardia; S, shock.

Table 39.3 Examples of common permanent pacemaker modes: fixed-rate pacing (AOO, VOO and DOO) is rarely used in permanent pacemakers

Code	Indication	Function
AAI	Sinus node disease Normal A-V conduction	Demand atrial pacing
VVI	Bradycardia without need for preserved A-V conduction (e.g. AF)	Demand ventricular pacing
DDD	Bradycardia Impaired A-V conduction	Maintains A-V concordance
DDDR	Bradycardia Impaired A-V conduction	Maintains A-V concordance Exercise response

(Table 39.3). Some PPMs have the ability to automatically switch pacing mode. These may be of use in patients with paroxysmal AF where the device will switch from DDD to VVIR or DDIR mode.

Cardiac resynchronization therapy

Cardiac resynchronization therapy (CRT) is used in advanced heart failure and requires an additional lead positioned via the coronary sinus designed to pace the

Table 39.4 Indications for ICD therapy

Primary prevention of sudden cardiac death

Coronary artery disease

Non-ischemic dilated cardiomyopathy

Long QT syndrome

Hypertrophic cardiomyopathy

Arrhythmogenic RV dysplasia/cardiomyopathy

Noncompaction of the LV

Primary electrical disease (idiopathic VF, short-QT and Brugada syndromes, and catecholaminergic polymorphic VT)

Idiopathic VT

Advanced heart failure and cardiac transplantation

Secondary prevention of sudden cardiac death

Sustained VT

Coronary artery disease

Non-ischemic dilated cardiomyopathy

Hypertrophic cardiomyopathy

Arrhythmogenic RV dysplasia/cardiomyopathy

Genetic arrhythmia syndromes
Syncope with inducible sustained VT

Source: American College of Cardiology/American Heart Association/Heart Rhythm Society 2008 Guidelines for Device-Based Therapy of Cardiac Rhythm Abnormalities (*Circulation* 2008;117: e350–408).

LV with a predetermined delay from the RV in an attempt to resynchronize LV and RV contraction and improve cardiac function. ICDs can be used in combination with CRT.

Implantable cardiac defibrillators

ICDs are complex devices that have the ability to differentiate cardiac rhythms and deliver anti-tachycardia pacing therapy as well as DC shocks to cardiovert or defibrillate the myocardium. The external casing is most commonly made from titanium (Figure 39.1). The UK National Institute for Health and Clinical Excellence (NICE) Guidelines have reinforced the increasing role of these devices in the prevention of "sudden cardiac death". Battery life is highly dependent on the number of shocks delivered. The indications for ICD therapy are summarized in Table 39.4.

Device implantation

Most PPM and ICD implants are performed under local anesthesia with conscious sedation, typically using a combination of a benzodiazepine and opioid. The subclavian, cephalic or axillary veins are commonly used for lead insertion. Leads are placed and secured in the cardiac chambers and the device is usually positioned subcutaneously in the left or right pre-pectoral region or in the sub-pectoral space.

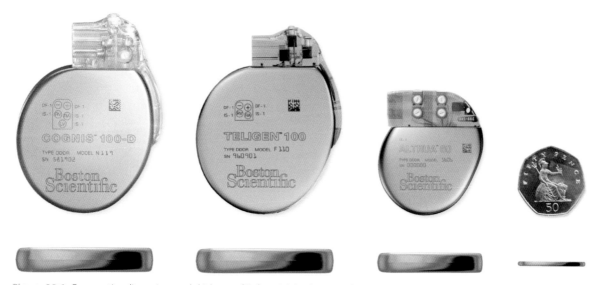

Figure 39.1 Comparative dimensions and thickness of (left to right) a biventricular ICD, dual-chamber ICD, and dual-chamber pacemaker (left to right). Images courtesy of Boston Scientific.

Implantation of ICDs is more complex – because of both the nature of the devices (thicker leads and larger devices – Figure 39.2) and the population of patients encountered. Introduction of smaller devices has allowed electrophysiologists to implant ICDs without surgical assistance. Conscious sedation is preferred to general anesthesia in many centers. Invasive arterial monitoring should be considered in all cases. Device testing requires induction of VF and measurement of the minimally effective defibrillation energy threshold (DFT). Most ICDs deliver a biphasic waveform of up to 30 joules, which provides a considerable margin of safety over the usual DFT of ∼10–15 joules. Standard inhalational anesthetic techniques increase DFT by ∼4 joules, whereas techniques using subcutaneous lidocaine have minimal impact on DFT.

Recent clinical trials support the administration of a prophylactic, broad-spectrum antibiotic immediately prior to device implantation. The use of antibiotics is mandatory in cases of pacemaker infection, lead-related endocarditis and prior to extraction of infected leads.

The complications of PPM and ICD implantation are summarized in Table 39.5.

Cardiac surgery

Perioperative considerations for patients with PPMs and ICDs are shown in Table 39.6. Because external PPM and ICD interrogation and programming devices

Table 39.5 Complications of PPM and ICD implantation

Early complications

Venous access	Pneumothorax, hemothorax, air embolus
Lead Related	Perforation, malposition, dislodgement
Pocket	Hematoma, infection

Delayed complications

Lead	Thrombosis, infection, insulation failure
Generator	Erosion, migration, external damage

Device function issues

Pacing/ sensing	Oversensing, undersensing, crosstalk
ICD-specific	Failure to deliver shock, ineffective, inappropriate

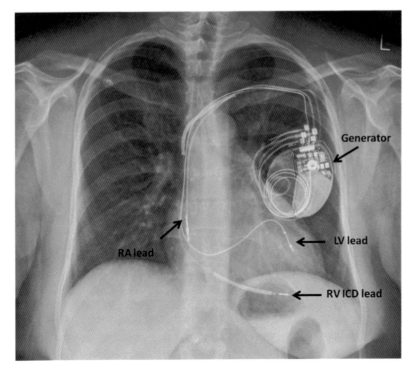

Figure 39.2 Posteroanterior CXR of a biventricular ICD.

Table 39.6 Perioperative considerations for patients with PPMs and ICDs

Original indications for implantation	Medical history and pre-pacemaker symptoms
Device type and manufacturer	PPM/ICD identification card carried by patient
Current mode of function	Device may be identified on plain CXR
Is device functioning properly?	Recent PPM/ICD checks? Recurrence of pre-pacemaker symptoms – particularly during exercise CXR: location, type and continuity of leads
Is patient pacemaker dependent?	ECG: evidence of pacing spikes and capture?
Is reprogramming necessary before surgery?	PPM usually reprogrammed to fixed rate pacing prior to induction of anesthesia for cardiac surgery
What are likely effects of anesthesia and surgery on device?	Electromagnetic interference (EMI)
	Diathermy may cause reprogramming to VVI or VOO Drugs, electrolytes, defibrillation
What are likely effects of device on anesthesia and surgery?	Bipolar diathermy where possible, smallest possible currents, avoid unnecessary cautery <5 cm from device

are manufacturer-specific and non-interchangeable, it is essential to determine the manufacturer and model. Current ASA guidelines on the management of patients with "rhythm management devices" recommend preoperative device interrogation. Implantable loop recorders (ILR) are occasionally encountered in the perioperative setting. While their role is purely diagnostic they should be interrogated preoperatively as electromagnetic interference (EMI) can permanently delete valuable diagnostic information.

A routine preoperative ECG should be obtained in all patients with PPMs and ICDs undergoing anesthesia. A CXR is not usually required but should be considered in heart failure patients with biventricular PPMs, as LV leads are especially susceptible to

dislodgement with intravascular interventions (e.g. insertion of central venous lines). Other investigations should be considered on a case by case basis. The anesthesiologist must be aware that PPMs are occasionally sited in unexpected locations, such as the anterior abdominal wall or axilla.

Patients with end-stage heart failure may require epicardial LV lead placement during the course of a palliative cardiac surgical procedure. These patients have little or no cardiac reserve and frequently have multi-organ system impairment, and require strict preoperative medical optimization.

Reprogramming

The need to alter PPM function during the perioperative period is determined by the underlying cardiac rhythm, hemodynamic state, the type of surgery being undertaken and likelihood of EMI. Rate-responsive or adaptive PPMs should have these features disabled during cardiac surgery. Passive body movements (e.g. patient positioning), drug-induced myoclonus, fasciculation or vibration (e.g. oscillating saws) would otherwise result in the abrupt onset of an inappropriate, paced tachycardia.

ICD antiarrhythmic features (i.e. anti-tachycardia pacing and defibrillation) can be disabled to prevent inappropriate discharge in response to EMI. Antiarrhythmic features (e.g. anti-tachycardia pacing and defibrillation) should be disabled for the duration of cardiac surgery.

Application of a magnet

Placing a permanent magnet over a PPM typically activates a predetermined pacing behavior (e.g. VOO) which varies according to battery state. This feature was originally incorporated to demonstrate remaining battery life and was never intended as a means to treat pacemaker-related emergencies secondary to EMI. It should be borne in mind that magnet responses are device- and manufacturer-specific, and can be altered from original factory settings or even deactivated by device reprogramming. It is essential that the magnet response of an implanted device be determined before surgery and early pacemaker technician referral is advised.

Application of a magnet over an ICD will generally disable the device by inhibiting arrhythmia detection. Prolonged magnet application may permanently disable some devices. Application of a magnet without knowledge of its effects is not recommended and is best avoided.

Central venous access

Insertion of central venous lines or right heart catheters in the perioperative period needs to take account of the location and course of pacing leads. Blind insertion of a central line risks lead dislodgement or damage, which may cause problems with sensing or pacing. Recently inserted right heart leads (<1 year) and LV leads are particularly prone to dislodgement. The presence of multiple leads in the same vein (e.g. subclavian) is associated with venous stenosis and thrombosis. The operative report from the pacemaker insertion or a CXR will reveal the course of the lead. A venogram or contrast CT may occasionally be required.

External pacing and defibrillation

An external defibrillator, ideally one with pacing functionality, must be available. External adhesive pads should be applied before induction of anesthesia. Defibrillation pads should be placed in both axillae, at least 10 cm from the PPM or ICD generator to prevent unintended hardware damage or reprogramming.

Preoperative antibiotic use

The risk of pacemaker lead-related infective endocarditis is low during cardiac procedures and cardiac surgery. The revised AHA guidelines recommend that antibiotic prophylaxis be reserved for patients with prosthetic cardiac valves or a history of infective endocarditis and those with complex congenital heart disease. The presence of PPM or ICD is not, by itself, an indication for antibiotic prophylaxis.

Monitoring

In order for pacing potentials ("spikes") to be visible on an intraoperative ECG monitor, high-frequency (low pass) filtering must be disabled. Other parameters, such as arterial pressure and pulse oximetry waveforms, should be used to confirm HR.

Electromagnetic interference

All electronic devices are potentially susceptible to electromagnetic or radiofrequency interference. In the clinical setting, the principal sources of EMI are electrocautery (diathermy), radiofrequency ablation

devices and MRI. Diagnostic, low-energy X-rays usually have no significant impact on PPM or ICD function. Although ultrasonic (harmonic) scalpels do not emit EMI, they are more than capable of cutting through pacemaker lead insulation and connectors.

Other sources of EMI that may be encountered in cardiac anesthesia include internal or external temporary pacing that may compete with an implanted device, external defibrillation, transcutaneous electrical nerve stimulation and evoked potential monitoring equipment.

Diathermy

Diathermy activation causes EMI, which is most commonly interpreted by PPMs as cardiac electrical activity. This can result in inappropriate inhibition of pacing or the onset of asynchronous pacing (a feature of a "noise reversion mode"). Unipolar diathermy is used most commonly in cardiac surgery. To minimize EMI, the diathermy grounding pad should be positioned as far away from the generator as possible or bipolar diathermy should be used instead. There are, however, reported cases of pacemaker-mediated tachycardia even with the use of bipolar diathermy at sites remote from the pacemaker. In the presence of ICDs, diathermy interference is interpreted as VF, and inappropriate shocks could be delivered if the ICD is not deactivated.

Diathermy generates tissue heating which can damage lead insulation and should be avoided in the vicinity of leads. Direct contact with the PPM or ICD generator must be avoided at all times. Diathermy use should be limited to short bursts with continuous hemodynamic monitoring, and discontinued immediately should hemodynamic compromise occur.

Radiofrequency ablation

Radiofrequency ablation devices can also interfere with ICD or PPM function. Furthermore, conduction of the ablation current along the leads can cause arrhythmias or unintended myocardial damage.

Magnetic resonance imaging

As mentioned above, magnetic interference can have unpredictable effects on PPM and ICD function. MRI may induce significant heating in leads and electrodes, culminating in electrical failure and direct myocardial damage. Because deaths have been reported when patients with PPMs have been exposed to MRI, all such exposure should be avoided. A new

Table 39.7 Common perioperative temporary pacing problems

Problem	ECG	Cause	Action
Failure to pace	No A or V pacing spikes	Connection problem Lead problem Pacing box	Check each in turn
Failure to capture	Pacing spikes present	High pacing threshold	Increase output ? Reposition leads
Failure to sense	Asynchronous pacing	Sensitivity too low *(Voltage too high)*	*Reduce* voltage on dial to increase sensitivity
Oversensing	Inappropriate output suppression	Artifacts or T waves may be mistaken for R waves	*Increase* voltage on dial to reduce sensitivity
Crosstalk	May inhibit V output	High A output V sensitivity too high	Reduce A output Reduce V sensitivity

generation of MRI-compatible rhythm management devices are becoming available.

Effects of anesthesia

Changes in plasma K^+ concentration may interfere with both pacing and defibrillation thresholds. Myopotentials secondary to drug-induced fasciculation (e.g. suxamethonium) or hypothermia-induced shivering could result in pacing inhibition or inappropriate antitachycardia therapy. The effects of general anesthesia on cardiac electrophysiology are discussed elsewhere.

Lead and device extraction

The increasing prevalence of implantable devices has inevitably increased the incidence of infective complications, and the need for lead and device extraction. Device extraction should be performed in an operating room or hybrid catheter laboratory room. The anesthesiologist must be familiar with the range of methods used and the potential complications. Serious, life-threatening complications include vascular injury, hemorrhage, damage to intracardiac structures and pericardial tamponade. For these reasons facilities for open cardiac surgery and CPB should be available.

Postoperative considerations

PPMs and ICDs should be checked postoperatively to ensure that they have sustained no intraoperative damage. Devices are typically reset to their original setting or reprogrammed to a new appropriate configuration.

Temporary pacing

Temporary pacing via wires attached to the epicardial surface of the RA and RV may cause problems. Fixed-rate pacing (e.g. DOO) should almost invariably be converted to demand mode (e.g. DDD) at the end of surgery (Chapter 29). Anesthesiologists need to become familiar with both the single-chamber and dual-chamber pacing systems (pulse generators) used in their institution. Traditionally, atrial wires are brought out through the right chest and ventricular wires through the left chest wall. Patients with long-standing chronic AF usually only have ventricular epicardial wires.

When a pacing problem is suspected, all connections should be checked to ensure that they are secure, and that atrial and ventricular outputs are connected to the correct epicardial wires! The presence of prominent or canon *a*-waves on the CVP pressure waveform may indicate ventricular activation secondary to an excessively high atrial voltage, selection of an inappropriately short A-V interval or transposed atrial and ventricular leads. Loss of atrial pacing is a common postoperative problem and is usually caused by atrial wire dislodgement.

Key points

- Patients with implantable devices should be identified and referred to a cardiac technician at an early stage.
- Application of a magnet without knowledge of its effects is not recommended and is best avoided.

- ICDs should be deactivated before surgery.
- Facilities for external defibrillation should be immediately available for the duration that ICD is disabled.
- Devices need to be checked and reprogrammed after surgery.

Further reading

American Society of Anesthesiologists Task Force on Perioperative Management of Patients with Cardiac Rhythm Management Devices. Practice advisory for the perioperative management of patients with cardiac rhythm management devices: pacemakers and implantable cardioverter-defibrillators: a report by the American Society of Anesthesiologists Task Force on Perioperative Management of Patients with Cardiac Rhythm Management Devices. *Anesthesiology* 2005; **103**(1): 186–98.

de Oliveira JC, Martinelli M, Nishioka SA, *et al.* Efficacy of antibiotic prophylaxis before the implantation of pacemakers and cardioverter-defibrillators: results of a large, prospective, randomized, double-blinded, placebo-controlled trial. *Circ Arrhythm Electrophysiol* 2009; **2**(1): 29–34.

Epstein AE, DiMarco JP, Ellenbogen KA, *et al.* ACC/AHA/HRS 2008 Guidelines for Device-Based Therapy of Cardiac Rhythm Abnormalities: a report of the American College of Cardiology/American Heart Association Task Force on Practice Guidelines (Writing Committee to Revise the ACC/AHA/NASPE 2002 Guideline Update for Implantation of Cardiac Pacemakers and Antiarrhythmia Devices) developed in collaboration with the American Association for Thoracic Surgery and Society of Thoracic Surgeons. *J Am Coll Cardiol* 2008; **51**(21): e1–62.

Wilson W, Taubert K A, Gewitz M, *et al.* Prevention of infective endocarditis: guidelines from the American Heart Association: a guideline from the American Heart Association Rheumatic Fever, Endocarditis, and Kawasaki Disease Committee, Council on Cardiovascular Disease in the Young, and the Council on Clinical Cardiology, Council on Cardiovascular Surgery and Anesthesia, and the Quality of Care and Outcomes Research Interdisciplinary Working Group. *Circulation* 2007; **116**(15): 1736–54.

Anesthesia and electrophysiological disorders

Andrew J. Richardson and J. M. Tom Pierce

Although the anesthesiologist's involvement with electrophysiological (EP) disorders includes managing such conditions within the operating room and ICU, this chapter will concentrate on anesthesia for procedures in the electrophysiology laboratory. Given the shift in the treatment of cardiac dysrhythmias, from pharmacological therapy to implantable devices, catheter-based ablation and surgical ablation, the cardiac anesthesiologist is increasingly involved in caring for patients with cardiac rhythm disturbances.

Spectrum of electrophysiological disorders

Table 40.1 Classification of electrophysiological disorders

Congenital
Acquired

Anatomic
Physiological

Disordered impulse generation
Disordered impulse conduction
Disordered action potential

Congenital anatomic disorders

With the increasing survival of patients born with congenital heart disease (CHD), greater numbers of patients with structurally abnormal hearts are presenting with cardiac rhythm disturbances. The most frequently seen dysrhythmias in adults with CHD include:

- macro re-entry tachycardia (associated with thrombosis and sudden death)
- atrial fibrillation
- ventricular arrhythmias (often in the setting of ventricular incision and scarring, and associated with sudden death)

- sinus node dysfunction (associated with paroxysmal atrial tachycardia)
- heart block (associated with surgery to the ventricular septum)
- pre-excitation syndromes (associated with Ebstein's anomaly).

Procedures undertaken for transposition of the great arteries (e.g. Senning, Mustard), functionally univentricular heart (e.g. Fontan) and Fallot's tetralogy are particularly associated with the late development of dysrhythmias (Chapter 51).

Various substrates may act to initiate dysrhythmias. These include myocardium subjected to chronic pressure and volume overload, hypertrophied myocardium, myocardial fibrosis and surgical scars. As dysrhythmias worsen cardiac function and vice versa, a vicious cycle of clinical deterioration may ensue.

Congenital physiological disorders

Pre-excitation syndromes

The presence of accessory conducting pathways that bypass or short-circuit the atrioventricular (A-V) node results in an abnormally short PR interval. The term pre-excitation includes conditions such as the Wolff-Parkinson-White (WPW) and Lown-Ganong-Levine syndromes. The differing relative refractory periods of the normal and accessory pathways predispose to the development of re-entrant circuits. Ablation of the accessory pathway may be fully curative.

Long QT syndromes

The normal QT interval (from the onset of the QRS to the end of the T wave) is normally 350–440 ms. Prolongation of the QT interval >440 ms increases susceptibility to the R on T phenomenon. Because the QT interval is inversely proportional to HR, it is usual

(a)

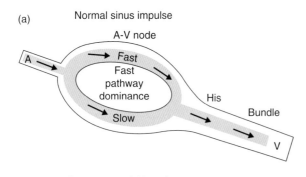

(b)

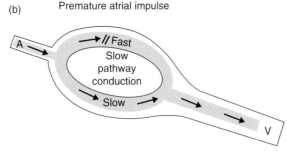

(c)

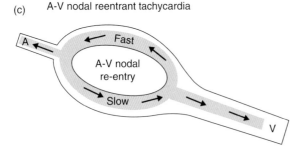

Figure 40.1 In WPW syndrome the accessory pathway may conduct APs retrogradely from the His-Purkinje system to the RA (orthodromic conduction). (a) If an atrial extrasystole reaches the AV node and accessory pathway when the accessory pathway is still in its refractory period, the AP is conducted to the His-Purkinje system via the A-V node. (b,c) If the accessory pathway is no longer refractory when the impulse reaches the His-Purkinje system, it can be conducted retrogradely into the atria, triggering a self-sustaining re-entrant loop that results in tachycardia.

to express the QT interval corrected for HR (QTc) using Bazett's formula:

$$QTc = QT/ \sqrt{RR \text{ interval}}$$

Inherited ion channel disorders (channelopathies) may predispose to malignant dysrhythmias and sudden cardiac death. It is now known that a large, and increasing, number of genetic disorders give rise to QT interval prolongation. Importantly, in these patients, drugs such as amiodarone may paradoxically enhance arrhythmogenesis. Acquired causes of QT

Table 40.2 Causes of QT interval prolongation

Inherited	Romano Ward syndrome (autosomal dominant) Jervell and Lange-Nielson syndrome (autosomal recessive)
Acquired	Myocardial infarction, complete heart block, cardiomyopathy, rheumatic fever Hypokalemia, hypocalcemia, hypomagnesemia
Drug-induced	Class Ia and Ic antiarrhythmics: procainamide, flecainide Class III antiarrhythmics: amiodarone, sotalol Antipsychotics: droperidol, thioridazine, risperidone Antidepressants: fluoxetine, sertraline Antimicrobials: erythromycin, clarithromycin Prokinetics: cisapride (withdrawn in many countries) Antihistamines: terfenadine

interval prolongation include drug therapy, acute MI and electrolyte abnormalities (e.g. hypokalemia, hypomagnesemia and hypocalcemia). Although long QT syndromes are not amenable to ablation therapy, patients may be offered implantable cardiodefibrillators (ICD).

Acquired disorders
Tachydysrhythmias

These include supraventricular dysrhythmias (e.g. atrial fibrillation, atrial flutter, A-V nodal re-entrant tachycardia and A-V re-entrant tachycardia) and ventricular dysrhythmias (e.g. extrasystoles, VT, VF and torsades des pointes).

Atrial fibrillation

AF is the commonest cardiac arrhythmia, affecting 10% of the population over 75 years of age. Although often associated with structural heart disease, it can occur with no detectable cause (lone AF). There is a particularly high incidence of AF after cardiac surgery. The condition affects over a third of patients undergoing CABG surgery and up to half undergoing valve surgery. Other causes include ischemic and congenital heart disease (especially atrial septal defects), LVH, alcohol, myocarditis, pericarditis, pulmonary embolism and respiratory tract infection (Table 40.3).

Table 40.3 Causes of atrial fibrillation
Ischemic heart disease
Atrial enlargement (e.g. mitral disease)
Hyperthyroidism
Idiopathic
Pulmonary embolism
Cardiomyopathy
Other – fever, infection, stroke, trauma

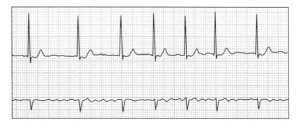

Figure 40.2 Atrial fibrillation.

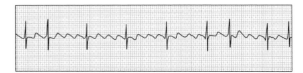

Figure 40.3 Atrial Flutter with variable AV conduction.

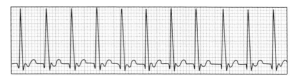

Figure 40.4 Supraventricular tachycardia.

Enhanced automaticity in atrial tissue within the pulmonary veins or vena cavae may trigger AF by generating multiple atrial ectopics, with multiple random re-entry circuits maintaining the dysrhythmia. Over time, electrical and structural remodeling occurs, leading to shortened refractory periods and a greater propensity to rhythm disturbance. AF is characterized by complete absence of coordinated atrial activity, with fibrillatory waves replacing P waves on the ECG. The ventricular response is irregular and frequently rapid if atrioventricular conduction is intact. Where there is a rapid or irregular broad QRS complex tachycardia, consideration should be given to the possibility of AF in the presence of conduction block or an accessory pathway. Ventricular filling is diminished through loss of atrial contraction and diastolic shortening, resulting in reduced CO, especially in patients with impaired ventricular compliance. Treatment of AF aims to restore normal sinus rhythm (NSR) or, if this is not possible, to control ventricular response rate. Other considerations include prevention of recurrent rhythm disturbance and the avoidance of thromboembolic complications.

Atrial flutter

An atrial ectopic beat can initiate a re-entrant atrial "loop" which discharges at ~300 beats per minute. The ventricular response rate is dependent on A-V nodal conduction, which typically varies between $150 \ min^{-1}$ (2:1 block) and $60 \ min^{-1}$ (5:1 block). Flutter waves can be difficult to distinguish amongst QRS complexes if ventricular response is rapid. However, a narrow complex tachycardia of ~150 beats per minute should be considered to be atrial flutter until proven otherwise. Maneuvers that increase A-V block (e.g. carotid sinus massage or adenosine) may be

diagnostic and therapeutic. In difficult cases (e.g. flutter with aberrant conduction) an atrial ECG may be helpful. Overdrive pacing, DC cardioversion or anti-arrhythmics may be used to restore NSR. Digoxin may convert atrial flutter to AF.

Supraventricular tachycardia (SVT)

This paroxysmal tachycardia is caused by a rapidly firing ectopic focus in the SA node, atria or A-V node. It may occur in the absence of organic disease or in association with hyperthyroidism, alcohol or caffeine intoxication, and pre-excitation syndromes. The ventricular rate ranges from 140 to 240 min^{-1}, with narrow QRS complexes in the absence of bundle branch block.

Cardioversion may be achieved with vagal maneuvers, DC cardioversion, drugs (e.g. adenosine, esmolol, amiodarone) or overdrive pacing. Digoxin and verapamil should not be used unless it is certain the patient does not have WPW syndrome.

Ventricular tachyarrhythmias

Ventricular extrasystoles are relatively common and usually benign. They may be a normal variant or secondary to IHD, hypoxemia, hypercapnea, electrolyte imbalance or drugs (e.g. halothane,

251

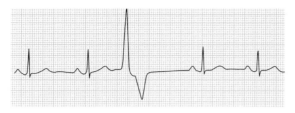

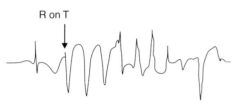

R on T

Figure 40.5 (Left) Ventricular extrasystole. (Right) R on T phenomenon triggering torsades des pointes.

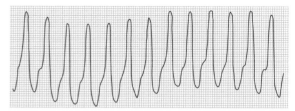

Figure 40.6 Ventricular tachycardia.

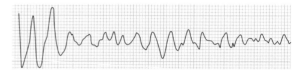

Figure 40.7 Degeneration of VT into coarse VF.

antiarrhythmics). The presence of two or more ectopic foci (i.e. multifocal extrasystoles) is of more concern. They rarely require treatment unless the R-wave coincides with the previous T-wave (R on T phenomenon), when other arrhythmias may be triggered.

A run of three or more consecutive ventricular extrasystoles constitutes VT or torsades des pointes. The rhythm is sustained by a rapidly discharging ventricular focus. If there is no CO, immediate DC cardioversion is indicated. If the patient remains conscious, however, DC cardioversion should be undertaken under general anesthesia. In the relatively asymptomatic patient, overdrive pacing, lidocaine or amiodarone may be considered.

Degeneration of the rhythm to VF is an indication for immediate DC cardioversion. No anesthetic is required!

Bradydysrhythmias

Bradycardias result from abnormalities of AP generation or conduction. Causes include sinus node dysfunction, drugs (e.g. β-blockers) and heart block. (See Chapter 14.)

A-V (heart) block commonly indicates the presence of ischemic or structural heart disease. It is important to identify patients with block that may progress to complete heart block and cardiovascular collapse (e.g. bifascicular block or LBBB with first-degree heart block). Although these patients are at high risk of developing bradyarrhythmias with hemodynamic compromise, progression to complete heart block is independent of

whether first-degree block is present and not as common as previously thought. Historically transvenous pacing was considered necessary before anesthesia. Nowadays it is recommended that bradyarrhythmias be treated with chronotropic drugs, with facilities for temporary pacing on "standby".

Anesthesia for electrophysiological procedures

Preoperative assessment

The following questions must be answered:

- What is the rhythm disturbance and what compromise results from it?
- Is the cardiac anatomy normal?
- If the anatomy is not normal, is there any history of progression of heart failure, cyanosis or chronic pulmonary disease?
- What is the ventricular performance?
- Are there are any implanted devices?
- What is the anti-coagulation status?
- Are serum electrolyte concentrations (especially potassium and magnesium) within acceptable ranges?
- What procedure is intended?

The patient population ranges between two extremes. At one end of the spectrum is the asymptomatic or minimally compromised patient with a structurally and functionally normal heart, who does not require specialized perioperative care. Fortunately more rarely is the grossly compromised patient with palliated complex congenital heart disease who requires

Table 40.4 Pitfalls of elective DC cardioversion (DCC)

Situation	Pitfall	Solution
Ever present risk of LA thrombus in longstanding AF	Embolization and stroke	Therapeutic anticoagulation for 3 weeks prior to DCC or TEE to exclude LA thrombus
Paroxysmal AF	Patient may be in NSR on arrival	Scrutinize monitored ECG Abandon procedure
Atrial flutter	Easy to convert to NSR	Start with 30 J biphasic shock
Presence of PPM or ICD	Interpretation of ECG may be difficult Potential device damage with DCC	DCC and expect ventricular depolarization change DCC in an axis perpendicular to that of the lead system Post DCC PPM/ICD check
Obesity	Anterolateral electrode position may result in reduced trans-myocardial current	Position electrodes between scapulae and over left precordium
After cardioversion	Hypotension in the setting of NSR	IV fluids
Slow ventricular response rate	Profound bradycardia after cardioversion	Temporary external pacing facility incorporated into the defibrillator

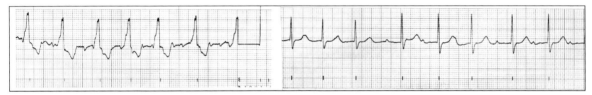

Figure 40.8 ECG recording from a patient with AF undergoing elective DC cardioversion. Conversion to sinus rhythm eventually required a 200 J monophasic shock. The aberrant ventricular conduction (left) is at least in part due to the presence of a VVI pacemaker (pacemaker impulses not visible), making interpretation difficult. After successful cardioversion the QRS complex is of normal width although the PR interval is long.

full invasive cardiovascular monitoring and post-operative admission to the intensive care unit.

Some procedures may last several hours, making general anesthesia more desirable than prolonged conscious sedation. Exact practice in this regard varies between centers. Pediatric and many grown-up CHD (GUCH) patients require general anesthesia.

DC cardioversion

This is the most commonly performed electrophysiological intervention and is often performed on a day-case basis. The anesthesiologist is frequently the most senior doctor present. In the vast majority of cases the underlying rhythm disturbance is either atrial fibrillation (90%) or atrial flutter. Common pitfalls are described in Table 40.4.

Accurate identification of the underlying cardiac rhythm in the presence of a permanent pacemaker may be challenging (Figure 40.8). Elective cardioversion requires a minimum period of 3 weeks therapeutic anticoagulation and protocols dictate a plasma potassium concentration ≥ 4.5 mmol l^{-1}. Practical considerations include the application of "hands-free" adhesive electrodes and scrutiny of the monitored ECG to confirm the dysrhythmia *before* induction of anesthesia. Anteroposterior electrode positioning may increase the likelihood of success in the obese patient. Following pre-oxygenation, intravenous propofol 1–2 mg/kg and spontaneous respiration with oxygen provide both a rapid loss of consciousness and rapid recovery. In comparison to monophasic waveforms, biphasic energy waveforms achieve higher rates of cardioversion at lower energies and cause fewer skin burns. All patients undergoing cardioversion should have a post-procedure 12-lead ECG recorded. Patients with a PPM or ICD should undergo a device check.

253

Mapping and radiofrequency ablation

This is performed to characterize and treat supraventricular and ventricular tachydysrhythmias. The procedure typically entails deliberate triggering of the dysrhythmia, in order to identify the foci and circuits involved and guide ablation. Whilst many procedures are performed under conscious sedation, general anesthesia is preferred for children and elderly patients undergoing lengthy procedures during which radiofrequency-induced pericardial pain is likely. General anesthesia eliminates restlessness and reduces the risk of hypoxia, hypercarbia and aspiration.

Transcutaneous cardioversion/defibrillation pads are placed pre-induction. The preferred routes of cardiological access are the subclavian and femoral routes: if central venous cannulation is indicated for anesthetic reasons care should be taken to avoid these sites and to keep the tip well away from the heart. Not infrequently the cardiologist will site a femoral arterial catheter for continuous monitoring. A detailed discussion of the electrophysiological techniques involved during ablation (Figure 40.9) is beyond the scope of this chapter; however, Figure 40.10 describes in some detail the intracardiac electrode configuration and the interpretation.

Effects of anesthetic agents on cardiac conduction

The interaction of both intravenous and volatile anesthetic agents with the cardiac conduction system is complex and incompletely understood, in terms of both the effects themselves and the clinical significance of such effects.

In isolated heart preparations, thiopental has been shown to significantly prolong the atrial refractory period in a concentration-dependent manner, whilst propofol and ketamine have no effect on atrial refractoriness. However, ketamine causes a dose-dependent decrease in atrial conduction velocity, not seen with propofol and thiopental. All three drugs produce a concentration-dependent decrease in A-V node conduction and an increase in A-V node effective refractory period, with propofol being more potent in this regard than the other two agents. By contrast, some in vivo studies have shown that propofol has no clinically significant effect on atrial-His interval, His-ventricular interval, corrected sinus node recovery time, A-V node refractory period and atrial effective refractory period.

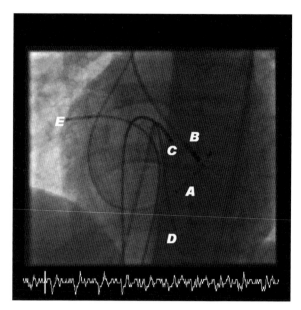

Figure 40.9 Electrophysiology catheters in the right anterior oblique (RAO) view: surface ECG electrodes are marked with yellow arrows. The decapolar catheter, introduced via the jugular vein, is situated in the coronary sinus (CS). The electrodes are numbered from 1 to 10 in a distal to proximal fashion so that the distal pair is 1–2 and the proximal pair is 9–10. The distal electrodes record the potential from the LA. The quadripolar catheter is placed anteriorly and pointed inferiorly in the RV.

Opioids, when used in combination with a benzodiazepine (e.g. alfentanil + midazolam or sufentanil + lorazepam) have no significant effect on either the normal cardiac conduction tissue or accessory pathways found in Wolff-Parkinson-White syndrome.

The evidence for the effects of volatile agents on cardiac conduction is conflicting. Halothane in vitro depresses atrial conduction more than other agents, but has no effect on atrial refractoriness. Desflurane at 2 MAC shortens atrial AP duration and the effective atrial refractory period. Isoflurane prolongs the atrial refractory period and delays ventricular repolarization. In vivo, enflurane, isoflurane and halothane increase refractoriness within normal A-V and accessory pathway tissue. In Wolff-Parkinson-White syndrome sevoflurane <1 MAC increases intra-atrial conduction but has no effect on conduction in the normal A-V or accessory conducting pathways. Neither propofol nor isoflurane alters SAN or A-V node function compared to the combination of alfentanil and midazolam.

In summary, therefore, it seems that both intravenous and volatile anesthetic agents have effects on the cardiac conduction system, which vary between and

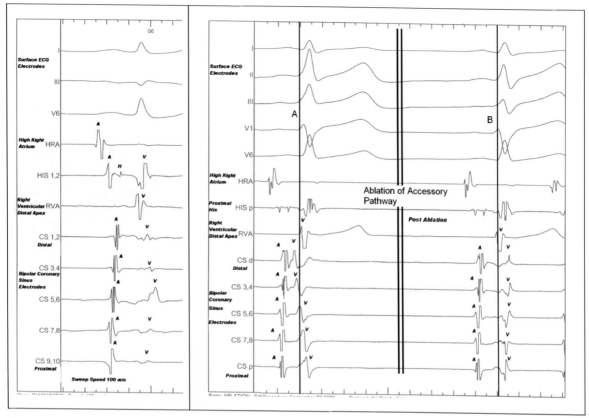

Figure 40.10 (Left) The pattern of electrical activation through the cardiac conducting system in normal sinus rhythm recorded during an electrophysiological study. (Right) Sinus rhythm in Wolff-Parkinson-White syndrome with a left lateral accessory pathway. At time point A it can be seen that accessory pathway conduction causes the V wave in the distal coronary sinus (CS d) to precede the surface electrode QRS complex, producing a shortened A-V interval. After ablation, at time point B, the V wave in all the coronary sinus electrodes occurs after the surface electrode QRS complex, showing loss of conduction down the accessory pathway. The coronary sinus electrodes are numbered from 1 to 10 in a distal to proximal fashion so that the distal pair is 1–2 and the proximal pair is 9–10.

within class of drug. These effects appear to be of little or no clinical significance, leading many to suggest that both isoflurane- and propofol-based anesthesia are suitable for patients undergoing electrophysiological studies and radiofrequency catheter ablation.

Geographic considerations

Cardiac operating room

Patients with chronic AF presenting for cardiac surgery may also undergo concomitant ablation using radio-frequency energy, cryotherapy, laser, high-intensity focused ultrasound or surgical incision. These produce full-thickness scarring and prevent the passage of late circus re-entrant dysrhythmias. In paroxysmal AF the pulmonary veins are isolated from the body of the LA and for persistent AF an atrial maze is created. While these interventions increase complexity they do not usually unduly prolong the cardiac surgical procedure. The efficacy of the procedure may not be apparent until several weeks later.

Cardiac catheter laboratory

The majority of cardiological interventions are undertaken in cardiac catheter laboratories. These are frequently located outside the main operating suite and, from the anesthesiologist's perspective, are potentially hostile environments. Specific challenges for the anesthesiologist include:

- working with staff unfamiliar with routine operating room procedures and practice
- lack of an area for patient preparation and induction of anesthesia
- the presence of imaging and other electronic equipment which may limit access to the airway and vascular lines

255

- moving patient and equipment with the potential to dislodge tracheal tube and vascular access
- exposure of staff and patient to ionizing radiation
- temperature control and avoidance of hypothermia
- ECG lead positioning to avoid interference with imaging.

Potential pitfalls

- Unsynchronized DC shocks may induce ventricular fibrillation. Inexperienced cardiology trainees sent to perform the cardioversion list may forget to depress the synchronized shock button. Conversely, when attempting defibrillation, the "synchronize" setting must be turned off.
- Some dysrhythmias occur more frequently in association with cardiac anomalies (e.g. WPW syndrome and Ebstein's anomaly) or genetic syndromes (e.g. WPW syndrome and Leber's Hereditary Optic Neuropathy variants). The cardiac function may be severely impaired as a consequence of the structural abnormalities rather than the dysrhythmia, and other issues, such as a difficult airway, may make the safe administration of general anesthesia and post-anesthesia care challenging.
- When testing ICDs after implantation facilities to provide back-up emergency cardioversion must be immediately to hand.
- The anesthesiologist needs an awareness of the potential immediate adverse effects of certain anti-dysrhythmic drugs. The administration of AV node blocking drugs in the setting of AF in the presence of an accessory pathway may prove catastrophic, due to ultra-rapid conduction of impulses down the accessory pathway, leading to ventricular fibrillation (VF). Likewise, Class III anti-dysrhythmic drugs will worsen the occurrence of long QT-induced dysrhythmias, and flecainide in the setting of myocardial scarring, ischemia or conduction delay may be associated with life-threatening intractable dysrhythmias.

Key points

- A broad complex tachycardia may indicate SVT with aberrant A-V conduction.
- Digoxin and verapamil should not be used to treat SVT unless WPW syndrome has been excluded.
- Perioperative progression of chronic bifasicular block or LBBB to complete heart block is rare. Routine prophylactic insertion of a temporary pacemaker is rarely indicated.
- An undiagnosed conduction abnormality may become apparent during the course of general anesthesia for a non-cardiac surgical procedure.
- Anesthesia in the cardiac catheter laboratory brings its own set of challenges for which the anesthesiologist must be fully prepared.
- Whilst both intravenous and volatile anesthetic agents have effects on the cardiac conduction system, these effects are of little clinical significance and play no role in determining the anesthetic technique.

Further reading

Erb TO, Kanter RJ, Hall JM, Tong JG, Kern FH, Schulman SR. Comparison of electrophysiologic effects of propofol and isoflurane-based anesthetics in children undergoing radiofrequetncy catheter ablation for supraventricular tachycardia. *Anesthesiology* 2002; **96**: 1386–94.

Acute myocardial ischemia and infarction

Andrew Neitzel and Bevan Hughes

According to the World Health Organization, cardio-vascular disease is the leading cause of death. Coronary artery disease (CAD) is responsible for 40% of these deaths, principally as a result of complications associated with the acute coronary syndrome (ACS). The cardiothoracic anesthesiologist plays a key role in the management of some of these high-risk patients and as such requires an in-depth understanding of the pathogenesis, presentation and complications of the disease process.

Pathogenesis

Atherosclerosis is a chronic inflammatory process that results in the formation of atheroma (plaques) on the arterial intima. It is a progressive process characterized by intimal thickening which gradually reduces the intraluminal caliber of the vessel, impeding blood flow and myocardial perfusion. It is believed that an occult injury to the vascular endothelium is often the initiating event in atherogenesis. Subsequent to this, infiltration of the vascular wall by inflammatory cells (monocytes and macrophages) begins a process involving digestion of oxidized low-density lipoproteins and the formation of foam cells. These intramural fatty streaks in turn provoke the proliferation of smooth muscle and the appearance of atheromatous plaques. The plaques are encapsulated by a meshwork of connective tissue that provides a relatively smooth intraluminal surface. Degradation of this fibrous cap compromises plaque stability and ultimately may lead to plaque rupture and complete occlusion of the vessel.

Exposure of the sub-endothelial matrix after plaque rupture causes platelet adhesion, activation and aggregation with subsequent thrombus formation. Platelet-rich thrombus (white clot) forms in areas of high shear stress and generally only partially occludes the vessel, whereas fibrin-rich thrombus (red clot) often results in complete obstruction to arterial flow. Thrombus formation is central to the pathogenesis of ACS and is most commonly the final pathway between ischemia and infarction.

It is now recognized that vasoconstriction plays an important role in myocardial ischemia. Endothelial dysfunction secondary to plaque formation results in reduced production of vasodilators such as nitric oxide and prostacyclin, whereas platelet-derived vasoactive moieties increase vascular tone.

Acute coronary syndrome

ACS refers to a spectrum of conditions, ranging from chest pain to frank myocardial necrosis, associated with impaired coronary perfusion and myocardial ischemia. Depending on the extent of tissue ischemia, ACS may present as unstable angina (UA), non-ST-elevation MI (NSTEMI), ST-elevation MI (STEMI) or sudden death.

Unstable angina

Patients with acute myocardial ischemia typically present with central chest pain – the clinical manifestation of a mismatch between myocardial oxygen supply (MDO_2) and demand (MVO_2). Unstable angina is defined as angina that exhibits one or more clinical features (Table 41.1). By definition, the myocardial ischemia associated with UA does not cause myocardial necrosis or release of laboratory biomarkers (e.g. troponins or creatine kinase).

Non-ST-elevation myocardial infarction

UA and NSTEMI are closely related conditions. A diagnosis of NSTEMI is generally made when

Core Topics in Cardiac Anesthesia, Second Edition, ed. Jonathan H. Mackay and Joseph E. Arrowsmith. Published by Cambridge University Press. © Cambridge University Press 2012.

Table 41.1 Symptoms of unstable (CCS Class IV) angina

Angina occurring at rest (or with minimal exertion) lasting longer than 20 min

Angina which is severe and of new onset (within the last 8 weeks)

Angina with a crescendo pattern; increasing intensity, frequency or duration

Table 41.2 Localization of culprit lesion in STEMI

Infarction	ST elevation	Vessel
Inferior	II, III, aVF	Right coronary artery
Antero-septal	V_1, V_2	Left anterior descending
Antero-apical	V_3, V_4	Distal left anterior descending
Antero-lateral	V_5, V_6	Circumflex

Table 41.3 Common arrhythmias associated with ACS

Arrhythmia	Incidence	Etiology
Atrial fibrillation	10%	Atrial ischemia Increased LA pressure
Ventricular tachycardia	3–5% (within first 4 h)	Ischemia
Ventricular fibrillation	2–4%	Ischemia
Bradycardia	Up to 20% with inferior infarction	Inferior wall infarction Ischemia of SA and A-V nodes High vagal tone

myocardial ischemia is associated with a detectable increase in circulating biomarkers. The ECG changes associated with NSTEMI are generally nonspecific and may include ST segment depression or T wave inversion.

ST-elevation myocardial infarction

A diagnosis of STEMI is made when characteristic ECG changes accompany elevated circulating levels of biomarkers. These include ST segment elevation of ≥ 2 mm (0.2 mV) in two or more contiguous ECG leads or new-onset left bundle branch block (LBBB). The majority of patients with ST elevation have ST depression in reciprocal leads. By identifying the changes in specific leads, the culprit vessel can often be identified using only the ECG (Table 41.2).

Anesthetic management

When atherosclerotic narrowing of the coronary vasculature significantly limits blood flow, perfusion must be urgently restored to prevent irreversible myocardial damage. In ACS with occlusive thrombus, this can be achieved either pharmacologically using a thrombolytic agent, or by physically restoring flow. The latter is achieved using either percutaneous intervention (PCI; angioplasty and stenting) or CABG surgery. PCI is preferable in the acute setting as general anesthesia and surgery are associated with significant morbidity and mortality. Compared to thrombolysis, emergency PCI provides a survival benefit in STEMI and is recommended as a first-line intervention.

When providing anesthesia for a patient undergoing myocardial revascularization surgery, it is important to understand the impact of drugs and IPPV on MDO_2 and MVO_2 (Figures 5.3 and 31.4). The fundamental goals are maximizing MDO_2 and minimizing MVO_2 by maintaining coronary perfusion pressure, and avoiding anemia, hypoxemia, ventricular

distension, increased LVEDP, tachycardia and excessive inotropy. For these reasons insertion of an IABP before induction of anesthesia may be advantageous (Figure 56.1).

While some anesthesiologists find CO monitors helpful in this situation, there is little doubt that TEE assessment of preload, myocardial contractility and valvular function is extremely valuable. Cases with significant risk of myocardial ischemia and hemodynamic instability are a class I indication for TEE.

Complications
Arrhythmias

Rhythm disturbances are common and one of the main causes of mortality in the early post-infarction period. They often indicate ongoing ischemia or direct disruption of the conduction system, and may be exacerbated by acidosis, electrolyte disturbances, congestive heart failure or cardiogenic shock. While hemodynamically insignificant ECG changes (e.g. unifocal ventricular ectopics) do not usually require treatment, the possibility of severe hypotension due to dysrhythmia requires vigilance in the peri-infarct period. Timely intervention to restore normal sinus rhythm, using either electrical cardioversion or appropriate antiarrhythmic agents, is crucial to avoid circulatory collapse (Table 41.3).

Pericarditis

This is a common complication after ACS, particularly in patients with inferior wall infarction (Table 41.4). In severe cases it may precipitate the development of a hemodynamically significant pericardial effusion. In rare cases this may be large enough to induce tamponade physiology.

Table 41.4 Clinical presentation of pericarditis

Symptoms

Chest pain, radiating to the back
Exacerbated by deep inspiration
Relieved by sitting forward

Signs

Pericardial friction rub

ECG

Diffuse ST and T wave changes

Ventricular septal rupture

Ventricular septal rupture (VSR) is an infrequent (0.2%) but lethal complication of ACS and is typically associated with an extensive transmural infarction. Approximately 60% of VSRs are associated with anterior MI, and 40% with posterior or inferior MI. Most cases occur within 48–72 hours of infarction and, without treatment, most patients die within a week. The primary physical finding is a new, harsh holosystolic ejection murmur audible over the entire precordium that is often accompanied by a palpable thrill. Ultimately, echocardiography is used to delineate the extent and precise location of the septal rupture.

VSR creates a sudden left → right intracardiac shunt with RV overload and increased pulmonary blood flow. This may cause acute RV failure, pulmonary edema and hemodynamic collapse. Management of these patients is challenging – while reducing LV afterload reduces left → right shunt, it does so at the expense of reduced coronary perfusion pressure. The definitive treatment is surgical but precisely when to

Table 41.5 Ventricular free wall rupture

Type	Pathology	Clinical features
Acute	Full-thickness free wall rupture	Sudden-onset chest pain, hypotension, jugular venous distension, tamponade, electromechanical dissociation and death
Sub-acute	Slow pericardial leak	Progressive symptoms of tamponade with ventricular failure and cardiogenic shock
Pseudo-aneurysm	Contained within layers of pericardium (Figure 43.3)	Features imitate those of acute ventricular aneurysm with heart failure, arrhythmias and persistent ST-segment elevation

operate remains controversial. An IABP is a helpful adjunct regardless of the timing of surgery.

Ventricular free wall rupture

Ventricular free wall rupture (VWR) occurs in less than 1% of patients with acute MI and of these up to half present with sudden death. It most commonly occurs early; 40% occurring in the first 24 hours and 85% within the first week. There are several types of VWR with characteristic features (Table 41.5).

Complete rupture can cause a hemopericardium with acute tamponade, electromechanical dissociation and sudden death. Typical symptoms include recurrent chest pain, repeated emesis, agitation and syncope. This presentation may be difficult to distinguish from persistent myocardial ischemia and may even exhibit similar rhythm and ST segment changes. Urgent echocardiography is required to make the diagnosis.

Papillary muscle rupture

Mitral regurgitation after MI can occur as a result of several mechanisms (Table 41.6) and is associated with poor prognosis. Papillary muscle rupture (PMR) occurs most commonly after an inferior MI and often involves the postero-medial papillary muscle because of its singular blood supply. The occurrence of PMR is still rare, but when it happens it results in rapidly progressive pulmonary edema and cardiogenic shock. Physical examination typically reveals a harsh, pansystolic murmur and diffuse

259

Table 41.6 Mechanisms of post-infarction mitral regurgitation

Worsening of pre-existing MR

Rupture of chordae tendinae or papillary muscle

Dilated MV annulus due to LV failure

Restricted leaflet movement due to papillary muscle dysfunction

inspiratory pulmonary crackles. Although the ECG and CXR are helpful, definitive diagnosis is best made with echocardiography.

Emergency valve repair or, more usually, replacement is the definitive treatment for these patients and concomitant revascularization improves long-term survival. The anesthetic goals are summarized in Table 32.2. Maintaining coronary perfusion takes precedence over both reducing LV afterload and increasing effective LV stroke volume. Inotropic and chronotropic support is usually required, albeit at the expense of increased MVO_2. The use of an IABP may be especially effective as it simultaneously promotes antegrade LV ejection and improves coronary perfusion without increasing MVO_2.

Left ventricular outflow tract obstruction

Dynamic LV outflow tract (LVOT) obstruction is an uncommon complication of anteroapical MI. It occurs in the presence of an infarcted or hypokinetic LV apex. A compensatory increase in basal and middle-segment LV contractility reduces the cross-sectional area of the LVOT during systole. As in other cases of LVOT obstruction, the situation is further complicated by acute MR secondary to systolic anterior motion (SAM) of the anterior mitral leaflet. LV end-diastolic volume is significantly increased leading to a vicious cycle – LV dilatation, increased LV wall stress and worsening ischemia.

Treatment is focused on reducing both myocardial contractility and HR while judiciously expanding intravascular volume and maintaining adequate afterload. The goals of this therapy are to optimize intraventricular dimensions and to reduce LVOT obstruction and blood flow velocity. As such, β-blockers (e.g. esmolol) and vasoconstrictors (e.g. phenyephrine) are potentially beneficial, although in cases of impending cardiogenic shock their use may be contraindicated. The IABP, inotropes and vasodilators are ineffective and may exacerbate LVOT obstruction.

Table 41.7 Clinical presentation of LVOT obstruction

Outflow tract obstruction

New systolic ejection murmur heard best at the left upper sternal edge with radiation to the neck

Systolic anterior motion of AML

New holosystolic murmur heard best at the apex with radiation to the axilla

Congestive heart failure

S_3 gallop, pulmonary crackles, hypotension and tachycardia

Key points

- ACS results from a mismatch between myocardial oxygen supply and demand, often as a result of atherosclerotic plaque rupture.
- Surgical revascularization following ACS is often postponed until after stabilization and restoration of adequate perfusion to ischemic myocardium.
- Ventricular rupture after transmural infarction is potentially catastrophic and can lead to intracardiac shunt or tamponade.
- Acute mitral regurgitation after MI is associated with poor prognosis.

Further reading

Antman EM, Anbe DT, Armstrong PW, *et al.* ACC/AHA guidelines for the management of patients with ST-elevation myocardial infarction – executive summary. A report of the American College of Cardiology/American Heart Association Task Force on Practice Guidelines (Writing Committee to revise the 1999 guidelines for the management of patients with acute myocardial infarction). *J Am Coll Cardiol* 2004; **44**(3): 671–719.

Brown C, Joshi B, Faraday N, *et al.* Emergency cardiac surgery in patients with acute coronary syndromes: a review of the evidence and perioperative implications of medical and mechanical therapeutics. *Anesth Analg* 2011; **112**(4): 777–99.

de Silva R, Fox KM. The changing horizon of acute coronary syndrome. *Lancet* 2009; **374**(9696): 1125–7.

Wilansky S, Moreno CA, Lester SJ. Complications of myocardial infarction. *Crit Care Med* 2007; **35**(8 Suppl): S348–54.

42

Miscellaneous catheter laboratory procedures

Tom Rawlings and Jean-Pierre van Besouw

Recent advances in percutaneous endovascular techniques mean that some cardiac anesthesiologists are spending more time in the cardiac catheter laboratory. These techniques typically require the use of high-definition fluoroscopic X-ray imaging and, more often than not, transesophageal echocardiography. Endovascular interventions can be broadly divided into two categories, coronary and intracardiac, the latter of which will be discussed in this chapter. Intracardiac procedures can be further divided into those which deal with stenotic valvular lesions and those that deal with an anatomical defect.

Stenotic lesions

In theory, stenosis of any of the cardiac valves can be ameliorated by percutaneous balloon valvuloplasty. In adult practice, however, the procedure is generally reserved for mitral or aortic stenosis.

Balloon mitral valvuloplasty

The principal clinical indication for mitral valvuloplasty is symptomatic isolated mitral stenosis with impaired LV function and pulmonary edema. The mitral area should be less than 1.5 cm^2, there should be no significant mitral regurgitation and there should be no LA thrombus. The likelihood of success is greatest when echocardiographic assessment yields a so-called "splitability score" of <8 (Table 42.1).

The MV is usually instrumented via a femoral vein using an antegrade transseptal approach. A flexible guidewire is introduced into the LA and steered through the stenosed valve using TEE and fluoroscopy. A balloon catheter is then advanced over the guidewire through the LA into the LV, such that the mid-point of the balloon lies at the level of the MV leaflets. The balloon is then inflated to a predetermined volume using radio-opaque contrast, which results in dilatation of the valve along the fused commissures. The procedure has a 95% success rate with a reported procedural mortality of 1–2%. Atrial or, rarely, ventricular perforation may cause cardiac tamponade. Other complications, including new-onset mitral regurgitation secondary to valve leaflet tearing or chordal rupture and embolic stroke, are more likely in patients with unfavorable valvular anatomy.

Table 42.1 Abbreviated scoring system to assess suitability for mitral valvuloplasty based on valve morphology and leaflet mobility. The descriptions for scoring grades 1 and 3 have been omitted for simplicity

Score	0	2	4
Mobility of leaflets	Normal	Normal mobility of middle and base portions	No or minimal forward movement in diastole
Thickening of leaflets	Normal	Marked thickening (5–8 mm) of margins, but mid portions normal	Gross thickening (8–10 mm) of entire leaflet
Subvalvular thickening	Normal	Thickening of chordae involving up to one third of chordal length	Extensive thickening and shortening of chordal structures extending to papillary muscles
Calcification of leaflets	Normal	Scatters areas of brightness confined to leaflet margins	Extensive brightness throughout leaflet tissue

Reproduced from Wilkins *et al. Br Heart J* 1988; 60: 299–308 with permission from BMJ Publishing Group Ltd.

Core Topics in Cardiac Anesthesia, Second Edition, ed. Jonathan H. Mackay and Joseph E. Arrowsmith. Published by Cambridge University Press. © Cambridge University Press 2012.

Balloon aortic valvuloplasty

Balloon dilatation of a stenotic AV is rarely undertaken nowadays and is generally reserved for those patients in whom AV replacement is either contraindicated or considered to be too risky. The valve is approached in a retrograde fashion via a femoral artery under local anesthesia. A fluid-filled balloon is inflated within the valve to a high pressure for 30–60 s and then rapidly deflated. The aim of the procedure is to reduce the transvalvular (peak to peak) gradient to <30 mmHg. As well as transient loss of cardiac output during balloon inflation, complications of the procedure include aortic regurgitation and cardiac tamponade.

Cardiac defect occlusion devices

The longest-established percutaneous devices were developed for the closure of atrial septal defects. First-generation devices were cumbersome to use and difficult to deploy. These problems were largely eliminated by the use of *nitinol*; an alloy of nickel and titanium with the unique properties of shape memory and superelasticity. Percutaneous closure is suitable for lesions that are not too large, that can be crossed with a guidewire and that have a sufficient rim of tissue at their margin. Although these devices are most commonly used to close ASDs and PFOs, the range of indications has increased to include small congenital VSDs, ischemic VSDs and paraprosthetic valvular regurgitation.

Patent foramen ovale (PFO)

Indications for closure

PFO closure was initially described in children. It is only since the mid 1990s that interest in adult closure has grown. Percutaneous PFO closure has been shown to have a protective effect on stroke or transient ischemic attack (TIA) occurrence compared to medical therapy. Percutaneous PFO closure is therefore indicated to reduce the risk of embolic stroke. Percutaneous closure has also been advocated as a treatment for other conditions such as migraine and to prevent paradoxical embolization in decompression illness.

Types of device

At least seven types of percutaneous PFO closure device are currently available (Figure 42.1). The most commonly used devices are the Amplatzer, Cardio-SEAL-STARFlex and Helex occluder.

Deployment techniques

Percutaneous PFO closure is undertaken in conjunction with fluoroscopy and TEE guidance. Although individual devices vary – most devices comprise two interconnected discs or plates – deployment techniques are very similar. A guidewire is used to position the delivery catheter in the body of the LA. The distal (LA) disc is then deployed and pulled against the LA wall of the septum after which the proximal (RA) disc is deployed. The discs now lie either side of the septum, thus closing the defect. Once the position and efficacy of the closure device has been confirmed, the delivery cable is mechanically disengaged from the device.

Medium-term outcomes

In comparison to untreated PFO, the risk of peripheral embolization with neurologic sequelae is reduced from 5% to 2% per year after PFO closure. Medium-term complications include device thrombosis and paroxysmal AF.

Atrial septal defect (ASD)

Indications for closure

The first percutaneous ASD closure was performed in 1974. Because an ASD can lead to significant pulmonary hypertension in later life, absence of symptoms is not an indication for conservative management. A significant shunt with RV volume overload is an indication for closure before PA systolic pressure reaches 40 mmHg. Normal life expectancy can be achieved if closure is performed at <25 years of age. Percutaneous ASD closure is only indicated in secundum defects with a tissue margin sufficient to prevent compression and distortion of nearby structures – the vena cavae and atrioventricular valves. Echocardiography is particularly useful for delineating the location and size of the defect, quantifying the degree of shunt, assessing the severity of pulmonary hypertension and documenting underlying cardiac function.

Types of device

Two main types of device are commonly used: the Amplatzer septal occluder and the Helex septal occluder (Figure 42.1). The Amplatzer device consists of two discs made of polyester fabric in a nitinol wire

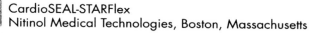
Figure 42.1 Devices for percutaneous ASD and PFO closure.

CardioSEAL-STARFlex
Nitinol Medical Technologies, Boston, Massachusetts

CardioSEAL
Nitinol Medical Technologies, Boston, Massachusetts

Amplatzer PFO Occluder
AGA Medical, Golden Valley, Minnesota

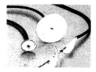

Helex Occluder
W.L. Gore and Associates, Inc, Flagstaff, Arizona

PFO-Star
CARDIA, Burnsville, Minnesota

Guardian Angel
Microvena Corporation, White Bear Lake, Minnesota

Sideris Buttoned Device
Custom Medical Devices, Amarillo, Texas

mesh whilst the Helex occluder device comprises a Gore-Tex® membrane covering a nitinol wire frame.

Deployment techniques

The static diameter of the defect is assessed using echocardiography and the stretched diameter with a sizing balloon. They are deployed in the same way as the PFO occlusion devices.

Medium-term outcome

Following percutaneous ASD closure, patients face an increased risk of developing AF, the incidence of which is age-dependent. Evidence of AF, TIA, stroke, worsening RV function or worsening pulmonary hypertension following repair all require further investigation.

Evidence suggests that, in comparison to surgical closure, percutaneous closure results in a greater preservation of cardiac function, a significantly lower complication rate and shorter length of hospital stay.

Ventricular septal defect (VSD)
Indications for closure

VSDs are more common than ASDs. Left untreated, VSDs inevitably lead to pulmonary hypertension and RV failure. Studies indicate that patients do equally well if treated surgically or by percutaneous closure. Percutaneous closure can provide an alternative means of

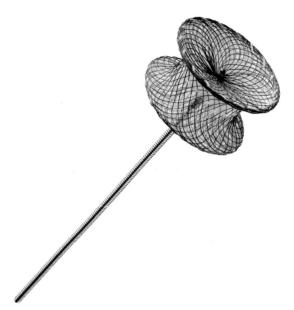

Figure 42.2 The Amplatzer® Muscular P.I. VSD Occluder. Courtesy of St. Jude Medical, Inc., Plymouth, MN, USA.

Table 42.2 Potential advantages of transcatheter aortic valve insertion

No need for sternotomy	Faster recovery Less postoperative pain Reduced wound infection Avoidance of re-sternotomy and damage to adherent structures, including patent coronary grafts
No need for CPB	Reduced neurologic complications? No activation of coagulation cascade, reduced bleeding and blood transfusion Reduced myocardial dysfunction after cross-clamp/cardioplegia
Reduced use of resources	Avoidance of ICU admission Shorter ICU and hospital stay cost offset at present by increased prosthetic valve cost

Modified from: Klein *et al. Br J Anaesth* 2009;103(6):792–9 by permission of Oxford University Press.
AVR, aortic valve replacement; CPB, cardiopulmonary bypass; ICU, intensive care unit.

treatment for those patients considered unfit, unstable or unwilling to undergo open cardiac surgery. It may have a role to play in the treatment of post MI, residual or iatrogenic VSD. Patients considered unsuitable for percutaneous VSD closure include infants under 3 kg of weight, those in whom the edge of the defect is <4 mm from a valve, and those with high PVR or sepsis.

Types of device

The Amplatzer muscular VSD occluder (Figure 42.2), a double-disc device, is the most commonly used and has the best results; a number of other devices are in development.

Deployment techniques

The trabeculae of the RV make crossing a VSD using a venous approach difficult. For this reason a double-catheter approach is often used for a percutaneous VSD repair. This may actually involve cannulation of the right internal jugular vein as well as a femoral artery and vein. The double-disk device is then positioned in a similar fashion to that for PFO/ASD closure, using a combination of echocardiography and fluoroscopy.

Medium-term outcome

A large prospective study comparing surgical and percutaneous VSD closure demonstrated no difference in outcomes. The percutaneous closure was associated with shorter hospital stay, fewer blood transfusions and fewer complications. It was also noted that percutaneous VSD closure was associated with improved ventricular reverse remodeling.

Percutaneous valve devices

Transcatheter aortic valve implantation

Indications

Untreated aortic stenosis is associated with high morbidity and mortality (Chapter 31). Patients considered, by virtue of advanced age and comorbidities, to be at too great a risk for conventional valve replacement surgery may be offered transcatheter AV implantation (TAVI). The criteria for selecting TAVI in preference to open surgery include poor LV function, previous sternotomy for coronary revascularization, diabetes mellitus, renal dysfunction, peripheral vascular disease and advanced age. In the absence of a TAVI-specific risk model, conventional scoring systems (e.g. Euro-SCORE) are used to estimate perioperative risk.

Types of device

There are two devices currently available for TAVI in the UK (Figure 42.3). The Edwards-SAPIEN valve (Edwards Life Sciences, USA) is a balloon expandable

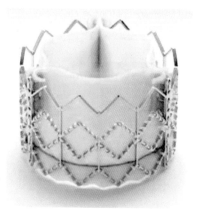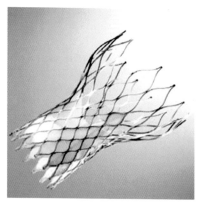

Figure 42.3 Transcatheter aortic valves. (Left) Edwards-Sapien aortic valve (Edwards LifeSciences Inc, USA). (Right) CoreValve aortic valve (Medtronic Inc USA).

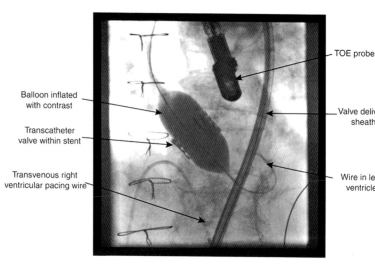

Balloon inflated with contrast

Transcatheter valve within stent

Transvenous right ventricular pacing wire

TOE probe

Valve delivery sheath

Wire in left ventricle

Figure 42.4 Fluorogram taken during transfemoral TAVI in a patient who has had a previous sternotomy. The balloon is inflated to expand the Edwards-Sapien valve during deployment. Reproduced from: Klein *et al. Br J Anaesth* 2009; 103(6): 792–9, with permission from Oxford University Press.

prosthesis. A bovine pericardial tri-leaflet valve mounted in a stainless steel stent is delivered over a balloon catheter and inflated to deploy the valve. The second device is the CoreValve (Medtronic Inc.); a nitinol framework encases a tri-leaflet porcine pericardial valve. The nitinol framework is malleable when cooled but when deployed and warmed to body temperature unravels, becoming rigid to assume its predetermined shape.

Deployment techniques

Both types of valves can be deployed via a femoral arterial sheath. The Edwards valve may also be implanted via a transapical approach. The transapical approach requires a small anterior thoracotomy to access the LV apex and is the favored mode of deployment for those with advanced aorto-iliac disease, which precludes the femoral approach.

A guide wire is advanced across the diseased AV and balloon valvuloplasty carried out prior to deployment of the prosthesis. To facilitate deployment rapid ventricular pacing is used to minimize LV ejection.

Patients are pre-treated with anti-platelet therapy and heparinized intraoperatively.

Para-valvular leak and LV perforation with the guide wire leading to cardiac tamponade are potential early complications.

Medium-term outcome

Following the introduction of TAVI in 2002 a number of groups have looked at outcome (Table 42.4). In survivors, clinical and hemodynamic improvement was seen 2 years after TAVI in patients with severe aortic stenosis. Long-term outcome data are awaited.

265

Table 42.3 Immediate complications of TAVI

Poor recovery of cardiac function after rapid ventricular pacing

Hemodynamic instability

Incorrect stent placement
  too high may impair coronary flow, leading to myocardial ischemia and infarction
  too low may lead to device embolization

Embolization of aortic material or air, leading to neurologic dysfunction

Aortic regurgitation, especially paravalvular
  may need further device dilatation to improve molding of device to aorta

Complete heart block

Transfemoral approach
  Vascular access damage (femoral/iliac artery or aorta), including dissection, rupture, and hemorrhage

Transapical approach
  Difficulty closing ventricular apex, leading to hemorrhage

Post-thoracotomy pain

Modified from: Klein *et al. Br J Anaesth* 2009;103(6):792–9 by permission of Oxford University Press.

Table 42.4 Intermediate and late complications of TAVI

Mortality at 30 days	5–18%
Mild to moderate paravalvular leak	50%
Vascular complications	10–15%
Acute myocardial infarction	2–11%
Stroke	3–9%
Atrioventricular block	4–8%
Prosthesis embolization	1%
Coronary occlusion	1%

Source: European Association of Cardio-thoracic Surgery and European Society of Cardiology.

Mitral valve procedures

Due to its more complex anatomic architecture the development of devices to repair or replace the mitral valve via a percutaneous approach has been more protracted.

Where MR is the primary problem, a percutaneous approach to MV repair has been described using an Alfieri-like "edge to edge" technique. The Mitra-Clip (Evalve Inc. USA) device is used to staple the tips of anterior and posterior leaflets to create a double-orifice MV.

Where functional MR is present, secondary either to degenerative or ischemic heart disease, the degree of regurgitation may be reduced by annuloplasty. A percutaneous approach, involving the deployment of reshaping devices in the coronary sinus to reduce MV annulus size, has also been trialled. In the near future it is possible that a patient with functional MR will be treated by a combination of transcatheter leaflet repair and coronary sinus annuloplasty.

At the development stage are a variety of percutaneous approaches to redo MV replacement. In many cases this has involved so-called "valve in valve" placement in which the transcatheter valve is implanted *within* an existing deficient prosthetic valve. The rationale for this approach is that the existing prosthetic annulus acts as a framework to support the new valve upon deployment.

Anesthetic considerations

The increasing complexity of percutaneous cardiological interventions has necessitated the development of hybrid environments that combine the features of a diagnostic imaging suite with those of an operating room. Despite the best design intentions these environments are typically more crowded, noisy and hazardous than traditional operating rooms.

Preoperative assessment

It is increasingly recognized that complex, catheter laboratory-based procedures under general anesthesia require a multi-disciplinary approach. Planning decisions, such as the choice of anesthesia, intraoperative monitoring, postoperative care and whether to institute CPB or convert to an open procedure in the event of complications, should be made well in advance of the procedure.

Anesthetic management

Although the spectrum of anesthetic involvement ranges from light sedation to invasively monitored general anesthesia for CPB the general principle of maintaining hemodynamic stability remains unchanged.

The need for intraoperative TEE during procedures that can normally be undertaken under sedation usually dictates the use of general anesthesia and endotracheal intubation. Additional relative indications for general anesthesia include: orthopnea, procedures expected to last more than 90 minutes, procedures known to be associated with significant hemodynamic instability and where the likelihood of conversion to open surgery with or without CPB is high.

The choice of anesthetic technique and airway management device is largely a matter of institutional protocol and personal preference. Volatile anesthetic agents are best avoided in the absence of active scavenging facilities. That said, a technique that facilitates early tracheal extubation and rapid recovery is highly desirable. Patients undergoing transapical procedures typically require a combination of simple oral analgesics, intercostal nerve blocks and patient-controlled opioid analgesia.

Key points

- Complex, catheter laboratory-based procedures require a multi-disciplinary approach.
- Despite the best design intentions, hybrid operating rooms are typically more crowded, noisy and hazardous than traditional operating rooms.
- Favorable long-term outcomes after TAVI may significantly reduce the number of patients with aortic stenosis considered unsuitable for valve replacement.

Further reading

Chiam PT, Ruiz CE. Percutaneous transcatheter aortic valve implantation: evolution of the technology. *Am Heart J* 2009; **157**(2): 229–42.

Goldberg SL, Feldman T. Percutaneous mitral valve interventions: overview of new approaches. *Curr Cardiol Rep* 2010; **12**(5): 404–12.

Klein AA, Webb ST, Tsui S, Sudarshan C, Shapiro L, Densem C. Transcatheter aortic valve insertion: anaesthetic implications of emerging new technology. *Br J Anaesth* 2009; **103**(6): 792–9.

Rosengart TK, Feldman T, Borger MA, *et al.* Percutaneous and minimally invasive valve procedures: a scientific statement from the American Heart Association Council on Cardiovascular Surgery and Anesthesia, Council on Clinical Cardiology, Functional Genomics and Translational Biology Interdisciplinary Working Group, and Quality of Care and Outcomes Research Interdisciplinary Working Group. *Circulation* 2008; **117**(13): 1750–67.

Cardiomyopathies and constrictive pericarditis

Florian Falter and Jonathan H. Mackay

Hypertrophic obstructive cardiomyopathy

Hypertrophic obstructive cardiomyopathy (HOCM) is a progressive disease, also referred to as idiopathic hypertrophic subaortic stenosis (IHSS) or asymmetrical septal hypertrophy (ASH). It is usually caused by a mutation in one of the nine sarcomeric genes; its inheritance is autosomal dominant with heterogeneous phenotypes in some families. The incidence is 0.2–0.5%.

Pathology

The predominant lesion is a ventricular septal hypertrophy with LVOT narrowing. The LV free wall, in comparison, remains relatively thin.

Clinical features

The most common presentation is sudden death in previously asymptomatic and often athletic individuals. A small number of patients develop symptoms similar to those of AS – typically breathlessness, angina and syncope/pre-syncope on exertion. Atrial and ventricular dysrhythmias are common.

Pathophysiology

HOCM causes dynamic LVOT obstruction, functional AS and dynamic MR. These lead to a secondary increase in LA pressure (LAP), reduced CO and hypotension.

Narrowing of the LVOT during systole leads to increased systolic ejection velocity, creating a Venturi effect, which draws the anterior mitral leaflet (AMVL) towards the hypertrophied septum. Simultaneously, systolic anterior motion (SAM) brings the AMVL in contact with the septum, leading to LVOT obstruction and MR secondary to distortion of the MV in

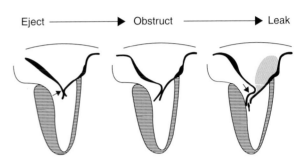

Eject ———▶ Obstruct ———▶ Leak

Figure 43.1 Systolic anterior motion of the anterior mitral leaflet, dynamic LVOT obstruction and mitral regurgitation in obstructive hypertrophic cardiomyopathy. Adapted from Grigg *et al. J Am Coll Cardiol* 1992; 20: 42–52.

mid to late systole. This sequence of events is summarized in Figure 43.1.

Increased muscle mass, decreased LV volume and myocardial fibrosis lead to decreased compliance and diastolic dysfunction. Reduced Ca^{2+} uptake by the sarcoplasmatic reticulum increases myoplasmic Ca^{2+} concentration, further contributing to impaired relaxation. Factors influencing the systolic LVOT pressure gradient and obstruction are summarized in Table 43.1.

Table 43.1 Factors determining LVOT obstruction in HOCM

Factors increasing	Factors decreasing
↓ Arterial blood pressure	↑ Arterial blood pressure
↓ Preload	↑ LV volume
↑ Blood flow velocity – inotropes	↓ Blood flow velocity – β-blockers/verapamil
↓ SVR	↑ SVR

Investigations

- *2D echo* This determines end-diastolic septal thickness and LVOT diameter, characterizes SAM and identifies the AMVL–septum contact point.

Core Topics in Cardiac Anesthesia, Second Edition, ed. Jonathan H. Mackay and Joseph E. Arrowsmith. Published by Cambridge University Press. © Cambridge University Press 2012.

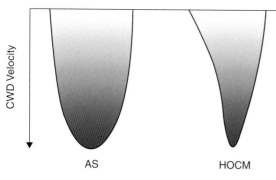

Figure 43.2 Continuous-wave Doppler in AS and HOCM.

Table 43.2 Anesthetic considerations in HOCM

Preload	Better full than empty
HR	Rather 60 than 80 bpm
Rhythm	Preserve NSR
Contractility	Maintain (most will tolerate mild depression as long as they are well filled)
SVR	Maintain or slightly ↑ to preserve coronary perfusion

The goals are very similar to those for AS.

- *Color Doppler* Shows characteristic systolic turbulence in LVOT with posteriorly directed MR jet.
- *CWD* Characteristic "shark tooth" velocity contour differs from AS (Figure 43.2). Velocity increases during systole due to SAM.
- *PWD* Determining the transmitral and pulmonary venous blood flow velocities allows assessment of impaired LV relaxation (see Chapter 25).
- *Cardiac catheterization* Continuously measuring pressure while withdrawing a catheter from the LV into the ascending aorta allows determination of the pressure differentials within the LVOT (so-called "pull-back" gradients).
- *Cardiac MRI* Functional imaging of LVOT obstruction during the cardiac cycle.

While imaging is the basis of investigation in HOCM, genetic testing should be considered especially in patients with a family history of unexplained sudden death.

Management

Most patients can be managed conservatively.

- *Medical* β-Blockers are the first-line treatment. If the LVOT gradient and symptoms persist a calcium channel antagonist of the verapamil type should be substituted. Implantation of a DDD pacing device can improve symptoms. Patients thought to be at high risk of sudden death should be considered for a combined pacemaker and ICD.
- *Interventional* Septal myectomy through the AV orifice can be performed in patients with poor symptom control despite maximum medical therapy. It focuses on relieving the LVOT

obstruction. In a select group of patients septal ablation, achieved by injecting alcohol into the septal branches of the LAD, may yield a similar result.

Anesthetic goals

The basic rule is to avoid any hemodynamic derangements that worsen LVOT obstruction. Surgery for the relief of dynamic LVOT obstruction is considered a category 1 indication for perioperative TEE (Chapter 24).

Complications after surgery

These include residual LVOT obstruction, VSD and conduction abnormalities requiring permanent pacing.

Restrictive cardiomyopathy

Restrictive or obliterative cardiomyopathy is a rare cause of severe diastolic dysfunction.

Pathology

The condition is characterized by increasing stiffness of the ventricular myocardium and endocardial thrombosis, leading to poor diastolic filling. The myocardium is not normally thickened. The causes can be divided in primary and secondary.

- Primary
  - Löffler's endocarditis
  - Endocardial fibroelastosis
- Secondary
  - Amyloidosis
  - Sarcoidosis
  - Hemochromatosis
  - Carcinoid

- Glycogen storage diseases
- Post radiation fibrosis
- Tropical endomyocardial fibrosis

Clinical features

Patients usually present with signs and symptoms of biventricular failure: shortness of breath, palpitations and edema. Signs of right heart failure tend to predominate. Chest pain and syncope are less common.

Pathophysiology

There are many similarities to constrictive pericarditis. Severe myocardial stiffening and very poor ventricular compliance cause the characteristic pattern of rapid but early diastolic filling.

Investigations

2D echo Shows normal systolic function but restricted diastolic relaxation. Biatrial dilatation is common.

PWD Shows restrictive filling pattern (see Figure 25.9)

Cardiac MRI Can detect accumulation or infiltration with amyloid or iron.

Cardiac catheterization Allows endomyocardial biopsy and measurement of pressure in cardiac chambers.

Management

Seventy percent of patients with restrictive cardiomyopathy die within 5 years of the onset of symptoms. Standard heart failure treatment is not helpful as it lowers venous return and reduces systemic blood pressure. On occasion, diuretics are indicated to relieve edema.

Anesthetic goals

See Table 43.3.

Table 43.3 Anesthetic considerations in restrictive cardiomyopathy

Preload	High
HR	High – in view of fixed SV
Rhythm	NSR preferred – but little dependent on late diastolic filling
Contractility	Maintain – inotropic support invariably needed
SVR	Maintain – in view of fixed SV

Dilated cardiomyopathy

Dilated cardiomyopathy (DCM) is the most common form of cardiomyopathy. It is most common in males between the ages of 20 and 60 years and is responsible for up to a third of all cases of congestive heart failure.

Pathology

DCM is characterized by four-chamber cardiac enlargement, cardiomyocyte hypertrophy and a propensity towards formation of intra-cardiac thrombi. Cardiomyopathy secondary to myocardial ischemia may be limited to the LV.

DCM is likely to be the result of damage to the myocardium by toxic, infectious or metabolic agents. However, in many cases the etiology will remain unknown. Between 20 and 40% of patients have a familial form of the disease, transmission typically being autosomal dominant.

- Primary
  - Idiopathic
  - Sickle cell disease
  - Duchenne muscular dystrophy
- Secondary
  - Ischemia
  - Infection (viral, trypanosomal)
  - Toxins (ethanol, doxorubicin, cobalt, ionizing radiation)
  - Stimulants (amphetamine)
  - Thyroid disease (myxedema)
  - Uncontrolled, persistent tachycardia
  - Morbid obesity
  - Peripartum

Clinical features

DCM is characterized by progressive left, right or biventricular failure and declining functional status. Ventricular dysrhythmias are common. Patients are at risk of pulmonary and arterial embolism from intracardiac thrombi if inadequately anticoagulated.

Pathophysiology

Impaired systolic and diastolic function, low CO and an elevated LVEDP are typical in DCM. Subsequent A-V valve regurgitation worsens atrial enlargement, increasing the likelihood of AF. Ventricular compliance is reduced. Measuring diastolic transmitral blood flow velocity reveals impaired relaxation very early in the disease process (see Figure 25.9).

Investigations

DCM is usually diagnosed on the basis of echocardiographic examination. 2D echo shows dilatation of all four chambers and poor ventricular contractility. Other investigations such as MRI and cardiac catheterization are rarely of additional diagnostic value, although the latter may reveal coronary artery and valvular disease that may be amenable to surgery.

Management

Patients are treated with standard heart failure therapy, comprising ACE inhibitors, diuretics and possibly digoxin. A pacemaker or ICD should be considered in patients with conduction abnormalities or arrhythmias. Despite medical therapy, a significant number of patients die within 3 years of the onset of symptoms. Mechanical ventricular assist devices and cardiac transplantation are of proven prognostic benefit (see Chapter 57).

Anesthetic goals

See Table 43.4.

Table 43.4 Anesthetic considerations in DCM

Preload	Already high, avoid overfilling
HR	Avoid tachycardia – impaired ventricular relaxation
Rhythm	NSR preferred –little dependence on late diastolic filling
Contractility	Maintain – inotropic support invariably needed
SVR	Maintain or slight decrease – increase poorly tolerated

Ventricular aneurysm

It is important to distinguish between false and true LV aneurysms. A false ventricular aneurysm or ventricular pseudoaneurysm is a rupture of the ventricular free wall contained by the surrounding pericardium (Figure 43.3) Ventricular rupture following myocardial infarction has a peak incidence 5–10 days after the event (Chapter 41). As the likelihood of further rupture and tamponade is high, surgical

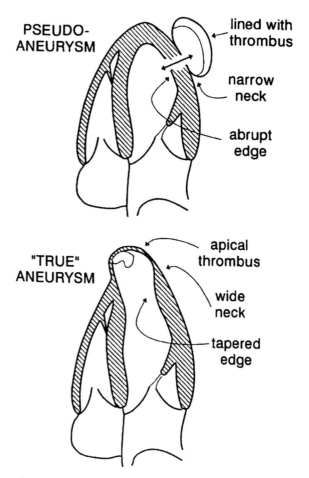

Figure 43.3 False and true aneurysm of the LV. (From Otto CM. *Textbook of Clinical Echocardiography*, 2nd edn. Philadelphia: WB Saunders; 2000. p. 221.)

repair is indicated. Ventricular pseudoaneurysm may also occur following MV, AV and congenital heart surgery.

A true ventricular aneurysm is an area of the ventricle where thin stretched scar tissue has replaced muscle. During diastole the aneurysm appears as a protruding segment of ventricular wall beyond the expected outline of the ventricular cavity. During systole the segment appears either akinetic or dyskinetic (Figure 43.4).

- The overwhelming majority of LV aneurysms are secondary to coronary artery disease (CAD).
- More than 80% of LV aneurysms involve the anterior wall or apex and are associated with occlusion or high-grade stenosis of the LAD.
- An LV aneurysm may be evident on ventriculography within 2 weeks of transmural MI.

271

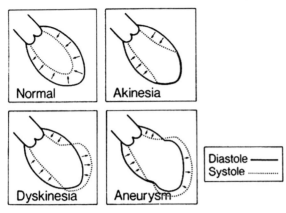

Figure 43.4 The natural history of a true left ventricular aneurysm. (From Grondin P, Kretz JG, Bical O, *et al.* Natural history of saccular aneurysms of the left ventricle. *J Thorac Cardiovasc Surg* 1979; 77: 57–64.)

Approximately 8% of patients with coronary artery disease referred for coronary angiography have an LV aneurysm. Mitral regurgitation is a frequent finding. Ventricular arrhythmias and LV failure are the commonest causes of death. Although the overall risk of thromboembolic events is small, patients with mural thrombus or low LVEF (i.e. <25%) should be anticoagulated.

Indications for surgery

Patients with LV aneurysm who are asymptomatic have a good prognosis without surgical intervention. In patients with triple-vessel CAD, surgery improves both symptoms and prognosis. LV aneurysm repair is, therefore, often performed together with coronary revascularization.

There is currently a trend toward more aggressive management of LV aneurysm – a more detailed discussion about the decision to plicate, resect or ignore the LV aneurysm is beyond the scope of this chapter. The generic term "Laplace operations" has been applied to these procedures, which all reduce ventricular size and, thus, wall stress.

Constrictive pericarditis

Constrictive pericarditis is an uncommon cause of diastolic dysfunction.

Pathology

Pericardial inflammation leads to fibrosis and calcification. The fibrous tissue contracts over years,

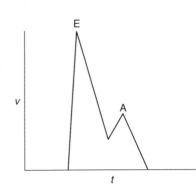

Figure 43.5 Transmitral diastolic flow pattern in constrictive pericarditis. Note the high-velocity E-wave and short deceleration time.

ultimately encasing the heart in a non-compliant sac. This prevents normal diastolic filling and the transmission of intra-thoracic pressure changes to the cardiac chambers.

Tuberculosis (TB) used to be the most common cause of chronic pericarditis, but now only accounts for about 2% of cases in developed countries. Frequently the etiology of constrictive pericarditis is unknown. Frequently suspected causes include:

- infection (viral, TB, fungal)
- radiotherapy to the chest
- connective tissue disorders (rheumatoid arthritis, systemic lupus erythematosus)
- previous blunt chest trauma
- previous cardiac surgery
- chronic renal failure.

Clinical features

Signs of impaired RV filling predominate. Patients usually present with hepatomegaly and ascites rather than peripheral edema. In the latter stages of the disease patients often appear cachectic and jaundiced. Although it may be difficult to distinguish constrictive pericarditis from restrictive cardiomyopathy, it is important to make the correct diagnosis as treatment is very different (Table 43.4).

Pathophysiology

Constriction gives rise to rapid early diastolic filling, which ceases abruptly when the limits of ventricular expansion are reached (Figures 43.5 and 43.6). End-diastolic pressures are virtually the same in all four cardiac chambers. Overall cardiac volume is fixed, which leads to exaggerated ventricular interdependence. There is dissociation between intrathoracic and intracardiac pressures.

Table 43.5 Differential diagnosis of constrictive pericarditis and restrictive cardiomyopathy

	Constrictive pericarditis	Restrictive cardiomyopathy
CXR	Diffuse calcification of pericardium	Normal heart size
CVP	Prominent $y \gg x$ descents	Elevated. Prominent cv-wave in the presence of tricuspid regurgitation
PA catheter	PA systolic pressure normally <40 mmHg	PA systolic pressure $\geq$50 mmHg
LV catheter	"Square root" sign RVEDP = LVEDP RV systolic pressure $\leq$50 mmHg	LVEDP – RVEDP >5 mmHg RV systolic $\geq$50 mmHg
2D echo	Pericardial thickening and effusion	Normal pericardium
Doppler echo	Restrictive pattern Respiratory swing >25% variation peak mitral velocities during inspiration	Little respiratory swing in velocities
CT and MRI	Pericardial thickness >4 mm	Pericardial thickness <4 mm

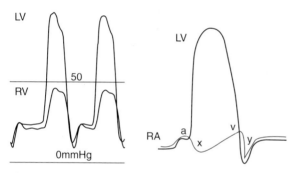

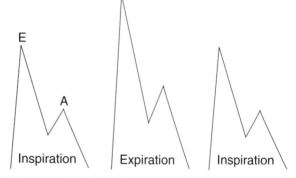

Figure 43.6 Typical pressure waveforms in constrictive pericarditis. (Left) The pathognomonic "square root sign" can be seen in both the LV and RV pressure traces. (Right) Rapid, unimpeded early diastolic filling gives rise to a deep y-descent in the RA pressure trace. The short duration of the y-descent is due to abrupt cessation of early diastolic filling.

Figure 43.7 The effect of spontaneous respiration on diastolic LV filling in constrictive pericarditis.

During normal spontaneous respiration, inspiration increases venous return to the right heart with a slight shift of the interventricular septum to the left. In contrast, increased pulmonary capacitance (fall in PAWP > fall in LVEDP) reduces venous return to the left heart, resulting in a fall in systemic arterial pressure by up to 10 mmHg. As changes in intrathoracic pressure are not transmitted in constrictive pericarditis, this respiratory paradox is exaggerated and LV filling can vary by more than 25% throughout the respiratory cycle (Figure 43.7).

Investigations
Diagnosis is often difficult and needs a high index of suspicion.

Management
Mild pericardial constriction may be amenable to diuretic therapy aimed at lowering venous filling pressure. Definitive treatment requires open surgery to remove the pericardium. The procedure carries a significant risk, with a reported mortality of up to 6%. Patients are often in poor physiological condition, and are prone to major hemorrhage and hemodynamic instability during dissection. Unstable cases may need CPB standby.

273

Most surgeons use median sternotomy as it provides better exposure and makes cannulation easier. If an anterolateral thoracotomy is used, lung isolation is usually required. Because institution of positive-pressure ventilation is associated with a significant reduction in LV filling and profound hypotension, airway pressure should be kept to a minimum and PEEP should be avoided. Pressure-controlled ventilation is often preferable to volume-controlled ventilation.

Unlike pericardial tamponade, pericardiectomy in the setting of constrictive pericarditis does not usually result in instantaneous reversal of pathophysiology and improvement in cardiovascular parameters.

Anesthetic goals

Anesthetic considerations are similar to those for cardiac tamponade. Both conditions are associated with impaired diastolic filling, increased atrial pressures, tachycardia and reduced SV. In constrictive pericarditis, however, ventricular filling occurs in early diastole, whereas in tamponade ventricular filling occurs predominantly in late diastole.

Arrhythmogenic right ventricular cardiomyopathy

Formerly known as arrhythmogenic RV dysplasia, this inherited cardiomyopathy (ARVC) is characterized by gradual replacement of RV myocardium with fat fibrous tissue which provides an excellent substrate for arrhythmias. The majority of cases present in early adolescence with syncope, monomorphic VT or sudden cardiac death. A family history of syncope or sudden cardiac death should elevate the degree of suspicion. The diagnosis is made using RV angiography, echocardiography and MRI. Fortunately, drugs used for general anesthesia do not appear to increase arrhythmogenicity.

Table 43.6 Anesthetic considerations in pericardial constriction

Preload	Increased
HR	High – in view of fixed SV
Rhythm	NSR preferred –little dependence on late diastolic filling
Contractility	Maintain – inotropic support may be needed
SVR	Maintain

Non-compaction cardiomyopathy

Non-compaction cardiomyopathy (NCC) or spongiform cardiomyopathy is a rare and relatively recently described congenital myocardial abnormality. The condition may occur in isolation or in association with other cardiac abnormalities. NCC may be completely asymptomatic, present acutely with ventricular tachyarrythmia or thromboembolic phenomena, or present with symptoms of progressive cardiac failure. The diagnosis, confirmed when the trabeculations are more than twice the thickness of the underlying venticular wall, is typically made using echocardiography and MRI.

Key points

- Strategies to reduce LVOT obstruction in HOCM include increasing preload and afterload, and reducing myocardial contractility.
- A false ventricular aneurysm is a ventricular free rupture wall contained by the pericardium.
- The differentiation between constrictive pericarditis and restrictive cardiomyopathy can be difficult.
- Pressure-controlled ventilation and avoidance of PEEP are preferable in constrictive pericarditis.

Chapter

44

Cardiac transplantation

Clive J. Lewis

Historical perspective

A number of landmark events led Christiaan Barnard to perform the world's first heart transplant in 1967, including development of surgical techniques and understanding the immunological basis of transplantation. The last 40 years have seen an evolution in this understanding and the organization of transplantation to allow appropriate organ allocation and a mechanism for registering the results of transplantation around the world. Despite the increasing longevity of patients with long-term ventricular assist device (VAD) support, cardiac transplantation remains the only real long-term treatment for patients with end-stage heart failure receiving optimal medical and device therapy.

Heart transplant significantly improves both long-term survival and quality of life, with 50% of patients surviving for 10 years and 20% for 20 years (Figure 44.1). Initial results were disappointing and only improved following the introduction of ciclosporin. Despite improvements in care and the introduction of newer drugs, cardiac transplantation remains a palliative procedure, with the majority of patients dying from allograft vasculopathy and other complications of long-term immunosuppression.

Transplant volume

The International Society for Heart and Lung Transplantation registry shows that the number of cardiac transplants peaked at around 4000 per year in the mid 1990s and has fallen to a relatively stable level of around 3000 procedures per year since. The number of transplants is limited by the supply of organs and, thus, the number of suitable organ donors. Improved road safety and neurosurgical intensive care are, at least in part, responsible for a decrease in the number of suitable donors. The shortage of organs has necessitated the use of resuscitated "marginal donors" whose organs would previously have been considered unsuitable for transplantation.

The overwhelming majority of cardiac transplants take place in North America and Europe. Experience is concentrated in relatively few centers, with 79% of these performing fewer than 20 transplants each year. The relative risk for 1-year mortality is inversely proportional to volume.

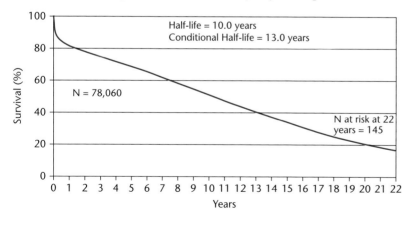

Figure 44.1 Kaplan-Meier survival curve for cardiac transplantation from data submitted to the International Society of Heart and Lung transplantation (January 1982 – June 2007). Conditional half-life is the time to 50% survival for those recipients surviving the first year post transplantation. Reproduced with permission from: Taylor DO, Stehlik J, Edwards LB, et al. 2009. © Elsevier 2009.

Core Topics in Cardiac Anesthesia, Second Edition, ed. Jonathan H. Mackay and Joseph E. Arrowsmith. Published by Cambridge University Press. © Cambridge University Press 2012.

Indications for transplantation

Cardiac transplantation should be considered in any patient with end-stage heart failure, NYHA class III or IV symptoms and significant limitation of activity despite maximal medical or device therapy. Survival in this group of patients, estimated using the Seattle heart failure model, is <2 years. Other indications include recurrent refractory life-threatening arrhythmia and intractable angina in patients considered unsuitable for conventional revascularization. Cardiomyopathy (predominantly dilated forms) and coronary artery disease make up almost 90% of all patients accepted for transplantation, with the latter decreasing in recent years. Other indications include hypertrophic cardiomyopathy, restrictive cardiomyopathy, arrhythmogenic right ventricular cardiomyopathy, congenital heart disease, valvular heart disease, peripartum cardiomyopathy and, perhaps controversially, re-transplantation.

Contraindications

Good candidates for cardiac transplantation have single organ failure and no significant comorbidity. General contraindications are the presence of any non-cardiac condition which would shorten life expectancy or increase risk of death after transplantation (Table 44.1).

Pulmonary hypertension, secondary to elevated LAP, is common. Pulmonary vascular resistance (PVR) and transpulmonary gradient (TPG) are key determinants of outcome.

$$\textbf{TPG} = \textbf{Mean PAP} - \textbf{PAWP}$$

$$\textbf{PVR} = \textbf{TPG/CO}$$

A normal TPG is ~6 mmHg, therefore a normal PVR is 6 mmHg/5 l min^{-1} = 1.2 Wood units (1.2 mmHg/l min^{-1} ~ 96 dyne s cm^{-5}). An irreversible PVR >5 Wood units and/or TPG >15 mmHg is associated with an increased incidence of post transplantation RV failure. If PVR falls below 5 Wood units with medical treatment, the risk may be considered acceptable. A TPG >15 mmHg is associated with unacceptably high mortality and is an absolute contraindication to heart transplantation. In contrast to LV failure, where there is elevation of both PA diastolic (PAD) and LV end-diastolic pressure, only PAD pressure is elevated in pulmonary hypertension and there may be a large gradient between PAD pressure and LVEDP (Figure 44.2).

Table 44.1 Contraindications to cardiac transplantation

Absolute	Relative
Significant pulmonary hypertension systolic PA pressure >60 mmHg raised PVR (>5 Wood units) or trans-pulmonary gradient (>15 mmHg)	Older age (>65 years)
Advanced lung disease (FEV$_1$ < 50%)	Peripheral or cerebral vascular disease
Diabetes mellitus with significant end organ damage	Obesity (BMI >30 kg m^{-2})
Advanced liver disease bilirubin >2.5 mg dl^{-1} (43 μmol l^{-1})	Osteoporosis
Renal dysfunction estimated GFR <40–50 ml min^{-1} 1.73 m^{-2}	Psychosocial factors leading to non-adherence
Infection (active sepsis, HIV, active hepatitis B/C)	Previous malignancy with risk of recurrence
Recent PE, CVA or malignancy	Bleeding risk (diverticulitis, peptic ulcer disease)
Active alcohol, smoking or other substance misuse	Mechanical ventilator dependence

FEV1, forced expiratory volume in 1 second; GFR, glomerular filtration rate; HIV, human immunodeficiency virus; BMI, body mass index.

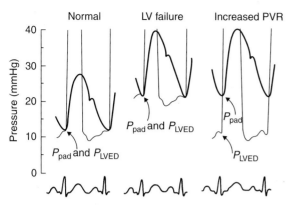

Figure 44.2 LV and PA pressure waveforms. In LV failure the PA diastolic (PAD) and LV end-diastolic (LVEDP) pressures are elevated, whereas increased PVR results in a large pressure gradient (i.e. PAD > LVEDP) From: Benumof JL. *Anesthesia for Thoracic Surgery*, 2nd edn. Philadelphia: WB Saunders; 1995.

Assessment and recipient selection

Selection of patients for cardiac transplantation requires a specialist multidisciplinary approach. Many countries maintain two waiting lists ("elective" and "urgent") for cardiac transplantation to allow prioritization of scarce resources. The clinical spectrum of expectant recipients ranges from the patient at home to the inpatient requiring mechanical ventricular support on an ICU. Patients considered too "well" for transplant and those already accepted for transplantation must undergo regular evaluation, particularly if there has been a worsening of symptoms. A recommended evaluation protocol is shown in Table 44.2.

Donor selection

When a donor heart is offered for transplantation, matching the donor organ to a recipient takes into account the following:

- ABO blood group compatibility
- HLA antibodies
- height and weight of both donor and recipient (aim for mismatch <10%)
- clinical priority of recipient
- potential duration of organ ischemic – interval between application of aortic cross-clamp in the donor to release of aortic cross-clamp in recipient (aim for <4 h).

Estimation of the likely duration of organ ischemia is often difficult, being influenced by the geographic location of the recipient and donor, transportation issues and even the weather!

Table 44.2 Evaluation protocol for cardiac transplantation

General	History and examination Nutritional status – body mass index
Immunology	Blood group HLA antibody screening
Cardiovascular function	ECG and CXR 6 min walk (<300 meters) Echocardiogram Cardiopulmonary exercise testing – VO_2max <14 ml kg^{-1} min^{-1} Right heart catheterization for PAP, PVR, TPG Consider left heart catheterization/imaging for viability
Other organ function	Routine biochemistry, hematology, coagulation Urinalysis and 24 h urine collection for proteinuria and GFR Lung function – pulmonary function tests
Infectious disease screening	Serology for Epstein-Barr, cytomegalovirus, hepatitis B and C, HIV, toxoplasma, rubella, varicella zoster, herpes simplex viruses Update vaccination for hepatitis B, influenza, pneumococcus
Preventive and malignancy	Prostate-specific antigen Fecal occult blood Mammography Cervical smear Dental review Neuropsychosocial evaluation Consider further imaging Carotid/peripheral Doppler, chest/abdominal CT

The donor management team is responsible for the assessment of the donor heart. Their role is optimization of hemodynamics and maximizing the chances of successful organ procurement from marginal donors. Factors affecting donor selection at the time of organ retrieval include:

- donor age (<65 years)
- cardiac function (ideally ECG and echocardiogram)
- significant coronary artery disease
- comorbidity, e.g. diabetes mellitus, extracranial malignancy
- known or suspected substance abuse
- history of cardiac arrest, mode of death
- untreated sepsis.

Surgical considerations

Orthotopic heart transplantation was first described by Lower and Shumway using a biatrial anastomosis using cuffs of LA (containing pulmonary veins) and RA (with both SVC and IVC). Nowadays, most surgeons use bicaval anastomosis, a technique associated with lower mortality, lower postoperative RA pressures, less tricuspid regurgitation and a greater chance of normal sinus rhythm. Special consideration should be given to patients undergoing re-sternotomy, VAD explantation and those with complex anatomy in congenital heart disease.

Anesthetic considerations

Many aspects of the perioperative anesthetic and critical management of heart transplant surgery patients are similar to those of conventional cardiac surgery. The overall approach is the same as that for a patient with severely impaired LV function undergoing conventional cardiac surgery (Table 44.3). Use of an 8F central venous sheath allows rapid fluid administration and facilitates subsequent PAFC insertion. Given that the RIJ will be used for obtaining biopsies to monitor rejection, in some centers use of the LIJ vein is preferred for the operation. The maintenance of cerebral, renal and

Table 44.3 Anesthetic and critical care considerations in cardiac transplantation

Preoperative	Fasting status – it is unusual to meet patients who have been fasting for <3 h
	History of previous instrumentation of central veins – in some centers the right internal jugular vein is preserved for postoperative endocardial biopsy
	Presence of permanent pacemaker/ICD (see Chapter 39)
	Preoperative anticoagulation and need for blood products
	Perioperative administration of immunosuppressants according to local protocols
	Prophylactic antibiotics
	Induction and maintenance of anesthesia in the context of pulmonary hypertension
Cardiac function	Hemodynamic monitoring e.g. intraoperative TEE
	PAFC – there is little point advancing the catheter until after implantation
	Inotropic support early after transplant e.g. epinephrine, isoproterenol, dopamine, and (increasingly) phosphodiesterase inhibitors
	Donor organ dysfunction
	LV dysfunction – consider if low MAP/CO despite moderate doses of inotropes, failure to wean from CPB or rising LA pressure
	Use vasoconstrictors, IABP and mechanical support
	RV dysfunction – consider if RA >15 mmHg and raised PVR/PAP (especially if pre-existing)
	Use inotropic support for RV and adjust RV preload
	Consider pulmonary selective vasodilators e.g. prostacyclin (epoprostenol 2–50 ng kg^{-1} min^{-1}), nitric oxide (up to 20 ppm) and RV assist device
	Avoid hypoxemia, hypercarbia, and metabolic acidosis
	Management of vasoplegia – persistent hypotension secondary to ↓SVR despite use of vasoconstrictors
	Assess graft function for 8–12 h prior to tracheal extubation
Disturbance of heart rate/rhythm	Donor sinus node dysfunction and pacing
	Transplanted heart denervation
	Arrhythmia management
Maintenance of renal function	Often impaired preoperatively due to low CO and drug therapy
	Primary determinant of good cardiac function
	Consider early renal replacement therapy for inadequate urine output
	Delay initiation of calcineurin inhibitors
Prevention of infection	Continuing prophylactic antibiotics
	Prophylactic antivirals (especially cytomegalovirus)
	Prophylactic antiprotozoals (e.g. toxoplasma, pneumocystis)
Additional considerations	Avoid transfusion unless necessary – may increase PVR and risk of sensitization
	Careful fluid balance management

splanchnic perfusion is of greater importance than balancing myocardial oxygen demand and supply. Post-induction hypotension is common and should be treated aggressively with a combination of fluids, vasopressors and inotropes. It should be borne in mind that myocardial sensitivity to inotropes may be reduced.

The use of a PAFC before explantation is not routine as it rarely alters management. The catheter may be difficult to insert, may cause significant dysrhythmia, and must be withdrawn to <15 cm before explantation. TEE offers major advantages over the PAFC during surgery and provides valuable information about donor heart function. PAFC monitoring of mixed venous oxygen is particularly useful in the early postoperative period.

Immediately following implantation, de-airing and reperfusion of the donor heart, isoproterenol (5–10 µg kg^{-1} min^{-1} for up to 5 days) is used to provide chronotropic support (target HR ~100) and mild pulmonary vasodilatation. As the output of the donor heart is largely rate-dependent, epicardial atrioventricular sequential pacing should be initiated if isoproterenol is ineffective. Taking care not to disrupt surgical anastamoses, a PAFC may be advanced at this stage with the help of the surgeon. Persistent hypotension in the presence of normal or elevated filling pressures should be treated with further inotropic support.

Patients with established pulmonary hypertension are at increased risk of donor heart dysfunction. TEE will reveal RV dilatation and a small, hyperkinetic LV. The therapeutic approach consists of inotropic support and vasodilatation. Hypoxia, hypercarbia and metabolic acidosis must be avoided. Because of its effect on PVR, enoximone or milrinone are useful adjuncts. Inhaled NO (up to 20 ppm) or epoprostenol (prostacyclin – PGI2; 2–50 ng kg^{-1} min^{-1}) may be considered in refractory cases.

If ventricular failure persists despite maximal inotropic and vasodilator therapy, mechanical circulatory (i.e. IABP) or ventricular assist (i.e. VAD) should be considered as a "bridge to recovery".

An increasing proportion of patients presenting for heart transplantation will have been taking anticoagulants before surgery. It is, therefore, important to have blood products (red cells, FFP and/or platelets) readily available after CPB.

The transplanted heart is initially denervated. In the absence of adrenergic and vagal efferents, the Frank-Starling mechanism and levels of circulating catecholamines and metabolites (e.g. lactate, H$^+$) dictate cardiac performance. Resting heart rate is usually higher than normal and rises to a lesser degree during exercise. Paradoxically, ischemic injury to the sino-atrial or atrioventricular nodes may produce severe bradycardia. Up to 20% of transplanted patients will require a permanent pacemaker.

Management of immunosuppression

Induction refers to the administration of immuno-suppressants at the time of transplant in order to establish an immunological environment for graft acceptance. In addition to high-dose corticosteroids (e.g. methylprednisolone) and other maintenance immunosuppressants, drugs directed against thymocytes (T cells) are used in 50% of transplant centers. In an effort to preserve renal function, polyclonal antibodies (e.g. rabbit anti-thymocyte globulin) or interleukin-2 receptor antagonists (e.g. basiliximab) are often used to delay the introduction of calcineurin inhibitors. Use of this approach, however, is associated with increased late infection and post transplant lymphoproliferative disease (PTLD).

Maintenance immunosuppression usually consists of a combination of a calcineurin inhibitor (or a TOR inhibitor if there is renal dysfunction), an anti-proliferative agent and corticosteroid. This allows enhanced immunosuppressant efficacy whilst reducing organ toxicities (Table 44.4).

Post transplant complications and surveillance

Acute rejection

This may be cellular or antibody-mediated. Both can result in allograft dysfunction but may be asymptomatic. Symptoms include pyrexia, arrhythmia, fluid retention and dyspnea. Acute rejection is responsible for 12% of deaths between months 1 and 12 after transplantation. Surveillance myocardial biopsy is performed weekly immediately post transplantation, or following emergence of symptoms of rejection. Biopsy frequency is reduced to 2–3 monthly by 12 months, after which many centers do not routinely perform biopsies. Rejection treatment includes high-dose corticosteroids, augmentation of maintenance immunosuppression, anti T-cell antibodies, interleukin-2 inhibitors, plasmapheresis and total lymphoid irradiation.

Table 44.4 Immunosuppressants commonly used in cardiac transplantation

Corticosteroids	Inhibit T-cell cytokine production
	Methylprednisolone 1 mg kg^{-1} reducing to maintenance 0.2 mg kg^{-1} by 3 weeks
	70% of patients at 1 year and 50% at 5 years remain on steroids
Calcineurin inhibitors	Prevent T-cell activation
	Ciclosporin (1–3 mg kg^{-1} day^{-1}) and tacrolimus (0.15–0.3 mg kg^{-1} day^{-1})
	Initiation should be delayed until renal function has normalized and dose adjustment by trough blood level monitoring
	Metabolized by cytochrome P450: care with co-administered drugs
	Toxicity includes nephrotoxicity, hypertension, dyslipidemia, hyperkalemia, hypomagnesemia, hyperuricemia and neurologic effects
Anti-proliferative agents	Inhibit lymphocyte proliferation
	Azathioprine (2–4 mg kg^{-1}), mycophenolate mofetil (2–3 g day^{-1})
	Toxicity includes myelosuppression and gastrointestinal disturbance
Target of rapamycin (TOR) inhibitors	Prevent T and B-cell activation
	Sirolimus (2–5 mg.day^{-1}) is usually used *de novo* or late after transplant for renal dysfunction (minimal nephrotoxicity)

Allograft vasculopathy

This is also termed chronic rejection – an accelerated coronary vasculopathy common in the first decade after transplantation (affecting 30% by 5 years and 55% by 10 years). It is the leading cause of late death (4% by 10 years) and graft dysfunction (9% by 10 years) after transplantation. The phenomenon is probably immune-mediated. The characteristic concentric intimal proliferation involves the whole length of the vessel, making revascularization virtually impossible. Surveillance is by invasive coronary angiography, yearly in some centers, and intra-vascular ultrasound. There is no effective treatment apart from statins and re-transplantation.

Infection

Common infections include respiratory viruses and bacteria, fungi, cytomegalovirus, toxoplasmosis and pneumocystis.

Malignancy

Up to 30% of transplant recipients develop immuno-suppression-related malignancy by 10 years. Common types include skin (85%) and PTLD (2–3%).

Renal dysfunction

This may be classed as severe in 5% of cases. Long-term renal replacement therapy is required in 1–2% of cases. Renal transplantation takes place in 0.3% patients by 5 years.

Other problems

These include hypertension (90% by 5 years), dyslipidemia (90% by 5 years), diabetes mellitus (40% by 5 years), osteoporosis, gout and late tricuspid regurgitation. It is not unusual, therefore, for patients to be taking aspirin, statins, anti-hypertensives, calcium and vitamin D supplements, bisphosphonates, allopurinol and hypoglycemics in addition to routine immunosuppression.

Key points

- RV failure is likely to occur if a heart is transplanted into a recipient with PVR >5 Wood units.
- A TPG >15 mmHg is associated with higher postoperative mortality.
- Maintaining perfusion pressure and oxygen delivery to the key organs is the primary goal in the pre-CPB period.
- The two key determinants of outcome are absence of pulmonary hypertension in the recipient and quality of myocardial protection of the implanted heart.
- The proportions of heart transplant recipients surviving 1, 5, and 10 years are approximately 90%, 70%, and 50% respectively.

Further reading

Kirklin JK, Young JB, McGiffin DC (Eds.). *Heart Transplantation*. Philadelphia: Churchill Livingstone; 2009.

Madsen JC, Klein A, Lewis C (Eds.). *Organ Transplantation: A Clinical Guide*. Cambridge: Cambridge University Press; 2011.

Taylor DO, Stehlik J, Edwards LB, *et al.* Registry of the International Society for Heart and Lung Transplantation: Twenty-sixth Official Adult Heart Transplant Report-2009. *J Heart Lung Transplant* 2009; **28**(10): 1007–22.

Pulmonary vascular disease

Cameron Graydon and Roger M. O. Hall

Patients with pulmonary vascular disease (PVD) and pulmonary hypertension (PHT) may present for anesthesia as part of treatment or investigation of PHT, or for unrelated procedures. PHT is a manifestation of a heterogeneous group of diseases. It is defined as a mean PA pressure >25 mmHg at rest. The diagnostic criterion of PA pressure >30 mmHg on exercise is now depreciated. A mean PA pressure of 20 mmHg is considered to be the upper normal.

Classification

The latest clinical classification of PHT, the result of the 4th World Symposium, is shown in Table 45.1.

Table 45.1 Updated clinical classification of pulmonary hypertension. The 2008 Dana Point Classification

1. Pulmonary arterial hypertension (PAH) – precapillary vasculopathy

Idiopathic (IPAH)
Heritable
Drug-induced
Associated with
    collagen vascular disease
    HIV infection
    portal hypertension
    congenital heart disease
    schistosomiasis
    chronic hemolytic anemia
Persistent pulmonary hypertension of the newborn

1. Pulmonary veno-occlusive disease (PVOD) and/or pulmonary capillary hemangiomatosis (PCH)

2. Pulmonary hypertension owing to left heart disease

Systolic dysfunction
Diastolic dysfunction
Valvular disease

3. Pulmonary hypertension owing to lung diseases and/or hypoxia

Chronic obstructive pulmonary disease (COPD)
Interstitial lung disease
Other pulmonary diseases with mixed restrictive and
    obstructive patterns
Sleep-disordered breathing
Alveolar hypoventilation disorders
Chronic exposure to high altitude
Developmental abnormalities

4. Chronic thromboembolic pulmonary hypertension (CTEPH)

5. Pulmonary hypertension with unclear multifactorial mechanisms

Hematological (e.g. myeloproliferative disorders)
Systemic disorders (e.g. sarcoidosis)
Metabolic disorders (e.g. Gaucher disease)
Other (e.g. chronic renal failure)

J Am Coll Cardiol 2009; 54(1 Suppl): S43–54.

Pathophysiology

Pulmonary vascular tone is normally regulated through the complex interaction of vasoactive factors, growth inhibitors and mitogens (Figure 45.1). The release or activity of these factors is altered by an initiating event, for example inflammation or increased endothelial shear stress. Whatever the initial

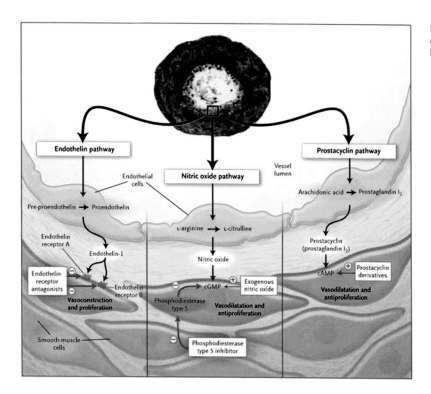

Figure 45.1 Targets for current or emerging therapies in pulmonary arterial hypertension. *N Engl J Med* 2004; 351(14): 1425–36.

pathology, the vascular response is similar with varying degrees of vasoconstriction, remodeling (smooth muscle proliferation and intimal fibrosis) and *in situ* thrombosis resulting in characteristic plexiform lesions with the physiological consequence of braised PVR. An increased understanding of the interplay of these vasoactive factors has led to the development of targeted therapies for PHT.

Right heart pathophysiology

The consequence of elevated PVR is increased RV afterload. The normal RV is a thin-walled chamber typically exposed to only modest increases in afterload during exercise. For this reason, the RV is very vulnerable to an acute increase in PVR (e.g. following acute massive PE) which precipitates lethal RV failure. In contrast, a gradual increase in PVR leads to compensatory RV hypertrophy and dilatation, and ultimately RV failure. Severe exercise limitation in patients with chronic PHT is the clinical manifestation of the inability of the RV to generate an increased CO. In health, RV coronary perfusion occurs throughout the cardiac cycle. In PHT, however, RV coronary perfusion becomes phasic and is predominantly diastolic – i.e. similar to normal LV

coronary perfusion. As a consequence, patients with PHT are vulnerable to acute RV dysfunction when there is an imbalance between myocardial oxygen supply and demand, for example in arterial hypotension and elevated RV end-diastolic pressure (RVEDP). Patients with severe PHT (mean PA pressure >50 mmHg) have a poor prognosis – 2 year survival <50%.

Clinical features

It is widely recognized that PHT is under-diagnosed. The onset of symptoms and signs is often insidious and it is not unusual for patients to be treated for "asthma" and other common respiratory disorders for up to 3 years before a definitive diagnosis is made. A high degree of clinical suspicion is required in conditions known to be strongly associated with PHT (e.g. collagen vascular disorders, sickle cell disease, uncorrected congenital heart disease, severe MR, chronic LV failure, severe COPD, morbid obesity and severe portal hypertension).

Patients often present with exertional dyspnea, and nonspecific symptoms such as non-productive cough, presyncope and exertional syncope. In advanced cases there may be hemoptysis, ascites, peripheral edema, atypical chest pain or angina from RV ischemia. Rarely an enlarged PA may produce hoarseness secondary to recurrent laryngeal nerve compression and angina secondary to left coronary artery compression.

Clinical signs of PHT include: cyanosis, hepatomegaly, ascites, peripheral edema, elevated jugular central venous pressure, RV heave, loud P_2, RV S_4 gallop and a pansystolic TR murmur.

Investigations

The aims are confirmation of the diagnosis of PHT, assessment of the severity and, where possible, determination of the underlying cause. In patients with chronic thromboembolic PHT (CTEPH) further evaluation is required to determine suitability for surgery.

ECG: signs of RV or RA hypertrophy and dilatation (Figure 45.2).

CXR: enlarged proximal pulmonary arteries and peripheral oligemia ("pruning").

Pulmonary function tests: should be performed to assess parenchymal lung function. Patients with IPAH, however, often have a mild to moderate decrease in pulmonary function. The 6-minute walk distance and formal cardiopulmonary exercise testing provide objective measures of exercise tolerance.

2-dimensional TTE: signs of RV pressure or volume overload (RVH, dilated intrahepatic veins), dilatation of PA, thrombus in proximal PA. Signs of underlying left heart disease may be present.

Pulsed-wave Doppler: regurgitant TR jet velocity can be used to estimate RV and PA systolic pressure. The sensitivity of echocardiography as a diagnostic test for PHT is reduced in the absence of TR.

CT/MRI: is used to assess the distribution of disease and suitability for surgery.

Cardiac catheterization: used to measure PA pressure and CO, and to perform PVR partitioning prior to pulmonary endarterectomy. Coronary angiography is usually required in surgical candidates to exclude significant coronary artery disease.

Miscellaneous: specific blood testing can be considered to exclude inherited thrombophilias if CTEPH is suspected, auto-antibodies, HIV serology, thyroid and liver function tests, and ABG analysis. Brain-natriuretic peptide or its degradation products may be a useful marker of both disease progression and prognosis.

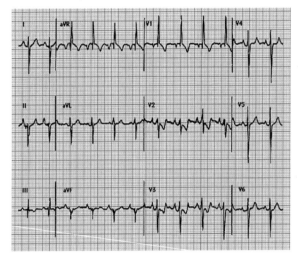

Figure 45.2 ECG in pulmonary hypertension. Criteria for RVH include: a tall R-wave (>7 mm) and a small S-wave in V1 (<2 mm) and R-wave:S-wave ratio >1; a tall S-wave and a small R-wave in V5/V6 (R-wave:S-wave ratio <1); and right axis deviation. Complete or partial RBBB, ST segment depression and T-wave inversion in the anterior leads (V1-V4) suggest severe right heart strain. RA enlargement is suggested by P-waves >2.5 mm in the inferior leads (II, III, aVF).

Management

The management of PHT is complex and largely governed by the underlying etiology. Treatments provide symptomatic relief, prognostic benefit or both.

Primary therapy

This is directed at the underlying disease process. Patients with PHT secondary to cardiac disease (Dana Point Group 2) are managed by treating the underlying cardiac lesion, for example MV surgery, coronary revascularization or closure of a VSD. The success or failure of this approach depends on whether changes in the pulmonary vasculature have become irreversible, as in Eisenmenger's syndrome. In patients with CTEPH (Dana Point Group 4), pulmonary endarterectomy (PEA) may provide significant symptomatic and prognostic benefit.

Conventional therapy

This includes graded exercise regimens, anticoagulation, supplemental oxygen, diuretics, calcium channel blockers and digitalis. Anticoagulation reduces the risk of secondary pulmonary thromboembolism, which is commonly seen in PHT. A combination of

Table 45.2 Advanced therapies in pulmonary hypertension

Second messenger	Selective	Non-selective
cAMP	**Prostaglandins and prostanoids** • Epoprostenol (prostacyclin, PGI_2) inhaled and IV – usual doses do not produce hypotension from "spillover" • Treprostinil (SC, inhaled), beraprost (oral), iloprost (inhaled) • Prostin (PGE_1)	**Beta-adrenergic receptor agonists** • Isoproterenol, dobutamine • Epinephrine (<0.05 µg kg^{-1} min^{-1}), dopamine (<5 µg kg^{-1} min^{-1}) • Mixed α/β – at low doses β predominates and causes pulmonary vasodilatation
	Endothelin antagonists • Bosentan, tezosantan (non-selective) • Ambrisentan, sitaxsentan (endothelin receptor ET_A selective)	**Nitrovasodilators** • Hydralazine, glyceryl trinitrate, sodium nitroprusside
	Adenosine • Infusion favors pulmonary vasodiliation	**Calcium channel blockers** • Nifedipine, nicardipine
cGMP	**Inhaled nitric oxide**	**Phosphodiesterase inhibitors** • PDE_3 – milrinone, amrinone, enoximone • PDE_5 – sildenafil, dipyridamole

SC, subcutaneous; PDE, phosphodiesterase; ET, endothelin.

diuretics may be required to treat peripheral edema and ascites associated with RV failure. Calcium channel blockers are reserved for patients with PAH who demonstrate a significant decrease in PA pressure at right heart catheterization in response to this therapy. Atrial septostomy is occasionally performed to permit right → left shunting and increase CO. This is usually considered a palliative or salvage procedure as it worsens cyanosis and is associated with high operative mortality. Lung transplantation remains the treatment of last resort in a small number of suitable patients.

Advanced therapy

This aims to reduce PVR by dilating the pulmonary arterioles. Pulmonary vasodilators may be selective or non-selective; the latter having pulmonary and systemic effects. Newer therapies may have additional anti-proliferative or anti-thrombotic properties. Most act via an increase in cAMP or cGMP, or a decrease in cytoplasmic calcium concentration in arteriolar smooth muscle (Table 45.2). Virtually every vasodilator has been used at some time to treat PHT. Their usefulness is largely dependent on the absence of systemic hypotensive effects. The following drugs have, through trial and error, found a role in improving symptoms and occasionally prognosis.

Prostaglandins

Prostacyclin (PGI_2) is a naturally occurring vasodilator. Its usefulness is limited by a short half-life, which necessitates continuous intravenous infusion. PGI_2 analogs with longer half-lives, such as iloprost, can be administered by nebulizer 3 hourly (Chapter 9).

Endothelin antagonists

Endothelin (ET) acts on ET receptors to increase pulmonary vascular tone. Selective ET_1 receptor blockade using ET_1 blockers such as bosentan reduces PA pressure in some patients.

Phosphodiesterase inhibitors

Inodilators, such as milrinone and enoximone, have widespread systemic and pulmonary effects (Chapter 9). Because the PDE_5 isoenzyme is highly expressed in lung tissue, selective PDE_5 inhibitors, such as sildenafil, are increasingly being used in the treatment of PHT.

Inhaled nitric oxide

Inhaled NO is the only true pulmonary vasodilator – its very short biological half-life prevents any systemic effects (Chapter 9). It is, however, a difficult drug to deliver, particularly to patients who are not intubated. In addition, toxic metabolites (e.g. NO_2) may cause harm. With the

285

Table 45.3 Management of pulmonary hypertensive crisis

Treatment	Rationale
Administer 100% O_2	Increasing P_AO_2 and PaO_2 can decrease PVR
Hyperventilate to induce respiratory alkalosis	PAP is directly related to $PaCO_2$
Correct metabolic acidosis	PVR is directly related to H^+ concentration
Administer pulmonary vasodilators	NO requires machine to deliver and should be readily available
Support cardiac output and perfusion	Adequate inotropic support and perfusion pressures
Attenuate noxious stimuli	Noxious stimuli can increase PAP and are attenuated by opioids

Adapted from: Friesen and Williams. *Paediatr Anaesth* 2008; 18(3): 208–16 with kind permission of John Wiley and Sons.

possible exception of persistent PHT of the newborn, inhaled NO is unsuitable for long-term therapy.

Anesthetic considerations

Patients with PHT undergoing non-cardiac surgery are at risk of significant morbidity and mortality. Perioperative risk is greatest in patients with a mean PA pressure >50 mmHg. For this reason, surgery should be reserved for life-threatening or severely disabling conditions.

Clinical assessment

Patients with established PHT are best managed using a multidisciplinary team approach. A careful review of prior investigations is essential. An abrupt change in symptoms should not be unquestioningly attributed to worsening PHT until other remedial causes (e.g. aortic stenosis) have been actively excluded.

Anesthetic drugs

Numerous studies have investigated the effects of anesthetic drugs on vascular tone. These are summarized in Tables 7.2 and 7.3.

The commonest cause of decompensation during anesthesia is acute RV dysfunction. The choice of anesthetic technique must, therefore, be guided by the need to preserve RV perfusion and function. RV ischemia may be caused by arterial hypotension or excessively elevated RVEDP secondary to volume overload.

Because PVR in patients with PHT is relatively fixed, it is uncommon for an acute deterioration during anesthesia to be caused by a change in pulmonary vascular tone. For these reasons, neuraxial anesthesia must be used with extreme caution and should perhaps be avoided altogether in favor of general anesthesia. The choice of anesthetic agent is largely guided by personal preference and institutional protocol. The anesthesiologist should resist the temptation to use drugs with which they are unfamiliar in the belief that they may provide a "safer" anesthetic. It may be prudent to administer a modest dose of an inotrope (e.g. dopamine 3–5 µg kg^{-1} min^{-1}) to improve RV contractility and reduce the likelihood and severity of hypotension. If the patient develops hypotension then norepinephrine has theoretical advantages in protecting the RV. Intravenous fluid should not be administered unless there is objective evidence of hypovolemia, as this may worsen RV function.

While most anesthesiologists would invasively monitor arterial and central venous pressure, there is no advantage in measuring PA pressure in most cases. It should be borne in mind that the risk of PAFC-induced PA rupture is greater in the PHT. The PAFC may, however, be of use during PEA to document changes in PVR and CO. While the use of TEE is superficially appealing, the same caveats apply.

Postoperative management

Hypoxemia and sympathetic stimulation (untreated pain) place patients with PHT at particular risk in the postoperative period. For these reasons, patients are best managed in a closely monitored environment. Although neuraxial anesthesia should be used with extreme caution, regional anesthesia (e.g. plexus blockade) should be used where possible to minimize the impact of general anesthetic and analgesic drugs.

Key points

- It is widely recognized that PHT is under-diagnosed.
- Virtually every vasodilator has been used at some time to treat PHT.

- The usefulness of pulmonary vasodilators is largely dependent on the absence of systemic hypotensive effects.
- RV ischemia in PHT is the commonest cause of acute decompensation during anesthesia.
- Pulmonary endarterectomy may provide significant symptomatic and prognostic benefit in patients with chronic thromboembolic PHT.

Further reading

Friesen RH, Williams GD. Anesthetic management of children with pulmonary arterial hypertension. *Paediatr Anaesth* 2008; **18**(3): 208–16.

Galiè N, Hoeper MM, Humbert M, *et al.* Guidelines for the diagnosis and treatment of pulmonary hypertension: the Task Force for the Diagnosis and Treatment of Pulmonary Hypertension of the European Society of Cardiology (ESC) and the European Respiratory Society (ERS), endorsed by the International Society of Heart and Lung Transplantation (ISHLT). *Eur Heart J* 2009; **30**(20): 2493–537.

Humbert M, Sitbon O, Simonneau G. Treatment of pulmonary arterial hypertension. *N Engl J Med* 2004; **351**(14): 1425–36.

MacKnight B, Martinez EA, Simon BA. Anesthetic management of patients with pulmonary hypertension. *Semin Cardiothorac Vasc Anesth* 2008; **12**(2): 91–6.

Simonneau G, Robbins IM, Beghetti M, *et al.* Updated clinical classification of pulmonary hypertension. *J Am Coll Cardiol* 2009; **54**(1 Suppl): S43–54.

Subramaniam K, Yared J-P. Management of pulmonary hypertension in the operating room. *Semin Cardiothorac Vasc Anesth* 2007; **11**(2): 119–36.

Chapter

46

Cardiac tumors

Nigel Farnum and Joseph E. Arrowsmith

Patients with cardiac tumors typically present with constitutional or cardiovascular symptoms. Many are discovered incidentally during investigation of an unrelated condition or at autopsy. The incidence of metastatic tumors of the heart is at least two orders of magnitude greater than that of primary tumors.

The overwhelming majority of primary tumors are histologically benign and not directly fatal. Complete heart block or other dysrhythmia, secondary to direct extension into the conduction system, and embolization of a tumor fragment or associated thrombus, may have lethal sequelae. Malignant tumors of the heart have a poor prognosis. The classification of cardiac masses is shown in Table 46.1 and the anatomic distribution of cardiac masses in Table 46.2.

Neoplastic tumors

Benign primary tumors

Myxoma

Myxomas account for half of all primary cardiac neoplasms. They are usually solitary and arise from or near the interatrial septum (LA 75%, RA 15–20%). More than half express neuroendocrine biomarkers, suggesting that myxomas have an endocardial neural origin. They occur in all age groups and are more common in women. Familial myxomas (autosomal dominant) account for <10% cases and may form part of the Carney syndrome.

Myxomas are typically compact and polypoid in appearance, range from 1–15 cm in diameter, and have a smooth or slightly lobulated surface. Larger tumors may contain cystic, necrotic or hemorrhagic

Table 46.1 Classification of cardiac masses

Neoplastic		Non-neoplastic
Primary	**Secondary**	
Benign	Direct	Hamartomas
Myoxoma, papillary fibroelastoma, lipoma, hemangioma, teratoma, mesothelioma	Breast, lung, esophagus, mediastinal tumor	Rhabdomyoma, fibroma, papillary fibroelastoma
Malignant	Hematogenous	Age-related growths
Angiosarcoma, rhabdomyosarcoma, mesothelioma, fibrosarcoma, osteosarcoma, lymphoma, neurogenic sarcoma	Melanoma, lung, breast, genitourinary, gastrointestinal	Lipomatous hypertrophy
	Venous	Reactive proliferation
	Renal, adrenal, thyroid, lung, hepatoma	Llambl's excrescence, papillary fibroelastoma
	Lymphatic	Other
	Lymphoma, leukemia	Thrombus, vegetation, calcified amorphous tumor, normal structure, imaging artifact

Papillary fibroelastoma may arise *de novo*, following endocardial injury or in the setting of hypertrophic obstructive cardiomyopathy. Adapted from Bruce CJ. *Heart* 2011; 97(2): 151–60. Adapted by permission from BMJ Publishing Group Limited.

288   *Core Topics in Cardiac Anesthesia, Second Edition*, ed. Jonathan H. Mackay and Joseph E. Arrowsmith. Published by Cambridge University Press. © Cambridge University Press 2012.

Table 46.2 The anatomic distribution and pathological characteristics of cardiac masses according to intracardiac attachment site in 75 consecutive patients undergoing surgery for cardiac mass removal at the Mayo Clinic; more than a third were atrial myxomas

Right heart	Left heart
Right atrium – SVC Thyroid (1), inflammatory pseudotumor (1)	**Left atrium** Myxoma (24), thrombus (6), sarcoma (3), rhabdomyoma (1)
Right atrium Myxoma (5), thrombus (2), melanoma (1), adrenocortical carcinoma (1)	**Left atrial appendage** Fibroelastoma (1)
Right atrium – IVC Hypernephroma (7), rhabdomyoma (1), hepatoma (1)	**Mitral valve** Fibroelastoma (3)
Tricuspid valve Fibroelastoma (1)	**Aortic valve** Fibroelastoma (5)
Right ventricle Myxoma (2), echinococcus cyst (1), thrombus (1), melanoma (1)	**Left ventricle** Thrombus (3), fibroma (2), metastatic breast carcinoma (1)

Reprinted from: Dujardin KS, et al. J Am Soc Echocardiogr 2000; 13: 1080–3 with permission from Elsevier.

areas. Papillary and villous myxomas are less compact and more prone to fragmentation than the more common polypoid variety.

The clinical presentation is largely dictated by anatomic location, size and mobility. Although small sessile myxomas may be asymptomatic, the majority of patients present with vague constitutional symptoms, an embolic event (e.g. stroke) or intra-cardiac obstruction. Myxoma-derived interleukin-6 is thought to underlie common clinical features such as fever, rash, arthralgia, cachexia and clubbing. Laboratory findings such as thrombocytopenia, antimyocardial antibodies and elevated C-reactive protein often lead to an incorrect diagnosis of collagen vascular disease. A systemic embolic event widens the differential diagnosis to include other vasculitides and infectious endocarditis.

Echocardiography is used to confirm the diagnosis and to define the anatomic and physiological characteristics of the lesion. Contrast-enhanced CT or MRI may be of use in selected cases.

In most cases, surgical resection is curative. Recurrence is more common with familial myxomas than with sporadic myxomas. The timing of surgery remains controversial. It is not usual for an otherwise fit and healthy patient to be referred for emergency surgery upon discovery of a myxoma on the grounds that they are at risk of stroke. While the reality is that the myxoma has been present for months, if not years, few anesthesiologists would welcome the responsibility for a stroke occurring in the period between referral

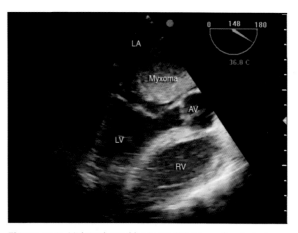

Figure 46.1 Midesophageal long-axis TEE image showing a large left atrial (LA) myxoma. The highly mobile tumor was seen to prolapse through the mitral valve during diastole.

and a suitable elective operating room vacancy. The timing of surgery following embolic stroke is problematic – the risks of intracerebral hemorrhage secondary to systemic anticoagulation for CPB have to be balanced against the risk of further tumor embolization.

Papillary fibroelastoma

These small (<1 cm diameter) solitary endocardial "flower-like" papillomas account for ~10% of primary cardiac tumors and are the second most common primary tumor. They predominantly affect the cardiac valves (in an equal distribution), occur in all age groups and are usually asymptomatic. They

289

are often found in association with hypertrophic obstructive cardiomyopathy (HOCM) and trauma. The most common clinical presentation is systemic embolization of an attached thrombus.

Surgical excision is usually reserved for large (>1 cm) and mobile tumors that liberate emboli or cause hemodynamic obstruction and patients with other operable lesions (e.g. ASD). In other cases, antiplatelet therapy and regular follow-up are recommended.

Other benign primary tumors

Rhabdomyomas arise from the ventricles and atrioventricular valves. They are invariably multiple and commonly associated with tuberous sclerosis. They may be 3–30 mm in diameter and, if pedunculated, can obstruct ventricular blood flow. There is a high incidence of tachydysrhythmias – typically ventricular pre-excitation syndromes. They are typically diagnosed in utero or in early childhood. A characteristic feature is spontaneous regression before 4 years of age. For this reason surgical resection is rarely required.

Fibromas are well circumscribed solitary lesions, often with central calcification, that affect the ventricles. The incidence is greatest in children, with a third under 1 year of age at the time of presentation. The prevalence is greater in patients with the autosomal dominant Gorlin syndrome. Typical clinical features include syncope, chest pain, dysrhythmia and sudden death. Cardiac imaging may reveal a homogeneous, non-contractile mass that mimics septal hypertrophy or HOCM. Surgical resection is advised, even in asymptomatic patients, where technically feasible.

Lipomas account for <5% primary cardiac tumors. They are encapsulated fatty tumors that typically arise from the epicardium and extend into the pericardial space. Subendocardial lipomas are usually small and sessile – protruding into the adjacent cardiac chamber. Lipomas are usually asymptomatic unless they cause dysrhythmias or compression of local structures.

Lipomatous hypertrophy of interatrial septum is caused by adipocyte hyperplasia and associated with obesity and increasing age. Despite their characteristic appearance on echocardiography, they are often confused with more sinister entities.

Malignant primary tumors

About 15–20% of primary cardiac tumors are histologically malignant. The majority (90–95%) are sarcomas, arising from malignant transformation of (connective) tissues derived from embryonic mesoderm. They affect males and females equally and may occur at any age, although most present between the ages of 20 and 40 years. Angiosarcomas and rhabdomyosarcomas account for the majority. Symptoms and signs are largely dictated by anatomic location, local infiltration and metastatic spread. Despite surgical resection, cardiac reconstruction, transplantation, chemotherapy and radiotherapy the prognosis is universally poor, the majority of patients dying within 2 years of presentation.

Secondary tumors

Although secondary or metastatic tumors account for the majority of cardiac tumors, most are clinically silent and only detected at autopsy. Cardiac involvement should, however, be suspected if a patient with known malignancy develops a pericardial effusion, cardiac failure, arrhythmia or heart block, or a new murmur. The differential diagnosis includes radiation-induced myocardial damage, cardiotoxic chemotherapeutic agents such as anthracyclines (e.g. doxorubicin), monoclonal antibodies (e.g. trastuzumab – Herceptin[r]) and tyrosine kinase inhibitors (e.g. imatinib), and infective endocarditis secondary to immunosuppression.

While long-term prognosis is usually dictated by that of the underlying primary malignancy, direct or metastatic cardiac involvement typically represents terminal disease progression. Treatment of cardiac involvement is typically directed at the control of symptoms secondary to heart failure or dysrhythmia and drainage of malignant pericardial effusion by pericardiocentesis or pericardial window.

Non-neoplastic tumors

Non-neoplastic cardiac tumors include hamartomas (tissue malformations that grow at the same rate as normal tissue), fibroelastomas and Llambl's excrescences (endocardial fronds that form on valve margins at the sites of valve closure). While historically benign they may be associated with dysrhythmias and thromboembolism.

Other cardiac masses

Intracardiac thrombus and vegetations are the commonest cardiac masses. Anatomic variants (e.g. prominent atrial pectinate muscle trabeculation,

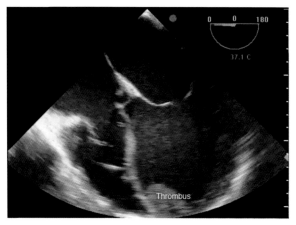

Figure 46.2 Midesophageal five-chamber TEE image showing a LV apical thrombus in a patient with ischemic cardiomyopathy.

moderator bands, a large Eustachian valve, Chiari networks, false ventricular tendons, fatty infiltration of TV annulus, fat within pericardium, and prominent atrial suture lines post cardiac transplantation) and echocardiographic imaging artifacts are commonly mistaken for pathological lesions.

Management

The commonest cardiac masses are thrombi and vegetations. In most cases the diagnosis can be made on the basis of the clinical presentation, i.e. myocardial infarction, mitral stenosis, atrial fibrillation, infective endocarditis. Thrombi tend to be discrete and somewhat spherical in appearance or laminated

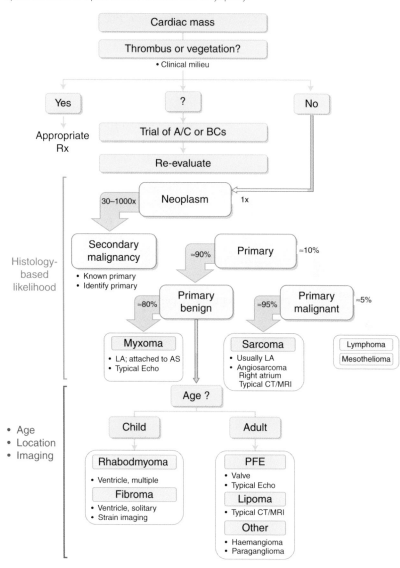

Figure 46.3 Diagnostic algorithm for evaluation of a cardiac mass based on histology-based likelihood, age, location and imaging characteristics. A/C, anticoagulation; AS, atrial septum; BCs, blood cultures; LA, left atrium; PFE, papillary fibroelastoma; Rx, treatment. From Bruce CJ. *Heart* 2011; 97(2): 151–60 with modification. Adapted by permission from BMJ Publishing Group Limited.

upon an atrial or LV apical wall. In contrast, vegetations are usually irregular, have their attachment on the "upstream" surface of a valve and are associated with valvular regurgitation. In a similar fashion, the likely etiology of a cardiac tumor can often be determined by considering the age of the patient at presentation, the likely histology based on known incidences, anatomic location, and echocardiographic, CT and MRI characteristics (Figure 46.3).

Key points

- Myxomas account for half of all primary cardiac neoplasms.
- The timing of surgery following embolic stroke is problematic – the risks of intracerebral hemorrhage secondary to systemic

anticoagulation for CPB have to be balanced against the risk of further tumor embolization.
- Intracardiac thrombus and vegetations are the commonest cardiac masses.

Further reading

Bruce CJ. Cardiac tumours: diagnosis and management. *Heart* 2011; **97**(2): 151–60.

Duwe BV, Sterman DH, Musani AI. Tumors of the mediastinum. *Chest* 2005; **128**(4): 2893–909.

Feneck R. Cardiac masses and pericardial disease. In Feneck R, Kneeshaw J, Ranucci M (Eds.), *Core Topics in Transesophageal Echocardiography*. Cambridge: Cambridge University Press; 2010. pp. 180–92.

Scheffel H, Baumueller S, Stolzmann P, *et al.* Atrial myxomas and thrombi: comparison of imaging features on CT. *Am J Roentgenol* 2009; **192**(3): 639–45.

Cardiothoracic trauma

Betsy Evans and John J. Dunning

Blunt or penetrating trauma may overcome the protection afforded to the heart, lungs and great vessels by the semi-rigid thorax. Life-threatening complications should be identified and treated immediately. The dynamic nature of thoracic injuries necessitates continuous reassessment, evaluation and immediate treatment. This chapter discusses the general principles of acute thoracic trauma with particular attention to the specific management of patients suffering trauma to the heart and great vessels.

Blunt trauma

Pathophysiology

Blunt injury to the chest can affect any component of the chest wall and thoracic cavity. Mortality is high because of associated multi-system injuries. The most important cause is high-speed road traffic accidents, due to deceleration injury and compression forces. Injuries associated with blunt trauma are listed in Table 47.1

Assessment

Although physical examination is the primary tool for diagnosis, obtaining a detailed history of the time and mechanism of injury is vital. Symptoms and physical signs of significant thoracic injury may be subtle or even absent. The process of physical examination (inspection, palpation, percussion and auscultation) should be concise and performed concurrently with resuscitation.

Primary survey: identify and treat immediate life-threatening conditions such as tension pneumothorax, open pneumothorax, massive hemothorax, cardiac tamponade and flail chest. The classic signs of distended neck veins and muffled heart sounds are

Table 47.1 Injuries associated with blunt trauma.

Rib fracture(s)
    Most common pathology

Flail chest
    When three or more ribs are fractured in two or more places

Sternal fracture

Tracheobronchial disruption

Pulmonary contusion

Hemothorax

Pneumothorax

Cardiac injuries and contusion

Great vessel injuries

Diaphragmatic rupture

Esophageal rupture

almost universally absent in traumatic cardiac tamponade.

Secondary survey: identify all injuries and plan further investigation and treatment.

Investigations

Adjuncts to clinical diagnosis are shown in Table 47.2.

Management

Many patients die because of inappropriate pre- and early in-hospital interventions resulting in delayed definitive surgical management. The majority of patients with blunt chest trauma do not require an operation; >80% require no more than an intercostal

Core Topics in Cardiac Anesthesia, Second Edition, ed. Jonathan H. Mackay and Joseph E. Arrowsmith. Published by Cambridge University Press. © Cambridge University Press 2012.

Table 47.2 Diagnostic adjuncts in blunt chest trauma

CXR	Plain anteroposterior CXR remains the standard initial investigation for chest trauma
ABG	Assess severity of gas exchange abnormalities and acid-base status
Troponin I	Elevated levels correlate with wall motion abnormalities on echocardiography
ECG	Tachyarrhythmias, conduction disturbances, ST segment elevation
FAST	Detect presence of intrapleural, intraperitoneal or pericardial blood
Spiral CT/aortography	Delineating location and extent of blunt aortic injuries
Bronchoscopy	Diagnose tracheobronchial injuries

FAST, focused abdominal sonogram for trauma. Studies suggest that FAST is quicker to perform and has better sensitivity and specificity than peritoneal lavage.

Table 47.3 Lesions caused by blunt thoracic trauma that require surgical intervention

	Immediate indications	Long-term indications
Chest wall and diaphragm	Traumatic thoracotomy Loss of chest wall integrity Diaphragmatic tears	Delayed recognition of blunt diaphragmatic injury Traumatic diaphragmatic hernia
Airway and GI tract	Tracheal, major bronchial or esophageal injury GI tract contents in the chest drain	Delayed recognition of tracheobronchial or esophageal injury Tracheo-esophageal fistula Persistent thoracic duct fistula/chylothorax
Pleural space	Massive air leak following chest drain insertion Massive hemothorax or continued high rate of blood loss via the chest drain	Chronic clotted hemothorax or fibrothorax Empyema
Lungs and heart	Cardiac tamponade	Traumatic lung abscess
Great vessels	Radiographic confirmation of a major vessel injury An embolism into the PA or heart	Late recognition of a major vessel injury, development of traumatic pseudo-aneurysm

drain or no invasive procedure at all. Lesions caused by blunt thoracic trauma that require surgical intervention are shown in Table 47.3.

Drainage of the pleural space is the commonest intervention following thoracic trauma, providing definitive treatment in the majority of cases. While a relatively simple procedure, it carries a significant complication rate (2–10%). Chest drain placement may be both diagnostic and therapeutic. During drain insertion a finger can be used to palpate the surfaces of the lung, diaphragm and pericardium to detect the contusions, lacerations and hemopericardium, respectively. The nature of the material draining from the tube is also important. Bright red (i.e. arterial) blood indicates that thoracotomy is more likely to be required. Intestinal contents implies an esophageal, gastric or bowel injury with diaphragmatic tear. A persistent air leak implies an underlying lung laceration. A large air leak may indicate tracheobronchial disruption.

Rib fractures

Ribs 4–10 are most frequently involved. Presentation is with inspiratory pleuritic chest pain, and local bony tenderness and crepitus over the site of the fracture. Fractures of ribs 8–12 are often associated with abdominal injuries. The finding of fractures of ribs 1–2 implies the delivery of considerable energy and is usually associated with cranial, major vascular, thoracic and abdominal injuries. A flail chest presents with paradoxical motion of the chest wall, dyspnea and tachycardia; pulmonary contusions are common. Treatment includes effective analgesia (intercostal, paravertebral or epidural blocks), to allow for early mobilization and physiotherapy. Endotracheal intubation and positive-pressure ventilation may be necessary.

Table 47.4 Indications for intercostal drain insertion and emergency thoracotomy following blunt chest trauma

	Indications	Complications

Intercostal chest drain	Absolute
	  Pneumothorax
	  Hemothorax
	  Traumatic arrest (bilateral)
	Relative
	  Rib fracture and PPV
	  Profound hypoxia, hypotension
	  Unilateral signs
		Hemothorax (damage to intercostal vessel)
		Lung laceration (adhesions)
		Diaphragm/Abdominal cavity penetration (drain too low)
		Stomach/colonic injury (diaphragmatic hernia not recognized)
		Ineffective drain (subcutaneous insertion)
		Pain (drain in too far)
		Blocked drain (clot, lung)
		Retained hemothorax
		Empyema
		Pneumothorax after drain removal

Thoracotomy	Massive hemorrhage (>1500 ml) after tube drain insertion Blood loss >500 ml in first hour, or >200 ml h^{-1} in subsequent hours Witnessed cardiac arrest	Hazards of general anesthesia Spinal cord damage following cervical injury Risk of worsening airway injury Risk of aspiration Masking signs of CNS deterioration Acute and chronic postoperative pain

Sternal fractures

Patients report pain, and dyspnea may be present. Examination reveals local tenderness, bruising, swelling or crepitus. Associated injuries, such as rib fractures, are common. Cardiac injuries are diagnosed in <20% of patients.

Diaphragmatic injuries

These should be considered following sudden compression of the abdomen (e.g. seat belt or blow) in a patient with dyspnea or respiratory distress. The left hemidiaphragm is more commonly affected because the liver protects the right. Hypovolemic shock may result from associated splenic or hepatic injuries. A diagnosis is usually made radiographically, with herniation of viscera into the chest. Laparotomy is required since 90% of cases have associated abdominal trauma.

Tracheobronchial injuries

Fractures, lacerations and disruptions are caused by severe rapid deceleration or compressive forces applied directly to the trachea. The results may be devastating and rapidly lethal. Patients surviving are typically in respiratory distress with stridor. Other signs include pneumothorax and subcutaneous emphysema. Flexible bronchoscopy may be required to assist securing the airway by endotracheal intubation.

Esophageal injuries

These are rare because of the posterior mediastinal location of the esophagus. Injuries are usually the result of a forceful blow to the epigastrium which leads to distal esophageal rupture and spillage of GI contents into the (usually left) chest. Associated injuries are common. Symptoms include upper abdominal and thoracic pain which is disproportionate to examination findings. Signs include cardiorespiratory compromise and subcutaneous emphysema. Surgery is required. Delayed presentation may result in systemic sepsis.

Pneumothorax

This is most frequently caused when a fractured rib penetrates the lung parenchyma and is often associated with some degree of hemothorax. Tension pneumothorax requires rapid diagnosis and treatment to prevent cardiovascular collapse. Immediate therapy includes decompression of the affected hemithorax by needle (16–14G) thoracostomy in the second intercostal space in the mid-clavicular line, followed by chest drain insertion. Persistent lung collapse with a massive air leak may be due to bronchial injury.

Hemothorax

Bleeding from the chest wall, lung parenchyma or major thoracic vessels manifests with varying degrees

295

of hemodynamic instability. Multiple chest drains may be required and drainage should be closely monitored. The need for surgery is based on initial and cumulative drainage. Large, clotted hemothoraces require surgical evacuation to allow full lung expansion and to prevent complications such as fibrothorax and empyema. Thoracoscopic approaches have been used successfully.

Pulmonary contusions

The transmission of external forces to the lung parenchyma typically results in edema and hemorrhage. Patients present with pain, dyspnea and hypoxia. An overlying chest wall injury is usually apparent. CXR changes may not become apparent for up to 48 h. Management is supportive, with careful fluid balance to avoid respiratory failure. If a large volume of lung parenchyma is involved, significant intrapulmonary shunting and dead space ventilation may necessitate endotracheal intubation and mechanical ventilation.

Cardiac injuries

The clinical spectrum ranges from contusion associated with transient arrhythmias to disruption of valves and interventricular septum, and myocardial rupture. Patients can be asymptomatic or have chest pain and signs of cardiac tamponade or cardiovascular collapse. Treatment ranges from simple analgesia and antiarrhythmic drugs to emergency surgical intervention. Tamponade requires rapid pericardiocentesis or creation of a sub-xiphistenal window. Disruption of intracardiac structures requires urgent evaluation (TEE may be particularly useful). Treatment is immediate surgical repair of the cardiac chamber or intracardiac structure. Unstable patients may benefit from insertion of an IABP. Patients with traumatic cardiac rupture usually die at the scene of injury.

Thoracic aorta and major arteries

Injuries often occur as a result of shearing forces during rapid deceleration. A significant number of patients die from exsanguination. Aortic transection is discussed in Chapter 38.

Proximal PA injuries are relatively easy to repair when in an anterior location. In contrast, repair of posterior PA injuries frequently requires CPB. Pulmonary hilar injuries present the possibility of rapid exsanguination and are best treated with pneumonectomy.

SVC and major thoracic veins

Isolated injuries of the major thoracic veins are rare. Management comprises urgent surgical repair. If repair proves to be difficult, the injured subclavian or azygous veins can be ligated. Injuries of the thoracic IVC or SVC may require CPB.

Penetrating trauma
Pathophysiology

Penetrating chest injuries may be low velocity (e.g. stabbing) or high velocity (e.g. gunshot). The pattern of injury is determined by the anatomic track, physical stability and kinetic energy of the penetrating object. While low-velocity gunshot wounds (GSWs) share many of the features of stabbing injuries, high-velocity GSWs generate considerable shearing forces, cavitation and tissue damage that extends well beyond the tract between entry and exit wounds.

Stab wounds have a far greater chance of survival than GSWs. Isolated thoracic stab wounds causing cardiac tamponade probably have the highest survival rate (~70%). In contrast, GSWs injuring more than one cardiac chamber and causing exsanguination have a much greater mortaility. Penetrating injuries involving the great vessels and pulmonary hila carry a high mortality.

Assessment

Unlike blunt chest injuries, penetrating injuries tend to occur in the young, are usually the result of violence and are commonly isolated – i.e. no associated head, neck or abdominal injury. While cardiac injury may follow any penetrating chest injury, the likelihood is greater if the entry/exit wound lies below the clavicles, above the costal margin and medial to the mid-clavicular lines – the so-called "cardiac box".

Physical examination is the primary diagnostic tool. Obtaining a detailed history rarely significantly alters management. Symptoms and physical signs of significant injury are usually obvious.

Primary survey: identify entry and exit wounds, and treat immediate life-threatening conditions.

Secondary survey: identify all injuries and plan further investigation and treatment.

Investigations

Extensive investigation is usually unnecessary and may delay definitive treatment. All patients with

GSWs between the neck and the pelvis/buttock area should have a CXR. Following penetrating trauma, an erect or semi-erect CXR should be obtained to increase the sensitivity of detecting a small hemothorax, pneumothorax or diaphragmatic injury. Ultrasound is increasingly being used as a diagnostic tool in the emergency department.

Management

Unlike blunt injuries, penetrating chest trauma patients often require surgical intervention as the definitive management strategy. An unstable patient with a penetrating chest wound should be taken directly to the operating room. A penetrating implement (e.g. knife) left *in situ* may paradoxically prevent exsanguination. For this reason it should not be removed before the patient is anesthetized, draped and ready for surgery.

Emergency thoracotomy should be reserved for patients with a spontaneous circulation and those who have sustained a recent, *witnessed* cardiac arrest. In traumatic arrest, internal cardiac massage should be started as soon as possible following relief of tamponade and control of hemorrhage.

Anesthetic management comprises substantial intravenous access, invasive arterial pressure monitoring and the facilities to rapidly administer warmed intravenous fluids. Management of the airway, in particular the requirement for lung isolation, should be discussed with the operating surgeon.

A supine anterolateral thoracotomy is the usual approach. Choice of side is dependent on injuries. It may be necessary to extend the incision across the sternum to aid access and vision (i.e. "clamshell" thoracotomy). The anterolateral thoracotomy incision, through the left fourth or fifth interspace, gives the best initial access to the pericardium, left pulmonary hilum and descending aorta, with flexibility for extension as the injury dictates. Median sternotomy is used when there is a high likelihood of cardiac injury. The groins and legs should be prepared in case CPB or a saphenous vein graft is required.

Cardiac tamponade

The pericardium is opened longitudinally to avoid damage to the phrenic nerve, which runs along its lateral border. Evacuation of blood and clots can be performed via either a median sternotomy or sub-xiphisternal approach.

Cardiac wounds

These should be controlled initially with direct finger pressure, prior to suturing or application of a stapling device. Large wounds may be controlled temporarily by the insertion of a Foley (urinary) catheter and inflation of the balloon. Vascular clamps can be placed across atrial wounds to control hemorrhage. With extensive cardiac damage it may be necessary to temporarily obstruct venous inflow to allow repair. CPB is rarely necessary.

Pulmonary and hilar injuries

Massive hemorrhage from the lungs or pulmonary hila can be temporarily controlled with finger pressure at the pulmonary hilum. This may be augmented by placement of a vascular clamp. In should be borne in mind that abrupt occlusion of the pulmonary hilum often leads to acute RV failure, particularly in young fit adults.

Great vessel injuries

Small aortic injuries can be controlled with digital pressure and sutured directly. Larger injuries, especially to the arch, may require temporary digital occlusion and insitution of CPB. Access to the vessels in the superior mediastinum via an anterolateral thoracotomy is difficult. Median sternotomy or a supraclavicular incision may be required to control hemorrhage from subclavian and innominate vessels. Again, control is achieved temporarily with digital pressure or proximal and distal clamp application prior to defintive repair.

Resuscitation

The primary causes of traumatic arrest are hypoxia, hypovolemia, tension pneumothorax and cardiac tamponade. Immediate treatment of traumatic arrest is directed at treating the cause of the traumatic arrest. Chest compressions in the trauma patient are generally ineffective, may increase cardiac trauma by causing blunt myocardial injury and obstruct access for performing definitive maneuvers. Administration of inotropes and vasopressors to the vasoconstricted hypovolemic patient may cause profound myocardial hypoxia and dysfunction.

Key points

- The heart, lungs and great vessels are normally well protected by the semi-rigid thorax.

- The vast majority of patients with blunt chest trauma require no more than an intercostal drain.
- A penetrating implement may paradoxically prevent exsanguination and should not be removed until the patient is in the operating room.
- Conventional advance life support (ALS) algorithms require modification in the setting of traumatic cardiac arrest.

Further reading

O'Connor JV, Adamski J. The diagnosis and treatment of non-cardiac thoracic trauma. *J R Army Med Corps* 2010; **156**(1): 5–14.

O'Connor J, Ditillo M, Scalea T. Penetrating cardiac injury. *J R Army Med Corps* 2009; **155**(3): 185–90.

Round JA, Mellor AJ. Anaesthetic and critical care management of thoracic injuries. *J R Army Med Corps* 2010; **156**(3): 145–9.

Tayal VS, Beatty MA, Marx JA, Tomaszewski CA, Thomason MH. FAST (focused assessment with sonography in trauma) accurate for cardiac and intraperitoneal injury in penetrating anterior chest trauma. *J Ultrasound Med* 2004; **23**(4): 467–72.

48

Cardiac surgery during pregnancy

Sarah Conolly and Khalid Khan

Cardiac disease was the most common cause of maternal deaths in the UK in the triennium 2006–2008 with 2.31 deaths per 100 000 maternities (20% of all maternal deaths). In contrast to the preceding triennium (2003–2005), where the leading cause of cardiac death was myocardial infarction, the commonest causes of cardiac death were sudden adult death syndrome (SADS) and peripartum cardiomyopathy (Table 48.1). A similar pattern is seen in North America. In the 8-year period between 1998 and 2005 the aggregate pregnancy-related mortality ratio was 14.5 per 100 000 live births. Bleeding, pulmonary thromboembolism, infection, pregnancy-associated hypertension, cardiomyopathy and other cardiovascular conditions each contributed 10% to 13% of deaths.

Physiological changes of pregnancy

There are numerous physiological changes that occur during pregnancy. A number of these changes cause exacerbation of co-existing cardiac disease. The most significant changes are a 40% increase in intravascular volume by 32 weeks and a 40% increase in CO. The CO increases further during labor and reaches its maximum immediately after delivery due to autotransfusion from the uterus and removal of the aortocaval compression by the fetus. These changes can lead to decompensation around the time of delivery and immediately afterwards. The other physiological changes are summarized in Table 48.2.

Labor and cesarean section

In those patients with cardiac disease who don't require cardiac surgery prior to delivery, the goals should be a monitored routine labor with vaginal delivery. Carefully titrated epidural analgesia is often beneficial due to the effects of vasodilatation and reduced pain.

Deterioration in cardiac function or other non-cardiac fetomaternal indication may prompt delivery by cesarean section. Regional analgesia and anesthesia can be used for the majority of patients with cardiac disease undergoing cesarean section when adequate assessment and monitoring is undertaken. Particular care does need to be taken with patients with severe stenotic valvular lesions when using regional anesthetic techniques because vasodilatation may cause catastrophic and irreversible hypotension. Combining spinal and epidural techniques allow the production of a more gradual onset of block. Invasive blood pressure monitoring is essential.

Cardiac surgery

The morbidity and mortality associated with cardiac surgery are greatly increased in pregnancy. Compared to non-pregnant females of a similar age there is at least a four-fold increase in complications following valvular surgery and 50% increase following repair of type A aortic dissection. For this reason surgery should be reserved for patients who fail to respond to medical therapy. Factors contributing to poorer outcomes in pregnant patients include:

- a history of TIAs, stroke or arrhythmia
- NYHA class III or IV heart failure prior to pregnancy
- left heart obstruction
  - MV orifice area <2 cm^2,
  - AV orifice area <1.5 cm^2 or
  - peak LVOT gradient >30 mmHg
- LV ejection fraction $<40\%$.

Core Topics in Cardiac Anesthesia, Second Edition, ed. Jonathan H. Mackay and Joseph E. Arrowsmith. Published by Cambridge University Press. © Cambridge University Press 2012.

Table 48.1 Causes of maternal death from cardiac disease in the United Kingdom (1994–2008)

Type and cause of death	1994–96	1997–99	2000–02	2003–05	2006–08
Acquired					
Aortic dissection	7	5	7	9	7
Myocardial infarction (MI)	6	5	8	12	6
Ischemic heart disease (no MI)	0	0	0	4	5
Sudden adult death syndrome (SADS)	0	0	4	3	10
Peripartum cardiomyopathy	4	7	4	0[a]	9[b]
Other cardiomyopathy	2	3	4	1	4
Myocarditis or myocardial fibrosis	3	2	3	5	4
Mitral stenosis or valve disease	0	0	3	3	0
Thrombosed aortic or tricuspid valve	1	0	0	0	2
Infective endocarditis	0	2	1	2	2
Right or left ventricular hypertrophy or hypertensive heart disease	1	2	2	2	1
Congenital					
Pulmonary hypertension (PHT)	7	7	4	3	2
Congenital heart disease (not PHT or thrombosed aortic valve)	3	2	2	3	1
Other	5	0	2	0	0
Total	39	35	44	48[c]	53

[a] Twelve *Late* deaths reported in 2003–05.
[b] Two *late* deaths reported in 2006–08.
[c] Includes one woman for whom information on cause was not available.
Source: The Eighth Report of the Confidential Enquiries into Maternal Deaths in the United Kingdom. *BJOG* 2011; **118**(Suppl 1):1–203. Reproduced with permission from John Wiley and Sons.

The MV is the valve most commonly requiring surgery during pregnancy. The underlying pathology is usually stenosis secondary to chronic rheumatic heart disease, which, although rare in developed countries, is increasing in prevalence as a result of population migration. Regurgitant lesions are often improved by the physiological reduction in SVR. By contrast, stenotic lesions are worsened during pregnancy due to the combination of increased HR, CO and circulating volume. When the MV orifice falls to <1.5 cm^2 the first intervention usually considered is percutaneous balloon valvotomy, which has a lower complication rate than open valve surgery. A significant number of these patients will, however, require replacement in the future.

Aortic stenotic lesions in this population are usually secondary to congenital bicuspid valves. Valve replacement during pregnancy is usually reserved for symptomatic patients and those with AV orifice area <1 cm^2.

The timing of surgery must consider the balance of risks to the expectant mother and the unborn fetus. From the fetal perspective, surgery in the first trimester of pregnancy should be avoided because of the increased risk of teratogenesis. In addition, the high fetal mortality associated with CPB (20–30%) dictates that cardiac surgery is best delayed until after delivery of a viable fetus. Fetal outcome is therefore improved if surgery is delayed until after delivery.

From the maternal perspective, available evidence suggests that mortality is similar in patients operated on during pregnancy, immediately after delivery or in the post-partum period. Morbidity,

Table 48.2 Normal physiological changes associated with pregnancy

Circulating volume
Blood volume ↑ 30–40%
Physiological anemia (plasma ↑ 45%/erythrocytes ↑ 20%)
↓↓ Colloid osmotic pressure ⇒ ↑ risk of pulmonary edema
Altered plasma protein binding of drugs
Neutrophilia
Hypercoagulable state

Cardiovascular
↑Sympathetic tone ⇒ SV ↑ 30% + HR ↑ 15% ⇒ CO ↑ 50%
↑Wall stress/contractility → ↑ myocardial O_2 consumption
CVP and PAWP unchanged (PVR and SVR ↓ 20%)
Systolic BP – unchanged
Diastolic BP – initially falls and then returns to normal at term
Aortocaval compression ⇒ ↓↓ CO
Increased vascularity of airway – especially nasal passages

Respiratory
Diaphragmatic splinting
Minute ventilation, ↑ RR, ↑ V$_T$ ↓ FRC
↓ Pa_{CO_2}, ↓ HCO_3^-, ↓ buffering capacity
Total body O_2 consumption ↑ 15–20%

Gastrointestinal
Delayed gastric emptying, constipation
Increased risk of gastro-esophageal reflux

Genitourinary
↑Renal blood flow and glomerular filtration rate
Increased risk of vesico-ureteric reflux/infection
Glycosuria (tubular transport maximum exceeded)
Proteinuria (up to 0.3 g day^{-1})

Metabolic and endocrine
↑↑Prolactin, ACTH, cortisol
↓ Growth hormone
↑Thyroid binding globulin, T_4 and T_3 (free-T_4 near normal)
↑Gastrin

ACTH, adrenocorticotrophic hormone; FRC, functional respiratory capacity.

however, is considerably greater if surgery is delayed until after delivery.

In the emergency setting, for example following acute type A aortic dissection, where discussion of the timing of surgery is academic, the well-being of the expectant mother takes precedence. Close liaison with obstetricians and pediatricians is essential.

Anesthetic management

All patients at >20 weeks of pregnancy should be placed in a left lateral tilt to minimize the impact of aortocaval compression. As with all cardiac cases, invasive monitoring is best instituted before induction of anesthesia. It should be noted that, because of the physiological changes of pregnancy, there is poor correlation between CVP and PAWP. For this reason TEE may provide a better assessment of LV filling than CVP. When using TEE it is important to remember that cardiac chamber enlargement, annular dilatation and valvular regurgitation – particularly of the right-sided valves – are normal findings in the late stages of pregnancy. In addition, PA pressure is significantly overestimated when measured using TEE compared to values obtained at cardiac catheterization.

Many anesthetic drugs and opioids readily cross the placenta and cause fetal depression and bradycardia. Although there is little evidence to suggest that any one drug is superior to another, propofol, thiopental, isoflurane, fentanyl and morphine have all been used safely for many years in obstetric anesthesia. Non-depolarizing muscle relaxants are unable to cross the placenta. Both unfractionated and low molecular weight heparins do not cross the placenta and are non-teratogenic. In contrast, warfarin does cross the placenta and is teratogenic in the first trimester of pregnancy.

Cardiopulmonary bypass

Fetal death during CPB is thought to be due to decreased uteroplacental blood flow. It is therefore important to monitor fetal HR throughout CPB. Signs such as fetal bradycardia, sinusoidal patterns and late decelerations all indicate fetal hypoxia. Reduced uteroplacental blood flow may be due to reduced maternal SVR, hemodilution, hypothermia, particulate or air embolism, obstruction of venous drainage during IVC cannulation, prolonged CPB and opioid administration. The following strategies are thought to improve fetal protection during CPB:

- pump flow rate >2.5 l min^{-1} m^{-2}
- perfusion pressure >70 mmHg
- hematocrit >28% to optimize O_2 carrying capacity
- normothermia
- pulsatile pump flow
- alpha stat blood gas management.

Key points

- Cardiac disease is the leading cause of maternal death in Europe and North America.
- An increase in the average age of expectant mothers is associated with an increase in the prevalence of pregnancy-associated cardiac disease.
- Cardiac surgery during pregnancy is associated with increased morbidity and mortality.
- Decompensation is most likely to occur during and immediately after delivery.
- Whenever possible, cardiac surgery should be delayed until after delivery of a viable fetus.

Further reading

Berg CJ, Callaghan WM, Syverson C, Henderson Z. Pregnancy-related mortality in the United States, 1998 to 2005. *Obstet Gynecol* 2010; **116**(6): 1302–9.

Chandrasekhar S, Cook CR, Collard CD. Cardiac surgery in the parturient. *Anesth Analg* 2009; **108**: 777–85.

Lewis G (Ed.). The Confidential Enquiry into Maternal and Child Health (CEMACH). *Saving Mothers' Lives: reviewing maternal deaths to make motherhood safer – 2006–2008. The Eighth Report on Confidential Enquiries into Maternal Deaths in the United Kingdom.* London: CEMACH. 2011. *BJOG* 2011; **118**(Suppl 1): 1–203.

General principles

Isabeau A. Walker and Jon H. Smith

Congenital heart disease occurs in approximately 8:1000 live births and may be associated with recognizable syndromes or chromosomal abnormalities in 25% of cases. Abnormalities are often complex, affecting structure and function. Surgery may be corrective or palliative and can be staged. Over half of these operations occur in the first year of life. The timing of surgery is dictated by the severity of the lesion, the need to avoid the development of pulmonary vascular disease or the complications of cyanotic heart disease.

There are significant differences in infant and adult physiology that have a bearing on the conduct of anesthesia for children with congenital heart disease. This chapter will address these differences in physiology and some general principles of anesthesia for pediatric cardiac surgery.

Normal neonatal physiology

Newborn infants have a high metabolic rate and oxygen consumption. This is reflected in a high resting RR and CI (neonate: 300 ml kg^{-1} min^{-1}, adult 70–80 ml kg^{-1} min^{-1}). They have limited capacity to increase SV in response to increased filling and the resting HR is near maximal (Table 49.1). Neonates are exquisitely sensitive to negative inotropic or chronotropic agents.

The sarcoplasmic reticulum in neonatal myocytes is poorly developed. Calcium for cardiac contraction is derived from the extracellular fluid and infants do not tolerate ionized hypocalcemia. There is a relative imbalance of sympathetic and parasympathetic nervous systems at birth and neonates are prone to vagal reflexes.

The infant lung is relatively non-compliant, the ribs horizontally placed and relatively compliant.

Table 49.1 Normal ranges for respiratory rate, heart rate and systolic blood pressure according to patient age

Age	Respiratory rate (breaths min^{-1})	Heart rate (beats min^{-1})	Systolic BP (mmHg)
Newborn	40–50	120–160	50–90
Infant (<1 year)	30–40	110–160	70–90
Pre-school (2–5 years)	20–30	95–140	80–100
Primary school (5–12 years)	15–20	80–120	90–110
Adolescent (>12 years)	12–16	60–100	100–120

The lower airways are small and easily obstructed by secretions. Infants are consequently prone to respiratory failure.

Other important factors to consider include immature renal function, temperature regulation, hepatic function and drug, particularly opiate, metabolism.

Transitional circulation

In utero blood bypasses the fetal lung via two shunts, the foramen ovale and the ductus arteriosus (DA). With the first few breaths, there is a dramatic reduction in PVR and closure of fetal shunts. Pulmonary vasodilatation continues during the first few weeks of life, due to thinning of smooth muscle in the media of the pulmonary arterioles. PVR reaches adult levels by a few weeks of age (Figure 49.1). During this time the pulmonary vasculature remains reactive and stimuli such as hypoxia, hypercarbia and acidosis will cause

Core Topics in Cardiac Anesthesia, Second Edition, ed. Jonathan H. Mackay and Joseph E. Arrowsmith. Published by Cambridge University Press. © Cambridge University Press 2012.

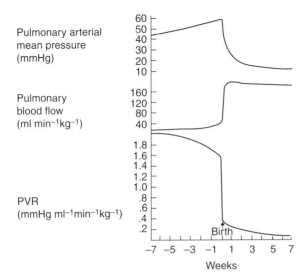

Pulmonary arterial mean pressure (mmHg)

Pulmonary blood flow (ml min⁻¹kg⁻¹)

PVR (mmHg ml⁻¹min⁻¹kg⁻¹)

Figure 49.1 Perinatal changes in pulmonary hemodynamics. Reprinted with permission from Rudolph *et al.*, 1996.

Table 49.2 Conditions dependent on continuing patency of the ductus arteriosus

Duct-dependent	Conditions
Systemic circulation	Critical coarctation, critical AS, HLHS
Pulmonary circulation	Pulmonary atresia, critical pulmonary stenosis, tricuspid atresia
"Mixing"	Transposition of the great arteries

HLHS; hypoplastic left heart syndrome.

pulmonary vasoconstriction and possibly reopen the ductus arteriosus (see below). Persistent pulmonary hypertension of the newborn (PPHN) may result; hypoxia may become critical and require treatment with inhaled nitric oxide or, in extreme cases, extracorporeal membrane oxygenation (ECMO).

Closure of the DA occurs in two phases. Functional closure occurs within 2–4 days in nearly all healthy infants under the influence of increasing PaO_2, falling $PaCO_2$ and prostaglandins. Anatomical closure of the DA due to fibrosis occurs within the first 3 weeks of life.

Continued ductal patency may occur due to prematurity (inadequate ductal smooth muscle) or in sick infants under the influence of excessive endogenous prostaglandin released in response to stimuli such as hypoxia (causing relaxation of ductal smooth muscle). A large duct may result in cardiac failure due to excessive pulmonary blood flow (PBF); diastolic BP will be low and may be associated with impaired renal or intestinal blood flow (possible renal impairment or necrotizing enterocolitis). Prostaglandin synthetase inhibitors such as indomethacin promote closure of the duct.

Duct-dependent circulation

In certain situations, continued ductal patency may be required for survival of the neonate (Table 49.2). In this situation prostaglandin E_2 infusion will be required and should be continued until definitive surgery. High doses of prostaglandin infusion can result in apneas, fevers and systemic vasodilatation. Where prostaglandin infusion has been continued long term (for instance, a premature neonate awaiting surgery), it should be remembered that prostaglandins are effective pulmonary vasodilators and may have to be weaned gradually post surgery.

Infants with a duct-dependent systemic circulation typically present with cardiac failure or collapse during the first week of life as the duct closes and shunting from the pulmonary to systemic circulation is lost. Treatment comprises resuscitation with inotropes and fluids, and institution of prostaglandin infusion prior to definitive surgery.

Infants with duct-dependent pulmonary circulation become cyanosed after duct closure and the loss of left → right shunting across the duct. Cyanosis will be unresponsive to increased FiO_2 and PBF must be restored with prostaglandin infusion before a definitive surgical procedure, for example valvotomy or systemic to pulmonary shunt, is performed.

Infants with duct-dependent "mixing" have two parallel closed-loop circulations and are dependent on mixing between the right and left side. Prostaglandin infusion and balloon atrial septostomy will be required where there is inadequate intracardiac mixing.

Balancing systemic and pulmonary circulations in neonates

Appropriate balance between systemic blood flow and PBF can be crucial, particularly in the neonate when alteration in direction of shunt blood flow may cause dramatic changes in saturation or CO.

Oxygen is a potent pulmonary vasodilator in neonates, while hypercarbia and acidosis cause pulmonary vasoconstriction. High FiO_2 and hyperventilation may be beneficial in infants with reduced PBF. Conversely, they may have a detrimental effect in infants with high PBF, or with balanced systemic and pulmonary shunts.

Exposure of neonates with large left → right shunts (e.g. large VSD) to high FiO_2 will cause pulmonary hyperemia and worsening cardiac failure. Infants in cardiac failure preoperatively should be given sufficient inspired oxygen to maintain SaO_2 in the low 90s only. Similarly, neonates with a duct-dependent systemic circulation (see above) or with high-volume, high-pressure shunts (e.g. A-V septal defect, truncus arteriosus, large Blalock-Taussig shunt) may have balanced shunts between systemic and pulmonary circulation. Ventilation with 100% oxygen may cause a marked fall in PVR, excessive left → right shunting and a fall in systemic perfusion leading to hypotension and metabolic acidosis. Strategies should be adopted to improve CO (e.g. fluids, inotropes) and reduce PBF. Mechanical ventilation in the operating room should be with air (or for cyanotic lesions, sufficient oxygen to maintain SaO_2 in the mid 80s), and with moderate hypercarbia. Conversely, a marked fall in SVR should be avoided as this may result in increased right → left shunting and critical cyanosis. Inotropic support may be required to increase SVR and CO, thus improving PBF. Similar principles should be followed postoperatively in the ICU, particularly after the first-stage Norwood procedure for hypoplastic left heart syndrome (HLHS).

SVR should be maintained in infants with large right → left shunts, such as tetralogy of Fallot. Excessive vasodilatation on induction of anesthesia may result in worsening cyanosis; vasoconstrictors may be required. Extreme right → left shunting is seen in the "spelling Fallot" due to spasm of the RVOT infundibulum in the presence of excess catecholamines. Measures to overcome infundibular spasm and increase PBF are required. These include adequate sedation, hyperventilation with 100% oxygen, a fluid bolus, bicarbonate or phenylephrine – the latter to reverse the direction of the shunt across the VSD and improve forward flow to the lungs. Propranolol may also be considered to reduce infundibular spasm.

SVR must be maintained in infants with left (or right) ventricular outflow obstruction. A fall in SVR may lead to critical hypoperfusion of the hypertrophied ventricle. A reduction in PVR may be beneficial in infants with RVH.

Cardiopulmonary interactions

Positive-pressure ventilation is generally beneficial to infants in cardiac failure due to poor myocardial function or left → right shunts (reduced work of breathing and afterload, improved oxygenation and CO_2 clearance), with attention to the FiO_2, as described above. However, hyperventilation at high airway pressures or lung volumes may increase PVR by distension of the lungs, disproportionately reducing the cross-sectional area of the pulmonary vasculature.

Spontaneous ventilation – where intra-pleural pressure is negative during inspiration – will augment systemic venous return to the right heart and improve PBF. This fact is utilized in the postoperative management of patients with cavo-pulmonary connections.

Surgical strategy

The timing of surgical repair is dictated by the functional impact of the cardiac lesion. Urgent balloon septostomy may be indicated in neonates with transposition of the great arteries (TGA). Duct-dependent lesions require corrective or palliative surgery within days of birth. Similarly, infants with obstructed total anomalous pulmonary venous drainage (TAPVD) may present with extreme cyanosis and cardiac failure requiring urgent corrective surgery.

Systemic arterial to pulmonary shunts such as the Blalock-Taussig (B-T; subclavian artery → main PA) shunt are performed in infancy for conditions associated with low PBF such as severe tetralogy of Fallot or pulmonary atresia. Definitive corrective surgery is performed, usually in the first year, after further growth of the pulmonary arteries.

Conditions involving left → right shunts increase PBF and cause cardiac failure and pulmonary hypertension (PHT). Typically, high-volume shunts cause heart failure as the PVR falls to adult levels at a few weeks of age (e.g. large VSD). Continued high PBF will result in irreversible changes in the pulmonary vasculature and will severely limit treatment options. Early surgery is therefore indicated. PA banding may be performed in infants with high PBF not suitable for early definitive surgery (e.g. multiple

VSDs). Low-volume shunts (e.g. ASD) may be closed when the child is older to avoid irreversible PHT in adult life.

Palliative surgery to create a univentricular circulation is performed in conditions where there is only a single functional ventricle or great vessel (univentricular A-V connection – double inlet ventricle, HLHS, tricuspid atresia or severe pulmonary atresia VSD). PBF may initially be provided with a B-T shunt in the neonatal period while the PVR remains high. Systemic venous shunts are performed after the PVR falls – initially a Glenn (SVC $\rightarrow$ PA) shunt, followed by an IVC $\rightarrow$ PA anstomosis to complete the Fontan circulation (or total cavopulmonary venous connection, TCPC) (see Chapter 51).

Closed cardiac surgery

Cardiac operations may be "closed" or "open". Open operations are performed on CPB and are discussed in the next chapter. Closed operations are usually performed on the great vessels and do not require CPB. The four commonest indications for closed operation in neonates and infants are:

- ligation of a patent ductus arteriosus (PDA) via left thoracotomy;
- repair of coarctation via left thoracotomy;
- PA banding via sternotomy or thoracotomy; PA banding is a temporary measure to prevent PHT and is reversed at the time of definitive surgery;
- systemic to pulmonary shunts; for example, B-T shunt via sternotomy or thoracotomy.

Cyanosis

Children with cyanotic heart disease maximize tissue oxygen delivery by becoming polycythemic and having a mild metabolic acidosis (causing right shift of the Hb-O_2 dissociation curve). Progression of cyanosis is reflected in an increase in hematocrit; venesection and hemodilution may be indicated. There is a risk of thromboembolism, including cerebral infarction, which is exacerbated by dehydration. Prolonged preoperative starvation must therefore be avoided. The prothrombotic tendency is partially compensated for by a mild coagulopathy – clotting factors should be available post CPB.

Key points

- Neonates have limited cardiopulmonary reserve and reactive pulmonary vasculature during the first weeks of life.
- Prostaglandin infusion is required for duct-dependent circulation prior to surgery.
- Manipulations of PVR and SVR have an important effect on balanced circulation; ventilation strategies should be carefully considered.
- Cardiac operations in children may be open or closed, depending on the abnormality.
- Children with cyanotic heart disease require careful perioperative care.

Further reading

James I, Walker I (Eds.). *Core Topics in Pediatric Anesthesia.* Cambridge: Cambridge University Press; 2012.

Rudolph AM, Rudolph CD, Hoffman JIE (Eds.). *Rudolph's Pediatrics*, 21st edition. Norwalk, Connecticut: Appleton and Lange; 1996.

Conduct of anesthesia

Jon H. Smith and Isabeau A. Walker

Pediatric cardiac anesthesiologists work as part of specialized multidisciplinary teams. The anesthesiologist requires a thorough understanding of congenital cardiac lesions, the planned surgery, the management of CPB and familiarity with anesthetizing small infants for major surgery. It is not for the occasional practitioner.

The anesthesia plan should be formulated in the light of all preoperative investigations and discussions. The predominant cardiac lesion should be considered on the basis of pathophysiology (Table 50.1),

myocardial reserve, and an assessment of the nature of shunt or obstructive lesions and the impact of alteration of SVR or PVR.

Children with uncomplicated procedures, such as closure of ASD, VSD or PDA, may be suitable candidates for a "fast track" approach and this should be taken into account in planning anesthesia. A child having a Fontan procedure (cavopulmonary connection) may benefit from early tracheal extubation as pulmonary blood flow (PBF) is improved with spontaneous ventilation. Children who are in cardiorespiratory

Table 50.1 Pathophysiology of congenital heart lesions

		Example	Comment
Acyanotic lesions	Left to right shunt		May lead to congestive cardiac failure and PHT, depending on the magnitude of the shunting
	Restrictive	Small ASD, VSD, PDA	
	Non-restrictive	Large ASD, VSD, PDA, A-VSD	
	Obstructive	Aortic stenosis, coarctation, interrupted aortic arch, HLHS, pulmonary stenosis, mitral stenosis, tricuspid stenosis	Severity of lesion determines age at presentation – neonates may be critically ill
	Regurgitant	Aortic regurgitation, mitral regurgitation, mitral valve prolapse, tricuspid regurgitation, pulmonary incompetence	
Cyanotic lesions	Transposition of the great arteries	With ASD, PDA or VSD, ±LVOT obstruction	May require BAS for survival if inadequate mixing. Presence of LVOT obstruction determines surgical options.
	Right to left shunt	Tetralogy of Fallot, critical pulmonary stenosis, pulmonary atresia (±VSD), tricuspid atresia	Severity of cyanosis depends on degree of obstruction through the right heart.
	Common mixing	TAPVD (+ASD, ±VSD, PDA, CoA), truncus arteriosus, double inlet ventricle ("single ventricle"), double outlet ventricle	Cyanosis may not be severe if lung blood flow unobstructed, but congestive heart failure will be present.

Modified from Archer and Burch, *Paediatric Cardiology: An Introduction.* Hodder Arnold; 1998.
ASD, atrial septal defect; VSD, ventricular septal defect; PDA, patent ductus arteriosus; CoA, coarctation of the aorta; TAPVD, total anomalous pulmonary venous drainage; BAS, balloon atrial septostomy.

Core Topics in Cardiac Anesthesia, Second Edition, ed. Jonathan H. Mackay and Joseph E. Arrowsmith. Published by Cambridge University Press. © Cambridge University Press 2012.

failure preoperatively, are unstable or who have large left to right shunts and are at risk for postoperative pulmonary hypertension (PHT) will require postoperative ventilation.

Preoperative assessment

The child must be evaluated carefully in the light of cardiological investigations. Symptoms of cardiac failure should be sought – poor feeding, sweating and grunting in young infants, recurrent chest infections, failure to thrive and poor exercise tolerance in older children. Signs of cardiac failure in young infants include tachycardia, tachypnea and hepatomegaly (but rarely edema). In children with cyanotic heart disease baseline SaO_2 should be recorded and a history suggestive of hypercyanotic episodes in children with tetralogy of Fallot should be sought. It is obviously important to exclude intercurrent infection as a cause of worsening symptoms.

Note should be made of associated congenital disorders, particularly those affecting the airway. Di George syndrome (22q11 deletion) causes 5% of cardiac anomalies, is associated particularly with truncus arteriosus and interrupted aortic arch and often results in thymic aplasia and neonatal hypocalcemia. The immunological defect necessitates the use of irradiated blood products to prevent graft versus host disease.

There should be a detailed and sympathetic discussion with the parents (and child if appropriate) concerning invasive monitoring, the need for postoperative intensive care, blood transfusion, analgesia and sedation. This is obviously a time of enormous stress for the family. It is our normal practice for the parents to accompany the child to the anesthetic room with a member of the nursing staff, if they wish – discussions should focus on their role and what to expect.

Premedication

Premedication of the young infant is not necessary, although chloral hydrate may be considered if the child has frequent hypercyanotic "spells". Older children may be premedicated with oral midazolam or temazepam, provided there are no contraindications, such as upper airway obstruction or limited cardiac reserve. Topical local anesthesia is routine; amethocaine gel (Ametop™) is suitable for infants from 6 weeks of age. No food or milk should be taken in the 6 hours prior to induction of anesthesia. Clear fluids, however, are permitted up to 2 hours prior to induction to reduce preoperative discomfort and intraoperative hypoglycemia.

Induction of anesthesia

Non-invasive monitoring is applied before induction; at minimum a SaO_2 monitor. Full monitoring should be applied as soon as the child will tolerate it. Infants who are unstable should be anesthetized in the operating room.

The choice of induction agent depends on the cardiac lesion. Children with less severe lesions (e.g. ASD, small VSD) will tolerate induction with judicious doses of propofol or thiopental. Inhalational induction with sevoflurane is routine for infants, although extreme care should be taken in sick infants with severe cyanosis or cardiac failure as they will not tolerate the myocardial depressant effects of volatile agents. Anesthesia may be maintained with isoflurane, and continued during CPB. Inhalational induction of anesthesia may be delayed in children with cyanotic heart lesions and be more rapid in children with left to right shunts, although this is of little clinical importance. Nitrous oxide is no longer used – it is a myocardial depressant and may increase PVR. Air must be available on the anesthetic machine as it is required for infants with balanced shunts.

Ketamine, a safe alternative to inhalational agents, is commonly used in sick patients. It causes an increase in cardiac index, SVR and PVR, although a rise in PVR may be avoided with effective airway control. It has a direct myocardial depressant effect that is usually offset by inhibition of norepinephrine uptake. The myocardial depressant effect may be evident in children on long-term inotrope therapy with depleted catecholamine stores.

High-dose fentanyl anesthesia is also suitable for infants with limited myocardial reserve. It will limit the stress response to surgery, but doses $>50\ \mu g\ kg^{-1}$ probably confer no additional benefit and may result in hypotension. Doses higher than $1–2\ \mu g\ kg^{-1}$ should only be given incrementally with invasive monitoring.

Uncuffed endotracheal tubes are traditionally used to secure the airway. Cuffed tubes are available down to size 3.0 and may be useful if lung compliance is poor, if there is a large leak around an uncuffed tube or if a thoracotomy is to be performed (coarctation repair, Blalock-Taussig shunt).

Some advocate regional anesthesia for pediatric cardiac surgery to reduce the stress response, improve postoperative recovery and reduce hospital costs. Others believe the risk of an epidural hematoma in a child who will be heparinized far outweighs the benefits. It is suggested that the risk of epidural hematoma is minimized by ensuring normal preoperative coagulation, abandoning difficult insertions or those where blood returns through the needle or epidural catheter. Heparin should be given at least 60 minutes after needle placement and the catheter removed only in the presence of normal coagulation.

Vascular access and monitoring

The long saphenous vein is useful for peripheral vascular access. Sites for arterial access may be the radial, femoral, axillary or brachial arteries. The arterial line and SaO_2 monitor should be sited in the right arm for coarctation repair. Monitoring from the ipsilateral arm during a B-T shunt should be avoided. Non-invasive blood pressure monitoring on the leg is useful after coarctation repair.

Central venous access is usually via the internal jugular vein (IJV). The authors use ultrasound guidance routinely. Double- or triple-lumen (4 Fr or 5 Fr) catheters are available in various lengths. The IJV should not be used in infants with univentricular physiology as thrombosis of the neck veins will make a subsequent Fontan procedure impossible. The femoral vein should be used as an alternative, with a small monitoring line in the IJV to reflect PA pressure. The left IJV should be avoided in children with a persistent left SVC as it commonly drains into the coronary sinus. Transthoracic lines are commonly used in the USA; they may be placed to measure LA or PA pressure post CPB; their routine use might spare the central veins and is said to be associated with a low incidence of bleeding once removed.

Core and peripheral temperatures are measured in all cases. The nasopharyngeal temperature gives a measure of brain temperature – a peripheral probe should be placed on the foot. Overhead radiant heaters may be useful in the anesthetic or induction room, if used, although overheating should be avoided and moderate hypothermia may be protective in infants undergoing coarctation repair.

Cardiopulmonary bypass

The difference in management of CPB in children compared to adults reflects differing physiology and complexity of intracardiac surgery. Cannulation will usually be bicaval for intra-cardiac surgery. Flow rates are relatively high, reflecting the increased metabolic rate of small infants. Perfusion pressures are maintained at 30–60 mmHg at normothermia and vasoconstrictors are rarely required. In the past, the volume of the pump prime was large relative to the circulating volume of infants; 800–1000 ml of prime relative to a blood volume of 250–300 ml. Citrated blood is added to the pump prime to avoid excessive hemodilution. Calcium is added to avoid hypocalcemia. In the current era there is much more emphasis on reducing the prime volume to minimize perioperative fluid overload. Pediatric oxygenators and cardiotomy reservoirs are smaller, the length and diameter of the bypass lines are reduced and, unlike most adult surgery, venous drainage is enhanced by applying negative pressure to the venous line.

Bypass may be conducted at normothermia, moderate hypothermia (25–32°C), deep hypothermia (15–20°C), or deep hypothermia with circulatory arrest (DHCA). Moderate hypothermia is mainly used in adolescents – SVC and IVC cannulae do not obstruct the surgeon's view of the intracardiac anatomy and full flows are maintained. DHCA is reserved for neonates and infants with complex lesions when the aortic and venous cannulae are removed to improve surgical access. DHCA also allows for periods of low flow to improve the surgical field.

There is significant risk of neurologic morbidity in infants undergoing DHCA, probably related to cellular ischemia. Periods of circulatory arrest are best combined with periods of low flow. Circulatory arrest of up to 30–40 min may be tolerated during deep hypothermia. Uniform cooling is important and inadequate cooling time (<18 min) is associated with worse outcomes. Vasodilatation during cooling may be useful. Cerebral protection may be improved using pH-stat acid-base management prior to circulatory arrest (associated with cerebral vasodilatation). Alpha-stat acid-base management, which preserves cerebral autoregulation, is used at other times. Icepacks are placed over the head during DHCA to prevent rewarming. Hyperglycemia should be avoided.

Weaning from cardiopulmonary bypass

Rewarming after aortic cross-clamp removal allows for spontaneous return of myocardial electrical activity. Ventricular fibrillation is uncommon in children

309

and, if persistent, may reflect poor myocardial preservation. Intracardiac de-airing should be meticulous to avoid coronary and cerebral air embolism – the lungs are ventilated and the venous line partially occluded to increase LA filling. As the heart starts to eject endotracheal suction is performed and ventilation recommended. Temporary pacing wires are routinely used as intracardiac surgery may affect the cardiac conducting system.

Vasodilators used to aid rewarming include sodium nitroprusside, phentolamine or in some centers phenoxybenzamine. Inotropic support is usual in infants and should be started when nasopharyngeal temperature reaches 30°C after removal of the cross-clamp. Epinephrine is the drug of choice, although dobutamine or a phosphodiesterase (PDE) inhibitor may be used if the PVR is increased. PDE inhibitors (e.g. milrinone) are commonly used when there is PHT or RV dysfunction. A loading dose is usually administered during CPB. The combination of a PDE inhibitor with epinephrine or dopamine is useful in the presence of poor ventricular function or after ventriculotomy (Table 50.2). Volume overload in the small non-compliant ventricle must be avoided.

The use of vasoconstrictors in children after cardiac surgery remains controversial. In the presence of systemic arterial hypotension and poor end organ perfusion in the setting of good cardiac function and oxygen delivery our preference is to use vasopressin at a dose of $0.0003-0.002$ U kg^{-1} min^{-1}. Vasoconstrictors should not be used in the context of low cardiac output where peripheral limb ischemia may result.

Measurement of mixed venous oxygen saturation (SvO_2), either by intermittent sampling of blood in the central veins or continuously using an oximeter that is integral to the central line, may be helpful in deducing adequacy of the cardiac output.

In the last 5 years, near infrared oximetry (NIRS) has been used to give an indication of the adequacy of cerebral, and occasionally visceral, oxygenation throughout the course of cardiac surgery requiring CPB. There are several devices available with some

Table 50.2 Common cardiac drug dosages in pediatric cardiac practice

Drug	Dilution	1 ml h⁻¹ =	Dose range
Dopamine	3 mg kg^{-1} in 50 ml 5% dextrose	1 μg kg^{-1} min^{-1}	5–10 μg kg^{-1} min^{-1}
Dobutamine	3 mg kg^{-1} in 50 ml 5% dextrose	1 μg kg^{-1} min^{-1}	5–10 μg kg^{-1} min^{-1}
Epinephrine	0.03 mg kg^{-1} in 50 ml 5% dextrose	0.01 μg kg^{-1} min^{-1}	0.005–0.1 μg kg^{-1} min^{-1}
Norepinephrine	0.03 mg kg^{-1} in 50 ml 5% dextrose	0.01 μg kg^{-1} min^{-1}	0.01–0.2 μg kg^{-1} min^{-1}
Milrinone	0.3 mg kg^{-1} in 50 ml 5% dextrose	0.1 μg kg min^{-1}	0.375–0.75 μg kg^{-1} min^{-1} Loading dose 50–100 μg kg^{-1} over 20 min
Isoprenaline	0.03 mg kg^{-1} in 50 ml 5% dextrose	0.01 μg kg min^{-1}	0.01–0.5 μg kg^{-1} min^{-1}
Sodium nitroprusside	3 mg kg^{-1} in 50 ml 5% dextrose	1 μg kg^{-1} min^{-1}	0.5–5 μg kg^{-1} min^{-1}
Glyceryl trinitrate	3 mg kg^{-1} in 50 ml 5% dextrose Maximum 1mg ml^{-1}	1 μg kg^{-1} min^{-1}	0.5–5 μg kg^{-1} min^{-1}
Calcium gluconate	10%		Bolus dose 0.1 ml kg^{-1}
Phenylephrine			Bolus dose 1 μg kg^{-1}
Vasopressin	3 U kg^{-1} in 50 ml 5% dextrose	0.001 U kg min^{-1}	

technical differences beyond the scope of this article. It is a proxy measure of cardiac output but is susceptible to changes in $PaCO_2$ and the perfusion pressure. Regional cerebral saturation <50% usually indicates that there is a major problem that requires intervention.

Management post bypass

Modified ultrafiltration

Modified ultrafiltration (MUF) is useful in children weighing <20 kg. It is started prior to protamine administration. Blood is taken from the aorta, passed through an ultrafilter and returned to the RA. The process usually takes 15–20 min and is continued until the hematocrit is ~40%. Between 150 and 500 ml fluid may be removed, depending on the prime volume and starting hematocrit. In addition to increasing hematocrit, MUF increases colloid osmotic pressure, removes extracellular water (including myocardial water), reduces transfusion requirements and improves hemodynamic function. It also reduces PVR, improves cerebral function and may reduce the levels of circulating vasoactive cytokines.

Hemostasis

Diffuse coagulopathy is common in neonates after CPB. This is due to a combination of immature hepatic function, hemodilution by the pump prime and activation of clotting by the large non-endothelialized surface of the bypass circuit. Operations tend to be long, may require DHCA, pump flow rates are high and relatively large volumes of blood are salvaged and returned to the bypass circuit. Thrombocytopenia and hypofibrinogenemia are common, and platelets and cryoprecipitate (or fresh frozen plasma) are ordered routinely. Mild coagulation defects are also common in children with cyanotic heart disease. CPB prime volumes have been reduced to limit the coagulation problems of neonatal bypass. It is now common to order a thromboelastogram in patients who continue to bleed after heparin reversal.

Aprotinin is now rarely used routinely, being reserved for complex transplants and re-operations (see Chapter 11). It may reduce bleeding after re-operation but its use in patients undergoing DHCA or venous shunts (e.g. bi-directional Glenn) is controversial. It may have a useful anti-inflammatory effect but a test dose should be given because of the risk of anaphylaxis. Tranexamic acid and epsilon aminocaproic acid may also be useful although there is some debate about the correct dose of tranexamic acid.

Transesophageal echocardiography

TEE is useful before the onset of CPB to exclude additional defects and in the post CPB period to assess myocardial contractility and the integrity of the surgical repair. Considerable expertise is required to interpret TEE images in the setting of complex lesions. Smaller infants should have epicardial echocardiography. Images should be obtained and stored routinely prior to leaving the operating room.

Delayed sternal closure

The chest may be left open after neonatal surgery or if there is evidence of cardiac tamponade after primary chest closure. Delayed primary closure is usually possible on the ICU after 24–72 h.

Pulmonary hypertensive crisis

All newborns and those with high PBF (e.g. truncus, A-V septal defect and anomalous pulmonary venous drainage) are at risk of postoperative PHT. For this reason, a monitoring line may be inserted into the PA during surgery. During a pulmonary hypertensive crisis there may be a sustained rise in PA pressure (>2/3 systemic) or PA pressure may be suprasystemic. It will usually respond to inhaled nitric oxide (20 ppm), although doses up to 80 ppm may be required. Standard management also includes moderate hypocapnia, avoidance of acidosis, ventilation with 100% oxygen and additional sedation and paralysis. The usual duration of therapy is 24–48 h.

Right heart failure

Right heart failure may be a consequence of surgical ventriculotomy, poor myocardial preservation (particularly with pre-existing RVH), transient PHT, raised transpulmonary gradient or anatomical problems subsequent to the surgery, such as an obstructed outflow tract. It is important to rule out the latter with on-table echocardiography or early postoperative right heart catheterization.

Treatment strategies include those for PHT, if indicated, careful volume loading (RA pressures 15–16 mmHg) and epinephrine combined with a PDE inhibitor. Failure to respond to high-dose inotropes may be an

311

indication for the use of extracorporeal membrane oxygenation or mechanical ventricular assist device.

Left heart failure

LV failure is due to acute or chronic ischemia (TGA, anomalous left coronary artery from the pulmonary artery), poor myocardial protection or preoperative dysfunction. Poor revascularization needs surgical revision. Low CO with high atrial pressures requires inotrope and vasodilator therapy. Should circulatory failure persist, mechanical support is used. ECMO supports both ventricles and the lungs. LVAD support may be used in the presence of normal or near normal RV function, PA pressure and pulmonary function.

Transfer to intensive care

Transfer of the child back to intensive care may be a hazardous process – lines may be displaced and hemodynamic instability may occur due to bleeding. The child should be fully monitored at all times. Finally, it is important that the anesthesiologist transfers the wealth of information they have gleaned about the patient during the perioperative period to the intensive care team in an effective manner.

Key points

- Conduct of anesthesia and CPB strategy are determined by patient age, the pathophysiology of the cardiac lesion and the planned surgical procedure.
- The surgical procedure frequently influences the location of monitoring site.
- Deep hypothermic circulatory arrest is often required in neonates with complex lesions.
- Recent advances include reduced pump priming volume and monitoring of tissue oxygenation.
- Modified ultrafiltration improves fluid balance and cardiac function after bypass in infants.
- Neonates with high pulmonary blood flow are at risk of pulmonary hypertensive crisis post bypass.

Further reading

Gaynor JW. Use of Ultrafiltration during and after cardiopulmonary bypass in children. *J Thorac Cardiovasc Surg* 2001; **122**(2): 209–11.

Goldman AP, Delius RE, Deanfield JE, Macrae DJ. Nitric oxide is superior to prostacyclin for pulmonary hypertension after cardiac operations. *Ann Thorac Surg* 1995; **60**: 300–6.

Hirsch JC, Charpie JR, Ohye RG, Gurney JG. Near-infrared spectroscopy: what we know and what we need to know – a systematic review of the congenital heart disease literature. *J Thorac Cardiovasc Surg* 2009; **137**: 154–9.

Laussen P. Optimal blood gas management during deep hypothermic paediatric cardiac surgery: alpha stat is easy, but pH stat may be preferable. *Paediatr Anaesth* 2002; **12**: 199–204.

Wypij D, Jonas RA, Bellinger DC, *et al.* The effect of hematocrit during hypothermic cardiopulmonary bypass in infant heart surgery: results from the combined Boston hematocrit trials. *J Thorac Cardiovasc Surg* 2008; **135**: 355–60.

Common congenital heart lesions

David J. Barron and Kevin P. Morris

Patent ductus arteriosus (PDA)

Incidence and associations

Common: persistence inversely proportional to gestational age. Incidence >80% in infants <1 kg birth weight. Associated with prematurity, diaphragmatic hernia, transposition of the great arteries (TGA), Fallot's tetralogy and pulmonary atresia

Anatomy

It is a remnant of the distal portion of the sixth left aortic arch. It connects the main PA to the descending thoracic aorta (Figure 51.1).

Physiology

Carries ~90% of RV output *in utero*. Left to right (L→R) shunt increases as PVR falls following birth. Functional (reversible) closure within 15 hours of birth. Permanent closure occurs within 3 weeks in term infants. Risk of endarteritis (often termed duct-related endocarditis). Hemodynamic impact of PDA dependent on size:

- Small PDA may go undetected.
- Large PDA may cause: severe heart failure. Excessive pulmonary blood flow (PBF) may exacerbate respiratory distress syndrome, precipitate pulmonary hemorrhage and compromise weaning from mechanical ventilation. "Run-off" from the aorta results in a low diastolic pressure and "steal" from the systemic circulation. Reduced mesenteric blood flow may result in necrotizing enterocolitis (NEC).

Diagnosis

Continuous machinery murmur. Echocardiography confirms duct and direction of shunting; LA:aortic diameter ratio reflects degree of L→R shunting.

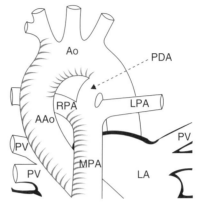

Figure 51.1
The patent ductus arteriosus. AAo, ascending aorta; MPA, main pulmonary artery; RPA, right pulmonary artery; LPA, left pulmonary artery.

Management

According to duct dependence (see Chapter 49).

- *Medical*: treatment with indomethacin or another NSAID may result in duct closure. Often combined with fluid restriction and diuretics.
- *Trans-catheter closure*: may be undertaken in the catheter laboratory in large infants or children.
- *Surgical*: necessary if medical treatment fails or is contraindicated (renal impairment, GI or other hemorrhage). Duct is ligated or closed with a clip via left thoracotomy without CPB. Pre and post ductal oximetry is required.

  - Complications: inadvertent ligation of left PA or descending aorta, damage to recurrent laryngeal nerve or thoracic duct, reduced pulmonary compliance, and LV failure. Inotropes rarely required for ventricular dysfunction and poor perfusion.

Coarctation of the aorta (CoA)

Incidence and associations

Six percent of all congenital heart disease. Associated with Turner's syndrome, bicuspid AV (up to 40%) and VSD.

Anatomy

Narrowing of aorta in the region of the ductal insertion, i.e. distal to the left subclavian artery. Can occasionally occur proximal to the left subclavian.

Physiology

Presentation depends on severity of narrowing.

- Severe CoA presents as a neonate as the duct closes. Aorta virtually occluded causing circulatory collapse, acute LV failure and loss of lower limb pulses.
- Moderate CoA presents more subtly with degree of LV failure in childhood (rare).
- Less severe CoA presents with chance finding of murmur or upper limb hypertension.

Management of the neonate

Prostaglandin E infusion. This reopens the duct and re-establishes flow to the lower body. Ductal tissue often involved in CoA, severity of CoA may also be reduced with PGE. Neonates usually have considerable heart failure. May require full resuscitation with ventilation/inotropic support. Condition can usually be stabilized with these measures. Rarely the duct will not reopen and surgery is required as an emergency.

Surgery

Via left thoracotomy. <1% perioperative mortality. Repaired either with resection and end-to-end anastamosis or with subclavian flap angioplasty. Both have excellent results; the former is regarded by most as the gold standard. Sacrificing the subclavian artery in the neonate does not cause limb ischemia and at worst may result in reduced limb growth. Repair of hypoplastic aortic arch may require CPB via sternotomy. Arterial line should be placed in right brachial/radial artery to ensure monitoring can be continued with clamp on aortic arch. Ideally two arterial lines, one in right arm and one femoral, can be placed.

- *Complications*: risk of recurrence 2–4%, majority can be successfully dilated with balloon angioplasty. Injury to recurrent laryngeal nerve or thoracic duct (rare). Risk of paraplegia (due to spinal ischemia <0.5% – virtually unknown in neonates). Core cooling to 35°C and keeping clamp time <30 min are protective. Full or partial CPB can be used allowing for deeper cooling.

Postoperative management

Monitor femoral pulses. Echocardiogram to assess LV function and confirm adequate arch repair. May have hypertension, requiring treatment (β-blocker). Record lower limb function when muscle relaxants are stopped.

Aortic interruption is an extreme form of CoA. Always associated with a VSD or, rarely, an aortopulmonary window and commonly associated with 22q11 deletion. Requires repair on CPB via sternotomy. Much higher risk condition.

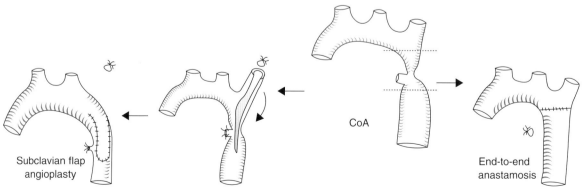

Subclavian flap angioplasty

CoA

End-to-end anastamosis

Figure 51.2 Surgery of coarctation of the aorta.

Atrial septal defect (ASD)

Incidence and associations

Eight percent of all congenital heart disease. Associated with Holt-Oram syndrome, maternal Rubella and Down's syndrome (primum only).

Anatomy

Defects occur at different sites (Figure 51.3).

- *Secundum ASDs* are the most common – the majority can be closed with a device in the catheter laboratory. Features making device closure unlikely are: very large defect, lack of inferior or lateral rim of tissue and relatively large defects in smaller children. All other types of defect require surgical closure.
- *Primum ASDs* are part of the spectrum of atrioventricular septal defects AVSDs

(Figure 51.6) and are more correctly called "partial AVSD". They are always associated with a cleft in the left A-V ("mitral") valve which is repaired as part of the procedure.

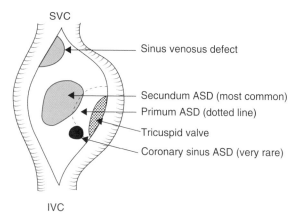

Figure 51.3 View inside right atrium.

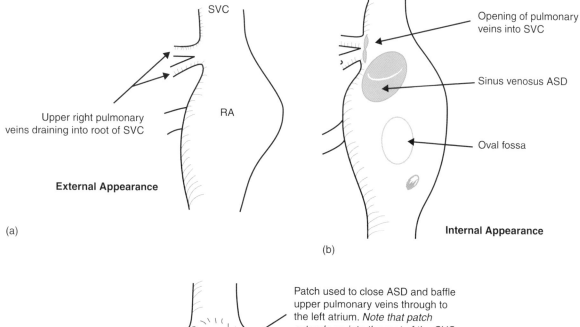

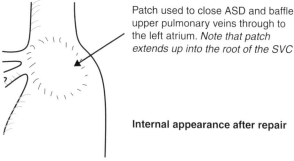

Figure 51.4 Surgical patch closure of sinus venosus ASD and baffling of right upper pulmonary vein into left atrium.

- *Sinus venosus ASDs* are associated with anomalous drainage of the upper right pulmonary veins into the root of the SVC (Figure 51.4a). These can be baffled back to the LA with a patch repair (Fig 51.4c).
- *Coronary sinus ASDs* are associated with unroofing of the coronary sinus, thus closing the defect leaves the CS draining into the LA creating a small, hemodynamically insignificant R→L shunt.

Physiology

L→R shunt causing volume load on pulmonary circulation. Most children are symptomless but plethoric lungs may predispose to chest infections and failure to thrive. Very large shunts may result in effort intolerance. PHT is *not* associated with isolated ASDs in children.

Surgery

Suture closure of small defects, autologous pericardium or prosthetic patch closure of large defects. Intraoperative echocardiography should focus on pulmonary venous drainage in sinus venosus ASD and on left A-V valve function in partial AVSD repair.

Postoperative care

Surgery is generally of low risk and children can be weaned from ventilation and extubated shortly after surgery. Sinus venosus ASD repair involves the root of the SVC and there is a risk of causing SVC obstruction. If the face looks plethoric or SVC pressure is high arrange echocardiographic or contrast evaluation. Nodal rhythms may occur with high atrial incisions (e.g. sinus venosus ASD).

Some units "fast-track" ASD repairs to a monitored "stepdown" facility on day of surgery.

Ventricular septal defect (VSD)

Incidence and associations

Thirty percent of all congenital heart disease. Associations include coarctation and the VACTERL syndrome (vertebral anomalies, anal atresia, cardiovascular anomalies, tracheoesophageal fistula, esophageal atresia, renal, limb defects). It should be borne in mind that many other complex forms of congenital heart disease include a VSD (e.g. truncus, pulmonary atresia, Fallot's).

Anatomy

A schematic view of the ventricular septum viewed from the right side is shown in Figure 51.5.

Physiology

The majority of VSDs do not require intervention and either close spontaneously or are so small as to not warrant closure. Perimembranous VSDs are unlikely to close spontaneously and are the most likely to need surgical closure. Large VSDs, causing heart failure and failure to thrive, are the commonest indication for repair.

"Unrestrictive" VSD means there is no Doppler gradient across the VSD on echocardiography. This means that the VSD must be large and that the pressure in the RV is at systemic level, leading to PHT. The PHT should completely reverse as long as the defect is closed before six months of age.

Less common indications for closure are:

- moderate VSDs in older children that have failed to close and continue to produce a significant shunt ($Q_P:Q_S > 1.5:1$)
- small VSDs that have been associated with an episode of endocarditis
- small perimembranous VSDs that have resulted in AV prolapse into the defect, with AR.

Surgery

The mortality rate is 1–2%. Most VSDs are closed via the RA using a prosthetic patch. Intraoperative echocardiography should focus on looking for any residual VSD, ensuring the LVOT is unobstructed and assessing TV function.

Postoperative management

Patients are usually neonates/young infants with considerable preoperative heart failure. Regular diuretics and vasodilators help offload the LV. *Check rhythm*: A-V node is adjacent to perimembranous VSDs and variable degrees of heart block can be seen. All patients should have atrial and ventricular pacing wires available. A-V block is usually transient (a few hours) but can be permanent (1–2%). Postoperative echocardiography should be used to reassess LV function, exclude any residual VSD and estimate RV pressure. Pulmonary hypertensive crises are a potential risk but uncommon after simple VSD repair, although older children (>6 months) with large VSDs are at a greater risk.

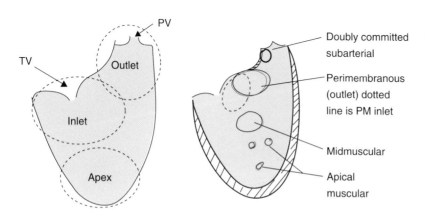

Figure 51.5 Schematic of ventricular septum viewed from right side. (a) The ventricular septum can be divided into inlet, apical and outlet portions. (b) Sites at which VSDs are found.

PV

TV

Outlet

Inlet

Apex

Doubly committed subarterial

Perimembranous (outlet) dotted line is PM inlet

Midmuscular

Apical muscular

Atrioventricular septal defect (AVSD)

Also called A-V canal defect or endocardial cushion defect. AVSDs may be complete (cAVSD) or partial (pAVSD).

Incidence and associations

Four percent of all congenital heart disease. Both cAVSD and pAVSD are strongly associated with Down's syndrome.

Anatomy

There is a defect in the center of the heart with a single valve (the common A-V valve) straddling both ventricles and a hole above and below it. In pAVSD the VSD component has closed, leaving only an ASD (Figure 51.6).

Physiology

- *Complete AVSD*: behaves like a large VSD (i.e. L→R shunt leading to high PBF and heart failure in neonates). In addition, the common A-V valve can be regurgitant, adding to the heart failure. All require surgical closure before 6 months of age.

Later repair is associated with significant risk of irreversible PHT.

- *Partial AVSD*: (also called primum ASD) the ventricular component has closed, there is less of L→R shunt and lower likelihood of heart failure. Repair is generally undertaken before 5 years of age.

Surgery

cAVSD ~ 5% perioperative mortality. pAVSD ~ 1% perioperative mortality. The VSD is closed with one patch, the ASD with another, sandwiching the valve between them. Surgery recreates two separate A-V valves. However, anatomically the valve between the LA and LV is not a true "mitral" valve and is referred to as the "left A-V valve" (Figure 51.7). The cleft in the left A-V valve is closed as part of the repair to create a competent valve. Repair of cAVSD in babies without Down's syndrome is typically more complicated (poor A-V valve function) compared to babies with Down's syndrome. Intraoperative echocardiography should focus on looking for any residual VSD, assessing left and right A-V valve function and ensuring that the LVOT is unobstructed.

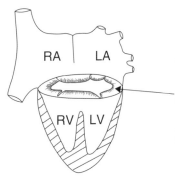

There is a defect in the center of the heart with a single valve (the common AV valve) straddling both ventricles and a hole above and below it. In partial AVSD the VSD component has closed leaving only an ASD
Common AV valve

Figure 51.6 Anatomy of atrioventricular septal defect.

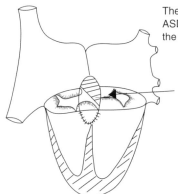

The VSD is closed with one patch, the ASD with another, sandwiching the valve between them

The cleft in the left AV valve is then closed to make the valve competent

Figure 51.7 Surgery for atrioventricular septal defect.

Postoperative management

LA line is useful and PA line is inserted where concern exists about PHT. Echocardiography is repeated to exclude residual VSD, and to assess ventricular and A-V valve function. Confirm rhythm, risk of heart block. Babies usually in marked heart failure preoperatively with pulmonary congestion may take time to wean from the ventilator. Risks and management of PHT are described in Chapter 53. Partial AVSD repairs are generally uncomplicated. All have had left A-V valve repair and should have an echocardiogram to document the result.

Fallot's tetralogy

It is also called tetralogy of Fallot, ToF and Fallot.

Incidence and associations

Six percent of all congenital heart disease. Fallot is associated with many syndromic conditions, affecting 20% of patients and include Di George syndrome/ 22q11 deletion, CHARGE (coloboma, heart defects, choanal atresia, retardation of growth or development, genital or urinary abnormalities, and ear abnormalities and deafness) association, VACTERL and Down's syndrome.

Anatomy

The key anatomical features, perimembranous VSD with aortic over-ride and multilevel RV outflow obstruction, are highlighted in Figure 51.8. The degree of right outflow tract obstruction is variable and tends to worsen with time as RVH progresses. Important variants are ToF with multiple VSDs and the presence of an anomalous left coronary artery (2–5%) – in the latter, repair requires a conduit to jump over the coronary as it crosses the outflow tract. Absent pulmonary valve syndrome is a rare type of Fallot with similar intracardiac anatomy but no true PV. The PAs beyond the valve have marked post-stenotic dilatation and may cause compression of the airways and bronchomalacia. Treatment is similar but involves plication of the aneurysmal central PAs and respiratory assessment.

Physiology

Management depends on the degree of cyanosis at presentation and associated lesions. Cyanotic neonates are usually palliated with a systemic-pulmonary shunt procedure, most commonly a B-T shunt. This is also used in patients with small/hypoplastic pulmonary arteries to encourage growth. An alternative is to use balloon dilatation or stenting of the RVOT.

Although some centers favor complete neonatal repair, the majority favor delaying surgery in stable infants until they are 6–9 months of age.

Cyanotic "spelling" typically develops in the first 6 months of life and is treated with β-blockers, which relieve infundibular muscle spasm and reduce the degree of cyanosis. Patients can "spell" severely on induction of anesthesia and if this fails to respond to oxygen therapy and volume infusion then a systemic vasoconstrictor (epinephrine/norepinephrine/phenylephrine) may be required to increase systemic afterload and so improve PBF.

Surgery

Early mortality is 3–4%. Muscle bundles in the RVOT are resected and the VSD is closed, usually via the RA. The PV and main PA usually need to be opened out and patched to enlarge the outflow tract sufficiently – requiring a transannular incision and patch. This relieves obstruction but leaves significant pulmonary regurgitation (Figure 51.9).

The presence of an anomalous LAD requires the placement of an RV → PA conduit to avoid the vessel. Intraoperative echocardiography should look for any residual VSD (or additional VSD) and carefully assess the RVOT looking for residual obstruction and quantify the degree of pulmonary regurgitation.

Postoperative management

Rhythm disturbances and low CO can occur. Junctional tachycardias are common and may be nodal or His bundle in origin. An atrial wire study may identify dissociated P-waves suggesting His bundle tachycardia. Management of junctional ectopic tachycardia is discussed in Chapter 53.

Restrictive physiology may lead to a low CO state and RV failure.

- A non-compliant, small RV chamber leads to predominantly diastolic dysfunction.
- A pathognomonic echocardiography finding is forward flow in the PA during ventricular diastole; atrial systole results in opening of the PV as a consequence of pressure transmission through the stiff, non-compliant RV.

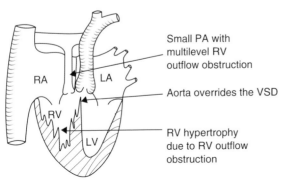

RA

LA

RV

LV

Small PA with multilevel RV outflow obstruction

Aorta overrides the VSD

RV hypertrophy due to RV outflow obstruction

Figure 51.8 Anatomy of tetralogy of Fallot.

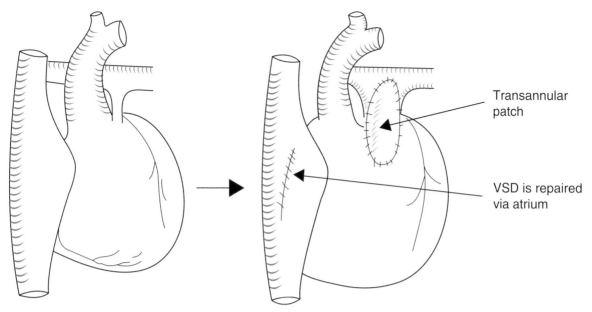

Figure 51.9 Surgery for tetralogy of Fallot.

- Residual structural RVOT obstruction must be excluded by echocardiography.
- Treatment is by increasing preload – RA pressure 10–15 mmHg.
- Inodilators such as milrinone are preferred to epinephrine, which may worsen RV diastolic function.
- PA forward flow and pulmonary regurgitation are adversely affected by positive-pressure ventilation; shorten inspiratory time relative to expiratory time, possible role for negative-pressure ventilation.
- Marked capillary leak often with high ascitic losses. Peritoneal dialysis may be needed.
- Consider return to operating room if residual RVOT obstruction cannot be overcome, placement of competent valve into RVOT or creation of an ASD to allow R→L shunt.

Pulmonary atresia

A complex group of conditions and may have areas of lung supplied by major aorto-pulmonary collateral arteries (MAPCAs). Can be divided into three groups:

(1) with intact ventricular septum

(2) with VSD, without MAPCAs

(3) with VSD and MAPCAs.

Incidence and associations

It constitutes 1.5% of all congenital heart disease. Associated with 22q11 deletion.

With intact ventricular septum

A "dead-end" ventricle which can vary in size from normal to hypoplastic. Management depends on size of RV.

- *Normal size*: perforation and balloon dilatation of PV (catheter laboratory) with or without surgical opening of RVOT.
- *Small*: modified B-T shunt with or without opening of RVOT to encourage forward flow through RV.
- *Very small (hypoplastic)*: modified B-T shunt.

Coronary fistulae or sinusoids – the "dead-end" ventricle leads to enormous intra-cavity pressures that may squeeze blood backwards into the coronaries and create fistulae. Fortunately rare, but if present cannot risk relieving the RVOT without causing coronary ischemia (RV-dependent coronary circulation).

With VSD, without MAPCAs

It is effectively an extreme form of tetralogy of Fallot. Duct-dependent at birth, requiring PGE infusion and modified B-T shunt. Postoperative management of a B-T shunt is detailed in Chapter 53. Complete repair is managed as per tetralogy of Fallot, using a RV → PA conduit.

Postoperative management

Majority follow single ventricle route, initially with modified B-T shunt. If RVOT has been opened beware of restrictive RV physiology (Figures 51.8 and 51.9).

With VSD and MAPCAs

- Pulmonary blood supply is from large collateral vessels arising from the aorta.
- Surgery aims to join the MAPCAs together (unifocalization), reconnect them to the native PAs (if present), insert an RV → PA conduit and close the VSD (Figure 51.10). This usually requires a combined thoracotomy and sternotomy.
- May require several staged procedures. VSD often left open until confident that PVR will be low enough for RV to cope.

Postoperative management

Will remain cyanotic postoperatively if VSD left open. Operated side may have considerable collapse or contusion of the lung. Previously poorly perfused areas may suffer reperfusion injury with localized edema, congestion and hemorrhage. Management includes positive end-expiratory pressure (PEEP) and diuretics. Any increase in PAP or PVR is usually a consequence of small PAs and is seldom reactive; i.e. unlikely to respond to inhaled NO. RV will be non-compliant and may show restrictive physiology.

(a)

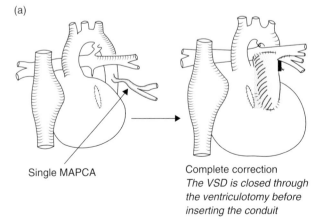

Single MAPCA

Complete correction
The VSD is closed through the ventriculotomy before inserting the conduit

(b)

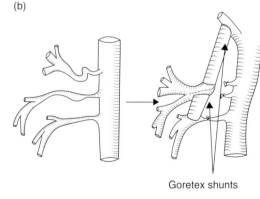

Goretex shunts

Figure 51.10 (a) Repair or PA/VSD with a single MAPCA. (b) Example of unifocalization of three MAPCAs to the right lung.

Transposition of the great arteries

It is also called "transposition" or TGA. D-TGA is the most common variety and the type requiring neonatal correction. L-TGA is very complex, often called congenitally corrected TGA (ccTGA) and not relevant to most practices.

Incidence

It constitutes 5% of all congenital heart disease.

Anatomy

Aorta arises from the RV and the PA arises from the LV. The great vessels usually lie in an anterior-posterior relationship with the aorta anterior and to the right. There are many associated features, but "simple" transposition (the commonest) implies the ventricular septum is intact (as opposed to TGA/VSD; Figure 51.11).

Circulations are in parallel rather than in series. Coronary arteries arise from the aorta from the sinuses that face the main PA and come off in a variety of patterns. Risk factors for a more complicated surgical course include:

- unusual coronary artery patterns, especially intramural coronaries, which run in the wall of the aorta in an oblique course and those with a single coronary origin;
- side-by-side great vessels (rather than anterior–posterior);
- presence of additional lesions, e.g. CoA or VSD;
- age >10 days slight risk. Age >42 days major risk.

Physiology

Cyanotic. Reliant on patent foramen ovale (PFO) and PDA to allow mixing. Presence of a VSD may improve mixing. In TGA with intact ventricular septum the LV muscle mass will begin to regress once PVR falls. Presence of VSD prevents this as ventricular pressures are both at systemic level. Rare combinations such as TGA/VSD/PS may be well-balanced cyanotic circulations and not require any early intervention.

Initial management

PGE infusion to maintain patency of PDA. May require mechanical ventilation. Cardiologists may perform balloon atrial septostomy, under echocardiographic guidance on the ICU, to enlarge PFO and improve mixing. In cases with an intact ventricular septum, the aim is to perform surgery within the first 10 days of life before LV muscle mass regresses. In late presentations (>4 weeks) PA banding may be considered to "train the LV" (i.e. increase muscle mass) prior to a switch procedure.

Surgery

The arterial switch procedure; a complex neonatal procedure with a 2–4% early mortality. The great arteries are divided and switched. The coronaries are transferred separately onto the neo-aorta. Note from Figure 51.12 that the PA ends up in front of the aorta (the so-called Lecompte maneuver). Additional lesions such as VSD or CoA are usually repaired at the same time, although this increases operative complexity and risk.

Intraoperative echocardiography should focus on LV and RV function. The LVOT and RVOT should be examined to assess the severity of any aortic and pulmonary regurgitation. An LA line is placed routinely.

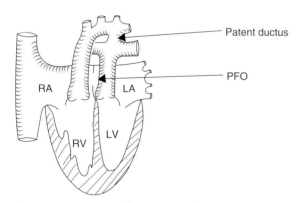

Figure 51.11 Anatomy of transposition of the great arteries.

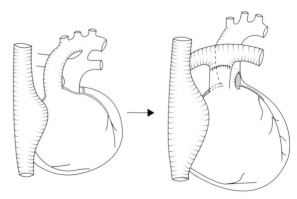

Figure 51.12 The arterial switch procedure.

Postoperative care

The LV tends to be non-compliant and small changes in preload cause marked changes in LA pressure. Kinking or malposition of the coronaries can result in coronary ischemia. If there are ST changes or rhythm problems, a 12-lead ECG should be performed. Echocardiography should be performed on return to ICU to:

- assess LV function and regional contractility

- examine LVOT and RVOT, and exclude any residual VSD
- exclude neo-aortic regurgitation.

Vasodilators may help a non-compliant LV to relax. Infants with large PDA may have had a high pre-operative PBF and require regular diuretics. Older switch patients (>4 weeks) may require prolonged inotropic support to "retrain" the LV. Branch PA stenosis may develop as a late complication.

Truncus arteriosus

It is also called common arterial trunk and "truncus".

Incidence and associations

It constitutes 1.5% of all congenital heart disease. Associated with 22q11 deletion (Di George syndrome).

Anatomy

Single ventricular outflow tract (arterial trunk) with a multi-leaflet truncal valve and VSD. PAs arise from the arterial trunk via a main PA (type 1) or via separate origins for right and left PAs (types 2 and 3) (Figure 51.13).

Complex variants include:

* truncus with interrupted arch
* disconnection of the left PA (supplied by a ductus).

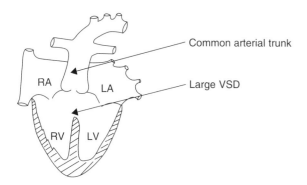

Figure 51.13 Anatomy of truncus arteriosus.

Physiology

Unrestricted PBF – causes heart failure in neonatal period. Cyanosis due to mixing of bloodstreams – this is usually mild because of high PBF.

Surgery

High-risk surgery with 10–15% early mortality. VSD closure, disconnection of PAs from trunk, RV → PA conduit (Figure 51.14).

Surgical risk factors include:

* regurgitant truncal valve
* presentation in severe heart failure
* complex variants.

Postoperative management

High-risk procedure, chest may be left open. LA and PA pressure monitoring lines are essential. Risk of PHT – aim for mean PA pressure <50% of mean systemic pressure. Management of PHT includes control of $PaCO_2$, inhaled NO and phenoxybenzamine, which may have been given perioperatively. Echocardiography should focus on: truncal valve regurgitation, any residual VSD and blood flow into the RV→PA conduit. Irradiated blood products should be used unless 22q11 deletion has been excluded. In the absence of a PA pressure monitoring line, PA pressure can be estimated from the velocity of a regurgitant TR jet and CVP (see Bernoulli equation in Chapter 24).

$$\text{PA Pressure} \approx \text{CVP} + \left(4 * \text{Velocity}_{TR}^2\right)$$

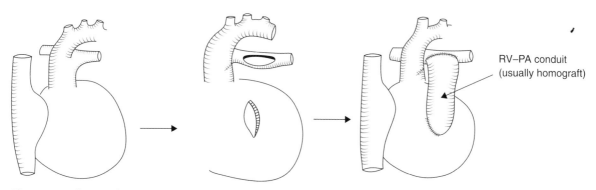

Figure 51.14 Surgery of truncus arteriosus.

Total anomalous pulmonary venous drainage

It is also called "TAPVD" or "TAPVC".

Incidence

It constitutes 1.5% of all congenital heart disease.

Anatomy

Pulmonary veins do not drain back to the LA, but to a separate collecting chamber that drains into the systemic venous circulation (Figure 51.15).

Physiology

Cyanotic. Kept alive due to a PFO allowing R→L flow. Key to the condition is whether or not the drainage is obstructive. When the pathway is unobstructed, the infant will be cyanosed but well. Obstructed pathways lead to PHT, pulmonary congestion (diffuse pulmonary edema on CXR), tachypnea and profound cyanosis.

Cor triatriatum is a condition in which there is a membrane within the LA between the pulmonary veins and the MV. If the opening in this membrane is small or absent, presentation in neonates will be similar to "TAPVD". Treatment is surgical resection of the membrane.

Management

Unobstructed cases are stable but cyanosed and need elective surgical repair. Obstructed cases present in the neonatal period; mechanical ventilation and urgent surgical decompression are often required.

Surgery

All types can be surgically repaired by restoring pulmonary vein → LA blood flow and dividing any superior or inferior draining vein. Early mortality is high (5–10%) and is dependent on the degree of obstruction. There is a risk of recurrent pulmonary vein stenosis, which is associated with poor outcome. Intraoperative echocardiography should focus on pulmonary venous blood flow, looking for stenotic turbulence.

Postoperative care

PHT is inevitable in obstructed cases, and is an additional operative risk. Consequently, it is an indication for PA pressure monitoring. The surgeon may leave a small PFO if there is concern about PHT; although the R→L shunt may reduce PA pressure it will lead to arterial desaturation. The LV tends to be non-compliant because it has not been exposed to a normal preload. For this reason, high LA pressures are generally required. Small fluid challenges, however, may produce a large increase in LA pressure. Obstruction at the level of the anastamosis will lead to pulmonary venous congestion. Re-operation should be considered if pulmonary vein (Doppler) flow appears obstructive.

(a) (b) (c)

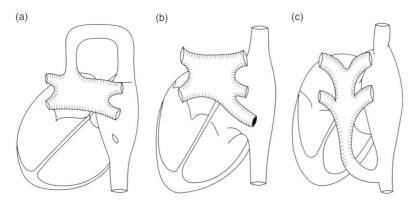

Figure 51.15 Three anatomical variants of TAPVD as seen from behind the heart. (a) Supracardiac: the most common, drain into an ascending vertical vein. (b) Cardiac: drain to coronary sinus; least likely to be obstructive. (c) Infracardiac (note not intracardiac): less common, drain into a descending vein usually below the diaphragm, most likely to get obstructed.

Hypoplastic left heart syndrome

This is also called "HLHS".

Incidence and associations

It constitutes 1.5% of all congenital heart disease, but accounts for 40% of all neonatal cardiac deaths. There are no proven associations, although potential gene loci have recently been identified.

Anatomy

Variety of subtypes with varying degrees of hypoplasia of the LV and LVOT. Classically occurs with mitral and aortic atresia.

Physiology

HLHS is characterized by an inability of the LV to support the systemic circulation. Thus the RV supports the systemic circulation via the PDA. The condition is fatal without surgery. Problems balancing parallel circulations are discussed in Chapters 53 and 54.

Preoperative management

Often present with profound circulatory collapse requiring preoperative mechanical ventilation, and inotropes and vasodilators to improve systemic circulation and limit PBF. A PGE infusion is often used to keep the PDA open. The goal is a balanced circulation (i.e. Qp:Qs = 1:1, aiming for $SaO_2 \approx 75$–80% if no forward flow through LVOT).

Surgery

The Norwood procedure (Figure 51.16): High risk: 25–30% perioperative mortality.

- RV supports both the systemic and pulmonary circulations. Surgery secures a controlled source of pulmonary blood supply via Gore-Tex® shunt and repairs any systemic outflow tract stenosis.
- Recent modification uses RV → PA conduit to supply PBF instead of modified B-T shunt (Sano modification). Maintains diastolic blood pressure.
- "Hybrid" technique is a further recent option placing bilateral PA bands and a stent in the PDA to mimic the Norwood circulation without the need for CPB. Some early success but longer-term outcomes awaited.

Postoperative management

Fragile postoperatively with chest usually left open. CVP line monitoring gives common atrial pressure. Avoid hyperventilation and high FiO_2 – these lead to pulmonary vasodilatation, increased $Q_P:Q_S$ and compromised systemic circulation. Aim for SaO_2 75–80%. Monitor blood lactate and central venous saturation

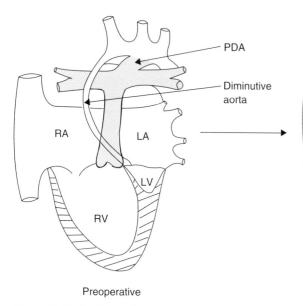

RA — LA — PDA — Diminutive aorta — LV — RV

Preoperative

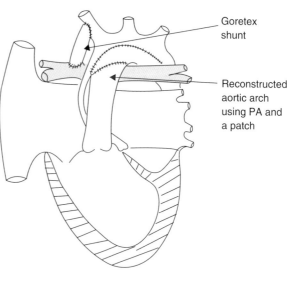

Goretex shunt — Reconstructed aortic arch using PA and a patch

Postoperative

Figure 51.16 The Norwood procedure.

Table 51.1 Interpretation of SaO$_2$ in the presence of different physiological states in patients with shunt

SaO$_2$	Physiological status	Consequences	Qp:Qs	Treatment
75%	Balanced Q$_P$ and Qs	None	~1:1	None
	↓CO	↑O$_2$ extraction, ↓SvO$_2$	>1:1	↑CO ↑PVR ↓SVR
	Lung disease	↓SpvO$_2$	>1:1	Optimize ventilation ↑PVR ↓SVR
>85%	Shunt too big	↑PBF	>1:1	↑PVR, revise shunt
<65%	Shunt too small or blocked	↓PBF	<1:1	Revise shunt
	↑PVR	↓PBF	<1:1	↓PVR ↑MAP
	↓CO	↑O$_2$ extraction, ↓SvO$_2$	~1:1	↑CO
	Lung disease	↓SpvO$_2$	~1:1	Optimize ventilation

SvO$_2$, mixed venous saturation; SpvO$_2$, pulmonary venous oxygen saturation.

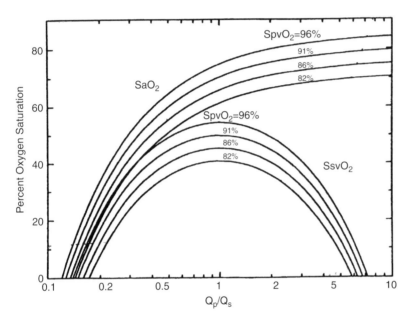

Figure 51.17 Balancing systemic and pulmonary flow in a Norwood circulation. The hyperbolic relationship between SaO$_2$ and Q$_P$:Q$_S$ and the parabolic relationship between systemic venous saturation (SsvO$_2$) and Q$_P$:Q$_S$ are not often appreciated. SaO$_2$ and SsvO$_2$ as a function of Q$_P$:Q$_S$ are shown for different values of pulmonary venous oxygen saturation (SpvO$_2$). It is often assumed that SaO$_2$ ~75% equates to the ideal Q$_P$:Q$_S$ of ~1:1. This will be the case if there is good systemic perfusion (oxygen extraction resulting in SvO$_2$ ~50%) and normal lung function (SpvO$_2$ ~100%). It is dangerous to infer Q$_P$:Q$_S$ from SaO$_2$ alone as SaO$_2$ of 75% may represent a Q$_P$:Q$_S$ >>1:1 in certain situations.

(SvO$_2$) to assess systemic perfusion. Aim for SvO$_2$ 45–60%, requires Q$_P$:Q$_S$ ≈ 1:1 (see Figure 51.17 and Table 51.1). Use vasodilators and inotropes to improve systemic perfusion. Echocardiography is required to assess RV function, the degree of TR and the arch repair. Do not manually ventilate with 100% oxygen. Always use air/oxygen mix to match FiO$_2$ used during mechanical ventilation. Chest closure can decrease RV compliance and cause deterioration over subsequent hours. Repeat echocardiography and maintain high vigilance following chest closure.

52

Common congenital heart operations

David J. Barron and Kevin P. Morris

Staged palliation of a functionally univentricular heart

A number of lesions are not suitable for a two-ventricle repair and are managed with a series of two or three palliative procedures. Examples include mitral atresia, tricuspid atresia, some forms of pulmonary atresia, double inlet LV and hypoplastic left heart syndrome (HLHS).

In the neonatal period surgery may be required to optimize pulmonary blood flow (PBF).

- If there is inadequate PBF or a duct dependent PBF, a pulmonary shunt may be inserted.

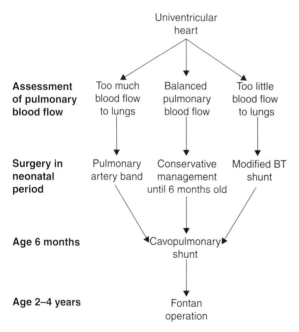

Figure 52.1 Pathways of palliative operations for a univentricular heart.

- If PBF is high, a band is placed around the PA and tightened to increase resistance and reduce flow to the lungs.

PVR is high in the newborn period and falls over the first few months of life.

If a cavopulmonary ("venous") shunt was created in the early neonatal period, the high PVR would result in excessively high SVC pressure and low PBF – hence an arterial (modified Blalock-Taussig, B-T) shunt is initially needed that provides a higher driving pressure and guarantees adequate PBF.

Pathways of palliative operations for a univentricular heart are summarized in Figure 52.1.

Arterial shunt

It is also called shunt, modified Blalock-Taussig (B-T) shunt, systemic→PA shunt and central shunt.

Physiology

Used to augment PBF in a variety of conditions with inadequate PBF. Some conditions have bi-ventricular anatomy (e.g. Fallot's, pulmonary atresia/VSD, TGA/VSD/PS). Others have functionally single ventricle anatomy (e.g. tricuspid atresia/TGA/PS, pulmonary atresia/intact ventricular septum). Behavior following the shunt is influenced by the underlying anatomy; patients with bi-ventricular anatomy are usually more stable and tolerate the volume load of the shunt better.

Many neonates are duct-dependent preoperatively and receiving a PGE infusion (see Chapter 49). The duct (PDA) will remain open for some time postoperatively even after the PGE infusion is stopped – this may have the effect of "flooding" the lungs until

Core Topics in Cardiac Anesthesia, Second Edition, ed. Jonathan H. Mackay and Joseph E. Arrowsmith. Published by Cambridge University Press. © Cambridge University Press 2012.

329

the duct closes. Blood flow through the shunt will be influenced by the shunt radius and length:

$$\text{Flow } \alpha \text{ radius}^4/\text{length.}$$

Typical shunt sizes are 3.5–4.0 mm in diameter, although these may need to be modified in light of PA size and PVR.

Surgery

A variety of approaches and techniques are described (Figure 52.2). Most common and most widely used is the modified B-T shunt performed via a left or right thoracotomy. Original description of B-T shunt divided subclavian artery and anastamosed it directly to PA. Generally performed on the side of the innominate artery (usually right) without CPB unless the child is very unstable or more complex repair required. Modification uses a synthetic graft between subclavian/innominate artery and PA.

Central shunt implies a shunt between the aorta and the PAs. This can be performed either via a thoracotomy (classic Waterstone/Potts) or a sternotomy, with or without CPB. Most common type of central shunt now is a modified type using a Gortex graft between the aorta and the central PAs.

Postoperative management

Establish the underlying anatomy.

- Single or bi-ventricular anatomy?
- Any other source of pulmonary blood supply other than the shunt?
- Duct still open?

Shunts that require CPB imply unstable hemodynamics and the need for careful monitoring. Shunts with underlying bi-ventricular anatomy tend to run a stable course. There is a need to balance Q_P:Q_S in functionally single ventricle. If the shunt is the only source of PBF, aim for SaO_2 ~75–80% and Q_P:Q_S = 1:1 (see Figure 51.17). Too small a shunt or an obstructed shunt results in hypoxemia; a trial of inhaled NO may be helpful in differentiating a structural shunt problem from elevated PVR. Only the latter is reactive and responds to inhaled NO. Too high a shunt flow leads to low diastolic pressure, pulmonary congestion and ventricular volume overload. Attempts to reduce PBF by increasing PVR are seldom effective. Lowering SVR with vasodilators is more effective at balancing Q_P:Q_S. Surgical revision of the shunt may be necessary.

Start heparin infusion on return to ICU when stabilized and not bleeding (10 units kg^{-1} h^{-1}).

Pulmonary artery banding

PA banding is performed in a variety of different conditions. The major indication is to limit PBF. The band protects the lungs from high pressure and flow in the following situations:

1. Bi-ventricular heart with multiple VSDs not suitable for surgical closure or for large VSD/ A-VSD in a neonate if felt to be high risk to repair.
2. CoA + VSD where the CoA is the critical lesion and is repaired via a thoracotomy. The band can also be placed via the thoracotomy.
3. Functionally single ventricle anatomy with excessive (unobstructed) PBF (e.g. tricuspid atresia with TGA/VSD). See "Staged palliation of a functionally univentricular heart".

Rarely PA banding is performed to "train" the sub-pulmonary ventricle in infants with TGA in preparation for an arterial switch procedure. This may be required in late presentations in which the LV muscle mass has

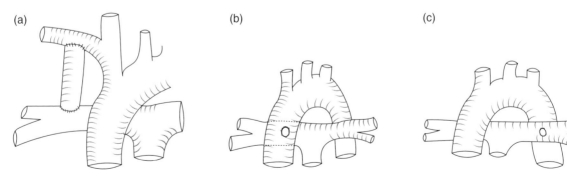

(a)   (b)   (c)

Figure 52.2 (a) Modified B-T shunt. (b) Waterstone shunt. (c) Potts shunt.

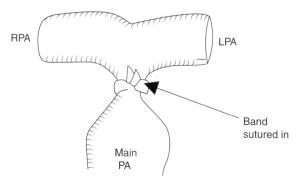

RPA

LPA

Band
sutured in

Main
PA

Figure 52.3 Pulmonary artery banding.

regressed. The band places an afterload on the ventricle and stimulates hypertrophy (Figure 52.3).

Physiology

Depends on the underlying anatomy. In groups 1 and 2 (above), the band reduces the degree of heart failure by reducing the L→R shunt across the VSD. Any shunting remains predominantly L→R and so SaO_2 will remain 95–100%. In group 3 (above), the band reduces PBF and so increases systemic flow at the expense of reducing SaO_2.

Surgery

Does not require CPB. Can be placed either via midline sternotomy or via left thoracotomy.

Postoperative management

Depends on underlying anatomy. In groups 1 and 2 (above) aim for SaO_2 95–100%. Generally well tolerated. Group 3 (above) will be cyanotic and may be hemodynamically unstable. Aim for SaO_2 75–80%. Echocardiography to look at: gradient across band, ventricular function (can cause rapid ventricular failure if band too tight) and atrioventricular valve function (band can increase atrioventricular valve regurgitation in AVSD). Bands placed for VSDs are tighter (Doppler flow velocity 3–4 m s^{-1}) than bands in the single ventricle setting (velocity 2.5–3 m s^{-1}). Babies with high PVR may show a deceptively small gradient because distal PA pressure is high rather than the PA band loose.

PA banding performed to "train" the LV in a baby with TGA may be complicated by hypoxemia due to a failure of mixing of systemic and pulmonary circulations. They may need the addition of a modified B-T

shunt. The stressed sub-pulmonary (left) ventricle may fail postoperatively as a result of excessive afterload. Echocardiography is used to assess the degree of ventricular dilatation and to monitor for a rise in LA pressure or signs of falling CO.

PA banding patients can be very unstable. Since the procedure is relatively minor, there is a tendency to regard the patients as low risk when the converse can be true.

Bi-directional cavopulmonary shunt and the Fontan procedure (total cavopulmonary connection)

Staged palliative procedures for children with a functionally single ventricle circulation, 5% of all congenital heart disease (e.g. tricuspid atresia, double inlet LV, HLHS, unbalanced A-VSD, PA/IVS).

Physiology

These procedures involve connecting the systemic veins directly into the pulmonary circulation, thus bypassing the right side of the heart completely. They rely on venous pressure to drive PBF and are only possible if PVR is low. A failing ventricle or a high PVR may preclude these procedures.

Bi-directional cavopulmonary shunt

Also called cavopulmonary (CP) shunt, modified Glenn, Hemi-Fontan. A bi-directional CP shunt is carried out around 6 months of age. The SVC is anastamosed to the PA, the IVC remains connected to the RA (Figure 52.4). If the patient has previously had an arterial shunt this is usually taken down. In other patient groups a decision is taken whether to ligate the main PA or to leave some antegrade PBF. The original Glenn operation involved direct anastamosis of SVC to isolated right PA.

Postoperative management

Arterial saturation typically 80–85%. SVC line and IVC (or common atrial) line. SVC pressure equates to PA pressure (typically 12–16 mmHg). The difference between PA pressure and atrial/IVC pressure gives the transpulmonary gradient (TPG). TPG of 8–10 mmHg generally implies low PVR and a favorable outcome. If TPG >15 mmHg a mechanical holdup (e.g. anastomotic narrowing, anastomotic

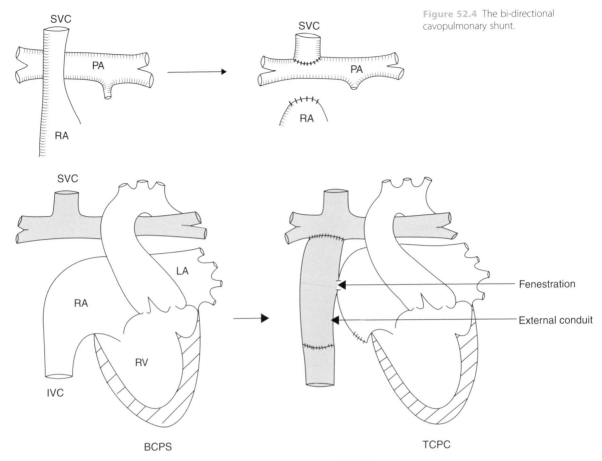

Figure 52.4 The bi-directional cavopulmonary shunt.

BCPS

TCPC

Fenestration

External conduit

Figure 52.5 Completion of a total cavopulmonary connection in a patient with HLHS.

thrombosis or PA narrowing) must be excluded before considering inhaled NO to reduce PVR. SVC and PA pressures may be elevated (>20 mmHg) with a normal TPG as a consequence of a high atrial pressure, secondary to ventricular dysfunction. Management is aimed at lowering atrial pressure (vasodilators, inotropes), which will lead to a lowering of SVC and PA pressures. Hemodynamics are generally good since the volume loading of the ventricle is substantially reduced by this procedure. Hypertension is common and may require treatment.

Ideally, infants are weaned from positive-pressure ventilation and the trachea extubated as soon as possible to reduce intrathoracic pressure and improve PBF. Any SVC line should be removed as soon as possible to reduce risk of thrombosis. High SVC pressure may result in pleural effusions (sometimes chylothorax), venous congestion of the head and neck, and headaches.

Total cavopulmonary connection

Also called TCPC or "Fontan". Children have almost always had a previous bi-directional CP shunt (BCPS). Very rarely performed as a single procedure. Early mortality is 5–7%.

The completion of the Fontan procedure, usually before school age, directs IVC blood flow to the PA. Surgery has evolved over time from the original Fontan (direct RA→ PA connection) to the TCPC, which is now achieved in one of two ways:

1. *Lateral tunnel TCPC*: a baffle is placed inside the atrium to redirect IVC blood into the PAs.
2. *External conduit TCPC*: a Gore-Tex™ tube is placed outside the atrium to divert IVC blood into the PAs.

The TCPC is usually fenestrated, which in the setting of high PVR preserves adequate ventricular output at the expense of a degree of hypoxemia (Figure 52.5).

Postoperative management

Similar principles to management of BCPS. SVC and IVC pressures are now equal and are equivalent to the PA pressure (typically 12–16 mmHg). A low PVR is essential and the TPG should ideally be <10 mmHg. SVC/IVC pressure is no longer a marker of ventricular preload and so all patients have direct atrial line to monitor filling pressure. These patients often require a lot of volume, which should be titrated to atrial pressure.

Fenestration causes some obligate R→L shunt, the degree of shunting being proportional to TPG and the size of the fenestration. Low PVR and favorable hemodynamics are generally associated with SaO_2 >90%.

Ideally, hemodynamically stable children should undergo early weaning from mechanical ventilation and tracheal extubation to decrease intrathoracic pressure and increase flow through the Fontan circuit, thus increasing CO. Hemodynamic instability, by contrast, is an indication for continued mechanical ventilation.

High PA pressure with low CO requires careful review – optimization of ventricular function and cardiac rhythm. A therapeutic trial of inhaled NO may be used, but is rarely effective. In this setting an urgent cardiac catheter may be required to assess flow

pathways and determine the need for enlargement of any fenestration or surgical revision.

Early postoperative anticoagulation is mandatory due to the sluggish nature of the venous circulation.

Echocardiography should be used to assess ventricular function, ensure non-obstructed pulmonary venous return and exclude any ventricular outflow tract obstruction (reduced ventricular volume load may unmask outflow tract obstruction).

The Ross procedure

Alternative type of aortic valve replacement using the patient's own pulmonary valve in the aortic position. Has the advantage of providing a living valve replacement that will grow with the child – thus, is suitable for infants and children.

Anatomy

Indications are similar to adult AVR; aortic regurgitation, stenosis or commonly a combination of both. Often related to a congenitally bicuspid aortic valve.

Significant aortic root dilatation is a contraindication to the Ross procedure as there is a risk that the new valve will also dilate.

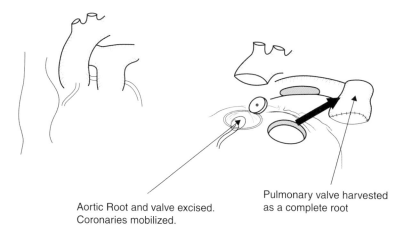

Figure 52.6 The Ross procedure (pulmonary autograft). (Above) Preoperative and intraoperative appearances. (Below) Completed appearance.

Aortic Root and valve excised. Coronaries mobilized.

Pulmonary valve harvested as a complete root

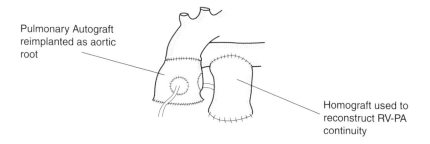

Pulmonary Autograft reimplanted as aortic root

Homograft used to reconstruct RV-PA continuity

Complex sub-aortic stenosis can also be addressed by extension of the procedure to widen the outflow septum – the so-called Ross-Konno procedure.

Surgery

Risk 2–3%. Complex procedure requiring excision of the pulmonary valve as a complete root and implanting this into the aortic position with reimplantation of the coronaries. The pulmonary valve is replaced with a homograft (allograft).

Intraoperative echocardiography should focus on regional ventricular wall function and on the new aortic valve to look for any regurgitation or stenosis.

Postoperative care

Usually have a LA line to monitor LV preload (avoid PAFC in the presence of a reconstructed RV outflow tract).

Check ECG for evidence of coronary ischemia.

Early echocardiography to assess ventricular function and new aortic valve function.

Extensive suture lines; so avoid hypertension and keep sedated and ventilated until all bleeding settled.

Long-term concerns over dilatation of the neo-aortic root have led to a decreasing enthusiasm for the procedure – but it remains a valuable technique in smaller children and infants where prosthetic valve replacement is not feasible.

Chapter

53

Postoperative care

Fiona E. Reynolds and Kevin P. Morris

This chapter highlights the similarities and differences between pediatric and adult cardiac critical care.

Routine postoperative care

Direct measurement of CO is rarely undertaken in pediatric critical care. If specific problems have been anticipated, direct LA and PA pressure monitoring may have been instituted during surgery. Indirect measures of CO and oxygen delivery (DO_2) (i.e. blood lactate and SVC/IVC SO_2) are more commonly utilized. Interpretation of blood lactate values (normal <2 mmol l^{-1}; 18 mg dl^{-1}) should take into account the complexity of surgery – elevated levels should normalize after surgery. Blood lactate >5 mmol l^{-1} (<45 mg dl^{-1}) implies inadequate DO_2 and is predictive of adverse outcome. Decline in mixed venous (or SVC or IVC) SO_2 should raise the suspicion of a low CO state (LCOS).

Blood transfusion may be required to ensure an optimal hemoglobin concentration. Aim for Hb >10 g dl^{-1} in children with non-cyanotic defects, and 12–14 g dl^{-1} in those with cyanotic heart defects. Chest drain blood loss should be <4 ml kg^{-1} in the first hour, <2 ml kg^{-1} in the second hour and <1 ml kg^{-1} h^{-1} thereafter. Re-exploration of the chest for excessive bleeding is infrequent in pediatric practice. Whenever possible, coagulopathy should be corrected prior to re-exploration.

Early postoperative transthoracic echocardiography is routinely performed in many pediatric units. The criteria for weaning from ventilatory support are broadly similar to those for adults. Tracheal extubation is considered once bleeding is minimal and the patient is warm and hemodynamically stable. IV opioids are typically used to provide postoperative analgesia.

Common problems

Low cardiac output state

LCOS may be the consequence of inadequate preload, impaired LV or RV function, high afterload or an abnormal heart rhythm. LCOS may manifest as hemodynamic instability, poor perfusion, oliguria, hyperlactatemia and metabolic acidosis. The presence of a residual cardiac defect must be excluded.

Preload: higher RA pressures may be required to maintain adequate CO following right-heart procedures (e.g. Fallot's tetralogy) because of reduced RV compliance. Similarly, a higher LA pressure is required following left-heart procedures (e.g. total anomalous pulmonary venous drainage). It is important to realize that the administration of small fluid volumes may result in large LA pressure changes.

Contractility: myocardial dysfunction may result from incomplete myocardial protection and the systemic inflammatory response to CPB. Metabolic derangements (acidosis, hypocalcemia) and injury to the conducting tissue, ventricular wall (e.g. ventriculotomy) or coronary arteries (e.g. Fallot's and arterial switch operations) may also impair cardiac function.

In adult myocardium, excitation–contraction coupling is mediated by the release of cytosolic (i.e. intracellular) Ca^{2+}, whereas in neonates cytosolic Ca^{2+} levels are lower and contraction is dependent on extracellular Ca^{2+}. For this reason neonates are particularly susceptible to hypocalcemia.

The choice of inotrope is dictated by the tone of the pulmonary and systemic circulations. Traditionally, dobutamine, dopamine or epinephrine have been the first-line choice, although the phosphodiesterase inhibitors are becoming increasingly popular.

Afterload: excessive vasoconstriction increases LV work and may reduce CO. Vasodilatation may be

Core Topics in Cardiac Anesthesia, Second Edition, ed. Jonathan H. Mackay and Joseph E. Arrowsmith. Published by Cambridge University Press. © Cambridge University Press 2012.

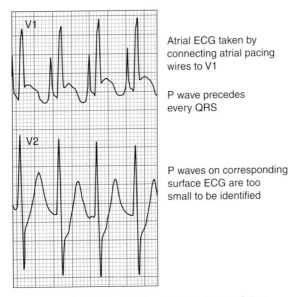

Atrial ECG taken by connecting atrial pacing wires to V1

P wave precedes every QRS

P waves on corresponding surface ECG are too small to be identified

Figure 53.1 Atrial (V1) and surface (V2) ECGs in normal sinus rhythm – P waves are amplified by atrial ECG.

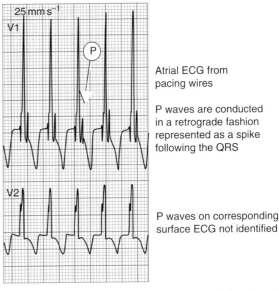

Atrial ECG from pacing wires

P waves are conducted in a retrograde fashion represented as a spike following the QRS

P waves on corresponding surface ECG not identified

Figure 53.2 Atrial (V1) and surface (V2) ECGs in nodal tachycardia. The retrograde P waves amplified by atrial ECG and are seen after the QRS complex.

achieved using GTN or SNP, although phenoxybenzamine (a non-competitive α-blocker with a long half-life) is still widely used in pediatric cardiac surgery.

If, despite maximal therapy, LCOS persists, further investigation to exclude a residual defect (i.e. echocardiography, cardiac catheterization) is mandatory. The following may be considered:

- chest reopening to reduce constriction of the heart and allow time for myocardial edema to resolve;
- cooling the patient to 34°C to reduce oxygen demand;
- extracorporeal membrane oxygenation (ECMO) or ventricular assist device (VAD);
- intra-aortic balloon counterpulsation.

Dysrhythmia

Bradycardia: surgery near conducting tissue, for example atrioventricular (A-V) septal defect repair, may result in bradycardia. Persistent complete heart block mandates permanent pacemaker insertion, whereas conduction defects secondary to edema usually only require temporary pacing.

Tachycardia: it may be the result of increased automaticity or re-entry phenomena. The risk is increased by metabolic abnormalities (K^+, Mg^{2+}, Ca^{2+} and PO_4^{2-}), pyrexia and sympathomimetic drugs.

Ventricular dysrhythmias: these are rare in pediatric practice and often reflect myocardial ischemia or ventricular dysfunction. Hemodynamically unstable VT or VF requires immediate direct current (DC) cardioversion.

SVT is more common. Accurate diagnosis is the key to determining appropriate therapy. A 12-lead ECG, supplemented with an atrial ECG (from temporary pacing wires), may yield the diagnosis. An atrial ECG amplifies atrial activity, allowing easier differentiation between atrial and ventricular excitation (Figures 53.1 and 53.2).

Adenosine, which slows or blocks A-V conduction, aids diagnosis and may terminate re-entrant tachycardias. Synchronized DC cardioversion or overdrive pacing may also be used.

Junctional ectopic tachycardia: results from increased automaticity with variable hemodynamic consequences. The diagnosis is confirmed by atrial ECG and lack of response to adenosine and overdrive pacing. Amiodarone may be required when hemodynamic compromise is significant, whereas a stable patient can be observed. Induced hypothermia may slow the rate and allow A-V sequential pacing at a greater rate.

Hemorrhage and tamponade

Causes and features of hemorrhage and tamponade are similar to adults (see Chapter 58). As in adults, echocardiography may fail to reveal tamponade and delay re-operation.

Neurologic injury

The mechanism of neurologic injury after cardiac surgery is multifactorial. It may present as seizure activity, encephalopathy or focal neurologic deficit. Seizures and chorea are more common in the pediatric population.

Renal dysfunction

Oliguria and renal impairment – leading to hyperkalemia, acidosis and fluid overload – are common after surgery. In contrast to the adult population, hemofiltration or hemodialysis are rarely required. Hyperkalemia and fluid overload usually respond to diuretic therapy. The combination of IV furosemide $(0.2–1.0 \text{ mg kg}^{-1} \text{ h}^{-1})$ and oral metolazone (a thiazide) is useful. The criteria for institution of renal replacement therapy (RRT) are the same as those for adults; however, peritoneal dialysis is more commonly used. A peritoneal catheter may be inserted at the time of surgery in high-risk infants. Mortality rate is increased in infants who require dialysis postoperatively.

Hypothermia

A high surface area to volume ratio makes children more vulnerable than adults to heat loss. Moderate and profound degrees of hypothermia are more commonly used in pediatric surgical practice, and immediate postoperative hypothermia is almost inevitable. Meticulous attention to the adequacy of rewarming and prevention of heat loss following CPB and during transport is necessary.

Controlled hypothermia may be used therapeutically to slow dysrhythmias, to limit oxygen demand in LCOS, or to ameliorate hypoxic ischemic brain injury following cardiac arrest. Hyperthermia should be avoided. Deleterious effects include tachycardia, increased metabolic rate and exacerbation of neurologic injury.

Pulmonary hypertension

Pulmonary hypertension (PHT) may complicate the postoperative course of some operations. It is particularly likely when a period of high pulmonary blood flow (PBF) has caused muscular hypertrophy of the

Table 53.1 Features of pulmonary hypertensive crisis

Rising PA pressure – exceeding systemic arterial pressure

Rising CVP

Falling LA pressure

Falling systemic blood pressure

Ventricular septal wall encroaching on LV cavity

PAs. The condition is characterized by an increase in PVR and increased PA and RV pressures resulting in RV dysfunction and worsening of any right → left shunt.

Therapy is directed at reducing PVR and supporting RV function. Adequate sedation and muscle relaxation should be ensured. Mechanical ventilation should be optimized to avoid hypoxemia and hypercarbia. Inhaled NO (5–20 ppm) may be beneficial. Although adverse effects at low NO concentrations are rare, methemoglobin and NO_2 concentrations must be monitored. Other drug treatments include prostacyclin, sildenafil, phenoxybenzamine and dipyridamole.

Ventilation

The general principles of mechanical ventilation are similar to those in adult practice, with attention to limiting FiO_2 and avoiding lung injury. In the absence of significant lung disease, positive end-expiratory pressure (PEEP) is usually set at 4–6 cmH$_2$O and tidal volume at 8–10 ml kg^{-1}. Respiratory rates are greater than those used routinely in adults and are age-dependent: neonates 25–35 bpm, infants 15–25 bpm, older child 12–20 bpm. Ventilation is adjusted to maintain normocapnia. Oxygenation may be problematic in the presence of a residual right → left shunt.

Control of $PaCO_2$ is particularly important in cases of PHT, in which an increase in $PaCO_2$ will increase PVR and may precipitate a pulmonary hypertensive crisis. In patients with PBF supplied by an arterial shunt (parallel circulation, e.g. Blalock-Taussig shunt) hyperventilation and a fall in $PaCO_2$ will lower PVR and increase PBF, potentially at the expense of systemic blood flow. In contrast, hypoventilation will increase PVR, lower PBF and result in increasing hypoxemia. In these groups of patients, volume-controlled ventilation produces a more stable

337

$PaCO_2$, as minute ventilation varies with lung compliance when pressure-controlled ventilation is used.

Following a bi-directional cavopulmonary shunt or Fontan procedure, PBF is dependent on the difference between systemic venous pressure and common atrial pressure, which in turn is very sensitive to changes in intrathoracic pressure. During mechanical ventilation, antegrade PBF may cease during inspiration. The optimum ventilation strategy includes a short inspiratory time (i.e. long I:E ratio), low/normal PEEP and the lowest achievable peak inspiratory pressure. As soon as the patient is stable they should be weaned and the trachea extubated. Negative-pressure ventilation has been used in difficult situations.

Malnutrition

In contrast to the average adult cardiac surgical patient, preoperative malnutrition or "failure to thrive" – secondary to heart failure and prolonged hospitalization – is common in pediatric patients. Postoperative fluid restriction, feed intolerance or necrotizing enterocolitis may further exacerbate the situation. Enteral feeding should be introduced as soon as practicable.

As in adults, total body water is increased following CPB. Modified ultrafiltration following CPB may be used in smaller children (see Chapter 50).

Infection

Gross sternal wound infection and mediastinitis are uncommon in the pediatric cardiac surgical patient. A prolonged delay before chest closure, with either opposed skin edges or a Gor-Tex™ membrane covering the heart, increases the potential for infection. Patients with a congenital defect of cellular or humoral immunity (e.g. Di George syndrome) are also at greater risk of infection.

Systemic inflammation

The systemic inflammatory response is associated with capillary leak, edema, and impaired pulmonary and renal function. Therapy is supportive and the patient may require ventilation and RRT until they resolve.

Outcome

Overall operative mortality for the correction of congenital heart disease is about 5% in developed countries. The perioperative mortality for surgical ASD closure is <1%, whereas mortality for first-stage palliation of hypoplastic left-heart syndrome is >25%. Co-existing congenital and acquired conditions are important co-determinants of outcome.

Key points

- Pediatric and adult cardiac surgical critical care have many facets in common. The variety of conditions encountered is much greater in pediatric practice.
- A detailed knowledge of anatomy and pathophysiology is needed, as management of individual complex lesions is very different.
- Management should be coordinated by the ICU team in close collaboration with cardiologists and surgeons.
- Low CO or deviation from expected clinical course should prompt exclusion of a residual lesion.

Further reading

Chang AC, Hanley FL, Wernovski G, Wessel DL. *Pediatric Cardiac Intensive Care*. Baltimore: Williams & Wilkins; 1998.

Appendix

Table 53.2 Pediatric resuscitation drug doses

- Epinephrine (1 in 10 000) 0.1 ml kg^{-1}
- Atropine 20 µg kg^{-1}
- Sodium bicarbonate 1 mmol kg^{-1} (2 ml kg^{-1} of 4.2% solution)
- 10% calcium gluconate 0.3 ml kg^{-1}
- Amiodarone 5 mg kg^{-1}
- 10% dextrose 5 ml kg^{-1}

54

Adult congenital heart disease

Craig R. Bailey and Helen M. Daly

Congenital heart disease occurs in 0.8% of newborns. In most developed countries there are more adults with congenital heart disease than children and the prevalence is increasing as more affected children survive to adulthood. Although the majority of patients will have undergone previous cardiothoracic surgery, some will have had no intervention or have undiagnosed lesions.

Patients with adult congenital heart disease (ACHD) require lifelong medical care. As children, decisions about treatment will have been made on their behalf and in their best interests. As adults,

patients with ACHD are expected to make their own informed decisions about therapy. Some find this transition very difficult – realizing the significance of their medical condition. Patients may be divided into those who have had corrective or palliative surgery and those with unoperated congenital heart disease. The focus of this chapter is anesthesia for moderate- and high-risk patients with ACHD, who should have surgery performed in a specialist center (Table 54.1).

Preoperative assessment

Assessment involves obtaining an accurate history, physical examination and analysis of appropriate investigations. The sheer volume of medical records that many of these patients accumulate over the years can make this both a challenging and a time-consuming process. Problems commonly encountered in ACHD patients are shown in Table 54.2. The questions that require consideration during preoperative assessment are listed in Table 54.3.

Table 54.1 Abnormalities best treated in specialist congenital heart unit

Valvular atresia

Double inlet/outlet ventricle

Malposition of great vessels

Fontan circulation

Single/common ventricle

Transposition of great arteries

Atrial switch procedure

Rastelli procedure

Eisenmenger syndrome

Pulmonary hypertension

Chronic hypoxemia

Qp:Qs > 2:1

Ventricular outflow gradient >50 mmHg

↑PVR

Secondary polycythemia

Table 54.2 Medical problems in adult congenital heart disease

Primary	Secondary
Shunts	Arrhythmias
Stenotic lesions	Cyanosis
Regurgitant lesions	Infective endocarditis
	Myocardial ischemia
	Paradoxical emboli
	Polycythemia
	Pulmonary hypertension
	Ventricular dysfunction

History

Details of previous surgical procedures, anesthetic records and the results of subsequent cardiological investigations should be reviewed. It is essential to understand the postoperative anatomy and the extent of any physiological adaptation and establish whether a shunt is present. Many patients are accustomed to poor exercise tolerance so it is important to determine what is normal for them. High-risk patients, such as those with Eisenmenger's syndrome, will have been advised not to exercise. The chances of encountering an adult with a Fontan circulation (Chapter 52) are increasing. The Fontan procedure is a procedure,

Table 54.3 Preoperative assessment of patients with adult congenital heart disease

What is the anatomy of any previous repair?

Are there any residual structural defects?

Is ventricular function normal?

Are there anatomic or physiological abnormalities of the pulmonary vasculature?

Is venous anatomy normal – connections, drainage and monitoring sites?

Are there residual ECG abnormalities?

What antibiotic prophylaxis is necessary?

Is anticoagulation therapy employed and when should it be withdrawn/reinstituted?

used to palliate patients with a univentricular heart, which diverts venous blood from the RA to the PA without it passing through the morphological RV. Patients are delicately balanced between inadequate blood supply to the lungs (causing cyanosis) and excessive pulmonary blood flow (PBF), which causes pulmonary edema.

Physical examination

Problems associated with the airway, combined with cyanotic ACHD or pulmonary hypertension (PHT), considerably increase perioperative risk. Previous cardiac surgery may have resulted in vocal cord damage, recurrent laryngeal or phrenic nerve damage or Horner's syndrome. Prolonged postoperative mechanical ventilation may have caused subglottic stenosis and there may be external vascular compression of the trachea which could compromise the airway on induction of anesthesia. Peripheral pulses may be unequal or absent following surgery or shunt placement. Neurologic assessment may reveal developmental delay secondary to congenital problems, hypoxia at birth or neurobehavioral abnormalities secondary to complex cardiac surgery with long CPB and deep hypothermic circulatory arrest (DHCA) times or prolonged ICU care.

Investigations

CXR: may show pleural effusions in the Fontan patient (requiring chest drainage), kyphoscoliosis,

Table 54.4 Common consequences of surgery for congenital heart disease

ASD	Residual shunt, septal aneurysm, device fracture
Coarctation of aorta	Systolic hypertension, residual gradient, inaccurate left arm BP (subclavian flap repair), aneurysm formation, dissection
PDA	Residual flow, recanalization, laryngeal nerve injury
TGA	
Atrial switch	Dysrhythmias, systemic ventricular dysfunction, baffle leak, venous pathway obstruction
Rastelli	Residual VSD, ventricular dysfunction, LVOT obstruction, conduit failure
Arterial switch	Supravalvar AS/PS, aortic regurgitation, ventricular dysfunction, coronary artery stenosis
Tetralogy of Fallot	Residual VSD, RVOT obstruction, RV dysfunction, pulmonary regurgitation, RBBB/A-V block, ventricular arrhythmias. B-T shunt → BP inaccurate
Single ventricle	Preload dependence, ventricular dysfunction, cyanosis (fenestration), protein-losing enteropathy, arrhythmias, diminished functional reserve

acute chest infection or pulmonary edema. A lateral CXR may reveal anterior mediastinal (retrosternal) calcification at the site of an RV conduit.

ECG: perioperative arrhythmias are common and may be symptomatic, especially in the failing heart. SVT is the commonest arrhythmia and may be caused by surgical scarring or previous arrhythmia ablation procedures. Patients with a Fontan circulation are especially susceptible to AF and are usually anticoagulated because they are prone to thrombus formation. Ventricular tachycardia is rare but may occur following ventriculotomy in patients with tetralogy of Fallot. Preoperative QRS prolongation indicates susceptibility to ventricular tachycardia.

Echocardiography: is used to document cardiac anatomy, assess ventricular and valvular function, and to evaluate flow in shunts and conduits. TEE may be required prior to DC cardioversion to rule out the presence of intra-atrial thrombus.

Angiography: the presence of large collateral arteries (e.g. bronchial) may induce systemic steal (L→L shunt) and ventricular distension during CPB. Selective angiography may be used to assess their anatomy and permits embolization prior to surgery. Although visualization may be difficult, they can be controlled or ligated before instituting CPB. Alternatively, DHCA or low-flow CPB with ventricular venting may be used.

MRI: may be required to accurately determine the anatomy prior to re-operation.

Hematology: polycythemia, a compensatory response to chronic hypoxemia, increases blood viscosity and renders the patient at increased risk of thromboembolic events. A hemoglobin concentration >18 g dl^{-1} may be an indication for venesection. Cyanotic ACHD is often associated with abnormal platelet function and reduced concentrations of circulating clotting factors.

Anesthetic management

Many patients are treated with antiplatelet drugs. In many cases, the advantages of withdrawing antiplatelet therapy before surgery are outweighed by the risk of thromboembolism. Those treated with warfarin should be "bridged" to surgery with heparin. The high incidences of previous transfusion and atypical antibodies mandate early cross-match.

Because polycythemic patients are at risk from dehydration, intravenous fluids are commenced the night before surgery. Preoperative venesection is performed for very high hematocrits, although usually only when symptomatic hyperviscosity is present. In the presence of diminished PBF, hypoxemia should be minimized by ensuring adequate hydration, maintaining systemic arterial BP, minimizing elevations in PVR and avoiding increases in O_2 consumption. Cardiac medications are typically continued until the time of surgery. Sedative premedication is popular, although caution must be exercised in the presence of hypoxemia.

Vascular access may present difficulties. There are a number of case reports that describe the successful, deliberate intra-arterial administration of anesthetic drugs (e.g. midazolam, fentanyl, vecuronium and atropine) in children with impossible venous access. Interruption of the IVC or thrombosis following previous instrumentation may preclude femoral vein cannulation. Placement of a PAFC may be technically difficult on account of anatomical abnormalities and might actually be dangerous in the presence of pulmonary reactivity. In the presence of a right subclavian to right PA (modified B-T) shunt, the left arm should be used for arterial pressure monitoring. Patients with cavopulmonary (e.g. Glenn and Fontan) shunts are at risk of venous thrombosis. Although PA pressure monitoring with an SVC line is often useful in these patients, a single-lumen line should be used and removed as early as possible to reduce the risk of thromboembolism. All intravenous lines, infusions and intravascular transducer monitors should be checked thoroughly to ensure no air bubbles are present and inline filters and non-return valves used to reduce the risk of air emboli. Meticulous care must be taken to avoid venous air entrainment in patients with shunt lesions as systemic embolization (i.e. stroke) can occur, even when shunting is predominantly L→R.

The selection of agents for induction and maintenance of anesthesia is a matter for individual choice. Although opioid-based techniques may be superior in patients with poor ventricular function, the choice of drugs is less important than the achievement of appropriate hemodynamic goals: maintenance of ventricular performance and avoidance of large alterations in Q_P:Q_S. When a shunt is present, blood leaving the heart may travel in one of two parallel circulations: either to the systemic circulation via the aorta or to the pulmonary circulation via the shunt. The SVR, PVR and the resistance of the shunt determine the flow through each vascular bed. In the perioperative period the goal is to balance the circulations (i.e. $Q_P:Q_S = 1:1$; see Chapter 51). Otherwise, the goals of anesthetic management are to avoid fluctuations in SVR and PVR, and to maintain preload, contractility and sinus rhythm.

Intravenous induction may be slowed if the circulation time is prolonged. R→L shunt theoretically prolongs inhalation induction, but this is rarely of clinical importance. Because of the adverse consequences of sympathetic stimulation, laryngoscopy should not be attempted before an adequate depth of anesthesia has been achieved. The presence of R→L shunt or common mixing will, however, cause end-tidal CO_2 monitoring to underestimate $PaCO_2$. Although vasodilatation during induction of anesthesia tends to increase R→L shunt and reduce SaO_2, this is partially offset by reduced metabolic rate. Narcotic-based anesthesia may be preferable in the presence of significant ventricular dysfunction. In the presence of maximal sympathetic stimulation, ketamine may paradoxically depress cardiac function. The hemodynamic impact of dynamic LVOT obstruction may be reduced by a modest depression of ventricular function.

External defibrillator pads are placed on patients undergoing reoperations, as access for internal paddles is usually impossible during chest opening. VT and VF are common during RV dissection. Exposure of the femoral vessels is usually obtained *before* resternotomy. If preoperative investigation indicates that a conduit is at risk, femoro-femoral CPB is instituted *before* sternotomy. Induction of hypothermia and circulatory arrest prior to sternotomy is occasionally necessary despite the risk of VF and ventricular distension. Ventricular decompression can be achieved by venting the left heart through the chest wall or by external cardiac massage.

Pulmonary vasodilators (e.g. NO) are required during ~5% of procedures. TEE is particularly useful in ACHD surgery to confirm preoperative findings and exclude previously undiagnosed lesions. In addition, TEE permits the assessment of ventricular performance, valvular function and blood flow velocity, and is essential for confirming adequate anatomical repair.

Invasive monitoring is not usually required for short or minor surgical procedures, even if the patient has cyanotic ACHD. However, the presence of severe PHT normally mandates the use of an arterial line regardless of the type of surgery planned.

General versus regional anesthesia

The majority of published reports describe the use of regional anesthesia in patients with ACHD undergoing elective cesarean section. Epidural anesthesia appears safe as long as invasive monitoring is undertaken and any reduction in SVR is treated promptly and aggressively. The difficulties encountered when considering neuraxial anesthesia in anticoagulated patients are discussed in Chapter 72.

Antibiotic prophylaxis

Antibiotic prophylaxis should be given according to international guidelines (Chapter 71). Patients with a history of infective endocarditis and those with complex congenital heart disease, prosthetic heart valves or surgically constructed shunts or conduits are all considered to be high-risk.

Balancing circulations

Excessively high PBF is usually achieved at the expense of systemic blood flow. Although SaO_2 remains high there is systemic hypotension, lactic acidosis and oliguria. Chronic elevation of PBF causes a reduction in lung compliance and increases the work of breathing. Treatment aims to increase CO, raise PVR and cause systemic vasodilatation. The principles underlying the management of the pulmonary and systemic circulations are discussed in Chapter 51.

Postoperative care

Many patients with moderate to severe ACHD do not require elective postoperative mechanical ventilation. Those with a Fontan circulation fare better breathing spontaneously but must not be allowed to become hypercarbic or develop post extubation airway obstruction. They must be alert, extubated and transferred to the recovery ward in a comfortable state or a decision should be made to continue ventilation until the patient is suitable for weaning and extubation on ICU.

All cardiac and major non-cardiac surgical patients should be managed in the ICU. If mechanical ventilation is continued postoperatively then PBF is less compromised if the inspiratory time is shortened, even if it is at the expense of higher peak inspiratory pressures. Nitric oxide should be available if there is PHT. Postoperative management should include patient-controlled analgesia, cardiological review, antibiotics, resumption of anticoagulants, continuation of oral pulmonary vasodilators (such as bosentan or sildenafil) and reintroduction of preoperative medications as required.

Key points

- Adults with congenital heart disease present a spectrum ranging from well patients with corrected minor defects to those with extreme deviations from normal physiology.
- Involvement of clinicians with experience of congenital heart disease is essential.
- Thought should be given to the appropriate placement of vascular catheters and avoidance of air embolism.

- A detailed understanding of the factors influencing pulmonary blood flow is essential.
- Antibiotic prophylaxis guidelines should be followed.

Further reading

Andropoulos DB, Stayer SA, Russell IA, Mossad EB (Eds.). *Anesthesia for Congenital Heart Disease*, 2nd edition. Singapore: Wiley-Blackwell; 2010.

Cannesson M, Earing MG, Collange V, Kersten JR. Anesthesia for noncardiac surgery in adults with congenital heart disease. *Anesthesiology* 2009; **111**(2): 432–40.

Joshi G, Tobias JD. Intentional use of intra-arterial medications when venous access is not available. *Paediatr Anaesth* 2007; **17**(12): 1198–202.

Cardiopulmonary bypass equipment

John Whitbread and Stephen J. Gray

"Surgery of the heart has probably reached the limits set by nature to all surgery; no new method, no new discovery can overcome the natural difficulties that attend a wound of the heart."

Stephen Paget, London Surgeon, 1896

History

Despite the introduction of novel percutaneous techniques, CPB retains its pre-eminent position in the management of complex cardiac disease. Current CPB systems bear little resemblance to the large device used by John H. Gibbon in Philadelphia over five decades ago. Table 55.1 outlines the key milestones in the development of CPB.

Modern CPB systems consist of numerous disposable components connected together with polycarbonate connectors and silicone, latex or polyvinyl chloride (PVC) tubing. The basic components of the system are illustrated in Figure 55.1. CPB systems for clinical use are considerably more complex (Figure 55.2).

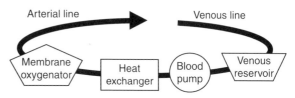

Figure 55.1 The basic components of a CPB system.

Table 55.1 Historical milestones in the development of cardiopulmonary bypass

1882	Von Schroder	Credited with introduction of bubble oxygenation
1885	Von Frey and Gruber	Devised the first artificial lung
1916	McLean	Heparin discovered. Protamine not discovered until 1937
1937	Gibbon	First use of CPB in cats
1948	Bjork	Devised first rotating disc oxygenator
1951	Lewis	Repaired ASD using surface cooling
1953	Gibbon	First successful human CPB using vertical screen oxygenator
1954	Lillehei	Correction of ASD using cross circulation technique
1955	Kirklin	Modifies Gibbon machine at the Mayo Clinic
1956	DeWall	Designs sigmamotor pump and disposable helical reservoir bubble oxygenator
1956	Melrose & Cross	Develop the Kay-Cross rotating disc oxygenator
1958	Melrose	Successfully completes UK's first open heart surgery
1970s		BioMedicus introduce centrifugal blood pumps
1980s		Hollow-fiber membrane oxygenators introduced

Core Topics in Cardiac Anesthesia, Second Edition, ed. Jonathan H. Mackay and Joseph E. Arrowsmith. Published by Cambridge University Press. © Cambridge University Press 2012.

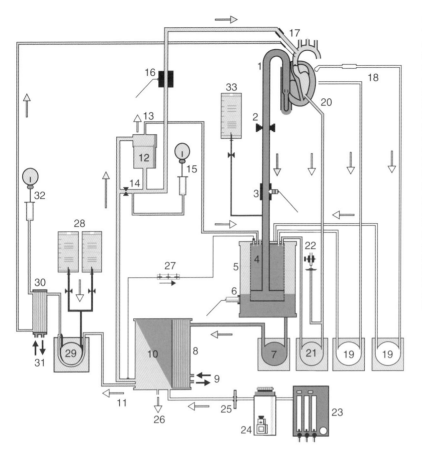

Figure 55.2 Schematic diagram of a typical CPB system: (1) venous line, (2) venous line clamp, (3) venous oxygen saturation meter, (4) cardiotomy filter, (5) venous reservoir, (6) reservoir-level detector, (7) main blood pump, (8) oxygenator heat exchanger, (9) water inlet and outlet for heat exchanger, (10) membrane oxygenator, (11) oxygenated blood outlets, (12) arterial line filter, (13) arterial filter vent, (14) arterial filter bypass, (15) arterial line pressure, (16) arterial bubble detector, (17) arterial line cannula, (18) sucker ends, (19) suction pumps, (20) vent, (21) vent pump, (22) vent suction controller, (23) gas supply and blender, (24) anesthetic vaporizer, (25) gas filter, (26) oxygenator gas outlet, (27) blood sample/injection ports, (28) cardioplegia solution, (29) cardioplegia pump, (30) cardioplegia heat exchanger, (31) cardioplegia water inlet and outlet, (32) cardioplegia pressure monitor and (33) fluid transfusion.

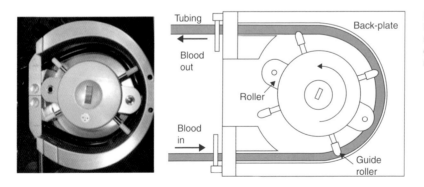

Figure 55.3 Twin-roller pump header. Note that in the photograph (left) the rollers remain in contact with the tubing enclosed in the "horseshoe-shaped" raceway for >180° of rotation.

Blood pumps

Two types of pumps are available, namely roller and centrifugal.

Roller pumps

Rollers remain in contact with the tubing in the pump head ("raceway") for 180–210° of travel. As the pump head rotates, the tubing is squeezed against a back-plate, propelling fluid forward. When stopped, these rollers act as a valve, preventing back-flow (Figure 55.3). Pump stroke volume is determined by (1) tubing internal diameter (ID) and (2) pump head diameter (Table 55.2). Pump flow (l min^{-1}) is the product of SV and pump speed in revolutions per minute (RPM). Most pumps are calibrated to display pump flow rather than RPM. The degree of tube compression is critical – excessive occlusion induces excessive shear, leading to hemolysis and increased tubing wear, whereas under-occlusion reduces the effective pump flow and permits regurgitation when the pump is stopped.

In addition to driving blood through the oxygenator, roller pumps are also used to provide variable cardiotomy suction (returning anticoagulated blood shed from the operative site to the venous reservoir) and to deliver cardioplegic solutions.

Centrifugal pumps

Two types of centrifugal pump are available, namely nested (stacked) cone constrained vortex (Figure 55.4) and vertical vaned impellor (Figure 55.5). The more commonly used vertical impellor is more energy efficient, generates less heat and requires a lower priming volume than the nested cone type. The BioMedicus® centrifugal blood pump (Figure 55.4), originally developed in the 1970s as a medium-term artificial heart, soon entered routine cardiac surgical practice.

A magnetic motor causes the cones to spin, inducing a constrained vortex effect, imparting kinetic energy to the blood, propelling it forward by vortex displacement. The center of the vortex is at a negative

Table 55.2 Relationship between internal tubing diameter and roller pump stroke volume

Internal diameter of pump tubing	Approximate volume displaced
1/2 inch (12.7 mm)	50 ml
3/8 inch (9.5 mm)	25 ml
1/4 inch (6.35 mm)	12.5 ml

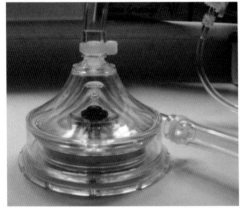

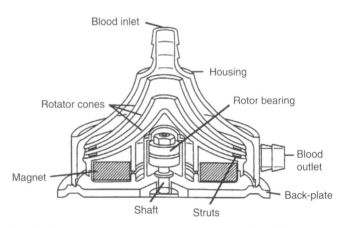

Figure 55.4 The Biomedicus nested or stacked cone centrifugal blood pump. The rotating cones create a constrained tornado-like vortex that sucks blood into the pump head from above and expels it outwards to the outlet.

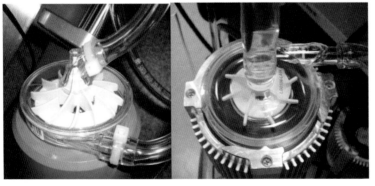

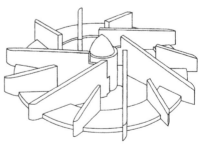

Figure 55.5 (Left) Sorin-Cobe Revolution spindle-held vaned centrifugal pump. (Center) Levitronix Centrig vaned head held by electromagnetic forces. (Right) Schematic diagram of vaned head.

pressure and "sucks" blood into the device. Some impellers have magnetic bearings, which reduce wear and clot formation.

Although the transmission of gases is impeded – because they receive much less kinetic energy than denser blood – potentially lethal gas embolism may still occur. As they are completely non-occlusive, fluid can flow in either direction; therefore, the arterial line must be clamped whenever the pump is not running.

Centrifugal pumps are both pre- and afterload dependent, that is their output is dependent upon filling and outflow impedance. This, at least in part, explains why there is no direct relationship between pump speed and pump output, and the requirement for an independent measure of flow, such as an electromagnetic flow sensor.

In contrast to roller pumps, centrifugal pumps cause less trauma to erythrocytes and platelets, and reduce the risk of embolization of damaged tubing fragments. These favorable characteristics have led to their use for short-term ventricular assist and mechanical (kinetic) assist for venous drainage in some specialized cardiac procedures.

Although the putative benefits of centrifugal pumps have not been translated into improved patient outcomes, they are commonly used for CPB procedures >3 hours in duration or for short-term extracorporeal support.

Oxygenators

In addition to oxygenating venous blood, oxygenators remove carbon dioxide (CO_2) and permit the administration of volatile anesthetic agents during CPB. The introduction of disposable bubble oxygenators in the 1950s rapidly led to the worldwide development of cardiac surgery. In the modern era, bubble oxygenators have largely been superseded by membrane oxygenators.

Bubble oxygenators

The contribution of De Wall in the early 1950s in developing a disposable bubble oxygenator should not be underestimated. The introduction of this disposable device undoubtedly accelerated the development of cardiac surgery worldwide. Gas exchange is achieved across the large blood–gas interface produced by "bubbling" oxygen directly through venous blood, creating a "froth of blood" where gas exchange takes place. Bubble size has an impact on the

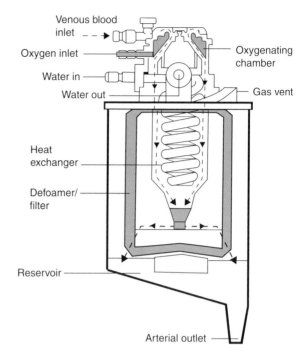

Figure 55.6 Cross section of a typical bubble oxygenator.

efficiency of both oxygenation and CO_2 removal. Oxygenation is improved with smaller bubbles (greater surface area to volume ratio) whereas CO_2 transfer is more efficient with larger bubbles (CO_2 tension rises faster in smaller bubbles). Bubble size selection is therefore a compromise. To avoid aeroembolism, the oxygenated blood "froth" is warmed and passed through a silicone anti-foam coated filter to remove bubbles before entering the arterial reservoir and being pumped back to the patient (Figure 55.6). The sheer number of smaller bubbles generated meant that it was impossible to completely remove them from arterialized blood. The ever-present risk of air embolism, embolism of anti-foam particles, and a tendency to greater hemolysis and complement activation have made this type of oxygenator obsolete.

Membrane oxygenators

Unlike the bubble oxygenator, the blood and gas phases in a membrane oxygenator are separated by a semi-permeable membrane – much like they are in the lung. Gas transfer is either by transmembrane diffusion or via micro-pores (<0.1 μm diameter) produced by stretching polypropylene. The membrane can take the form of flat sheets (100–150 μm thick) or hollow fibers (100–200 μm ID).

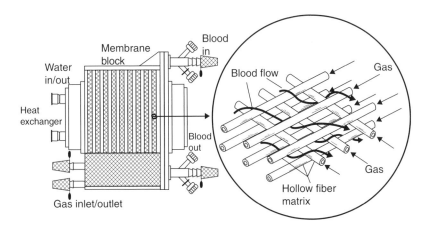

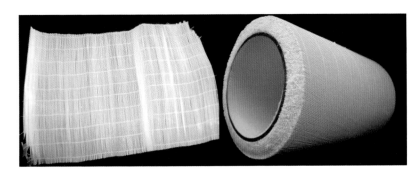

Figure 55.7 (Above) Cross section of typical membrane oxygenator block. The gas and blood phases move in opposite directions in a "counter-current" fashion. The micropores quickly become covered by a bridging protein layer, so decreasing the area of direct blood-gas contact. Should a single fiber rupture, blood contamination would only affect that one fiber, unlike the original designs where the whole phase could be compromised. (Below) Sheet of polypropylene fibers wrapped around one another to increase the blood/fiber contact.

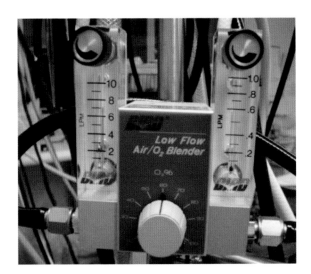

Figure 55.8 Example of a CPB sweep gas air/oxygen blender.

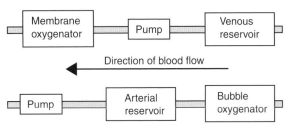

Figure 55.9 The contrasting arrangements of oxygenator, blood pump and reservoir in cardiopulmonary bypass systems employing membrane versus bubble oxygenator.

surface. Nitrogen is relatively insoluble and is therefore largely confined in the gas phase. A blender (Figure 55.8) is used to deliver the so-called "sweep gas" – an oxygen/air mixture. The O_2 concentration is used to regulate PaO_2, whereas the fresh gas flow determines $PaCO_2$. As the membrane oxygenator design imposes a much greater resistance to blood flow than bubble oxygenators, they must be placed after the blood pump (Figure 55.9).

During operation, micro-porous membranes quickly develop a proteinaceous coating once blood

In modern hollow-fiber oxygenators, the blood flows over the fibers (Figure 55.7) and a gas mixture is passed through them. Eddies induced in the blood continually bring more red cells to the gas exchange

349

comes into contact with them, preventing a direct blood–gas interface. With prolonged use, however, "plasma breakthrough" into the gas pathway reduces gas exchange efficiency, limiting device life to hours rather than days. In contrast, diffusion membranes may operate efficiently for several days or weeks.

The maximum O_2 transfer capacity of a membrane oxygenator is only 20–25% that of the lungs. It should be borne in mind, however, that this is achieved with an exchange surface area <6% that of the lungs.

Heat exchangers

Blood and cardioplegia solutions can be either warmed or cooled by passing them in a counter-current direction over corrugated aluminum sheets or stainless-steel tubes containing circulating water adjusted to the desired temperature.

The oxygenator heat exchanger is placed proximal to the gas exchange section to reduce the risk of gas rapidly coming out of solution when the oxygenated blood is heated. The cardioplegia heat exchanger is normally attached to a small bubble-trap device to remove any gaseous emboli. As heat exchangers use unsterile circulating water to alter blood temperatures, there exists a small risk of contamination (Figure 55.10).

Venous and cardiotomy reservoirs

A large-capacity (3000–4000 ml) reservoir is always positioned proximal to the main blood pump in any CPB circuit to buffer fluctuations in venous return. Reservoir volume mimics that of the patient's peripheral circulation (Figure 55.11).

Reservoirs are described as being either "open" or "closed" to the atmosphere. Hard-shell (open) reservoirs are more commonly used as they allow for the inclusion of a large capacity filter to manage cardiotomy suction and filter venous blood. Although collapsible bag (closed) reservoirs eliminate the blood–air interface present in open systems, a separate cardiotomy filter/reservoir is required, which increases both the blood contact surface area and the

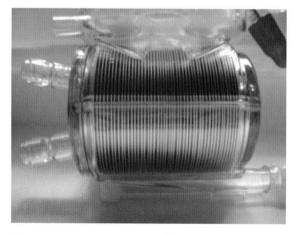

Figure 55.10 An integrated heat exchanger. Heat exchangers are normally built into oxygenators proximal to the membrane to minimize the risk of micro-bubble generation during rapid rewarming.

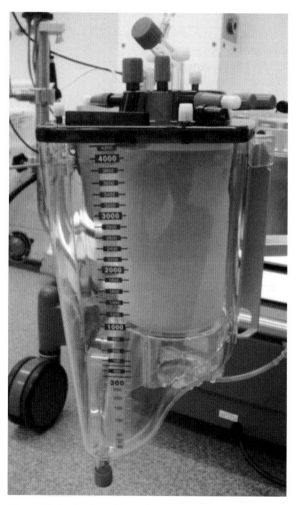

Figure 55.11 Combined (open, hard shell) venous reservoir and cardiotomy reservoir.

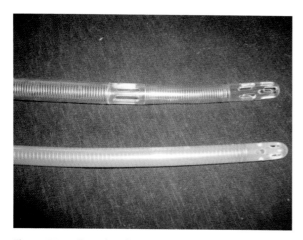

Figure 55.12 Examples of a two-stage (above) and single (below) venous cannulae. Owing to their size, venous cannulae are usually reinforced or armored with an integral wire spiral to prevent kinking.

Table 55.3 Examples of CPB tubing surface modifying agents

Carmeda®	Medtronic Inc. (covalently bonded heparin)
Duroflow II®	Baxter Inc. (ionic heparin bonding)
PMEA®	Terumo Med Inc.
SMART®	Cobe Cardiovascular Inc.
Trillium®	Medtronic Inc.

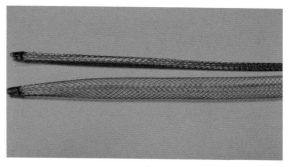

Figure 55.13 The Smartcannula® used in minimal-access surgery. The device is collapsed for insertion (above) and expands when engaged for use (below).

complexity of the circuit. Closed systems offer the advantage of protection against gross air entrainment but do not prevent air being pulled out of solution. Once gross air entrainment has occurred, it can be difficult to remove from the reservoir safely. This is discussed in more detail in the section on mini-bypass circuits.

Venous cannulae

Deoxygenated blood, which would normally enter the pulmonary circulation, is redirected to the CPB system using pipes inserted into the RA or vena cavae. For closed-heart cardiac surgery, such as CABG, a single two-stage venous cannula will suffice. This cannula has a short tapered distal section which is inserted down the IVC. Deoxygenated blood returning from the lower body drains through the tip. The main body of the cannula sits in the RA and a number of side holes proximal to the tapered section drain blood returning from the head and neck vessels.

If the surgical procedure requires the chambers of the heart to be opened with the risk of air entrainment (air-locks dramatically reduce venous return) then single-stage cannulae are inserted into the cavae. Each cava is then secured ("snugged") around the cannula so that all the venous blood (i.e. no air) is directed to the CPB venous reservoir. The drainage of venous blood is dependent on gravity. When the femoral vein is used for venous drainage a centrifugal pump or a vacuum applied to the venous reservoir may be

required to improve venous return. The growth of minimal-access open-heart techniques has triggered the development of new venous cannulae that do not obstruct the restricted surgical field (Figure 55.13).

Tubing

The diameter of CPB tubing is a trade-off between resistance to flow and priming volume. The choice of tubing sizes is determined by patient size, sites of cannulation and anticipated pressure drop. Venous tubing is invariably of larger diameter than arterial tubing to optimize passive venous drainage.

PVC and to a lesser extent silicone rubber are the most common types of tubing in use. Medical-grade PVC is tough, flexible and clear. It can be easily bonded to connectors and is resistant to chemical and solvent corrosion. The exceptionally smooth internal surface of PVC tubing allows maximum flow capabilities. Plasticizers contained within PVC promote flexibility, so enabling greater tubing manipulation between the operating field and the CPB system. Surface modifying additives, principally heparin, can be incorporated into the lining of the tubing to reduce thrombin formation.

351

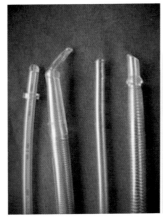
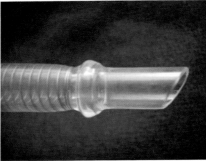
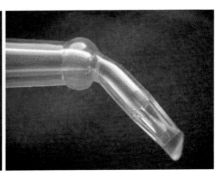

Figure 55.14 Arterial cannulae. (Left) From left to right; standard, armored curved-tip, percutaneous, wire reinforced. (Right above) Single end hole design. (Right below) Curved soft-flow side hole tip design.

The use of silicone tubing in roller pump raceways remains contentious. Although silicone is more malleable at lower temperatures than PVC, prolonged use can lead to spalation (shedding of the inner lining).

Arterial cannulae

The arterial cannula is a specialized, shaped tube designed to deliver oxygenated blood to the systemic circulation. There are numerous types of cannulae with differing profiles and flow characteristics. The choice of cannula is determined by the site and size of the vessel to be cannulated. For routine cardiac surgery the ascending aorta is the preferred cannulation site. For more complex surgical procedures it may be necessary to cannulate the femoral, iliac or innominate artery. Peripheral arterial cannulae are typically armored to reduce kinking. Long, tapered cannulae are available for minimal-access surgery. (Figure 55.14)

Arterial line filters and bubble traps

Screen filters (pore size 20–40 μm) provide a final stage of protection against systemic gas and particulate embolization. Although they provide excellent protection against gross air embolism, protection against micro-bubble embolism is dependent upon continuous venting of accumulated gas. The bubble-trapping properties of these devices are greatly aided by their architecture (Figure 55.15): the blood inlet is normally offset so that the blood flow creates a centrifugal effect, trapping the less dense air bubbles in the center long enough for them to rise to the top of

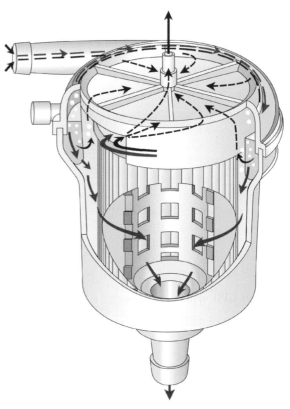

Figure 55.15 A typical auto-venting arterial line filter. Courtesy of Pall Biomedical, UK.

the filter to be removed. The "gas-free" blood then exits from the bottom of the device.

The incorporation of leukocyte-depleting filters has been shown to reduce the inflammatory response to CPB and the incidence of postoperative wound

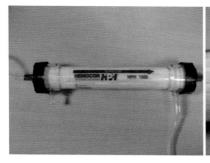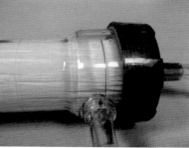

Figure 55.16 An arteriovenous hemofilter. (Right) Enlarged to show the hollow-fiber bundles.

infection. Leukocyte depletion of blood cardioplegia solutions may also limit free-radical-induced myocardial injury. Bubble traps that can be found on cardioplegia devices simply rely on the inlet and outlet being offset so that the less dense air bubbles naturally rise to the highest point of the system for removal.

Hemofilters

Hemofilters or hemoconcentrators utilize a pressure gradient across a semi-permeable membrane to filter excess fluid and metabolites from the circulating volume. Patients with renal impairment, pulmonary edema or hyperkalemia may benefit from hemofiltration. Because these devices typically filter molecules <20 kDa, close attention to anticoagulation (i.e. ACT) and blood biochemistry is absolutely essential. Recent reports suggest that hemofiltration removes inflammatory mediators such as C3a, C4a, C5a and IL-8. Pediatric centers use a modified ultrafiltration technique to reverse the deleterious effect of hemodilution.

Safety features

Modern CPB systems incorporate a number of features designed to protect both the patient and the circuit, and aid patient management during use. Several systems incorporate computerized record-keeping and can interface with hemodynamic monitors.

Additional ports permit:

- administration of crystalloids, colloids, blood products and drugs;
- arterial and venous blood sampling for blood gas and biochemical analysis;
- venting of blood to a secondary reservoir, if the primary reservoir overfills;
- incorporation of a hemoconcentrating device (e.g. hemofilter, see above);

- re-circulation of arterialized blood through the oxygenator (i.e. shunting) in certain clinical situations.

Monitors, which provide early warning of impending problems and may automatically alter pump controls, include:

- the venous oxygenator saturation monitor – providing a global estimate of CPB adequacy;
- the venous reservoir level detector/alarm – alerting the perfusionist to a fall in venous return and the risk of venous air entrainment;
- the arterial line pressure monitor/alarm – alerting the perfusionist to the risk of circuit/patient barotrauma; it may indicate clot formation or arterial cannula malposition; the monitor can also be used to measure proximal aortic pressure when the pump is not running;
- the arterial line bubble detector/alarm – alerting the perfusionist to the presence of air-embolism; it may indicate gross venous air entrainment, arterial line filter failure or loss of membrane integrity;
- an oxygen analyzer in the oxygenator gas supply line;
- venous and arterial line temperature monitors;
- In-line arterial blood-gas monitoring.

In the event of main power supply failure a battery backup or manual hand-crank can be used to maintain the output of the primary pump.

Mini-bypass circuits

The last decade has seen a drive to decrease the use of blood products by reducing prime volumes and the inflammatory complications of CPB. This has led to the emergence of so-called "mini-bypass" circuits with minimal priming volumes (600 ml vs. 1500 ml)

353

and the use of a cell saver for cardiotomy suction – all blood aspirated from the surgical field.

The components of a mini-bypass circuit include a soft-shell reservoir (removing the hard-shell reservoir substantially reduces the contact surface area for the blood), a centrifugal pump, a heat exchanger, an oxygenator, a cell saver and shorter circuit tubing.

Despite the putative advantages of reduced hemodilution and improved hemostasis, and emerging evidence of decreased cerebral microembolization and improved postoperative renal function, prospective studies have failed to show any difference in mortality.

Mini-bypass circuits are demanding for the perfusionist – the ever-present "air handling" issues are compounded by cell salvage, which inevitably delays the return of scavenged blood to the circulation.

Key points

- Centrifugal pumps are increasingly being used for more complex cases.
- Heat exchangers are normally built into oxygenators proximal to the membrane to minimize the risk of micro-bubble generation during rapid rewarming.

- Only diffusion membrane oxygenators have operational lives extending into days.
- Hemofilters on CPB circuits can remove large volumes of fluid and heparin.
- Mini-bypass circuits are starting to address the need for reduced prime volumes and improved hemostasis.

Further reading

Chilton V, Klein A. Equipment and monitoring. In Ghosh S, Falter F, Cook DJ (Eds.), *Cardiopulmonary Bypass*. Cambridge: Cambridge University Press; 2009. pp. 1–22.

DeBakey ME. John Gibbon and the heart-lung machine: a personal encounter and his impart for cardiovascular surgery. *Ann Thorac Surg* 2003; **76**(6): S2188–94.

Koivisto SP, Wistbacka JO, Rimpiläinen R, *et al.* Miniaturized versus conventional cardiopulmonary bypass in high-risk patients undergoing coronary artery bypass surgery. *Perfusion* 2010; **25**(2): 65–70.

Remadi JP, Marticho P, Butoi I, *et al.* Clinical experience with the mini-extracorporeal circulation system: an evolution or a revolution? *Ann Thorac Surg* 2004; 77(6): 2172–5.

56

Failure to wean from bypass

Simon Colah and Stephen J. Gray

Failure to wean a patient from CPB at the first attempt after routine, elective cardiac surgery is a relatively uncommon occurrence. By contrast, failure to wean after prolonged, complex or emergency surgery is relatively common. Fortunately, in most cases the underlying cause is remediable and the problem is temporary, merely delaying a successful clinical outcome. In the vast majority of cases, weaning difficulty can be attributed to myocardial ischemia secondary to prolonged aortic cross-clamp time, inadequate myocardial protection, coronary embolism or MI. Less common causes include extremes of vascular resistance, prosthetic valve malfunction, anastomotic strictures (e.g. in transplantation) and retained surgical swabs (e.g. atrial compression).

Regardless of etiology, the key to successful termination of CPB in this situation is the recognition that there is a problem, the identification of its causes and the timely institution of remedial therapy. In order to prevent ventricular distension and inadequate coronary perfusion, reinstitution of CPB should be considered. Generally speaking, conditions impeding successful weaning can be considered as either correctable or non-correctable by the anesthesiologist (Table 56.1).

Table 56.1 Causes of failure to wean from CPB: note that the anesthesiologist cannot correct some causes

Correctable by anesthesiologist or perfusionist

Impaired myocardial contractility

Air embolism

Dysrhythmia

Hypothermia

Metabolic/acid-base

Preload

Respiratory

Extremes of SVR and PVR

Profound hemorrhage

Gross anemia

Monitoring artifact

Non-correctable by anesthesiologist or perfusionist

Acute myocardial infarction

Inadequate surgical correction

New anatomical defect

Prosthetic valve malfunction

Correctable causes

Impaired ventricular performance

Dysfunction may be systolic or diastolic; effect LV or RV; and be regional or global. TEE is invaluable in assessing the extent and severity of ventricular dysfunction and the response to intervention. Myocardial stunning secondary to prolonged myocardial ischemia, or inadequate myocardial protection or revascularization, usually responds to a further period of CPB and inotropes. A minimum period of 10–15 minutes

of coronary reperfusion following removal of the aortic cross-clamp (AXC) should precede any attempt to wean from CPB. Spasm of native coronary arteries or arterial bypass conduits, which may cause significant ventricular dysfunction, usually responds to nitrates.

Air embolism

The incidence of air embolism is increased following procedures in which the left heart is opened

Core Topics in Cardiac Anesthesia, Second Edition, ed. Jonathan H. Mackay and Joseph E. Arrowsmith. Published by Cambridge University Press. © Cambridge University Press 2012.

Table 56.2 Diagnosing post CPB low cardiac output state

Cardiac index	$<2.0 \ l \ min^{-1} \ m^{-2}$
SVR	<5 Wood units (<400 dyne s cm^{-5})
	>20 Wood units (>1600 dyne s cm^{-5})
LA pressure/LVEDP	>20 mmHg
Urine output	$<0.3 \ ml \ kg^{-1} \ h^{-1}$

(e.g. aortic, MV, AV and LV aneurysm surgery). The right coronary artery (RCA) is more commonly affected as its anterior aortic ostium lies superiorly in the supine patient. RV distension and conduction abnormalities may be the first clinical indications of air embolism. TEE may reveal a regional wall motion abnormality (RWMA) and myocardial "air contrast" (increased echo reflectivity) in the RCA territory. In practice, vasopressors are used to treat mild myocardial dysfunction, whereas allowing the heart to eject while on partial CPB may be necessary if myocardial dysfunction is severe.

Dysrhythmia

It is futile attempting to terminate CPB in the presence of untreated asystole, bradycardia, VT or VF. Atropine and epicardial pacing are the first-line treatments for bradydysrhythmias. Persistent ventricular dysrhythmias require cardioversion in the first instance. An underlying physical or metabolic cause should be actively sought before resorting to an anti-dysrhythmic drug (e.g. lidocaine, amiodarone). New-onset AF or other SVT may respond to synchronized transatrial cardioversion, whereas unstable nodal rhythms may be converted to sinus rhythm by isoproterenol.

Hypothermia

Ventricular irritability, dysrhythmias and contractile dysfunction are more common at temperatures $<34°C$.

Metabolic

Increased or decreased $[K^+]$, decreased $[Mg^{2+}]$ and increased $[H^+]$ may induce dysrhythmia, impair myocardial contractility and increase PVR.

Preload

Inadequate ventricular preload leads to reduced CO. Overenthusiastic elevation of atrial pressures risks ventricular distension, MR, TR and cardiac failure. TEE assessment of LV end-diastolic area (LVEDA) is a better guide to preload optimization than CVP monitoring.

Respiratory

Inadvertent failure to restart mechanical ventilation may occur, particularly after repeated attempts to wean from CPB. Severe bronchospasm apparent at the termination of CPB is a rare but potentially lethal complication. The management of this complication requires continuation of CPB, avoidance of lung distension (which may damage a mammary artery graft), bronchoscopy (to exclude airway obstruction), aggressive treatment with several bronchodilators (e.g. isoflurane, epinephrine, β_2-agonists, aminophylline, ketamine, $MgSO_4$) and corticosteroids.

Extremes of SVR or PVR

CPB provides a ready opportunity to accurately calculate SVR (Table 56.3).

Assuming that SVR does not markedly change during weaning from CPB, an estimate of CO can be made using MAP, CVP and calculated SVR. A target SVR of 10–14 Wood units (800–1120 dyne s cm^{-5}) with a CVP of 5 mmHg will generate an MAP in the range 55–75 mmHg with a CO of 5 l min^{-1}. Reduced tissue perfusion and increased myocardial work secondary to excessive afterload (i.e. SVR >20 Wood units) may lead to acidosis and myocardial ischemia. In addition, increased vascular sheer stress may cause aortic dissection during decannulation and worsen bleeding from suture lines. An excessively low afterload (i.e. SVR <6 Wood units) may result in inadequate coronary perfusion and low CO.

Table 56.3 Estimation of SVR (in Wood units) during CPB

SVR = (MAP – CVP)/Pump flow

Wood units can be converted to dyne s cm^{-5} by multiplying by 80. For example; when MAP $= 65$ mmHg, CVP $= 5$ mmHg and pump flow $= 5$ l min^{-1}, the SVR $= 12$ Wood units or 960 dyne s cm^{-5}.

Profound hemorrhage

Bleeding from posterior structures or suture lines can be difficult to deal with. Elevating or rotating the heart around its base may impede venous return and dramatically reduce CO. Assessment and surgical repair may be more safely carried out on CPB.

Gross anemia

A hematocrit <20% is undesirable as low oxygen-carrying capacity coupled with low CO may lead to tissue hypoxia and acidosis. The hematocrit may be elevated by reducing crystalloid administration, red cell transfusion, diuretic administration or hemofiltration.

Monitoring artifact

Unexplained hypotension may be due to problems with invasive monitoring. Zero-drift, damping, line occlusion, transducer misplacement and other causes of inaccuracy must be excluded before the administration of vasoactive drugs. A large discrepancy between peripheral arterial pressure and CPB arterial line pressure (monitored by the perfusionist) should prompt the use of direct aortic pressure monitoring using a 21G needle and a separate manometer line and transducer.

Causes not correctable by anesthesiologist or perfusionist

Acute myocardial infarction

This is a difficult diagnosis to make intraoperatively. The diagnosis is suggested by persistent, new, severe RWMA (i.e. akinesia or dyskinesia) in a coronary artery territory. Causes include distal coronary embolization, graft occlusion and incomplete revascularization. The surgeon may consider further revascularization on CPB.

Inadequate surgical procedure

This is more common in surgery for congenital heart disease. Incomplete myocardial revascularization may cause problems, particularly in redo surgery.

New anatomical defect

Iatrogenic mitral stenosis, new ASD or LVOT obstruction may arise following MV surgery. Similarly, a basal VSD is a recognized complication of surgery for hypertrophic obstructive cardiomyopathy.

Prosthetic valve malfunction

Large paravalvular leaks, impeded leaflet opening due to prolapse of subvalvular tissue and inadvertent use of a mitral prosthesis in the aortic position (and vice versa) are rare causes of failure to wean from CPB following valve surgery.

Pharmacological support

Having excluded and treated reversible causes of failed weaning from CPB, administration of inotropic agents should be considered. Both SVR and PVR as well as institutional preference largely dictate drug selection. Inotropes are discussed in Chapter 9.

Mechanical support

Intra-aortic balloon counter-pulsation is a common intervention undertaken in all cardiac surgical centers. In contrast, the use of univentricular or biventricular mechanical assist and extracorporeal membrane oxygenation (discussed in Chapter 57) is usually restricted to designated specialist centers.

Intra-aortic balloon pump

The IABP may be used to augment pharmacological therapy or when drugs alone have resulted in failure to wean from CPB. The device consists of an inflatable, sausage-shaped balloon (30–40 ml), which is normally inserted into the descending thoracic aorta via the femoral artery such that the tip lies just distal to the left subclavian artery (Figure 56.1). Correct positioning may be confirmed by TEE or CXR. The device improves LV performance by augmenting coronary perfusion and reducing LVEDP (Figure 56.2).

Indications and contraindications

As the IABP does not interfere with cardiac surgery, insertion may be undertaken before induction of anesthesia in high-risk patients and in patients with angina despite maximal medical therapy. Other indications are summarized in Table 56.4.

Use of the IABP is contraindicated in the presence of moderate or severe aortic regurgitation and severe peripheral vascular disease.

Management

Use of an IABP usually requires systemic anticoagulation with unfractionated heparin to achieve an activated partial thromboplastin ratio of 1.5–2.0.

357

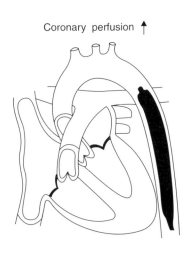

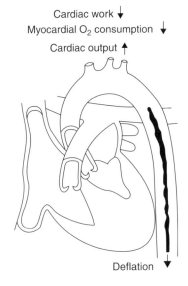

Cardiac work ↓
Myocardial O₂ consumption ↓
Cardiac output ↑

Coronary perfusion ↑

Deflation

Figure 56.1 The IABP. The balloon is positioned in the descending thoracic aorta just distal to the origin of the left subclavian artery. During diastole, the balloon is rapidly filled with helium and impedes blood flow to the distal aorta. The rise in proximal aortic pressure augments coronary perfusion pressure. The balloon is deflated at the end of diastole (*before* the onset of isovolumic LV contraction) resulting in reduced LVEDP. (Courtesy of Datascope Corp, NJ, USA.)

Table 56.4 Indications for intra-aortic balloon pump insertion

Ischemic myocardium

Structural complications of acute MI

Cardiogenic shock

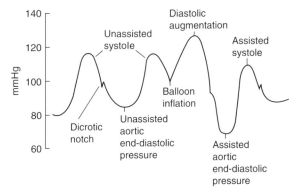

Figure 56.2 Proximal aortic pressure waveforms without and with IABP augmentation. Balloon inflation takes place at the dicrotic notch (AV closure). Balloon deflation takes place before AV opening so as not to impede LV ejection. (Courtesy of Datascope Corp, NJ, USA.)

The correct timing of balloon inflation and deflation is critical to optimal IABP use. On most IABP devices, timings can be derived from the ECG (R wave), pacemaker potentials or the arterial waveform, and adjusted manually. In addition the extent of balloon inflation ("augmentation") and the ratio of balloon inflations to heart rate (i.e. 1:1, 1:2 or 1:3) can be altered.

Excessive tachycardia and irregular cardiac rhythms (e.g. AF) reduce the effectiveness of the IABP.

Complications

Incorrect IABP positioning may result in left arm ischemia (balloon too high/proximal) or renal/gastrointestinal ischemia (balloon too low/distal). The most common complications are vascular injury (including dissection and pseudoaneurysm) and infection at the insertion site and lower limb ischemia.

Balloon rupture is not uncommon. The use of helium, which has high blood solubility, reduces the risks associated with gas embolism.

Thrombocytopenia is not uncommon and may be the result of mechanical platelet damage or inadequate anticoagulation, or may be heparin-induced.

Key points

- Myocardial stunning and inadequate myocardial protection or revascularization are common causes of failure to wean from CPB.
- Many of the causes of failure to wean from CPB are amenable to intervention by the anesthesiologist.
- Intraoperative myocardial infarction is difficult to diagnose with confidence.
- The IABP is contraindicated in the presence of significant aortic regurgitation.

Further reading

Maquet. *Intra-aortic Balloon Counterpulsation Therapy: Theory Program*. http://ca.maquet.com/file_assets/ educational_materials/e-learning/theory_program/ theory_program.html (accessed 23 November 2011).

Advanced mechanical support

Stephen J. Gray and Simon Colah

There are occasions when, having established optimal preload, instituted guided inotropic therapy and secured pacing, ventricular function still fails to maintain adequate organ perfusion. Mechanical strategies such as the IABP, ventricular assist devices (VADs) and extracorporeal membrane oxygenation (ECMO) can be used to facilitate separation from CPB.

Ventricular assist devices

Unlike the IABP, which only enhances LV function, VADs are mechanical pumps that can assist the LV, RV or both. These devices are inserted in parallel to one or both ventricles, effectively providing a bridge to transplant, bridge to recovery and destination therapy (long-term support). Indications and contraindications are summarized in Table 57.1.

Classification of devices

A number of differing classifications exist, although the most accepted is by "generation" of the device (Table 57.2).

Table 57.1 Indications and contraindication to VAD use

Indications

Severe heart failure with borderline hemodynamics despite inotropes and IABP.
Patients with severe heart failure deemed unsuitable for heart transplantation.
Post CPB (cardiotomy) shock and failure to wean from CPB.
Failed heart transplant.
Cardiac arrest refractory to conventional resuscitation.

Contraindications

Advanced age
Uncontrollable hemorrhage
Intractable metabolic acidosis
Other severe comorbidities

The first generation of mechanical pumps used positive displacement to produce pulsatile flow and were either pneumatically or electrically driven. Second-generation devices incorporate rotary pump designs, which produce continuous (i.e. non-pulsatile) flow. Third-generation devices incorporate magnetically suspended impellers, which also produced continuous flow. Many of the devices in this latter group are still under development. Examples of first-, second- and third-generation devices are shown in Figures 57.1–57.4. A more detailed description of this rapidly changing field is beyond the scope of this book.

Table 57.2 Classification of ventricular devices

Pump type (generation)

Displacement → pulsatile flow (1st)
Rotary → continuous flow (2nd)
Magnetically suspended impeller → continuous flow (3rd)

Anatomic location of pump

Intracardiac
Intracorporeal
Extracorporeal – pump distant from body
Paracorporeal – pump on body surface

Source of driving power

Pneumatic
Electrical

Ventricle supported

Left ventricle (LVAD)
Right ventricle (RVAD)
Both ventricles (BiVAD)

Intended duration of use

Bridge to recovery
Bridge to longer-term device
Bridge to transplant
Destination therapy (long-term support)

Core Topics in Cardiac Anesthesia, Second Edition, ed. Jonathan H. Mackay and Joseph E. Arrowsmith. Published by Cambridge University Press. © Cambridge University Press 2012.

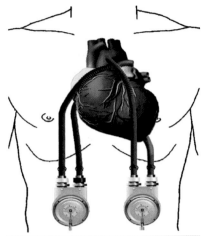

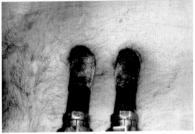

First generation, single chamber, pneumatically driven, pulsatile pump.

Inflow

From atrium or ventricular apex by passive or active means (vacuum). Fills blood pumping sac contained within translucent rigid plastic housing.

Outflow

To PA or aorta. Air from the pneumatic driver compresses the sac ejecting blood each cardiac cycle. Flows up to 6.5 l.min^{-1}.

Advantages

Suitable for LVAD, RVAD, BiVAD. No restriction on patient size. Biocompatible polmer chamber lining (Thoralon®). The extracorporeal location allows ease of exchange in the event of malfunction, thrombus formation and infection. Long term support.

Disadvantages

Inconvenience and discomfort of the extracorporeal location.

[Above] Configuration for biventricular support.
[Below] Subxiphisternal cannula exit sites.

Figure 57.1 Thoratec I (paracorporeal) VAD.

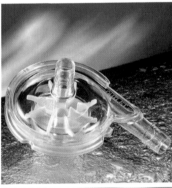

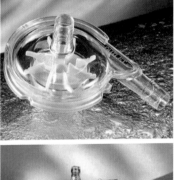

Second generation, extracorporeal, centrifugal flow, magnetically levitated impeller, electrically driven.

Inflow

Suction is created in the inflow line by the pump. Flow is directed towards the axis of the rotating impeller.

Outflow

Centrifugally (non-pulsatile) to PA or aorta. Flows up to 9.9 l.min^{-1}.

Advantages

Bearing-less pump—reduced risk of hemolysis and thrombus formation. Suitable for LVAD, RVAD, BiVAD.

Disadvantages

Preload and afterload dependent. Short term support. Risk of hemolysis.

[Above] Detailed view of Levitronix Centrimag disposable polycarbonate impeller unit. Blood enters the unit via a port above the rotor and leaves under centrifugal force via the tangential outlet port.
[Below] Disposable Levitronix Centri pump mounted in reusable motor (rotating magnet driver device). The motor is controlled using a primary console (not shown).

Figure 57.2 Levitronix Centrimag VAD.

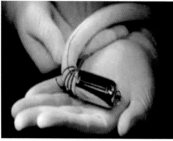

Second generation pump designed for destination therapy.
Axial flow, spinning titanium impeller, electrically driven.
Flows up to 7.0l/min.

Inflow
Intracardiac, the pump housing resides completely within the left ventricle.

Outflow
Fabric graft, channels blood from the pump to the aorta.

Advantages
Size: 2.5 × 5.5 cm, weighs 90 g. No size limitation, suitable for pediatric and adult patients. Implantation can be via median sternotomy or left thoracotomy with or without CPB. Available for long term support. Longest period of support ~7.5 years. Very portable.

Disadvantages
Thrombus formation in the ventricular apex and ascending aorta. Limited clinical experience.

[Above] The Jarvik 2000 blood pump (reprinted from Frazier OH. *J Congest Heart Failure Circ Suppl* 2000;1:107–11 with permission of Isis Medical Media, Oxford).
[Below] Diagram of insertion site and route of subcutaneous power cable used by the Oxford team (reprinted from Westaby *et al. J Thorac Cardiovasc Surg* 1997;114:467–74 with permission)

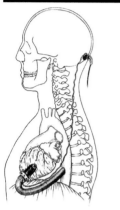

Figure 57.3 Jarvik 2000 VAD.

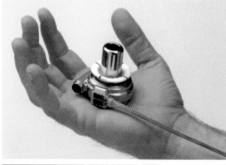

Third generation device currently undergoing clinical trials. Centrifugal flow device using the latest design feature of hydrodynamic bearings, eliminating heat from friction and reducing wear of components, hence optimizing biocompatibility and durability.

Inflow
Axial, ventricular apex

Outflow
Ascending aorta

Advantages
Much smaller size allows ease of positioning in a pre-peritoneal pocket with less surgical dissection reducing thrombus formation and infection.

Disadvantages
Limited clinical experience

[Above] HeartWare HVAD pump.
[Below] HVAD in pericardial space.
Courtesy of HeartWare International Inc.

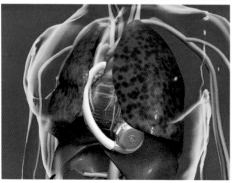

Figure 57.4 HeartWare VAD (HVAD).

VAD implantation

Surgical procedures that a patient requiring mechanical ventricular assist may undergo during hospital admission are shown in Table 57.3.

Initial assessment

Patients requiring VAD implantation include those with:

- clinically stable end-stage heart failure
- acute severe decompensated heart failure
- intractable post-cardiotomy shock.

Patients typically present in a fixed low-CO state, with minimal cardiopulmonary reserve and with markedly elevated filling pressures. Not infrequently there is evidence of pulmonary edema and hypertension, renal insufficiency, hepatic dysfunction, malnutrition, sepsis and, in some cases, depressed consciousness. Established therapy may include fluid restriction, diuretics, intropes, IABP, anti-dysrhythmics, implantable devices (pacemaker or cardiodefibrillator) and renal replacement therapy.

The anesthetic management of a patient undergoing VAD implantation is very similar to that of a patient undergoing cardiac transplantation (see Chapter 44). Initial assessment should include fasting status and documentation of risk factors known to be associated with adverse outcome: urine output <0.5 ml kg^{-1} h^{-1}, CVP >16 mmHg, mechanical ventilation, coagulopathy (prothrombin time >16 s), previous sternotomy and previous LVAD.

Induction

Invasive monitoring should be established before induction of anesthesia. When using an IV induction, the anesthesiologist should take into account an increased arm-brain circulation time and be prepared for the hemodynamic consequences of an abrupt reduction in sympathetic nervous system tone. An infusion of a vasopressor (e.g. norepinephrine, vasopressin) may be used as a precaution. In the presence of near-terminal circulatory collapse it should be borne in mind that femoro-femoral CPB can be established under local anesthesia *before* induction of anesthesia.

Antimicrobial prophylaxis

Infection remains the major cause of morbidity and death in VAD patients, with VAD-related infective episodes occurring in $>50\%$ patients. Local protocols

Table 57.3 Surgical procedures that patient requiring mechanical ventricular assist may undergo

VAD-related	Unrelated
VAD implantation	Tracheostomy
VAD revision/exchange	Thoracotomy for empyema
VAD explanatation to recovery	Craniotomy for hemorrhage
VAD explantation to transplantation	Cholecystectomy
Reoperations for hemostasis	Bowel resection
Reoperations for infective complications	Peripheral vascular surgery

typically include broad-spectrum antibacterial and antifungal agents.

Transesophageal echocardiography

TEE has become an indispensible diagnostic and monitoring tool both during and after VAD implantation. In addition to aiding the optimization of LV filling and assessment of RV function before CPB, TEE is used to exclude anatomic abnormalities that may interfere with VAD function. A patent foramen ovale (PFO) or other ASD will require repair to prevent hypoxia or paradoxical embolization following VAD activation. Similarly, conditions that may significantly impede VAD inflow (MS, TS, mural thrombus) or effective VAD output (AR, PR, MR, TR) must be excluded.

During CPB, TEE is used to assist the surgeon with optimal device and cannula positioning, and to confirm de-airing of the cardiac chambers. Following device activation, TEE is used to assess atrial and ventricular decompression, and exclude valvular regurgitation. During separation from CPB, TEE is useful for assessing RV function (when LVAD is used) and monitoring chamber decompression.

Conduct of bypass

With the exception of the implantation of transaortic devices (e.g. Abiomed Impella), the majority of cases are performed using conventional normothermic (atrio-aortic) CPB with continuous hemofiltration. Although most patients have some degree of preoperative coagulopathy, full anticoagulation (e.g. heparin 300–500 units kg^{-1}) is required. It is not unusual, however, to encounter heparin resistance and heparin-induced thrombocytopenia. Unlike conventional cardiac surgery with CPB, it is usual to continue mechanical ventilation of the lungs throughout the procedure to minimize any increase in PVR.

Preservation of RV function

Often the greatest challenge accompanying implantation of a VAD to support the LV is avoiding the need for implantation of an additional device to support the RV. Risk factors for RVAD implantation include: pre-existing RV dysfunction, pulmonary hypertension, elevated transpulmonary gradient, right coronary air embolism, impaired function of the interventricular septum and hemorrhage. Inhaled NO, phosphodiesterase inhibitors (e.g. milrinone, enoximone) and nebulized prostacyclin may be used before and after separation from CPB to improve RV function and reduce PVR. Although the need for concomitant RVAD implantation is associated with poorer outcome, current evidence suggests that early conversion from LVAD to BiVAD support improves outcome.

Hemostasis

The combination of hepatic dysfunction, previous cardiac surgery, extensive surgical dissection and anticoagulation for CPB make these patients particularly prone to excessive hemorrhage. It is undoubtedly true that VAD surgery has become more difficult in the post-aprotinin era. Measures to reduce hemorrhage and blood product use include correction of preoperative coagulopathy, antifibrinolytic therapy, avoidance of hypothermia and cell salvage.

Postoperative management

The sheer number of pieces of equipment that typically accompany the patient on their journey from the operating room to the ICU creates a number of potential hazards. Numerous personnel are required to ensure that tubes, drains, catheters, infusion lines and drive cables are not inadvertently damaged, disconnected or avulsed.

The VAD recipient

The commonest reasons for a VAD recipient to require further anesthesia is re-exploration for control of hemorrhage, relief of tamponade or explantation. In the patient with an isolated LVAD, preservation of RV function is of paramount importance. Similarly, maintenance of preload and afterload is vital.

VAD explantation

In most instances, VAD explantation is undertaken immediately prior to orthotopic cardiac transplantation. Allowance should be made for the additional time that may be required to establish vascular access and invasive monitoring. Patients with a non-pulsatile VAD may have no palpable pulses and central veins may be damaged from repeated cannulation or thrombosed. The pulse-less patient represents another indication for ultrasound (2D or Doppler) guided arterial and central venous cannulation.

VAD explantation following cardiac recovery is not without risk. Reducing or ceasing pump flow to assess underlying ventricular function exposes the patient to the risk of thromboembolic complications and a stopped device may not restart.

Extracorporeal membrane oxygenation

ECMO can provide either total cardiopulmonary support (venoarterial or VA-ECMO) or pulmonary support (venovenous or VV-ECMO). The technique effectively enables the use of CPB in an ICU setting. In adult practice, ECMO was initially reserved for patients with severe respiratory failure secondary to ARDS. ECMO in adults fell out of favor, largely because of poor outcomes. In pediatric practice, where outcomes are generally better, ECMO has remained in routine use for over three decades. Recent H1N1 ("swine flu") epidemics have led to a re-examination of the role of ECMO in adults with respiratory failure and a re-emergence of VV-ECMO. The recently published third report of the Interagency Registry for Mechanical Circulatory Support (INTERMACS) confirms a dramatic and sustained increase in the use of continuous-flow pump technology. Disposable, extracorporeal versions of this technology are particularly suited to short and medium-term ECMO. These devices are associated with significantly improved survival, fewer malfunctions, reduced bleeding during implantation and reduced infection rate. These factors may explain the trend from VAD to ECMO therapy in patients requiring short-term, post-cardiotomy cardiopulmonary support.

Indications

The broad indications for instituting ECMO are shown in Table 57.4.

Table 57.4 Indications for ECMO

Post-cardiotomy low cardiac output state

Persistent pulmonary hypertension (post pulmonary endarterectomy – PEA)

Fulminant respiratory failure

Intractable ventricular arrhythmias

Perioperative cardiac arrest

Equipment

A typical ECMO system comprises three principal components – a pump, an oxygenator and a heat exchanger – connected by polyvinyl chloride or silicone tubing. Unlike conventional CPB systems, ECMO systems are closed, have no venous reservoir or arterial line filter, and can be operated at lower levels of anticoagulation.

Oxygenator

Three types of so-called "membrane lungs" are used to oxygenate blood and remove CO_2. The original silicone spiral coil oxygenators have been largely superseded by polymethylpentene oxygenators.

Cannulation

Cannulation for VA-ECMO may be either central or peripheral. Failure to wean from CPB is an indication for central VA-ECMO, with the (RA $\rightarrow$ aorta) CPB cannulae being used for up to 72 h. If longer-term support is required, the patient will typically require VAD or peripheral ECMO support.

Peripheral VA-ECMO usually involves cannulation of a femoral or internal jugular vein and a femoral artery. Peripheral (femoro-jugular) cannulation is usually used for VV-ECMO. The availability of specialized cannulae (e.g. the Avalon Elite™ bi-caval dual-lumen catheter) in a range of sizes (e.g. 16–31Fr) has made peripheral cannulation a relatively straightforward bedside procedure. The distal (inlet) end is placed in the IVC, the proximal (inlet) is placed in the SVC and the outlet in the lower RA.

Management

Anticoagulation

Unless contraindicated, an infusion of unfractionated heparin is used for anticoagulation. The ACT is

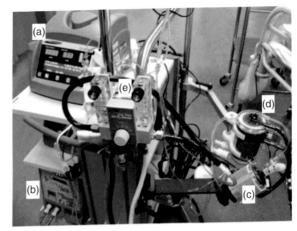

Figure 57.5 An example of an ECMO system employing a Levitronix Centrimag blood pump. (a) Pump control console. (b) Hot water supply for heat exchanger. (c) Disposable pump head mounted on pump motor. (d) Oxygenator with inbuilt heat exchanger. (e) Sweep gas blender.

maintained at 180–240 s. Thrombocytopenia and hemolysis are inevitable consequences of extracorporeal support. Erythrocytes and platelet transfusion are required to maintain a hematocrit of 40–45% and a platelet count $>80 \times 10^9 \, l^{-1}$.

Mechanical ventilation

Low tidal volume (<5 ml kg^{-1}), low rate (10 min^{-1}), low FiO_2 (<0.6) ventilation with PEEP (5–10 cmH_2O) is usually continued during ECMO support. This reduces the risk of barotrauma, volutrauma and pulmonary atelectasis.

Weaning

The timing of weaning from ECMO is largely dictated by the patient's clinical state. Weaning VA-ECMO support removes both respiratory and cardiac support. The patient should be hemodynamically stable with MAP >60 mmHg on minimal inotropic support and have adequate tissue perfusion (i.e. normal lactate, $SvO_2 >60\%$). After a bolus of heparin (5000 units), the pump flow rate is reduced in steps while TEE is used to assess cardiac function. Decannulation may be considered if the patient remains stable for a period of 60 min.

The effects of weaning VV-ECMO can be replicated by simply reducing "sweep" gas flow to the ECMO oxygenator. In adults, stable hemodynamics and acceptable ABGs on sweep gas FiO_2 0.3 are a prerequisite for considering weaning. Minimal acceptable ABGs without VV-ECMO on FiO_2 0.6 and at a respiratory

Table 57.5 Dealing with gross ECMO air entrainment (refer to Figure 57.6)

1. Clamp arterial line

2. Clamp venous line

3. Stop pump

4. Run crystalloid (e.g. Hartmann's solution) into circuit

5. Drain circuit in to empty 1000 ml IV infusion bag placed on floor (Purge Bag)

6. Remove disposable pump head from motor unit

7. Manually manipulate pump head to encourage air towards the oxygenator

Once air has drained onto the bag on the floor

8. Close tubing to IV infusion bag

9. Open the A–V bridge tubing (this connects the arterial and venous lines)

10. Place the pump back in the motor and recirculate blood at 3000 RPM

11. If no air seen, close the bridge and remove the clamps from the arterial and venous lines
Set pump speed at what it was before the incident

12. If air is detected, do not remove clamps and follow steps 3 to 9 again

13. Contact on-call perfusionist

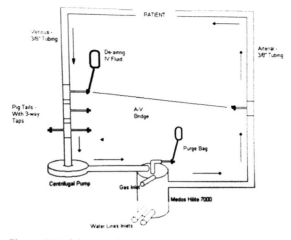

Figure 57.6 Schematic diagram of extracorporeal membrane oxygenation (ECMO) system incorporating an arteriovenous bypass to facilitate de-airing.

rate of 15 min^{-1} are: PaO_2 >8 kPa (60 mmHg) and $PaCO_2$ <6.5 kPa (50 mmHg).

Prevention and treatment of air entrainment

The very real and ever-present risk of air entrainment during ECMO support dictates the need for both emergency protocols and ongoing staff training. It should be borne in mind that indwelling venous catheters and hemofilters connected to the ECMO system are potential sources of air entrainment. A simplified treatment protocol for dealing with gross air entrainment is shown in Table 57.5 and Figure 57.6.

Key points

- Femoro-femoral CPB can be established under local anesthesia *before* induction of anesthesia.

- Inserting lines for invasive monitoring in a "pulse-less" VAD recipient can be very problematic.

- The use of ECMO to manage low cardiac output state post cardiac surgery is increasing.

Further reading

Bartakke AA, Peek GJ. Extracorporeal membrane oxygenation. In Ghosh S, Falter F, Cook DJ (Eds.), *Cardiopulmonary Bypass*. Cambridge: Cambridge University Press; 2009. pp. 176–86.

Kirklin JK, Naftel DC, Kormos RL, *et al.* Third INTERMACS Annual Report: the evolution of destination therapy in the United States. *J Heart Lung Transplant* 2011; **30**(2): 115–23.

Rao V, Oz MC, Flannery MA, Catanese KA, Argenziano M, Naka Y. Revised screening scale to predict survival after insertion of a left ventricular assist device. *J Thorac Cardiovasc Surg* 2003; **125**(4): 855–62.

Saravanan P, Arrowsmith JE. Extracorporeal circulation in the intensive care unit. In Robert R, Honoré P, Bastien O (Eds.), *Circulations extra-corporelles en réanimation*. Paris: Elsevier; 2006. pp. 421–35.

Thunberg CA, Gaitan BD, Arabia FA, Cole JD, Grigore AM. Ventricular Assist Devices Today and Tomorrow. *J Cardiothorac Vasc Anesth* 2010; **24**(4): 656–80.

58 Coagulopathy and blood conservation

David Cardone and Andrew A. Klein

Coagulation pathways

Models of coagulation

Coagulation is a complex and dynamic process involving enzymatic and cellular mechanisms, vascular and inflammatory processes and humoral responses. A new cell-based model of coagulation – involving initiation, amplification and propagation phases – has been proposed as an alternative to the classic model of extrinsic and intrinsic coagulation pathways leading to a final common pathway (Figure 58.1). The new model (Figure 58.2) attempts to account for the true "in vivo" complexities of the coagulation system.

The initiation phase of coagulation is triggered by vessel injury and exposure of subendothelial tissue factor. Circulating factor VIIa binds with exposed tissue factor to form a complex that activates factors IX and X in the presence of platelets.

The amplification phase occurs when platelet-bound Xa converts prothrombin to thrombin, which in turn activates platelets and factors XI, VIII and V.

The propagation phase leads to conversion of prothrombin to massive amounts of thrombin (the so-called thrombin burst) at the platelet surface. Thrombin then converts fibrinogen to fibrin, which is deposited at the site of vessel injury.

The arterial and venous circulations have differing hemostatic requirements. The high-pressure arterial system requires a rapid platelet-dominated hemostatic response at the time of vessel injury to prevent

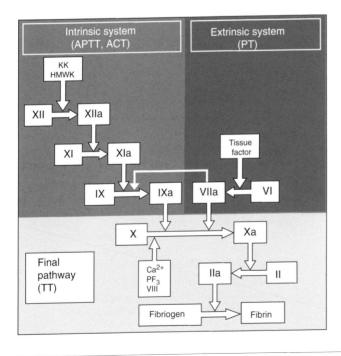

Figure 58.1 Simplified representation of the coagulation system. The intrinsic and extrinsic systems result in the formation of thrombin (factor IIa) and fibrin. APTT, activated partial thromboplastin time; PT, prothrombin time; ACT, activated clotting time; KK, kallikrein; HMWK, high-molecular-weight kininogen; PF3, platelet factor III.

Core Topics in Cardiac Anesthesia, Second Edition, ed. Jonathan H. Mackay and Joseph E. Arrowsmith. Published by Cambridge University Press. © Cambridge University Press 2012.

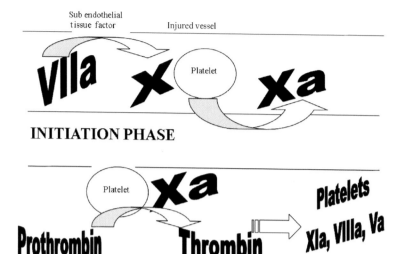

INITIATION PHASE

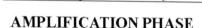

AMPLIFICATION PHASE

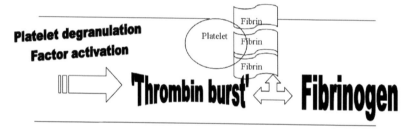

PROPOGATION PHASE

Figure 58.2 The cell-based model of coagulation.

significant blood loss. In contrast, hemostasis in the low-pressure venous system relies more on thrombin generation than platelets. These differences explain why antiplatelet agents are used to prevent coronary arterial thrombosis, whereas heparin and warfarin are used to prevent venous thrombosis.

Platelets

Platelets are disc-shaped enucleate cells derived from megakaryocytes, which circulate for approximately 7–10 days. They contain two types of granules (Table 58.1).

The classic platelet response consists of three steps: adhesion, activation and aggregation. In the presence of vascular injury and exposure of the subendothelium, circulating von Willebrand factor (vWF) binds glycoprotein Ib (GPIb) on the platelet surface and rapidly slows the platelet, tethering it to the subendothelium ("adhesion"). The vWF–GPIb interaction

causes platelet activation, resulting in degranulation and a conformational change in the platelet surface GPIIb/IIIa receptor. Platelet GPIIb/IIIa–vWF binding is somewhat stronger than the initial GP interaction and further embeds the platelets, forming a layer of activated platelets over the injured subendothelium. Activated platelets release ADP and serotonin from dense granules and thromboxane A_2 from the cytosol, resulting in recruitment and binding of additional platelets via GPIIb/IIIa–vWF or GPIIb/IIIa–fibrinogen interactions ("aggregation"). Once a stable platelet plug is formed the next stage is deposition of fibrin to conclude clot formation.

Endogenous anticoagulants and fibrinolysis

The extent and location of clot formation are determined by the delicate balance between endothelium-dependent (i.e. endogenous) coagulation

Table 58.1 The characteristics of platelets

General		2–3 μm diameter Nonadhesive surface (if undamaged) No nucleus – contain RNA but no DNA Half-life 9–10 days
Surface receptors	Glycoprotein (GP)	GP Ib: binds vWF GP Ia/IIa: binds collagen GP IIb/IIIa: binds fibrinogen and fibronectin
	Other	Thrombin, thromboxane, serotonin, α2-adrenergic
Contents	α granules	Procoagulants: PF4, βTG, factor V Anticoagulants: plasminogen Adhesive proteins: vWF, fibrinogen Growth factors: PDGF
	β granules	ATP, ADP, serotonin

vWF, von Willebrand factor; PF4, platelet factor 4; βTG, beta thromboglobulin; PDGF, platelet-derived growth factor.

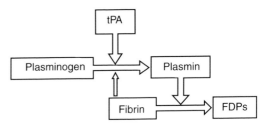

Figure 58.3 Fibrinolysis. The conversion of plasminogen to plasmin is catalyzed by activators such as tissue and urokinase plasminogen activators (tPA and uPA respectively). The rate of conversion is increased 500-fold in the presence of fibrin. FDPs, fibrin degradation (split) products.

and anticoagulation systems. The interaction of these complex cellular mechanisms permits a rapid but measured response to vascular injury, whilst avoiding spontaneous thrombus formation, excessive thrombus formation and prolonged hemorrhage.

Circulating anticoagulants include antithrombin, which inactivates thrombin, and activated protein C. Endothelium-derived anticoagulants, which act primarily on platelets, include NO and prostacyclin.

Fibrinolysis involves the proteolytic degradation of fibrin by plasmin. During clot formation, factor Xa and thrombin stimulate endothelial cells to release tissue plasminogen activator (t-PA) and urokinase plasminogen activator (u-PA). The balance between coagulation and fibrinolysis is determined by the rate at which plasminogen is converted to plasmin under the influence of t-PA and u-PA (Figure 58.3).

The lysine analogs – tranexamic acid and ε-aminocaproic acid – bind to plasminogen and inhibit its binding to fibrin, thus impairing fibrinolysis and reducing bleeding (Figure 58.4).

Coagulopathy in cardiac surgery

The coagulopathy associated with cardiac surgery is multifactorial in origin. The major hemostatic disturbances involve the coagulation, fibrinolytic and inflammatory enzyme cascades. Effective management requires an understanding of the factors involved. Contributory factors include the patient, surgery and CPB system (Table 58.2).

Bioincompatibility of the components of the CPB circuit results in "contact activation" and generation of inflammatory mediators (e.g. kallikrein, bradykinin) and procoagulants (e.g. factor XIIa) leading to significant thrombin and fibrin generation. CPB-activated endothelial cells induce fibrinolysis by release of t-PA and subsequent plasmin generation. Activation and sequestration of platelets on the subendothelium, CPB circuit and circulating monocytes causes thrombocytopenia. Complement activation of leukocyte activation causes cell-mediated fibrinolysis.

Diagnosis

The diagnosis of coagulopathy is usually made on the basis of clinical suspicion and the results of "near-patient" or "point-of-care" tests. Traditional laboratory tests (platelet count, APTT, PT, fibrinogen, and thrombin time; Table 58.3) may be used to guide management, but their value is often limited by the time taken to obtain results.

"Point-of-care" assays of coagulation include:

- activated clotting time
- thromboelastography (TEG)
- platelet function analyzers.

Perioperative use of blood components and the associated costs can be reduced by an appropriate coagulation management system. Algorithms for transfusion based on point-of-care testing permit goal-directed therapy of coagulation disorders.

Table 58.2 Causes of coagulopathy after cardiac surgery. The risk of coagulopathic bleeding is increased by endocarditis and prolonged CPB

Quantitative platelet problem	Destruction, hemodilution, sequestration, activation, consumption, use of cell salvage
Qualitative platelet problem	Damage, heparin, aspirin, clopidogrel, GP-IIb/IIIa inhibitors, NSAIDs, uremia, hypothermia, hypofibrinogenemia
Coagulation factor deficiency	Hemodilution, consumption, liver disease, congenital
Altered enzyme kinetics	Hypothermia
Anemia	Hemorrhage, hemodilution, hemolysis
Anticoagulants	Residual heparin, excessive protamine
Altered factor clearance	Hepatic and renal hypoperfusion, hypothermia

Table 58.3 Routine perioperative coagulation tests

Tests	Normal values
Platelets	
Platelet count	$150–400 \times 10^9 \ l^{-1}$
Coagulation	
Activated clotting time (ACT)	90–140 s
Prothrombin time (PT)	12–15 s (INR 1.0–1.3)
Activated partial thromboplastin time (APTT)	35–45 s
Thrombin time (TT)	<14 s
Fibrinogen	$>2 \ g \ l^{-1}$
Fibrinolysis	
Fibrin(ogen) split products	$<10 \ mg \ l^{-1}$
d-Dimers	Normally absent

INR, international normalized ratio.

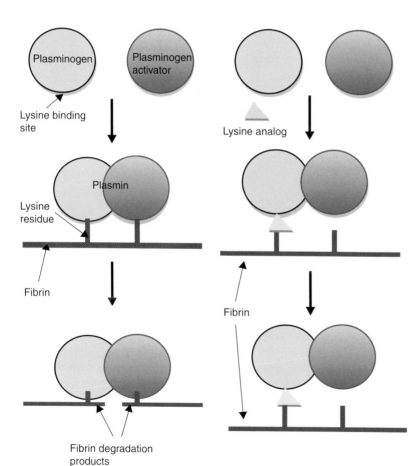

Figure 58.4 Mode of action of lysine analogs.

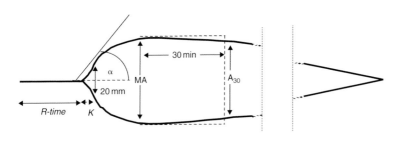

Figure 58.5 The thromboelastogram and derived parameters.

Parameter	Comments	Normal values
R	Reaction time: Time from start of the trace until oscillatory amplitude reaches 1mm Analogous to whole-blood clotting time Prolonged by anticoagulants and clotting factor deficiencies	6–8 min
K	The time from initiation of oscillatory movement to until oscillatory amplitude reaches 20mm A measure of the speed of clot formation Prolonged by thrombocytopaenia and hypofibrinogenaemia	4–6 min
α-angle	The angle of the tangent from R to K Reduced by thrombocytopaenia and hypofibrinogenaemia	50–60°
R + K	Sum of R time and K time represents the coagulation time	10–12 min
MA	Maximum amplitude: the point at which rotational torque is greatest Represents strength of clot formation Reduced by platelet dysfunction, hypofibrinogenaemia and heparin	50–60 mm
A_{30} and A_{60}	The rotational torque amplitude 30 and 60min after maximum amplitude reached A measure of clot stability and lysis	
MA/A_{60}	Whole blood clot lysis index Reduced by fibrinolysis	>0.85

Activated clotting time

ACT measures the integrity of intrinsic and common pathways. Activators (celite or kaolin) are added to whole blood to initiate coagulation. The major clinical application relates to assessment of heparin therapy during and after CPB. ACT measurement is simple, quick, inexpensive and reproducible.

Thromboelastography

TEG is a dynamic test of coagulation and fibrinolysis that assesses the viscoelastic properties of whole blood. It measures the speed, quality and stability of clot formation. Whole blood is placed in a cuvette, then a pin is lowered into the blood. Alternating rotational force is applied to the cuvette, and as clot formation occurs, the torque is transmitted from the pin to a torsion wire. Then as clot lyses and the fibrin strands linking clot and pin break down, the movement of pin and wire is reduced (i.e. torque reduces). The change in torsion over time is graphically displayed, and a number of parameters are derived (Figure 58.5).

The addition of reagents, such as heparinase, to the reaction cuvette allows detection of coagulation

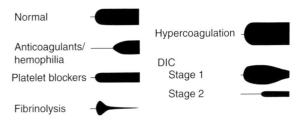

Figure 58.6 Normal and abnormal thromboelastograms.

abnormalities that may be masked by heparin. Many commercially available systems allow two or more samples (i.e. with and without heparinase) to be analysed simultaneously. This allows coagulation to be assessed during CPB. Following protamine administration, the presence of residual heparin produces a difference in the TEG R-times that is usually obvious within 10–12 min. Normal and abnormal TEGs are shown in Figure 58.6.

Platelet function analyzers

Reduced platelet function has been demonstrated within 20 min of the onset of CPB. Traditional laboratory platelet tests are purely quantitative, giving no indication of their functional state or contribution to coagulation.

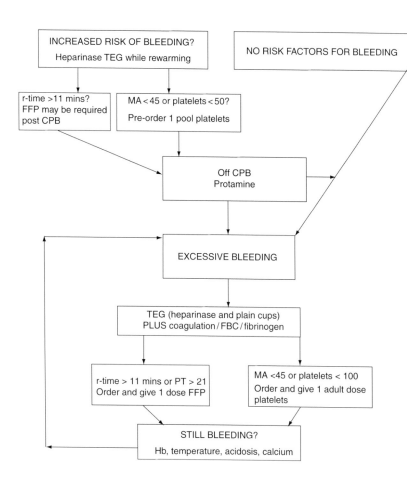

INCREASED RISK OF BLEEDING?
Heparinase TEG while rewarming

NO RISK FACTORS FOR BLEEDING

r-time >11 mins?
FFP may be required
post CPB

MA < 45 or platelets < 50?
Pre-order 1 pool platelets

Off CPB
Protamine

EXCESSIVE BLEEDING

TEG (heparinase and plain cups)
PLUS coagulation / FBC / fibrinogen

r-time > 11 mins or PT > 21
Order and give 1 dose FFP

MA <45 or platelets < 100
Order and give 1 adult dose
platelets

STILL BLEEDING?
Hb, temperature, acidosis, calcium

Figure 58.7 Protocol for using laboratory and point-of-care coagulation testing to guide blood component therapy. CCP, critical care (nurse) practitioner.

Although platelet function analyzers have existed for some time, it is only recently that systems suitable for "point-of-care" use have become available, including multiple electrode aggregometry-based devices.

Management

Blood product transfusion algorithms

Appropriate blood product administration based on objective measures of coagulation and locally derived algorithms is desirable. Point-of-care coagulation devices allow rapid assessment of coagulation and early therapeutic intervention (Figure 58.7).

Management of hypothermia

Coagulopathy and bleeding are exacerbated by hypothermia. Preventive measures should be made to ensure normothermia after CPB. These include adequate rewarming during CPB, warming of all intravenous fluids and use of active patient-warming devices (e.g. force air warmers).

Perioperative blood conservation

Blood transfusion is associated with increased morbidity and mortality, the latter being linearly related to the number of units transfused. Blood transfusion has many potential serious adverse effects. Immunological effects include hemolytic reactions (acute and delayed), immunomodulation and immunosuppression. Non-immunological effects include transmission of viruses and bacteria, increased infective complications and transfusion-related acute lung injury (TRALI). The reduction or even elimination of transfusion remains the subject of much research.

The most important blood conservation measures are, arguably, in the hands of the surgeon – careful surgery, attention to hemostasis and prompt arrest of hemorrhage. Despite extensive investigation, the efficacy of oxygen-carrying blood substitutes is unproven and none have entered clinical practice. While the practice of using pre-donated autologous blood is declining, perioperative cell salvage is increasing in popularity. A successful blood conservation program requires a multimodal approach supported by evidence-based guidelines, protocols, repeated audit and education. The Society of Thoracic Surgeons and Society of Cardiovascular Anesthesiologists have published comprehensive evidenced-based guidelines on blood conservation in cardiac surgery.

Pharmacological therapies

Hemostatic drugs can be used as both prophylaxis and treatment. These include the antifibrinolytics (tranexamic acid, ε-aminocaproic acid and aprotinin), desmopressin, recombinant factor VIIa, prothrombin complex concentrate and fibrinogen concentrate (see Chapter 11). Future pharmacological therapies aimed at reducing bleeding in the cardiac surgical patient may include individual factor replacement.

Prothrombin complex concentrate (PCC) is now licensed for warfarin reversal and should be used instead of fresh frozen plasma when warfarinized patients require urgent or emergency surgery. However, there are a number of published case series reporting successful use of PCC in bleeding secondary to coagulopathy caused by clotting factor deficiency, diagnosed by prolonged prothrombin time (laboratory) or R-time (TEG), and this is the subject of a number of ongoing trials in cardiac surgery.

Fibrinogen concentrate may also be used in place of cryoprecipitate when plasma fibrinogen levels are low (i.e. <1 g l^{-1}). There is some recent evidence that targeting higher fibrinogen concentration (e.g. > 1.5 g l^{-1}) may improve platelet function by promoting the formation of more stable platelet plugs and thus reduce postoperative bleeding, but the results of further research in this area are awaited.

Erythropoietin

Recombinant human erythropoietin (rEPO) has been used to stimulate erythropoiesis prior to preoperative autologous blood donation (PABD) and in refractory anemia. The effect of rEPO is rapid, yielding the equivalent of one unit of blood per week. The optimal dose to support a PABD program is unknown and its cost effectiveness is unproven. Supplementation with iron, vitamin B$_{12}$ and folate may also be necessary.

Autologolous blood transfusion

There are three types of autologous transfusion: preoperative blood donation, acute normovolemic

hemodilution and red cell salvage (intraoperative and postoperative).

Preoperative autologous blood donation

PABD involves the donation of one or more units of blood, 2–3 weeks before surgery. The blood is stored in a conventional blood bank, and is available for transfusion during or after surgery. Current recommendations limit the use of PABD to patients with rare blood groups, for whom allogeneic blood is difficult to obtain, and patients who refuse to consent to allogeneic transfusion.

Contraindications to PABD include: evidence of infection and risk of bacteremia, aortic stenosis, unstable angina, left main stem coronary artery disease, MI or CVA in the preceding 6 months, cyanotic heart disease and uncontrolled hypertension. Acceptable hemoglobin concentration ranges are required before considering PABD (males 11.0–14.5 g dl^{-1}, females 13.0–14.5 g dl^{-1}). Questions remain about cost effectiveness and safety.

Prophylactic iron is not recommended for iron replete patients undergoing PABD. Iron supplementation is, however, recommended for rEPO treated patients undergoing PABD. Iron deficiency – and importantly any underlying cause – should be investigated and treated before considering PABD.

Acute normovolemic hemodilution

Acute normovolemic hemodilution (ANH) is an autologous blood collection technique that involves the removal of whole blood immediately before surgery, with simultaneous crystalloid or colloid replacement to maintain normovolemia. Blood is collected in standard (CPDA1) blood bags; it remains in the operating room and is reinfused at an appropriate time during or after surgery. The rationale for ANH is that a lower hematocrit results in the loss of fewer red blood cells per unit volume of blood loss. The target hematocrit is ~25–30%.

Patients with a preoperative hemoglobin concentration ≥ 12 g dl^{-1} undergoing surgery with a high likelihood of transfusion may be suitable for ANH. The putative benefits of ANH include reduction of both costs and the risks associated with PABD. In addition PABD blood contains functional platelets and coagulation factors which will aid hemostasis. ANH appears to modestly reduce bleeding and the volume of allogeneic blood required.

Red cell salvage

Red cell salvage is a term that covers a range of techniques involving recovery and reinfusion of blood from the operative field. Cell salvage can be performed both during and after surgery. To remove non-cellular matter prior to reinfusion, some devices use centrifugal washing of the salvaged blood, while others use a countercurrent system similar to that used in hemofiltration. Processing shed blood in this way invariably removes platelets and plasma proteins, and contributes to a dilutional coagulopathy. The washing process can also lead to hemolysis, especially if suction pressures are not carefully regulated or the washing process is accelerated. Relative contraindications include the potential for aspiration of malignant cells, the presence of infection, gross bacterial contamination of the surgical field and the presence of other contaminants.

The majority of trials have demonstrated that cell salvage reduces blood transfusion in off-pump and in complex cardiac surgical procedures. In contrast, routine use of cell salvage in routine surgery (e.g. CABG, isolated valve surgery) has not been shown to reduce blood transfusion in the setting of a vigorous blood conservation program.

Blood recovered from surgical drains in the postoperative period is of variable quality – it is often dilute, partially hemolyzed and defibrinated, and may contain high concentrations of cytokines. The direct reinfusion of unwashed shed mediastinal blood is not recommended and may cause harm.

Surgical techniques

Off-pump CABG (OPCAB) surgery and other minimally invasive surgical techniques have obvious potential benefits in terms of reduced tissue trauma and bleeding. Off-pump surgery may avoid the need for full heparinization and the need for CPB. Randomized controlled trials have confirmed that, when compared to conventional CABG surgery, OPCAB results in reduced postoperative bleeding and allogeneic transfusion requirements. It is possible that similar results can be expected for minimal-access cardiac surgery; however, evidence from large randomized controlled trials is not available.

Topical hemostatic agents

Fibrin sealants are composed of human fibrinogen, human or bovine thrombin, or human factor VIII and bovine aprotinin. They are applied to aid hemostasis at sites of cannulation, laceration, and along suture lines.

Perfusion techniques

Perfusion strategies to reduce bleeding and transfusion requirements include use of biocompatible surface modification, closed venous reservoirs and mini-bypass circuits (see Chapter 55), and retrograde autologous priming.

Heparin anticoagulation management may have a significant impact on bleeding and transfusion requirements. There is anecdotal evidence that high-dose heparin (>500 units kg^{-1}) may better inhibit thrombin generation and reduce allogeneic blood transfusion in high-risk patients undergoing prolonged CPB.

Positive end-expiratory pressure

Increased end-expiratory airway pressure (PEEP) exerts mechanical pressure on the myocardium and may limit microvascular bleeding after surgery. A trial of therapeutic PEEP in the postoperative period to reduce excessive bleeding is not unreasonable. When PEEP is effective, the benefits are apparent within an hour. However, prophylactic PEEP to reduce hemorrhage is not recommended.

Key points

- Antiplatelet agents are used to prevent coronary *arterial* thrombosis, whereas heparin and warfarin are used to prevent *venous* thrombosis.
- Point-of-care testing and transfusion algorithms are both efficacious and cost-effective in limiting blood product transfusion.
- Perioperative cell salvage is of proven benefit in OPCAB and complex cardiac surgery.
- Clinical audit and education can be used to modify institutional practice and the behavior of individual physicians.

Further reading

Ferraris VA, Brown JR, Despotis GJ, *et al.* 2011 update to the Society of Thoracic Surgeons and the Society of Cardiovascular Anesthesiologists blood conservation clinical practice guidelines. *Ann Thorac Surg* 2011; **91**(3): 944–82.

Henry DA, Carless PA, Moxey AJ, *et al.* Anti-fibrinolytic use for minimising perioperative allogeneic blood transfusion. *Cochrane Database Syst Rev* 2011; **3**: CD001886.

Perry DJ, Fitzmaurice DA, Kitchen S, Mackie IJ, Mallett S. Point-of-care testing in haemostasis. *Br J Haematol* 2010; **150**(5): 501–14.

Chapter

59

The systemic inflammatory response to cardiopulmonary bypass

R. Clive Landis and Ravi J. De Silva

All patients undergoing cardiac surgery with CPB will, to some extent, exhibit features of the systemic inflammatory response syndrome and ~2% of these may suffer morbidity and mortality as a consequence. Surgical trauma, endotoxemia, the CPB system and ischemia-reperfusion injury (IRI) all contribute to the development of SIRS. While for most patients this produces mild and transient fever and diffuse tissue edema, SIRS can occasionally cause pathologic hemodynamic instability, coagulopathy and acute multiorgan system failure (MOF). This chapter focuses on the pathophysiology of SIRS, the reasons why some patients develop serious complications and interventions to reduce the incidence and severity of SIRS.

Definition

SIRS in the context of cardiac surgery has never been formally defined. It borrows its definition from the 1992 American College of Chest Physicians and Society of Critical Care Medicine Consensus Conference (Table 59.1).

The diagnostic criteria do not indicate causation and cannot, therefore, be used to guide therapy. The combined insult of operative stress and exposure of blood to the CPB circuit simultaneously activates multiple host defensive pathways (Table 59.2). While these responses are appropriate and desirable in the context of a localized injury or infection, they are not desirable systemically and contribute to morbidity and mortality.

The use of critical care criteria to diagnose SIRS may have led to an underestimate of the prevalence of the systemic inflammatory response in cardiac surgery and some degree of complacency. If we put aside the diagnostic criteria for a moment and consider instead whether systemic activation of host response

Table 59.1 Clinical diagnosis of the systemic inflammatory response syndrome

SIRS is diagnosed when two or more of the following are present:

Fever >38°C or temperature <36°C

Heart rate >90 beats per minute (not appropriate in children)

Respiratory rate >20 breaths per minute or a $PaCO_2$ <4.3 kPa (32 mmHg)

White blood cell count $<4 \times 10^9 \, l^{-1}$ or $>12 \times 10^9 \, l^{-1}$ or >10% bands

Table 59.2 Pathways that comprise the systemic inflammatory response

Complement	Coagulation	Kinins
Fibrinolysis	Hemolysis	Leukocye activation
Oxidative stress	Chemokines	Cyctokines

pathways (as defined in Table 59.2) has occurred, then we find overwhelming evidence in the literature for activation of all of these pathways, not just in occasional patients but broadly across the whole surgical population. It is therefore more appropriate to think of the systemic inflammatory response as occurring in *all patients*, linked to a range of mild, moderate to severe clinical outcomes, with frank SIRS and MOF at the extreme end of the spectrum being thankfully rare.

Pathophysiology

Contact activation

Blood–gas interfaces and exposure of blood to the foreign surfaces of the extracorporeal circuit result

Core Topics in Cardiac Anesthesia, Second Edition, ed. Jonathan H. Mackay and Joseph E. Arrowsmith. Published by Cambridge University Press. © Cambridge University Press 2012.

in activation of three interconnected plasma protease pathways, namely the kinin–kallikrein pathway, the fibrinolytic-coagulation pathway and the complement system.

Intrinsic coagulation and kinins

When bound to anionic surfaces, inert Hageman factor (factor XII) becomes factor XIIa and factor XIIf. In the presence of high-molecular-weight kininogen (HMWK), factor XIIa converts prekallikrein to kallikrein (KK), and generates more factor XIIa via a positive feedback mechanism. KK cleaves surface-bound HMWK to yield bradykinin, a potent vasodilator that promotes smooth muscle contraction and capillary permeability. This potentiates neutrophil-mediated endothelial permeability causing tissue edema. KK and factor XIIa cause neutrophil activation, resulting in reactive oxygen metabolite formation and neutrophil aggregation (Figure 59.1).

In the presence of KK and HMWK, factor XIIa cleaves factor XI to XIa, initiating the intrinsic pathway (also known as the contact pathway) of coagulation, eventually resulting in formation of thrombin (factor IIa). The extrinsic pathway of coagulation is also triggered during cardiac surgery when tissue factor, a membrane protein found subendothelially, is exposed to blood during surgery. Tissue factor acts with activated factor VIIa and phospholipid to promote activation of factor X to Xa, the entry into the common pathway of coagulation, again ending in production of thrombin. Thrombin's primary role in the final common pathway of coagulation is to promote formation of the hemostatic plug through conversion of fibrinogen to fibrin and to activate

platelets in consolidating the thrombus. Yet, thrombin is also a major crossing point into inflammatory pathways as a potent activator of endothelial cells and platelets via the protease activated receptor family.

Fibrinolytic pathway

Under normal conditions, fibrin clots formed at the site of surgical incision are eventually dispersed by plasmin. Bradykinin production during CPB promotes endothelial secretion of tissue plasminogen activator (tPA), which converts plasminogen to plasmin. In the presence of HMWK, KK cleaves pro-urokinase to yield urokinase. Urokinase activates urokinase plasminogen activator (uPA), resulting in increased plasmin formation. In the presence of plasmin, fibrin is proteolytically digested into pro-inflammatory fibrin split (degradation) products (FDPs). These inhibit further fibrin production and are implicated in platelet and endothelial dysfunction. Plasmin activation of factor XII completes a positive feedback loop (Figure 59.2).

Complement system

The complement system consists of over 20 plasma proteins. The host-defence functions include: chemotaxis, inflammation, opsonization, neutralization, lymphocyte activation, degranulation (mast cells, basophils and eosinophils) and lytic complex formation. Complement activation, leading to C3 cleavage, may occur by either "classical" or "alternative" pathways (Figure 59.3).

Cleavage of C3 leads to the production of C3a and C3b, which stimulate the release of histamine and other inflammatory mediators from mast cells, basophils and eosinophils, leading to increased vascular

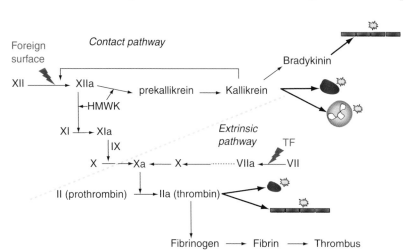

Figure 59.1 Contact activation of kinin and coagulation pathways. Also indicated is the extrinsic pathway of coagulation and points for cross-over into inflammatory activation. The interaction of plasma proteases during contact activation. (HMWK=high molecular weight kininogen; TF= tissue factor, points at which inflammatory activation occurs for platelets, endothelium and neutrophils are indicated)

375

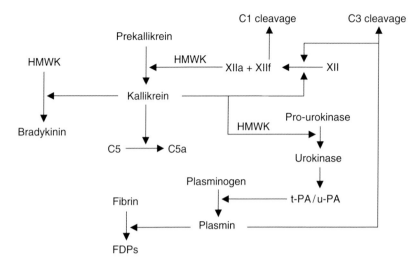

Figure 59.2 The interaction of plasma proteases during contact activation. HMWK = high molecular weight kininogen; t-PA = tissue plasminogen activator; u-PA = urokinase plasminogen activator, FDPs = fibrin degradation products.

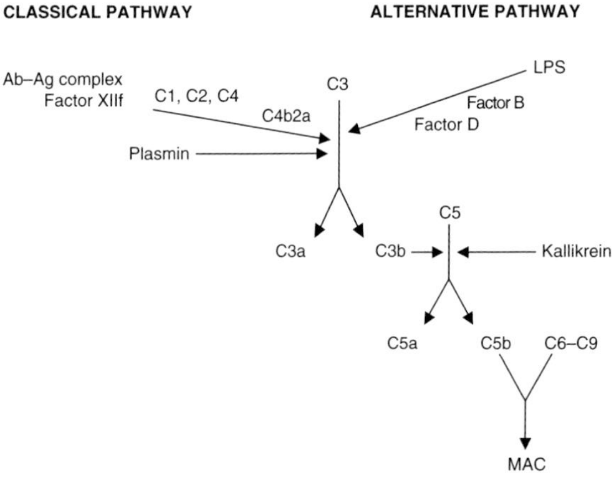

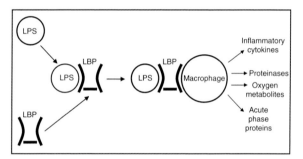

Figure 59.4 The role of endotoxemia in the inflammatory response to CPB. Circulating lipopolysaccharide (LPS) is bound to lipopolysaccharide binding protein (LBP). This complex activates macrophages, resulting in tumour necrosis factor (TNF) and protein kinase release.

Figure 59.3 Activation of the complement pathway. Factor XIIf (via C1 activation), plasmin and kallikrein can activate complement. C3a and C5a are so-called anaphylatoxins. MAC = membrane attack complex.

permeability and smooth muscle contraction. In addition, C3a is thought to cause tachycardia, coronary vasoconstriction and reduced cardiac contractility. C5a acts as a powerful chemo-attractant for neutrophils, as well as stimulating neutrophil aggregation, adhesion and activation. Due to their potent actions, C3a and C5a are also known as anaphylatoxins. C3b interacts with membrane-bound C5b and components C6–C9 to form the membrane attack complex, which has the ability to activate platelets and "punch" holes in bacterial cell walls.

Although CPB results in complement activation by the alternative pathway, protamine–heparin complexes may also activate complement by the classical pathway. Plasma levels of the products of complement activation rise within 2 minutes of the onset of CPB, and show a second peak after removal of the cross clamp and during rewarming. Levels return to normal 18–48 hours after uncomplicated surgery.

Endotoxemia

Plasma levels of endotoxins – lipopolysaccharides (LPS) derived from the cell membranes of Gram-negative bacteria – are known to rise during CPB. Splanchnic vasoconstriction leading to gut mucosal ischemia and bacterial translocation make the gut the most likely source of endotoxemia during CPB. The magnitude of endotoxin release is highly variable and may be related to CPB duration. Pulsatile CPB may be associated with lower levels of endotoxemia than non-pulsatile CPB.

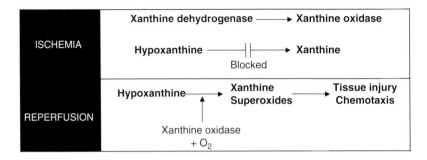

Figure 59.5 Hypoxanthine and xanthine oxidase accumulation during ischemia results in excessive superoxide anion production during reperfusion.

Once in the circulation, LPS is bound to LPS-binding protein (LBP), levels of which dramatically increase during endotoxemia. LPS–LBP complexes are a 1000 times more potent at activating macrophages than LPS alone. LPS-activated macrophages release a host of proinflammatory mediators, including acute-phase proteins (tumor necrosis factor alpha and interleukin [IL]-6), inflammatory cytokines (IL-1 and monocyte chemoattractant protein-1) and cytodestructive mediators (matrix metalloproteinases and reactive oxygen metabolites). Circulating LPS may synergize with local factors to activate vascular endothelium, such as ischemia reperfusion injury, malperfusion or physical handling injury, leading to leukocyte diapedesis at susceptible sites, tissue destruction and organ injury (Figure 59.4).

Ischemia–reperfusion injury

Myocardial and lung ischemia during CPB can be partially offset by the use of systemic hypothermia and cardioplegia. IRI describes tissue injury that paradoxically occurs after resumption of normal tissue perfusion following a period of ischemia. Neutrophils cause damage during IRI by the production of toxic substances during the metabolism of oxygen and the secretion of proteolytic enzymes from their granules. In order to cause this damage, activated neutrophils must first exit from the circulation through a sequential process of contact and adhesion with activated endothelium, extravasation and migration into the affected tissue. Intercellular adhesion molecules (ICAMs), selectins and chemoattractants, such as IL-8, all play an important part in this process. The observation that IRI-induced tissue injury is markedly reduced in neutrophil-depleted animals suggests a pivotal role for the neutrophil. Neutrophil depletion appears to have a much greater impact on late IRI (i.e. 4 hours after reperfusion) than early IRI (<30

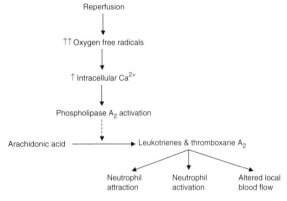

Figure 59.6 The role of products of arachidonic acid metabolism in neutrophil-mediated ischaemia-reperfusion injury.

minutes after reperfusion). This observation suggests a bimodal pattern of neutrophil involvement in this model, with early IRI occurring via a neutrophil-independent mechanism. Other cell types, such as mast cells, may in part mediate early IRI.

Reactive oxygen metabolites

Depletion of high-energy phosphates (i.e. adenosine triphosphate; ATP) in ischemic tissue leads to a build-up of reactive oxygen metabolites, such as hydrogen peroxide (H_2O_2), hypochlorous acid (HOCl) and the superoxide anion. Under normal conditions, hypoxanthine is oxidized to xanthine by xanthine dehydrogenase. In ischemic tissue, however, xanthine dehydrogenase is converted to xanthine oxidase and levels of hypoxanthine rise (Figure 59.5). Upon reperfusion, xanthine oxidase utilizes the now available oxygen to convert hypoxanthine to xanthine with the generation of large amounts of oxygen free radicals, which overwhelm endogenous scavenging systems and cause damage to cellular components. The resulting tissue injury leads to increased vascular permeability and chemotaxis.

377

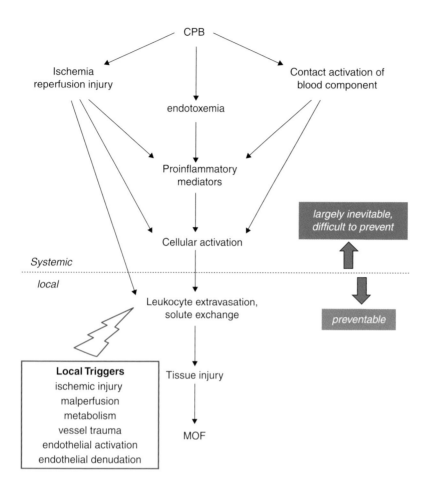

Figure 59.7 The concept of local and systemic triggers in the etiology of SIRS-induced organ injury.

Arachidonic acid metabolites

Arachidonic acid metabolites are generated as a consequence of free radical release and phospholipase A_2 activation (Figure 59.6). Leukotrienes and thromboxane A_2 result in further neutrophil attraction and activation, and produce local vasoconstriction.

Systemic factors + local triggers combine to cause organ injury

Figure 59.7 summarizes the interplay between endotoxemia, IR injury, contact-activation of plasma protease pathways in the CPB system, elaboration of inflammatory mediators and activation of inflammatory cells (leukocytes, endothelial cells and platelets) that results in the systemic inflammatory response. It is noteworthy that while concoction of this inflammatory soup in the systemic circulation is largely inevitable, translation into tissue injury and MOF is *not*

inevitable, but may be precipitated through perioperative procedures.

Gaining wider acceptance is the concept that the systemic release of inflammatory factors alone is insufficient to cause organ injury, and that local triggers are required (Figure 59.7). This concept allows interventions to be considered in two distinct categories: those aimed at reducing systemic activation (e.g. CPB system modifications and corticosteroids) or those aimed at protecting end-organs (e.g. changes in surgical or perfusion techniques to reduce endothelial denudation or anaerobic metabolism). The relative merit of each of these types of intervention is discussed.

Therapeutic intervention

Pharmacologic

The multifactorial etiology of SIRS invites the not unreasonable assumption that a combination of several interventions should form the basis of any therapeutic strategy. It is not surprising, therefore, that a large series of promising agents (e.g. anti-oxidant, anti-complement, anti-platelet and anti-protease) used as monotherapy have failed to demonstrate any clinical benefit. A recent evidence-based review has confirmed the paucity of clinically effective pharmacologic interventions. It was shown that in >96% of drug trials investigators were unable to link changes in biochemical markers of inflammation with clinical outcome. The use of corticosteroids and anti-fibrinolytic agents, however, is supported by Class IIa or equivocal (Class IIb) evidence.

It is ironic that the first meta-analysis of the anti-inflammatory properties of the protease inhibitor aprotinin should take place *after* the drug was withdrawn from the market. Putative anti-inflammatory benefits were promoted ahead of the scientific evidence base and ahead of more important clinical safety considerations, such as weight-based dosing. The rise and fall of aprotinin, therefore, stands as a cautionary tale for both clinicians and industry.

The challenges of designing a combinatorial intervention are undoubtedly formidable; large sample size, the high cost of clinical trials and the need for collaboration between companies. To mitigate such challenges a number of surrogate end-points of organ injury have been identified in the 2010 Outcomes Consensus Statement that are practical to measure and not too rare. These include clinical indicators as well as length of hospital stay and resource utilization. The harsh truth is that clinically effective pharmacologic interventions are still a long way off. The optimistic predictions made in the early 1990s have failed to materialize.

Circuit modification

The first evidence-based review carried out into the practice of CPB assigned Class IIa/Level B (see Appendix) to the use of modified CPB circuits, stating: "reduction of circuit surface area and the use of biocompatible surface–modified circuits might be useful-effective at attenuating the systemic inflammatory response to CPB and improving outcomes." The investigators in this study did not disaggregate data to produce individual recommendations for minimized circuits or specific types of biocompatible coating, limiting the practical usefulness of this recommendation. A detailed meta-analysis focussing on heparin-coated

circuits pointed out the limitations of such a coating strategy in reducing blood component activation, since the bulk of the intrinsic coagulation cascade occurs before the level of factor IIa (thrombin) – the main point at which heparin acts. The authors conclude that using biocompatible surfaces without other measures to limit blood activation resulted in limited clinical benefit.

New hope

End-organ injury results from the interaction between activation of systemic host defense pathways *and* localized injury to susceptible organs. Since many of the local triggers are generated inadvertently during surgery, the focus should be modification of surgical and perfusion practice.

Managing the aorta

There is considerable inter-center variation in the way the proximal aorta is managed during cardiac surgery. Rough palpation, "blind" cannulation and repeated cross-clamping of the proximal aorta may be associated with preventable atheroembolic complications. There is strong evidence that:

"In patients undergoing CPB at increased risk of adverse neurologic events, strong consideration should be given to intraoperative TEE or epiaortic ultrasonographic scanning of the aorta:

(1) to detect nonpalpable plaque (Class I, Level B) and (2) for reduction of cerebral emboli (Class IIa, Level B)."

Arterial line filters

To mitigate the effects of systemic embolization, arterial line filters have earned the strongest clinical recommendations:

"Arterial line filters should be incorporated in the CPB circuit to minimize the embolic load delivered to the patient. (Class I, Level A)."

Managing conduits

Saphenous vein grafts are particularly prone to endothelial denudation, which exposes the procoagulant subendothelium. It is the only variable independently associated with loss of graft patency in off-pump coronary revascularization.

Radial artery grafts, on the other hand, are prone to spasm and this may be linked to the type of harvest (open vs. closed harvest). Other practices such as saline distension or "pipe cleaning" of conduits should be avoided because they can disrupting the internal elastic lamina and causing gross endothelial denudation.

Despite the exquisite sensitivity of conduits to procurement injury, this critical aspect of surgery is often performed by the most junior and inexperienced members of the surgical team, and changes in surgical technique have failed to acknowledge the scientific evidence base. It cannot be emphasized sufficiently that the endothelium is the doorway that keeps the activated milieu in the systemic circulation away from the tissues and every effort must be made to preserve it intact. At a cellular level, endothelium should also be kept quiescent since it will otherwise promote solute exchange and trafficking of leukocytes into organs. Vascular endothelium in susceptible organ beds may become activated by periods of even modest ischemia and this should be taken into account when monitoring adequacy of perfusion in the tissues.

Adequacy of tissue perfusion

There is a growing appreciation that nomogram-derived CPB flow rates, which were originally established in healthy anesthetized volunteers, may not provide adequate tissue perfusion during CPB. The difficulty in maintaining adequate tissue perfusion in clinical practice is demonstrated by the fact that up to 20% of all cardiac surgical patients have hyperlactatemia at the end of CPB. Hyperlactatemia is a recognized indicator of suboptimal tissue perfusion and is a risk factor for adverse outcomes. Organ injury may be the result of direct organ hypoxia (particularly the renal medulla) or a more subtle form of IRI mediated via endothelial activation. Unlike quiescent endothelium, activated endothelium is prothrombotic, open to solute exchange and supports the trafficking of activated leukocytes into the organ. The key question is: how to maintain optimal tissue perfusion and prevent slippage into ischemia?

Maintaining optimal oxygen delivery (DO_2) is most probably the most important determinant for satisfying the metabolic needs of tissues during CPB. Although a specific cut-off value has not been determined, $DO_2 < 260$ ml min^{-1} m^{-2} has been linked with rises in peak blood lactate levels. However, hyperlactatemia per se is probably not the best marker to guide real-time interventions to minimize ischemic episodes, since the liberation of lactate into the circulation may lag hours behind its production in tissues. Carbon dioxide production may provide better real-time information on tissue perfusion, since physiologic buffering of lactic acid with bicarbonate produces CO_2. As a consequence, CO_2–derived parameters correlate well with tissue perfusion. Predictors of hyperlactatemia are CO_2 production (VCO_2) > 60 ml min^{-1} m^{-2}, a respiratory quotient > 0.9 and a DO_2:VCO_2 ratio < 5.

Continuous monitoring of DO_2 and CO_2-derived parameters during CPB may help to prevent the onset of anaerobic tissue metabolism and adverse clinical outcomes. Intraoperative cerebral oximetry may also provide invaluable feedback to allow rapid modification of perfusion characteristics. The brain as index organ for optimal perfusion has gained credence with publication of a randomized prospective study showing that maintaining cortical oxygen saturation at baseline levels resulted in significantly reduced length of ICU stay and morbidity (composite end-point of death, ventilation > 48 hours, CVA, MI, surgical re-exploration).

Perfusion registries and evidence-based practice supported by the International Consortium for Evidence Based Perfusion (ICEBP) and standardized reporting practices, like those promoted by the Outcomes Consensus Statement, will play an important role in the future to allow perfusionists to keep up with the evidence for improvements in perfusion practice.

Key points

- The systemic inflammatory response occurs to a greater or lesser extent in all patients.
- Up to 2% of patients may suffer morbidity and mortality as a consequence of SIRS.
- Surgical trauma, endotoxemia, ischemia-reperfusion injury and contact activation of numerous pathways combine in the systemic inflammatory response.
- Intact and quiescent endothelium provides an important barrier function to protect tissues from the systemically activated milieu.
- The neutrophil having gained access to the tissues is a principal mediator of cytodestruction.
- The impact of SIRS on individual organs is determined by susceptibility to ischemia and local triggers.
- The multifactorial etiology of SIRS suggests that monotherapy is unlikely to be of clinical benefit.

Further reading

Butler J, Rocker GM, Westaby S. Inflammatory response to cardiopulmonary bypass. *Ann Thorac Surg* 1993; **55**(2): 552–9.

De Somer F. Optimal versus suboptimal perfusion during cardiopulmonary bypass and the inflammatory response. *Semin Cardiothorac Vasc Anesth* 2009; **13**(2): 113–17.

Landis RC, Murkin JM, Stump DA, *et al.* Consensus statement: minimal criteria for reporting the systemic inflammatory response to cardiopulmonary bypass. *Heart Surg Forum* 2010; **13**(2): E116–23.

Murkin JM, Adams SJ, Novick RJ, *et al.* Monitoring brain oxygen saturation during coronary bypass surgery: a randomized, prospective study. *Anesth Analg* 2007; **104**(1): 51–8.

Ranucci M, Balduini A, Ditta A, Boncilli A, Brozzi S. A systematic review of biocompatible cardiopulmonary bypass circuits and clinical outcome. *Ann Thorac Surg* 2009; **87**(4): 1311–19.

Shann KG, Likosky DS, Murkin JM, *et al.* An evidence-based review of the practice of cardiopulmonary bypass in adults: a focus on neurologic injury, glycemic control, hemodilution, and the inflammatory response. *J Thorac Cardiovasc Surg* 2006; **132**(2): 283–90.

Temperature control, hypothermia and rewarming

Charles Willmott

Anesthetic agents impair thermoregulation. Despite active warming, prolonged exposure of skin and open wounds to ambient temperatures and the infusion of unwarmed fluids render cardiac surgical patients mildly hypothermic (34–36°C) during the perioperative period.

Control of temperature

In animals which maintain body temperature within a tight range (homeotherms), thermoregulation occurs as a result of the dynamic balance between heat production (thermogenesis) and heat loss. Stimulation of cutaneous cold receptors and temperature-sensitive neurons in the hypothalamus activates sympathetic autonomic (vasoconstriction), endocrine, adaptive behavioral and extra-pyramidal (shivering) mechanisms to maintain core temperature.

Inadvertent hypothermia

Hypothermia – defined as a core temperature <35°C – occurs when heat losses overwhelm thermoregulatory mechanisms (e.g. during cold immersion) or when thermoregulation is impaired by pathological conditions (e.g. stroke, trauma, endocrinopathy, sepsis, autonomic neuropathy, uremia) or drugs (e.g. anesthetic agents, barbiturates, benzodiazepines, phenothiazines, ethanol). Thanks to the early work of Currie and Rosomoff, and experience gained from managing accidental hypothermia, the physiological effects of hypothermia are well known (Table 60.1). An understanding of both normal physiological and pathological responses is essential when using deliberate or therapeutic hypothermia.

For the purposes of discussion, the human body may be considered to have a central, well-perfused core (head and torso) and a variably perfused periphery. In a normothermic patient, the former comprises two-thirds of body mass and the latter, one-third. Although the temperature within individual organs is not the same (liver >> testes), the mean core temperature is normally tightly regulated between 36.4°C and 37.4°C to preserve physiological and metabolic functions. Circadian variation, ovulation and exercise produce small, physiological changes in core temperature. At an ambient temperature of 20–22°C there is typically a 2–4°C core–periphery gradient.

In clinical cardiac surgical practice, core temperature is measured in the nasopharynx, distal esophagus and PA. Temperature monitoring in the bladder, rectum and tympanic membrane are less frequently used.

Excitation of peripheral thermoreceptors and temperature-sensitive neurons dispersed in the brainstem and spinal cord changes with temperature. Impulses are conveyed via the lateral spinothalamic tracts to the spinal cord, brainstem, midbrain and hypothalamus. Afferent impulses are modulated in regions such as the locus coeruleus and nuclear raphe magnus in the pons before ascending to the principal thermoregulatory center, the pre-optic anterior hypothalamus.

Vasoconstriction and vasodilatation are the earliest thermoregulatory responses in patients who cannot move, change their clothing or alter their environment. Most anesthetic techniques cause peripheral vasodilatation by both peripheral and central actions. Lowering of the central threshold for vasoconstriction in a cold environment (e.g. operating room) results in the transfer of heat from core–periphery and mild hypothermia of the core. The rate of heat loss is dependent on the core–periphery gradient. Later responses, such as non-shivering thermogenesis, shivering and sweating, are greatly affected by

Core Topics in Cardiac Anesthesia, Second Edition, ed. Jonathan H. Mackay and Joseph E. Arrowsmith. Published by Cambridge University Press. © Cambridge University Press 2012.

Table 60.1 The pathophysiology of hypothermia

	Mild (33–35°C)	Severe (<28°C)
Neurologic	Confusion Amnesia Apathy – Delayed anesthetic recovery Impaired judgment	Depressed consciousness Pupillary dilatation Coma Loss of autoregulation
Neuromuscular	Shivering Ataxia Dysarthria	Muscle and joint stiffening Muscle rigor
Cardiovascular	Tachycardia Vasoconstriction Increased BP, CO	Severe bradycardia Increased SVR, reduced CO ECG changes: J (Osborn) waves, QRS broadening, ST changes, T wave inversion, A-V block, QT prolongation VF → asystole
Respiratory	Tachypnea Left-shift HbO_2 curve	Bradypnea Bronchospasm Right-shift HbO_2 curve
Metabolic	Cold-induced diuresis	Reduced H^+ and glucose reabsorption
Gastrointestinal	Reduced drug metabolism	Metabolic (lactic) acidosis Ileus Gastric ulcers Hepatic dysfunction
Hematology	Increased blood viscosity and hemoconcentration (2% increase in hematocrit/°C)	Coagulopathy – inhibition of intrinsic/extrinsic pathway enzymes, platelet activation, thrombocytopenia (liver sequestration)
Immunologic	Increased infection risk	Leukocyte depletion, impaired neutrophil function and bacterial phagocytosis

anesthesia. Non-shivering thermogenesis is abolished, neuromuscular blockade prevents shivering and anticholinergics impair sweating.

Cold-induced platelet dysfunction and altered coagulation and fibrinolysis may worsen blood loss and increase transfusion requirements. Decreased skin and subcutaneous blood flow and impaired leukocyte function impair wound healing and increase the incidence of wound infection. The pharmacology of anesthetic drugs and muscle relaxants may be significantly altered and the increase in blood solubility of volatile agents at lower temperatures delays recovery.

Maintaining normothermia

Body heat is lost by conduction, convection, radiation and evaporation (Table 60.2). During surgery heat is lost by conduction to adjacent materials and through thin surgical drapes, convection of adjacent air and through open wounds, radiation of heat to enclosing surfaces and evaporation of liquid on the surface of tissues. Radiant losses, which are the most important, are dependent on the fourth power of the temperature difference (in °K) between the skin and enclosing surface. By virtue of their large surface area to volume ratio, neonates are more vulnerable to hypothermia.

Minimizing passive heat loss and active warming measures are required to maintain normothermia (Table 60.3). For patients undergoing anesthesia of <30 min duration, preoperative vasodilatation and active warming can prevent an intraoperative fall in core temperature. Active peripheral warming abolishes the temperature gradient between the core and peripheries, while vasodilatation increases the mass of tissues at core temperature. This strategy is largely

383

Table 60.2 Mechanisms of heat loss during anesthesia and surgery, and measures that may be used to reduce heat loss

Mechanism	Comments	Countermeasures
Conduction	Cold intravenous and irrigation fluids	Fluid warmer
Convection	Ventilation and laminar airflow ("wind-chill")	Surgical drapes and blankets
Radiation	Most significant factor – human skin is an efficient emitter of infrared energy	Reflective (foil) blanket
	Dependent on surface area:body mass ratio	Window blinds/curtains
Evaporation	Vaporization requires considerable energy	Heat and moisture exchanger
	Skin preparation solutions, surgical site and airway	

Table 60.3 Passive and active measures used during anesthesia and surgery to maintain normothermia

Thermal insulation (e.g. blankets)	Static air, trapped within a blanket, is a poor conductor of heat
	Limited ability to insulate the legs and torso in cardiac surgery
Forced air warmer	Prevent radiant heat loss by covering the body with a warm outer shell
	The contact of warm air and skin reduces convective > conductive losses
	Warming in proportion to the area of skin covered
	Considerably more effective than passive measures and heated mattresses
Heated mattress	Modern operating tables are well insulated; therefore most heat is lost through front of body
	Limited skin contact with mattress minimizes transfer of thermal energy
	Risk of pressure-heat necrosis (burns) at temperatures >38°C
Radiant heaters	Generate infrared energy. Most efficient when placed close to the body and when the direction of radiant energy is perpendicular to the body surface
	Allows heat transfer without the need for protective coverings
	Convective losses continue unimpeded
	Most commonly used in neonatal practice
Fluid warming	The effect of fluid warming is greatest for refrigerated fluids (e.g. blood) and the rapid administration of fluids at room temperature (i.e. 20°C)
	Warming of maintenance fluids (administered slowly) is of little benefit
	Packed red cells at 4°C represent a thermal stress of 120 k Jl^{-1} (30 kcal l^{-1})
	One unit of red cells at 4°C may reduce adult core temperature by ~0.25°C
Humidification	Respiratory tract heat losses account for ~10% of total
	Passive (i.e. heat and moisture exchangers) measures are less effective but more convenient to use than active humidification systems

ineffective for longer procedures as initial heat losses are increased by peripheral vasodilatation.

Cardiopulmonary bypass

CPB offers the facility to produce greater and more rapid changes in core temperature than can be achieved in any other type of surgery. Assuming that human tissue has an average specific heat capacity of ~3.5 kJ kg^{-1} $°C^{-1}$ (0.83 kcal kg^{-1} $°C^{-1}$), raising the temperature of a 70 kg adult from 30°C to 37°C requires an energy transfer of at least 1700 kJ (400 kcal). In practice, on-going heat losses during warming dictate that greater overall energy transfer will be required.

While rapid cooling can be achieved with few obvious deleterious effects, rewarming must be undertaken gradually with a smaller gradient between warmed oxygenated blood returning to the aorta and measured core temperature. Even when rewarming is performed slowly, heat is transferred to the core compartment more rapidly than it can be redistributed to the periphery, resulting in substantial core to peripheral gradients. Following the termination of CPB, heat

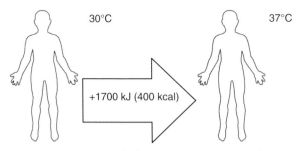

Figure 60.1 Energy transfer during rewarming. Assuming that human tissue has an average specific heat capacity of ~3.5 kJ kg^{-1} °C^{-1} (0.83 kcal kg^{-1} °C^{-1}), raising the temperature of a 70 kg adult from 30°C to 37°C requires a minimum energy transfer of ~1700 kJ (400 kcal) – the same energy required to raise the temperature of 5 liters of water from 20°C to 100°C.

Table 60.4 Factors influencing the magnitude of "after-drop"

Duration of rewarming

Relative masses of core and periphery

Core to peripheral temperature gradient

Core temperature during hypothermic CPB

Heat loss from open chest post CPB

Use of vasoactive agents

Active warming of peripheries

is transferred from the core to the inadequately warmed periphery, frequently resulting in core temperatures <35°C – a degree of postoperative hypothermia that would not be tolerated in the non-cardiac surgical setting. This redistribution of heat and subsequent core hypothermia following hypothermic CPB is known as "after-drop". Factors influencing the rate and magnitude of after-drop are shown in Table 60.4. In practice, the duration of rewarming after hypothermic CPB is the best measure of the adequacy of rewarming.

The use of vasodilators during the rewarming phase of CPB reduces the core–periphery temperature gradient and slows the rate at which core temperature rises. Although this technique results in a higher peripheral temperature at the end of CPB, the eventual impact that this has on after-drop is small (~0.3°C) and clinically unimportant. Forced air heating of the legs during rewarming and after CPB is more effective – reducing after-drop by as much as 0.7°C.

Despite the adverse consequences of mild postoperative hypothermia, it is known that even mild degrees of hyperthermia are more deleterious and should be avoided at all costs.

Traditionally both core and peripheral temperature have been measured on cardiac surgical ICUs, enabling trends in core to peripheral gradient to be observed. Since most clinical decisions (e.g. need for forced air rewarming, timing of tracheal extubation) are based on core temperature measurement, many centers have abandoned peripheral temperature measurement.

Therapeutic hypothermia

The findings of two large, multicenter studies demonstrating the efficacy of mild, deliberate hypothermia in the management of comatose patients after out-of-hospital cardiac arrest have stimulated both considerable research and changes in clinical practice. The goal of therapeutic hypothermia in this setting is improved neurologic outcome at hospital discharge.

Current indications include comatose patients who have a return of spontaneous circulation after either out-of-hospital or in-hospital cardiac arrest. Hypothermia must be induced as soon as practicably possible after return of spontaneous circulation. Surface techniques (e.g. cooling pads, cooling blankets and ice packs) or internal techniques (e.g. endovascular cooling device) are used to reduce core body temperature to 32–34°C for 12–24 h.

The risks of hemorrhage and infection may explain the relatively rare use of therapeutic hypothermia following cardiac arrest in cardiac surgical patients.

Key points

- The most significant cause of intraoperative hypothermia is radiant heat loss.
- Passive measures to prevent intraoperative heat loss are only successful for short procedures.
- Clinical decision-making should be based on core temperature rather than the gradient between core and peripheral temperatures.
- In practice, the duration of rewarming after hypothermic CPB is the best measure of the adequacy of rewarming.
- Therapeutic hypothermia may be of benefit in comatose survivors of cardiac arrest. There is less evidence for use after cardiac arrest from non-shockable rhythms.

385

- There is recognition that many of the accepted predictors of poor outcome in comatose survivors of cardiac arrest are unreliable, especially if the patient has been treated with therapeutic hypothermia.

Further reading

Ginsberg S, Solina A, Papp D, Krause T, Pantin E, Scott G, *et al.* A prospective comparison of three heat preservation methods for patients undergoing hypothermic cardiopulmonary bypass. *J Cardiothorac Vasc Anesth* 2000; **14**(5): 501–5.

Grigore AM, Murray CF, Ramakrishna H, Djaiani G. A core review of temperature regimens and neuroprotection during cardiopulmonary bypass: does rewarming rate matter? *Anesth Analg* 2009; **109**(6): 1741–51.

National Institute for Health and Clinical Excellence. *Clinical Guidance 65: Perioperative hypothermia (inadvertent).* April 2008. http://guidance.nice.org.uk/CG65/Guidance/pdf/English.

National Institute for Health and Clinical Excellence. *Intervention Practice Guideline 386: Therapeutic hypothermia following cardiac arrest.* March 2011. http://www.nice.org.uk/nicemedia/live/12990/53610/53610.pdf.

Rajek A, Lenhardt R, Sessler DI, Brunner G, Haisjackl M, Kastner J, *et al.* Efficacy of two methods for reducing postbypass afterdrop. *Anesthesiology* 2000; **92**(2): 447–56.

Sessler DI. Complications and treatment of mild hypothermia. *Anesthesiology* 2001; **95**(2): 531–43.

Chapter 61

Deep hypothermic circulatory arrest

Charles W. Hogue and Joseph E. Arrowsmith

The majority of cardiac surgical procedures are accomplished using cardioplegia-induced cardiac arrest, with CPB to maintain perfusion to other organs. However, in certain situations the nature of the surgical procedure or the pathology of the underlying condition necessitates complete cessation of blood flow (Table 61.1). Preservation of organ function during the period of total circulatory arrest can be achieved by reducing the core temperature of the body. The technique of core cooling combined with cessation of blood flow is termed "deep hypothermic circulatory arrest" (DHCA).

DHCA provides excellent operating conditions – albeit of limited duration – whilst ameliorating the major adverse consequences of organ ischemia. By reducing cellular metabolism, hypothermia preserves high-energy phosphate stores and protects organs from short periods of ischemia. The brain is the organ most vulnerable to injury, but may be protected if cooled to reduce oxygen-dependent neuronal metabolic activity and excitatory neurotransmitter release before and during the period of arrest. Similarly,

other organs that are less susceptible to ischemic damage may be protected by core cooling.

History

DHCA owes its existence to the pioneering work of Bigelow in the 1940s and to two overlapping eras; a brief period in the early 1950s when hypothermia was used as the sole method for organ protection during surgery, and the current epoch of CPB heralded by Gibbon in 1953. Subsequent modifications to the basic technique have extended both the duration of "safe" circulatory arrest and the range of surgical indications (Table 61.2).

Anesthesia

DHCA is commonly used in emergency, life-saving procedures. For this reason it may not be possible to undertake the usual battery of "routine" preoperative investigations. The presence of significant comorbidities (e.g. coronary artery disease, cerebrovascular disease, renal insufficiency, diabetes mellitus) should be anticipated on the basis of the clinical history and physical examination.

Invasive monitoring

Standard arterial, central venous and peripheral venous access is required in all cases. In anticipation of division of the innominate vein to improve surgical access, venous cannulae should be sited in the right arm or in the femoral vein. Cannulation of the right radial artery and a femoral artery permits arterial pressure monitoring both proximal and distal to the aortic arch. Cannulation of a femoral artery also serves as an anatomic marker for the surgeon should an IABP be required on separation from CPB. Whilst not considered mandatory, PA catheterization may aid management

Table 61.1 Cardiac and non-cardiac indications for DHCA

Cardiac

 Repair of complex congenital cardiac anomalies

 Aortic aneurysm, rupture or dissection

 Aortic arch reconstruction

Non-cardiac

 Hepatic and renal cell carcinoma

 Repair of giant cerebral aneurysms

 Resection of cerebral AV malformations

 Pulmonary (thrombo)endarterectomy

Table 61.2 Historical milestones in the development of DHCA

1940s	Bigelow demonstrated that a reduction in body temperature to 30°C increased the period of "safe" cerebral ischemia from 3 to 10 min
1950s	Lewis first successfully used hypothermic inflow (caval) occlusion in cardiac surgery
	Iced water bath for cooling, described by Swan
	The types of procedures that could be undertaken during inflow occlusion, however, were limited to atrial septal defect repair, valvotomy and valvectomy
	Drew and Lewis later described more profound degrees of hypothermia
	Despite spectacular successes, the incidence of death and complications such as hypothermia-induced VF, hemorrhage, myocardial failure and neurologic injury were high
1960s	CPB-induced hypothermia and DHCA in the management of aortic arch pathology described
1970s	Griepp demonstrates that DHCA offered a relatively simple and safe approach for aortic arch surgery

immediately after CPB and in the early postoperative period. Where available, and in the absence of contra-indications, TEE may be used to assess cardiac function and assist with cardiac de-airing.

Choice of anesthetic drugs

The choice of anesthetic drugs is largely a matter of personal and institutional preference. In theory, using propofol and opioid-based anesthesia in preference to volatile anesthetic agents reduces cerebral metabolism without uncoupling flow-metabolism relationships. The impact of hypothermia on drug metabolism and elimination should be considered and drug infusion rates adjusted accordingly.

Temperature management

Accurate temperature monitoring – at two or more sites – is crucial. Nasopharyngeal or tympanic membrane temperature monitoring provides an indication of brain temperature, whereas rectal or bladder temperature monitoring provides an indication of body core temperature. Whilst these devices are accurate at steady-state it should be borne in mind that, during both cooling and warming, thermal gradients may be generated in tissues and monitored temperature may lag behind actual tissue temperature by 2–5°C.

All measures should be taken to facilitate rewarming and prevent "after-drop" hypothermia following the termination of CPB. The use of a heated mattress, sterile forced-air blanket and an IV fluid warmer should be considered in all cases.

Other considerations

The long duration of surgery with DHCA mandates careful attention to prevent pressure sores and inadvertent damage to the eyes, nerve plexuses, peripheral nerves and pressure points. Cannulation sites, three-way taps, monitoring lines, the ETT connector and TEE probe should be padded to prevent pressure necrosis of the skin.

Surgery

In some cases, such as acute type A aortic dissection, femoral or right axillary arterial cannulation may initially be necessary together with femoral venous cannulation. Femoro-femoral or axillo-femoral CPB permits systemic cooling prior to sternotomy and affords a degree of organ protection should chest-opening be accompanied by inadvertent damage to the aorta or heart and exsanguination. After completion of the aortic repair placement of the arterial line directly into the prosthetic graft permits restoration of anterograde flow. Cannulation of the mid or distal aortic arch may be required in cases of degenerative aortic aneurysm to reduce the risk of atheroembolism associated with retrograde flow via femoral arterial cannulation.

The choice of venous drainage site and cannula type is largely dictated by surgical preference and the degree of access necessary. For example: bicaval cannulation is required if retrograde cerebral perfusion (RCP) is to be used with reversal of blood flow in the SVC. If selective anterograde cerebral perfusion (SACP) is to be used, with selective arterial cannulation of the carotid arterial circulation, then adequate cerebral venous drainage must be ensured, again using bi-caval cannulation, to optimize cerebral perfusion pressure and prevent cerebral edema. Removal of a renal tumor from the IVC requires the use of a right atrial basket – in preference to a caval or two-stage cannula – to permit full visualization of the cava and to prevent dislodged fragments of tumor from becoming impacted in the pulmonary circulation.

The use of DHCA during surgery of the distal aorta via left thoracotomy presents several problems. Access to the proximal aorta is limited and femoral arterial cannulation may be required initially. Access to the right atrium typically requires an extensive thoracotomy that traverses the sternum. Alternatively, venous drainage may be achieved using pulmonary artery cannulation or a long femoral cannula advanced into the right atrium.

Extracorporeal circulation

The nature of DHCA requires modifications to be made to the standard extracorporeal circuit:

- infusion bags for the storage of heparinized blood during hemodilution (see below);
- use of a centrifugal pump – in preference to a roller pump – to reduce damage to the cellular components of the circulation and reduce hemolysis;
- incorporation of a hemofilter to permit hemoconcentration during rewarming;
- incorporation of a leukocyte-depleting arterial line filter (see below);
- selection of a cardiotomy reservoir of sufficient capacity to accommodate the circulating volume during exsanguination immediate before DHCA;
- arteriovenous bypass and accessory arterial lines – to permit RCP or SACP (see below);
- an efficient heat exchanger; the energy required to warm a 70 kg adult from 20°C to 37 C is at least 4.2 MJ (1000 kcal) – the energy required to boil 12.5 liters of water;
- consideration of the use of heparin-bonded circuits; this is advocated in cases requiring prolonged CPB, despite lack of conclusive evidence of benefit.

Cooling

Following anticoagulation, CPB is instituted with a constant flow rate of 2.4 l min^{-1} m^{-2} and cooling immediately commenced with a water bath – blood temperature gradient of $<10°C$. The application of external ice packs or a cooling cap to the head assists cerebral cooling. Vasoconstrictors (e.g. phenylephrine, metaraminol) or vasodilators (e.g. glyceryl trinitrate, sodium nitroprusside) are used to ensure a MAP of 50–60 mmHg. The onset of hypothermia-induced VF signals the need for either application of an AXC and administration of cardioplegia, or more commonly insertion of a vent to prevent LV distention.

As much of the planned procedure (e.g. surgical dissection and preparation of any prosthetic grafts) is carried out as possible during the cooling phase prior to DHCA in order to minimize the duration of circulatory arrest.

Cooling continues until brain (i.e. nasopharygeal) and core body (i.e. bladder) temperatures have equilibrated at the target temperature for 10–15 min. In some centers continuous monitoring of the EEG, evoked potentials or jugular venous saturation is used as a guide to the adequacy of cerebral cooling.

Circulatory arrest

The operating table is then placed in a slightly head-down (Trendelenberg) position, the pump stopped and the patient partially exsanguinated into the venous reservoir. Once isolated from the patient, blood within the extracorporeal circuit is then recirculated via a connection between the arterial and venous lines in order to prevent stagnation and clotting. The surgical repair then proceeds with heed to the duration of circulatory arrest.

As the intravenous administration of drugs during DHCA is at best pointless and at worst potentially dangerous, all infusions should be discontinued when the CPB pump is switched off.

Removal of the AXC and opening the aorta to the atmosphere exposes both the coronary and cerebral arteries to the risk of air embolism. At the end of DHCA, therefore, adequate de-airing and measures such as head-down tilt and flooding of the surgical field with crystalloid at 4°C should be undertaken. At the end of DHCA, infusions of anesthetic agents should be restarted to avoid the risk of inadvertent awareness during rewarming.

Safe period of circulatory arrest

Determining the duration of DHCA that any particular patient will tolerate without sustaining disabling neurologic injury remains, at best, an inexact science. In general, however, neonates and infants tolerate longer periods of DHCA than adults. Current practice makes it difficult to separate the neurologic risks of the

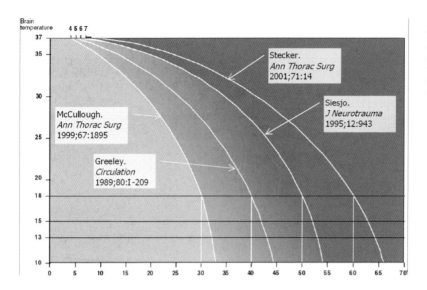

Brain temperature

Stecker.
Ann Thorac Surg
2001;71:14

Siesjo.
J Neurotrauma
1995;12:943

McCullough.
Ann Thorac Surg
1999;67:1895

Greeley.
Circulation
1989;80:I-209

Figure 61.1 The effect of brain temperature on reported safe duration of deep hypothermic circulatory arrest duration. Reproduced with permission from Ghosh S, Falter F, Cook DJ. *Cardiopulmonary Bypass*. Cambridge University Press; 2009.

prolonged CPB, reperfusion and rewarming – all unavoidable consequences of DHCA – from those of DHCA alone.

Most patients tolerate 30 min DHCA at 18°C. The incidence of neurologic injury rises sharply when DHCA exceeds 40 min and only three-quarters of patients tolerate 45 min of DHCA at this temperature. On the basis of animal experimentation and clinical observation, unmodified DHCA is typically limited to no more than 60 min at 18°C. Frustratingly, while some patients appear to tolerate DHCA >60 min without apparent injury, others sustain major brain injury after <20 min DHCA. The spectrum of neurologic injury following surgery with CPB and DHCA is similar to that following cardiac surgery (see Chapter 70). Seizures and choreoathetosis may occur in up to 20% of pediatric patients.

Rewarming

Animal evidence suggests that a period of 10–20 min "cold reperfusion" (i.e. rewarming delayed) at the end of DHCA may improve outcome. Excessively rapid rewarming, accompanied by a rise in cerebral arterio-venous O_2 difference, is known to worsen neurologic outcome. In patients undergoing CABG surgery, maintaining a temperature gradient of <2°C between inflow temperature and brain (nasopharyngeal) temperature has been shown to improve cognitive outcome. Inflow temperature should not exceed 37°C and CPB is terminated when core body temperature reaches 35.5–36.5°C. A significant "afterdrop" is inevitable and patients are sometimes admitted to the ICU with temperatures as low as 32°C. Using a slow rate of re-warming with adequate time for even distribution of heat between core and peripheral tissues helps to reduce the extent of this afterdrop.

During the period of re-warming attention should be given to the correction of metabolic abnormalities, particularly the metabolic acidosis that inevitably accompanies reperfusion following circulatory arrest. Correction of acid-base balance may require the titrated administration of sodium bicarbonate or use of hemofiltration (ultrafiltration).

Hemostasis

Prolonged CPB and hypothermia produce a coagulopathy. Hemostasis is facilitated by meticulous surgery, the use of predonated autologous blood and administration of donor blood components under the guidance of laboratory tests of coagulation and thromboelastography. Despite safety concerns, antifibrinolytic agents (e.g. tranexamic acid, ε-aminocaproic acid) and aprotinin have been shown to be efficacious in aortic arch surgery with DHCA.

Cerebral protection

Although hypothermia is the principal neuroprotectant during DHCA, additional strategies may be employed to reduce the likelihood of neurologic injury. These include acid-base management strategy, hemodilution, leukodepletion and glycemic control.

Surgical maneuvers, such as intermittent cerebral perfusion, SACP and RCP, may also be used to both protect the brain and extend the operating time available to the surgeon.

Temperature

Hypothermia remains the single most important mechanism of cerebral protection. Cerebral metabolism decreases by 6–7% for every 1°C fall in temperature below 37°C, with consciousness and autoregulation being lost at 30°C and 25°C respectively. At temperatures <20°C, ischemic tolerance is around ten times that at normothermia. DHCA at 15–20°C provides the longest safe period of circulatory arrest. The application of external ice packs or a cooling cap to the head delays brain rewarming during DHCA.

Hemodilution

The combination of vasoconstriction, increased plasma viscosity and reduced erythrocyte plasticity secondary to hypothermia leads to impairment of the microcirculation and ischemia. Progressive hemodilution during hypothermic CPB, typically to a hematocrit of 0.18–0.20, is thought to partially mitigate this phenomenon. In some centers, a degree of normovolemic hemodilution is undertaken prior to the onset of CPB. The optimal hematocrit for a particular individual at a specific temperature remains unclear. Gross anemia (i.e. hematocrit <0.10) may result in inadequate tissue oxygen delivery, particularly during re-warming. This approach is supported by the more recent observation that maintaining a higher hematocrit during deep hypothermic CPB did not impair the cerebral microcirculation.

Acid-base management

Cerebral vasodilatation associated with pH-stat blood-gas management improves brain cooling and ensures more homogeneous cooling of deeper brain structures. pH-stat may, however, induce a cerebral metabolic acidosis and increase microembolization secondary to increased cerebral blood flow (CBF). In the piglet model of DHCA, pH-stat management improves neurologic outcome. In neonates undergoing DHCA for repair of congenital heart defects, pH-stat management prior to DHCA appears to be associated with fewer complications than α-stat

management and better developmental outcome. In adults, however, the superiority of one strategy over another in the setting of DHCA remains unproven. On theoretical grounds, using pH-stat during cooling and α-stat during rewarming (the so-called "crossover" management) has some appeal.

Glucose management

Insulin resistance and hyperglycemia are common during cardiac surgery with DHCA. In animal models, hyperglycemia worsens outcome following cerebral infarction. Whilst tight glycemic control during cardiac surgery appears to reduce mortality and infective complications, any neuroprotective effect remains unproven.

Leukocyte depletion

The use of leukocyte-depleting arterial line filters is reported to moderate the systemic inflammatory response to CPB, reduce reperfusion injury and reduce postoperative infective complications. Evidence for cerebral protection by leukocyte depletion is lacking in humans, and animal experimentation has yielded conflicting results.

Pharmacological

Pharmacological protection from cerebral ischemia remains elusive and at present no drug is licensed for neuroprotection in cardiac surgery. Although various anesthetic agents (e.g. thiopental, propofol and isoflurane) can induce EEG burst suppression and profoundly decrease cerebral metabolic rate (for oxygen; $CMRO_2$), their neuroprotective properties remain unproven.

In many centers thiopental 15–30 mg kg^{-1} continues to be administered before DHCA despite any objective evidence of efficacy. The widely held belief that thiopental reduces neurologic injury in conventional cardiac surgery is not borne out by published evidence, although there is some suggestion that it reduces overall mortality. Animal evidence suggests that the administration of corticosteroids (e.g. methylprednisolone 15 mg kg^{-1}) prior to DHCA affords a degree of neuroprotection.

Selective antegrade cerebral perfusion

This technique involves selective cannulation of the brachiocephalic, axillary or carotid arteries.

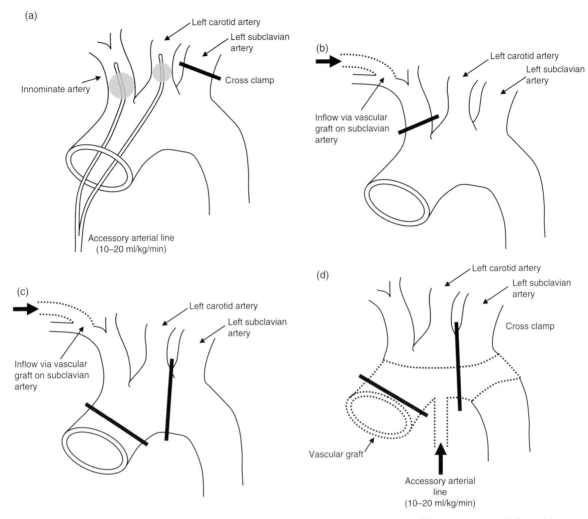

Figure 61.2 Examples of selective antegrade cerebral perfusion techniques. (a) Direct cannulation of the innominate and left carotid arteries. (b) Hemicranial perfusion via a left subclavian artery graft. (c) Bilateral cranial perfusion via a left subclavian artery graft. (d) Bilateral cranial perfusion via a sidearm on vascular graft. Reproduced from Hogue *et al.* 2006.

Oxygenated blood is pumped via a separate arterial line at 10–20 ml kg^{-1} to maintain a perfusion pressure – measured in the right radial artery – of 50–70 mmHg. Although SACP permits surgery to be conducted at lesser degrees of systemic hypothermia (e.g. 22–25°C) it often requires greater mobilization of the epiaortic vessels and division of the innominate vein. In addition to increasing complexity and crowding the surgical field with cannulae, SACP is accompanied by the risk of cerebral embolization. An intact circle of Willis is required when unilateral SACP is employed. A misplaced cannula may result in inadequate cerebral perfusion while giving a false sense of security.

Intermittent cerebral perfusion

Intermittent systemic perfusion punctuated by <20 min periods of DHCA has been used as an alternative strategy to prolong the total duration of DHCA. It is suggested that intermittent reperfusion preserves neurologic tissue by replenishing cerebral high-energy phosphates and removing accumulated waste products.

Retrograde cerebral perfusion

RCP, which relies on the fact that cerebral veins have no valves, involves the continuous administration of cold (10–15°C) oxygenated blood via a SVC cannula

Table 61.3 Potential problems associated with antegrade and retrograde cerebral perfusion during DHCA

Selective antegrade cerebral perfusion

Embolization of air or plaque

Cannula malposition and inadequate CBF

Unilateral flow requiring flow through circle of Willis to contralateral side

↑Complexity of surgery and crowding of the surgical field

Retrograde cerebral perfusion

↑Intracranial pressure

Cerebral edema

Low level of substrate supply

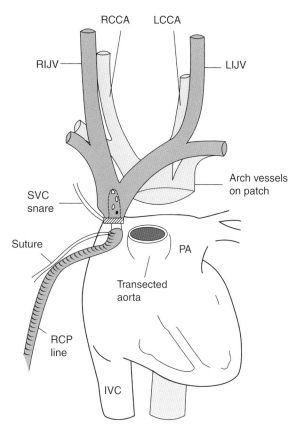

Figure 61.3 Retrograde cerebral perfusion via a cannula in the SVC. A purse string suture is used to hold the cannula in place and a circumferential snare is used to prevent reflux of blood into the RA. Other cannulae have been omitted for clarity.

(Figure 61.3). Blood flow to the brain is most likely to occur via the azygos veins because the internal jugular veins possess valves. The azygos vein has connections to the vertebral venous system and the venous plexus of the foramen magnum and intracranial sinuses. Massive shunting via the superficial and deep venous systems, including the internal and external jugular veins, may result in only a small fraction of the blood entering the SVC actually reaching the cerebral arteries. For this reason the exact levels of CBF and metabolic substrate delivery provided by RCP have yet to be defined (Table 61.3). Suggested blood flow rates for RCP are 200–300 ml min^{-1} with SVC pressure <25 mmHg. Interestingly, the use of multi-modal neurologic monitoring to guide RCP delivery at pressures as high as 40 mmHg – considered by many surgeons to be harmful and to cause cerebral edema – has been shown to be safe.

Theoretical advantages of RCP include: more homogeneous brain cooling; washout of air bubbles, embolic debris and metabolic waste products; prevention of cerebral blood cell microaggregates; and delivery of O_2 and metabolic substrates to the brain. The prolongation of safe DHCA that can be achieved with RCP is less than that with SACP. RCP for >60 min is a significant predictor of permanent neurologic dysfunction.

Spinal cord protection

Surgery involving the descending thoracic aorta may interrupt blood flow to the spinal cord via the anterior

spinal artery (of Adamkiewicz) and cause paraplegia. Spinal cord protection is discussed further in Chapter 38.

Neurologic monitoring

Until recently, the use of monitors of cerebral substrate delivery or neurologic function (see Chapter 26) has largely been confined to specialist centers, researchers and enthusiasts. It goes without saying that a monitor must prompt a corrective intervention before the onset of irreversible neurologic injury to be of any use. Cost and lack of level 1A evidence of efficacy means neurologic monitoring has yet to be universally adopted as "standard of care".

Postoperative care

Postoperative care is similar to that for any patient undergoing cardiac surgery. Every effort should be made to ameliorate the impact of secondary brain injury – hyperthermia, hypoxemia, hypotension and hypoperfusion should be aggressively treated. Even mild degrees of hyperthermia, a common occurrence after cardiac surgery, have been shown to be detrimental after DHCA.

The incidence and severity of postoperative complications associated with DHCA are largely determined by the pathology being treated, the presence of significant comorbidities and the urgency of surgery.

Key points

- Hypothermia is the single most important mechanism of cerebral protection during DHCA.
- Drugs with putative neuroprotective properties are still widely used prior to DHCA despite an absence of convincing evidence of efficacy.
- Hemodilution is used to improve microcirculation.

- The use of continuous or intermittent cerebral perfusion techniques during DHCA may prolong the safe duration of circulatory arrest.
- Infusions of anesthetic drugs should be discontinued prior to the onset of DHCA and restarted soon after the commencement of rewarming.

Further reading

Dorotta I, Kimball-Jones P, Applegate R 2nd. Deep hypothermia and circulatory arrest in adults. *Semin Cardiothorac Vasc Anesth* 2007; **11**(1): 66–76.

Hogue CW Jr, Palin CA, Arrowsmith JE. Cardiopulmonary bypass management and neurologic outcomes: an evidence-based appraisal of current practices. *Anesth Analg* 2006; **103**(1): 21–37.

Khaladj N, Shrestha M, Meck S, *et al.* Hypothermic circulatory arrest with selective antegrade cerebral perfusion in ascending aortic and aortic arch surgery: a risk factor analysis for adverse outcome in 501 patients. *J Thorac Cardiovasc Surg* 2008; **135**(4): 908–14.

chapter 62

Cardiopulmonary bypass emergencies

David J. Daly

Failure of tissue oxygenation represents an emergency during CPB. The principal causes are gaseous embolism, inadequate oxygenation and inadequate CPB flow.

Air (gas) embolism

There are two types of perfusionist...
those that have pumped air and those that will pump air.
Old perfusionists' proverb

Massive air embolism (AE) is defined as the witnessed or likely entry of air into the circulation. The quoted incidence is 1:1000 cases, which probably represents under-reporting. In 25% of recorded cases, massive AE leads to permanent injury or death.

Air can enter the circulation from the surgical field, from the CPB circuit and via indwelling venous and arterial cannulae. A degree of venous AE probably occurs in all patients undergoing CPB and appears to have few obvious consequences.

Surgical field entrainment

This is by far the most common source of significant AE. Air enters the circulation when the heart is opened or when a loose atrial suture allows air to be entrained via the venous cannula. The inadvertent delivery of air with cardioplegia solutions may lead to coronary embolism. An aortic root or pulmonary vein vent, at high negative pressure, can draw air into the ventricle via a coronary arteriotomy. Valve-less centrifugal pumps may allow retrograde siphoning of arterial blood and air entrainment via the arterial cannula.

Cardiopulmonary bypass air

The maintenance of an adequate volume in the CPB venous reservoir is a fundamental principle of perfusion. In the early days of CPB, without automatic reservoir level alarms, arterial line AE secondary to reservoir emptying was relatively common. Advances in CPB circuit design, monitoring and alarm systems have dramatically reduced the likelihood of this event. Nowadays, CPB equipment includes venous and arterial line bubble detectors, and a system that automatically shuts off the pump when the reservoir volume falls below a critical level.

The transition from bubble to membrane oxygenators has significantly reduced the amount of gas deliberately added to the circulation during oxygenation. Punctured or misconnected lines and loss of membrane integrity may, however, lead to significant gas embolism.

Anesthetic

Unprimed monitoring and intravenous infusion lines and the use of pressurized infusion devices may result in the inadvertent delivery of significant quantities of air. The practice of re-connecting partially used infusion bags greatly increases the risk of AE and should be avoided. AE of this type tends to occur before and after CPB, at times when the patient may already be hemodynamically unstable.

Physical principles

An understanding of the gas laws and the properties of air bubbles within the circulation is the key to successful management (Table 62.1).

Nitrogen and oxygen are the main constituents of air. As oxygen is readily absorbed, the challenge

Core Topics in Cardiac Anesthesia, Second Edition, ed. Jonathan H. Mackay and Joseph E. Arrowsmith. Published by Cambridge University Press. © Cambridge University Press 2012.

Table 62.1 The gas laws

Charles's law	States that at a constant pressure the volume of a given mass of gas varies directly with the absolute temperature
Boyle's law	States that at constant temperature the volume of a given mass varies inversely with the absolute pressure
Henry's law	States that at a particular temperature the amount of a given gas dissolved in a given liquid is directly proportional to the partial pressure of the gas in equilibrium with the liquid

Table 62.2 Basic principles of the management of massive air embolism during CPB

Make the diagnosis

Communicate the diagnosis

Prevent further air embolism

Identify the source of air embolism

Limit organ damage

Clear the CPB circuit of air

Expel air from the major arteries

Re-establish circulation

Table 62.3 The roles of surgeon, perfusionist and anesthesiologist in the management of massive air embolism during CPB

Perfusionist	Surgeon	Anesthesiologist
Stop CPB pump and clamp lines	Clamp aortic cannula Cut aortic cannula	Carotid compression Steep head-down position Ventilate with 100% O_2
Add cold fluid to reservoir	Prevent cardiac ejection	Cerebroprotectants?
Refill arterial line	Connect arterial line to RA	
RCP at 1–2 l min^{-1}	Initiate RCP at 20°C Vent air from aortic cannula	
Stop RCP	Reconnect arterial line to aorta	
Restart CPB & cool	Complete surgery	Maintain MAP ~80 mmHg
Slow partial rewarm		Consider hyperbaric O_2 Consider postoperative therapeutic hypothermia for 24–48 h

RCP, retrograde cerebral perfusion.

is the enhancement of nitrogen elimination. Hypothermia tends to reduce bubble size (Charles's law) and increase blood nitrogen solubility (Henry's law). Barometric and hydrostatic pressures (Boyle's law) prevent dissolved nitrogen leaving solution, while the partial pressure dictates any tendency to bubble formation (Henry's law). Self-contained underwater breathing apparatus (SCUBA) divers know that too rapid an ascent can lead to the formation of nitrogen bubbles, causing decompression illness (the bends).

The institution of hyperoxia ($PaO_2 \gg 13$ kPa) gradually leads to nitrogen displacement (denitrogenation). The arteriovenous oxygen difference (i.e. $PaO_2 - PvO_2$) reflects the gradient favoring nitrogen absorption. A nitrogen bubble, 4 mm in diameter (i.e. 0.025 ml), takes >10 h to be absorbed while breathing air, but <1 h while breathing 100% oxygen.

As with anesthetic gas elimination, the rate of denitrogenation is cardiac-output-dependent.

Management

As massive AE is rare, it is essential that anesthesiologists are aware of the possibility and the goals of management *before* they encounter the problem for the first time. For this reason many centers have developed their own management protocols with action plans for the anesthesiologist, surgeon and perfusionist. The clinical scenario also lends itself well to simulation (Tables 62.2 and 62.3).

The fundamental principles of good management are early diagnosis, good communication and rapid institution of measures of proven or likely benefit.

Most management plans include retrograde cerebral perfusion (RCP) on the grounds that cerebral AE will have occurred. After the CPB pump is stopped and the line clamped, the surgeon will usually clamp the aortic cannula, cut the arterial line close to the cannula and assist the perfusionist in refilling the line. This practice reduces the risk of aortic injury caused by decannulation and subsequent recannulation. The primed arterial line is then inserted into the RA or SVC, retrograde perfusion commenced at $1–2\ l\ min^{-1}$ and the "stump" of the cut aortic cannula unclamped to allow air to be vented from the aorta. Ideally, the IVC should be compressed or occluded to encourage cephalad blood flow and maximize the effectiveness of RCP. RCP is continued until no more bubbles are seen emerging in the aortic cannula. De-airing the ascending aorta and aortic arch may be monitored with TEE.

Gross air embolism occurring during atriofemoral CPB can be managed in a similar manner, although de-airing the aorta will require insertion of a vent into the ascending aorta or aortic arch – typically a cardioplegia administration cannula.

Gross air embolism occurring during femorofemoral CPB is more problematic, particularly if the chest has not been opened or dissection sufficient to permit central cannulation is incomplete. Because RCP from a femoral vein is ineffective, the likelihood of a successful outcome is determined by the volume of air administered and the accessibility of the RA and ascending aorta.

The theoretical benefits of intermittent carotid compression (to reduce antegrade cerebral air delivery and encourage air-flushing from the vertebral arteries during RCP) have to be balanced against the small risk of plaque fissuring and embolization.

The role of pharmacological neuroprotectants remains controversial. Although a number of agents are used in this setting, none have demonstrated unequivocal efficacy and none are licensed for this specific indication (Table 62.4).

Table 62.4 Putative neuroprotectants used after cerebral air embolism

Therapeutic hypothermia

Corticosteroids

Antioxidants

Free radical scavengers

General anesthetic agents

Local anesthetics

Inadequate oxygenation

Inadequate oxygenation of blood during CPB can occur as a result of failure of the gas delivery system or the oxygenator. The presenting features are darkening of arterial blood and reduced SvO_2, which may be associated with a rising transmembrane pressure gradient. ABG analysis is used to confirm the clinical diagnosis. As a temporizing measure the pump flow rate can be increased and some of the arterial flow can be diverted (i.e. shunted) back to the venous reservoir, thus increasing SvO_2. The sequence of checks given in Table 62.5 is suggested.

The use of point-of-care anticoagulation monitors means that oxygenator failure due to coagulation is exceedingly rare. In addition to falling PaO_2 and rising $PaCO_2$, the presence of "frothy" pink fluid in the gas exit port (the result of protein and water entering the gas phase of membrane) may signal impending oxygenator failure. Changing an oxygenator during CPB requires at least two perfusionists and a period of circulatory arrest; it should therefore be considered an intervention of

Table 62.5 Checklist for inadequate oxygenation during CPB

Gas supply	Gas delivery circuit not compromised
	Gas source connected to gas inlet port of oxygenator
	Gas flow $>0.5\ l\ min^{-1}$ (visual and by back-pressure in line)
	No leak from vaporizer manifold
	Ensure adequate F_iO_2 via in-line oxygen analyzer
	Gas scavenging system (if used) not obstructed
Blood flow	Ensure adequate blood flow through oxygenator
	Ensure adequate anticoagulation
Patient factors	Ensure depth of anesthesia is adequate (vaporizer leak)
	Check for hyperthermia ($\uparrow$ CMRO$_2$)
	Cold agglutinins
	Anaphylaxis
Surgical factors	Severe AR
	Over-venting the heart without adequate forward flow
	Unsecured cava snares without lung ventilation (creates an effective R→L shunt)

CMRO$_2$, cerebral metabolic rate for oxygen.

397

Table 62.6 Abbreviated example of an oxygenator changeout protocol

Perfusionist #1	Perfusionist #2
Shouts "coming off bypass" Stops pump and clamps venous and arterial lines Starts timer	
Cuts venous line from reservoir Removes pump boot and level sensor	Divides arterial line with sterile shears between two clamps Disconnects heat exchanger water pipes Removes old oxygenator Installs new oxygenator
Connects venous line	Connects arterial line and de-airs tubing Reservoir level sensor reattached
Installs pump boot in roller pump Recirculates reservoir contents through arterial line filter Shouts "back on bypass" Starts pump Stops timer	Connects heat exchanger water pipes to oxygenator Reconnects cardiotomy suckers to cardiotomy reservoir Complete and file critical incident report

Table 62.7 Causes of inadequate CPB flow

Electrical pump failure	Impact minimized by uninterruptible power supply Back-up generators and emergency back-up batteries incorporated in pump
Mechanical pump failure	Roller head under occlusion
Venous return	Air locks, lifting heart
Cannula problem	Total obstruction: retained clamp Partial obstruction: small size, kinking
Aortic dissection	↑ line pressure and ↓ patient arterial pressure

last resort. A discussion of this unusual procedure is shown below.

Oxygenator changeout during CPB

Changing the core components of the CPB system during the course of CPB is a major undertaking. Ideally this should be performed as a planned "urgent" procedure under hypothermia. The perfusionist must alert both surgeon and anesthesiologist of impending CPB system failure.

Inadequate flow

Inadequate flow can result from electrical or mechanical pump failure, a venous "air lock", cannula obstruction (e.g. kinking, malposition and clamping), covert circulating volume loss and aortic dissection (Table 62.7).

By its very nature, electrical power failure during CPB is a rare and unpredictable event. An uninterruptible power supply combined with an on-site backup generator should make total electrical failure in the operating room an extremely rare occurrence. Modern CPB pumps have emergency battery backup, which can be used to drive the pump and critical monitors. Although roller pump heads can be manually cranked during total power loss, this procedure is tiring and requires two individuals if undertaken for more than 5 min. Total power loss causes heater unit failure, which makes rewarming virtually impossible.

As air entrainment interferes with a siphon, venous return to the reservoir may be halted by the presence of a sufficiently large volume of air – an "air lock". If elevation of the tubing in sections fails to rectify the problem the venous cannula is clamped, and the venous line disconnected and back-filled.

Cannula size determines the flow rate within the venous line. An inappropriately small cannula or kinks in the line will lead to decreased venous return, necessitating a reduction in pump flow. Obstruction to flow in the arterial line or oxygenator is confirmed by finding a high CPB flow line pressure and a low patient arterial pressure.

Aortic dissection is generally noticed when CPB is first commenced. CPB arterial line pressure is elevated while patient arterial pressure is low. The aorta may be flaccid on palpation with an obvious expanding mural hematoma. Unrecognized aortic dissection is associated with significant morbidity and mortality. The extent and impact of aortic dissection can be minimized by prompt diagnosis, discontinuation of CPB and repositioning of the aortic cannula. Despite this approach, many surgeons will opt for formal ascending aortic repair (e.g. an interposition graft).

Key points

- Emergencies during CPB are uncommon but potentially catastrophic.
- All staff should be familiar with the management of massive air embolism during CPB.
- Retrograde cerebral perfusion is used in the management of air embolism during CPB on the grounds that cerebral air embolism will have occurred.
- Therapeutic postoperative hypothermia (24–48 h) should be considered after significant air embolism during CPB.

Further reading

Mills NL, Ochsner JL. Massive air embolus during CPB: causes, prevention and management. *J Thorac Cardiovasc Surg* 1980; **80**(5): 708–17.

Tovar EA, Del Campo C, Borsari A, Webb RP, Dell JR, Weinstien PB. Postoperative management of cerebral air embolism: gas physiology for surgeons. *Ann Thorac Surg* 1995; **60**(4): 1138–42.

von Segesser LK. Unusual problems in cardiopulmonary bypass. In Gravlee GP, Davis RF, Stammers AH, Ungerleider RM (Eds.), *Cardiopulmonary Bypass: Principles and Practice*, 3rd edition. London: Lippincott Williams & Wilkins; 2008. pp. 608–13.

Controversies in cardiopulmonary bypass

63

Christiana C. Burt and Florian Falter

Despite six decades of clinical experience and considerable research, the characteristics of "optimal" CPB remain imprecisely defined. This chapter discusses the main areas of controversy (Table 63.1).

Pressure versus flow

There is no doubt that prolonged periods of hypotension and hypoperfusion are deleterious, and that the brain is the organ most at risk. Despite the fact that routine CPB perfusion pressures of 40–60 mmHg represent deliberate hypotension, the vast majority of patients appear to survive without evidence of significant neurologic injury. When pressure falls below this range an increase in either pump flow rate or administration of a vasoconstrictor to increase SVR is the usual response. The question of whether the perfusion pressure or the perfusion flow rate is more important for organ preservation remains unanswered.

At normocarbia, cerebral autoregulation maintains cerebral blood flow (CBF) over a wide range of perfusion pressures (50–150 mmHg). During hypothermic CPB the lower limit of cerebral autoregulation falls to as low as 30 mmHg. Children appear to tolerate pressures even lower than this. It follows, therefore, that in the absence of significant cerebrovascular disease, cerebral hypoperfusion will be unlikely with MAP >40 mmHg and this remains the lowest acceptable pressure in adult practice. There is general agreement that a target of perfusion pressure of 50–60 mmHg is safe in the majority of cases.

Cerebral autoregulation is altered by a number of disease processes (e.g. hypertension, diabetes mellitus) and, to a lesser extent, drugs such as volatile anesthetic agents and vasodilators. It has long been argued that two groups of patients might benefit from

Table 63.1 Controversies in CPB management

CPB perfusion characteristics	Optimum perfusion pressure
	Pressure versus flow
	Pulsatile versus non-pulsatile
Temperature	Normothermia versus hypothermia
Acid-base management	pH-stat versus α-stat
Hemoglobin	Minimum hematocrit on CPB
Blood glucose	Glycemic control
CPB equipment	Pump characteristics
	Circuit surface modification
	Reservoir characteristics
	Processing cardiotomy blood

increased perfusion pressure (i.e. 70–80 mmHg) during CPB – those with altered cerebral autoregulation and those with cerebrovascular disease. (Table 63.2)

In 1995, a randomized trial of higher (80–100 mmHg) versus lower (50–60 mmHg) CPB perfusion pressure in 248 CABG patients showed that *combined* neurologic and cardiac outcomes 6 months after surgery were significantly better in the higher-pressure group. The study was criticized for analyzing combined outcomes, using multiple comparisons, the high stroke rate (7.2%) in the lower pressure (control) group and being insufficiently powered to detect a 50% reduction in stroke rate. The following year, TEE findings in 75% of these patients were published and it became apparent that the incidence of high-grade aortic atheroma was greater in the lower-pressure group (~30% versus 40%). From this intriguing and provocative study, it can be tentatively concluded that higher perfusion pressures may reduce

Core Topics in Cardiac Anesthesia, Second Edition, ed. Jonathan H. Mackay and Joseph E. Arrowsmith. Published by Cambridge University Press. © Cambridge University Press 2012.

Table 63.2 Patient groups which may benefit from a higher CPB perfusion pressure

Advanced atherosclerosis

Severe (grade IV and V) atheromatous disease of the descending thoracic aorta (visible on TEE) is a good marker of atheromatous disease near the aortic cannulation site, which is not well visualized with TEE.

Chronic hypertension

In patients with chronic, poorly controlled hypertension the pressure-flow autoregulation curve is shifted to the right, therefore a mean perfusion pressure >50 mmHg is required to maintain flow.

Cerebrovascular disease

Patients with cerebrovascular disease and those with a history of stroke may have impaired regional cerebral autoregulation and are at greater risk of neurologic injury.

Diabetes mellitus

These patients appear to have an impaired metabolism-flow coupling during CPB with possibly some loss of pressure-flow regulation. It has therefore been postulated, but not proven, that a higher perfusion pressure would be required during rewarming or during normothermic CPB.

Age >70 years

Increasing age does not affect cerebral autoregulation per se. However, there may be slower vasodilatation of cerebral resistance vessels during rewarming leading to transient episodes of metabolism-flow mismatch with resultant ischemia. Unless there is coexisting atherosclerotic or hypertensive disease there is, as yet, no evidence that age per se is a reason for using high perfusion pressures.

Table 63.3 Proposed advantages and disadvantages of low and high CPB perfusion pressure

Perfusion pressure	Advantages	Disadvantages
Lower (< 60 mmHg)	↓ Incidence of emboli ↓ Hematological trauma ↓ Collateral warming of the heart Less blood in operative field	Cerebral and renal hypoperfusion
Higher (> 80 mmHg)	Vital organ perfusion maintained In event of cerebral injury secondary to emboli, collateral flow is said to be pressure-dependent	↑Hematological trauma ↑Risk of emboli ↑Bleeding complications

the risk of stroke in patients with severe aortic atheroma (Table 63.3).

By contrast, a retrospective study of ~3000 patients undergoing CABG surgery demonstrated a significant inverse relationship between CPB perfusion pressure and postoperative stroke or coma. This finding might indicate that patients deemed to be at higher risk were managed using higher perfusion pressures. Alternatively, it might be concluded that higher perfusion pressure during CPB is not without risk.

Studies examining the influence of CPB flow rate on CBF and metabolism have produced conflicting results – the principal study design flaw being failure to control for hematocrit. The only conclusion that can be drawn is that, within the bounds of usual clinical practice, modest changes in flow rate have little impact on CBF at normocarbia.

It should be borne in mind that:

- tissue oxygen delivery is a function of pump flow rate, SaO_2 and hematocrit, and
- pump flow rate gives no indication of regional organ perfusion.

The only organ amenable to flow modification at a constant pressure is the brain (by changing $PaCO_2$). Evidence of inadequate tissue perfusion includes reduced SvO2, metabolic acidosis and lactatemia. Assuming a normal Hb concentration, the recommended pump flow rate at normothermia is 2.2 l min^{-1} m^{-2}. The reduction in metabolic rate that accompanies hypothermia (50% for every 7°C) permits flow rates to be reduced.

Normothermia versus hypothermia

Hypothermic CPB was widely practiced until the mid 1990s. Studies suggesting that normothermic cardioplegia and CPB may improve myocardial protection during cardiac surgery led to the adoption of so-called "warm-heart" or normothermic techniques for some cardiac surgical procedures. The principal concern is that improved myocardial outcome is achieved at the expense of decreasing the margin of safety afforded by hypothermia and increasing the risk of neurologic injury.

In 1994, the Toronto Warm Heart Investigators reported no increase in adverse neurologic outcomes in patients maintained at normothermia (33–37°C versus 25–30°C) during CPB, whereas the Atlanta group reported a marked increase in neurologic injury. Based on patient numbers, however, evidence accumulated in subsequent studies suggests that the avoidance of hypothermia during CPB does not increase the risk of adverse neurologic outcomes (Table 63.4).

The majority of published randomized trials comparing warm versus cold temperature management during CPB have suffered from poor study design and have been insufficiently powered to detect differences in mortality and major morbidity.

Published in 2001, a Cochrane review of 17 studies revealed that hypothermia was associated with a *trend* towards a reduction in non-fatal strokes and a *trend* towards an increase in non-stroke-related perioperative deaths. In addition hypothermia was associated with a higher incidence of myocardial damage and low CO syndrome, although temperature management strategy appeared to have no impact on the incidence of non-fatal MI. The authors concluded that there was no definite advantage of hypothermia over normothermia in the incidence of clinical events. Because cognitive function testing was only undertaken in 4/17 studies, no conclusions could be made regarding the effect of normothermia on cognitive outcomes.

Pulsatile versus non-pulsatile flow

It has long been thought that pulsatile CPB is beneficial by virtue of the fact that it is more physiological. The additional energy present in pulsatile flow increases capillary perfusion and enhances lymphatic drainage. A pulsatile flow profile can be generated either with a programmable roller pump or with an IABP during non-pulsatile CPB (Table 63.5). The contradictory conclusions of clinical studies may in part be explained by differences in the pressure–flow characteristics of pulsatile CPB employed.

In patients with pre-existing renal insufficiency, pulsatile CPB appears to be associated with improved postoperative renal function. The application of an AXC denies the ischemic heart any potential benefit from pulsatile CPB. Any improvement in myocardial outcome may be solely due to the higher perfusion pressures generated during pulsatile CPB. Published in 1995, a Canadian study of 316 CABG patients demonstrated that pulsatile CPB was associated with lower mortality and cardiovascular morbidity but no improvement in neurologic and cognitive outcomes. One reason why subsequent investigations may have failed to replicate these findings is the lack of definition of what constitutes pulsatile flow and how to quantify it. The amount of hemodynamic

Table 63.4 Reasons for failure to demonstrate hypothermic neuroprotection

Normothermic CPB in many cases meant a temperature of 35.5°C, which may have conferred a degree of neuroprotection

Inadvertent cerebral hyperthermia during rewarming during hypothermic CPB

Patients in both hypothermic and normothermic CPB groups were relatively normothermic at times of greatest cerebral vulnerability – aortic cannulation/ decannulation and onset/offset of CPB

Table 63.5 Putative benefits of pulsatile and non-pulsatile CPB

Pulsatile

↑Myocardial (subendocardial) perfusion, oxygenation and contractility
↑Renal (cortical) blood flow and urine output
↑Cerebral perfusion
↓ Catecholamine, renin, angiotensin, aldosterone and lactate levels
Preserved baroreceptor function
Maintenance of pancreatic β cell function

Non-pulsatile

↓ Hemolysis
↓ Platelet damage
Less complex CPB system

Table 63.6 The differences between the clinical applications of α-stat and pH-stat blood-gas management strategies

α-stat	pH-stat
Derives its name because the ionization state of enzymatic α-histidine-imidazole groups is maintained constant	So called because pH is maintained at ~7.4 regardless of blood temperature
Blood gas analysis results *not* corrected for temperature	Blood gas analysis results corrected for temperature
Target = "normal" blood gases at 37°C	Target = "normal" blood gases at *blood temperature*
Temperature-corrected hypocarbia and alkalosis tolerated	Temperature-uncorrected hypercarbia and acidosis tolerated
No additional CO_2 administered to patient	Additional CO_2 administered to patient

Table 63.7 Putative advantages and disadvantages of α-stat and pH-stat blood-gas management strategies

	Advantages	Disadvantages
α-stat	Cerebral autoregulation preserved ↓ Cerebral microembolization Improved neurologic outcomes ↓ Cerebral injury post-DHCA Improved myocardial function	Risk of cerebral hypoperfusion
pH-stat	More uniform cerebral cooling ↑H^+ reduces organ metabolism HbO_2 dissociation curve right shifted	Pressure passive CBF ↑Cerebral microembolization ↑Free-radical-induced tissue damage

energy delivered by different pulsatile pumps can vary widely and the pressure waveform can be affected by other components of the bypass system. A recent review called for future investigators to standardize CPB systems and conduct when investigating this question.

Alpha-stat versus pH-stat

The solubility of a gas in a liquid is inversely proportional to temperature. As temperature falls, the total gas content remains unchanged but the proportion of dissolved gas in equilibrium with the gas phase (i.e. the partial pressure) falls. For this reason automated blood-gas analysis, which is performed at 37°C, masks a fall in PaO_2 and $PaCO_2$ during hypothermia. In the case of CO_2, the $PaCO_2$ is reduced by 4.4% for every 1°C decrease in temperature. When temperature-corrected blood-gas measurements are used, hypothermic patients appear hypocarbic and alkalotic.

In nature, two blood-gas management strategies have emerged to maintain normal physiology during hypothermia. Poikilotherms (e.g. fish and reptiles) exhibit "alpha-stat" blood-gas changes when exposed to different environmental temperatures. In contrast, hibernating mammals (e.g. bears) exhibit "pH-stat" blood gases during hypothermic hibernation (Table 63.6).

During hypothermic CPB, blood vessels maintain their responsiveness to CO_2 and modulate organ blood flow accordingly. The impact of blood-gas management strategy on neurologic, cardiac and renal outcomes following hypothermic CPB has generated considerable debate (Table 63.7).

Based on the results of laboratory and clinical studies, α-stat is recommended for adults undergoing uninterrupted hypothermic CPB, while pH-stat should probably be used during hypothermic CPB prior to deep hypothermic circulatory arrest (DHCA). The risk of neurologic injury during DHCA appears, at least in part, to be due to incomplete brain cooling and insufficient metabolic rate reduction in the early part of cooling. As cerebral autoregulation is lost as temperature falls, blood-gas management strategy has progressively less influence on CBF.

Table 63.8 STS and SCA practice guidelines for blood transfusion during CPB

Indication class	LOE	Indication
IIa	C	Trigger Hb = 6 g dl^{-1} unless patient is at risk for decreased cerebral O_2 delivery (previous CVA, diabetes mellitus, carotid stenosis, cerebrovascular disease)
IIa	C	Transfusion above Hb 6 g dl^{-1} needs to be guided by patient factors (age, severity of illness, cardiac function, risk of critical end-organ ischemia) laboratory parameters such as hematocrit or SvO_2
IIb	C	It is not unreasonable to keep patients at risk for critical end-organ injury at Hb >7 g dl^{-1}

STS, Society of Thoracic Surgeons; SCA, Society of Cardiovascular Anesthesiologists; LOE, level of evidence.

The reduction in organ metabolism (O_2 consumption) associated with increased H^+ concentration during pH-stat is attributed to acidosis-induced intracellular enzyme dysfunction and impaired O_2 utilization.

Glucose

There is now consensus that hyperglycemia prior to DHCA is deleterious and should be avoided. Debate continues regarding the continued use of CPB priming solutions containing glucose for patients undergoing CPB without circulatory arrest. Supporters of glucose-containing priming solutions argue that hyperglcemia is unlikely to worsen permanent focal ischemia caused by embolization of atheromatous debris. Adding glucose to priming solutions results in less subsequent crystalloid administration, reduced perioperative fluid retention and enhanced diuresis – all of which may improve lung function after surgery. Opponents argue that most neurologic injuries involve some degree of reperfusion injury and that hyperglycemia worsens ischemic intracellular acidosis, neuronal regulation and mitochondrial ATP generation, thus exacerbating neurologic injury.

Recent evidence that tight glucose control improves outcomes in critically ill patients poses a simple question: is the problem adding glucose or failing to manage hyperglycemia? If the latter is true, patients may enjoy the benefits of glucose, insulin and potassium therapy without additional cerebral risk.

Finally, the normothermic brain is likely to be more sensitive to the deleterious effects of hyperglycemia than the hypothermic brain. It has been suggested that the hyperglycemia and cerebral hyperthermia contributed to the higher incidence of adverse neurologic outcomes in the Atlanta warm heart study.

Hematocrit

Blood viscosity is inversely related to temperature, and is a positive exponential function of hematocrit. Hypothermia increases overall blood viscosity – plasma viscosity increases and red cell membrane plasticity decreases. It was widely believed that the reduction in blood viscosity associated with hemodilution improved tissue perfusion during hypothermic CPB – counteracting the negative impact of anemia. Consequently, severe anemia (hematocrit <20%) during CPB was commonplace until the end of the 1990s.

While the majority of patients undergoing hypothermic CPB tolerate dilutional anemia, the use of normothermic perfusion techniques has forced reconsideration of the minimum acceptable hematocrit during CPB. Early observational studies suggested that the severity of anemia during CPB correlated with failure to wean from CPB, IABP use and mortality. One prospective study, in which patients were randomized to a minimum hematocrit of either 27% or ~16%, was halted by the safety monitoring committee because of the excess adverse events in the lower hematocrit group. Other investigators have demonstrated a similar relationship between lowest hematocrit during CPB and early (in-hospital) mortality, late mortality, stroke, low CO syndrome, cardiac arrest, pulmonary dysfunction, renal dysfunction and sepsis. The cut-off value for the lowest acceptable hematocrit on CPB is often dictated by the use of hypothermia and appears to be in the range of 21–25%.

Blood transfusion during CPB

Inadequate DO_2 during CPB – evidenced by metabolic acidosis and low SvO_2 – in the presence of SaO_2 >95% and a low hematocrit should prompt consideration of RBC transfusion. In 2007 the Society of Thoracic Surgeons (STS) and the Society of Cardiovascular Anesthesiologists (SCA) jointly released a clinical practice guideline addressing the issue of perioperative blood transfusion and blood conservation in cardiac surgery. Within these guidelines, specific reference is made to the indications for transfusion during CPB (Table 63.8). Interestingly, the practice guideline does not address the possibility of increasing pump flow to increase DO_2 to compensate for a low hemoglobin concentration.

Key points

- Higher perfusion pressures may reduce the risk of stroke in patients with diabetes mellitus, chronic hypertension or severe aortic atheroma.
- Patients are relatively normothermic at times of greatest cerebral vulnerability during cardiac surgery with hypothermic CPB.
- Alpha-stat is recommended for adults undergoing uninterrupted hypothermic CPB.
- The minimum acceptable hematocrit during CPB should be dictated by adequacy of tissue oxygenation.

Further reading

Gold JP, Charlson ME, Williams-Russo P, et al. Improvement of outcomes after coronary artery bypass: a randomized trial comparing intraoperative high versus low mean arterial pressure. *J Thorac Cardiovasc Surg* 1995; **110**(5): 1302–14.

Grigore AM, Mathew J, Grocott HP, et al. Prospective randomized trial of normothermic versus hypothermic cardiopulmonary bypass on cognitive function after coronary artery bypass graft surgery. *Anesthesiology* 2001; **95**(5): 1110–19.

Martin TD, Craver JM, Gott JP, et al. Prospective randomised trial of retrograde warm cardioplegia: myocardial benefit and neurological threat. *Ann Thorac Surg* 1994; **57**(2): 298–304.

Murkin JM, Martzke JS, Buchan AM, et al. A randomized study of the influence of perfusion technique and pH management strategy in 316 patients undergoing coronary artery bypass surgery. II. Neurologic and cognitive outcomes. *J Thorac Cardiovasc Surg* 1995; **110**(2): 349–62.

O'Dwyer C, Prough DS, Johnston WE. Determinants of cerebral perfusion during cardiopulmonary bypass. *J Cardiothorac Vasc Anesth* 1996; **10**(1): 54–64.

Patel RL, Turtle MR, Chambers DJ, James DN, Newman S, Venn GE. Alpha-stat acid–base regulation during cardiopulmonary bypass improves neuropsychologic outcome in patients undergoing coronary artery bypass grafting. *J Thorac Cardiovasc Surg* 1996; **111**(6): 1267–79.

Rees K, Beranek-Stanley M, Burke M, Ebrahim S. Hypothermia to reduce neurological damage following coronary artery bypass surgery. *Cochrane Database Syst Revs* 2001; **1**: CD002138.

The Warm Heart Investigators. Randomised trial of normothermic versus hypothermic coronary bypass surgery. *Lancet* 1994; **343**(8897): 559–63.

van Wermeskerken GK, Lardenoye JW, Hill SE, et al. Intraoperative physiologic variables and outcome in cardiac surgery: Part II. Neurologic outcome. *Ann Thorac Surg* 2000; **69**(4): 1077–83.

Chapter

64

Non-cardiac applications of cardiopulmonary bypass

Joseph E. Arrowsmith and Jonathan H. Mackay

Since its introduction into clinical practice in the early 1950s, the indications for CPB have broadened, from operations on or within the heart, to include non-cardiac thoracic, abdominal and neurologic procedures. The indications for CPB for non-cardiac surgery are shown in Table 64.1.

Anesthetic considerations

Similar principles apply to the application of CPB in both cardiac and non-cardiac surgery. In practice, however, there are a number of important factors that must be considered. With the exception of thoracic aortic surgery, non-cardiac CPB procedures are performed rarely and frequently involve staff who have little or no regular experience of CPB. Moreover, non-cardiac surgeons do not routinely operate on fully anticoagulated patients. Published case series and experience gained in previous cases should form the basis of detailed protocols for future reference.

Femoro-femoral CPB, which avoids the need for sternotomy or thoracotomy, is often employed in procedures that do not routinely involve chest opening. In this situation, there is retrograde perfusion of the aorta. Although the size of the femoral arterial cannula has minimal impact on CPB flow rates, a small femoral venous cannula may significantly reduce venous return. For this reason the maximal achievable flow rate may be insufficient at normothermia. To circumvent this problem, partial or incomplete CPB is initiated and lung ventilation continued until the degree of hypothermia is compatible with CPB at reduced flow rates. It is essential that hypothermia-induced VF does not occur before reaching this level of hypothermia.

The risk of CPB-related adverse events is the same, regardless of the clinical application. The basic

Table 64.1 Non-cardiac surgical applications of CPB

Thoracic	Surgery of the great vessels Pulmonary embolectomy/ endarterectomy Tracheobronchial reconstruction Resection of mediastinal tumors Lung transplantation Retrotracheal goitre
Abdominal	Resection of renal tumors with IVC extension
Neurologic	Arteriovenous malformations Basilar artery aneurysm
Resuscitation	Accidental hypothermia Patient transfer

principles of adequate anticoagulation, avoidance of air embolism and maintenance of vital organ perfusion are no less important. Femoral cannulation may result in lower limb ischemia or neurologic injury. In difficult cases it should be borne in mind that femoro-femoral CPB can be established under local anesthesia prior to the induction of general anesthesia.

Thoracic surgery

CPB for surgery on the ascending aorta and aortic arch is discussed in Chapters 36 and 37, respectively. Pulmonary embolectomy and (thrombo) endarterectomy, performed for acute and chronic pulmonary thromboembolic disease, respectively, requires CPB ± deep hypothermic circulatory arrest (DHCA).

In the past, resection of tracheal and carinal tumours was routinely performed with CPB. Advances in endoluminal intervention (e.g. stents, cryotherapy, lasers, etc.) have limited the indications for CPB to:

- patients at high risk of airway obstruction following induction of anesthesia
- repair of tracheal dehiscence following heart–lung transplantation
- resuscitation of patients suffering massive hemorrhage after pulmonary resection.

Mediastinal surgery

Patients with large anterior mediastinal tumors (e.g. teratoma, lymphoma or seminoma) may develop airway collapse and great vessel compression following induction of anesthesia. In addition, initiation of intermittent positive-pressure ventilation may cause distal air trapping. Although an inhalational induction and maintenance of spontaneous respiration is theoretically attractive, induction even with sevoflurane may be slow and hazardous. The left lateral position may be preferable as placing the patient in the supine position may lead to cardiac arrest from PA or SVC obstruction. Neither inhalational induction nor awake-intubation completely avoids the risk of airway obstruction distal to the ETT. If there is any doubt the groins should be prepared for femoral cannulation prior to induction of anesthesia.

Transplantation surgery

Although the majority of single- and double-lung transplants can be accomplished using standard thoracic anesthetic techniques without CPB, a perfusionist should always be immediately available. Induction of anesthesia and initiation of positive-pressure ventilation in patients with end-stage emphysema commonly result in severe hypotension. Air trapping and breath "stacking" have been likened to a tourniquet being applied to the right heart. If in doubt, the patient should be deliberately disconnected from the ventilator to let the trapped gas out. The patient with emphysematous lungs will *expire* if given insufficient time to *exhale*!

Intolerance of one-lung anesthesia, due to hemodynamic instability, severe hypercarbia or hypoxia, is the principal indication for CPB. Severe gas trapping in the dependent lung or, more rarely, a dependent pneumothorax may produce rapid decompensation. The choice of cannulation site is largely dictated by surgical approach (i.e. lateral thoracotomy, sternotomy or "clam shell") and expediency.

Urological surgery

The principal indication for CPB in this setting is resection of renal tumors (e.g. renal cell carcinoma or hypernephroma, nephroblastoma) with IVC extension. The aim of surgery is radical, curative resection with the operative approach being largely determined by the superior limit of caval extension. In advanced cases the tumor may prolapse through the TV and produce hemodynamic compromise. In this situation, sternotomy is required to establish CPB (i.e. SVC to ascending aorta) as IVC obstruction precludes femoro-femoral CPB. A short period of DHCA may be required for removal of tumor from the RA.

The anesthesiologist should be aware of the potential for massive hemorrhage, tumor fragmentation/embolism and paraneoplastic phenomena (e.g. hyperglycemia, hypertension, hypercalcemia and hypokalemia). Short central venous cannulae and TEE should be used, and PAFCs avoided.

Neurosurgery

First used in the late 1950s, DHCA was widely used for intracranial aneurysm surgery until the late 1960s. Extra-thoracic cannulation techniques largely overcame the need for simultaneous thoracotomy and craniotomy. Subsequent advances in neurosurgery led to the abandonment of DHCA for all but the most technically demanding cases, for example posterior fossa hemangioblastomas and giant basilar aneurysms.

Resuscitation

In the setting of cardiac surgery, surgical re-exploration and re-institution of CPB is a common means of dealing with cardiovascular collapse in the early postoperative period. CPB may also be of use in major trauma, particularly in the presence of airway disruption. The benefits of heparinization and CPB have to be carefully weighed against the risk of exsanguination or intracranial hemorrhage. Less commonly, CPB has been successfully used to treat accidental hypothermia and drug overdose (e.g. flecainide, bupivacaine). In practice, the logistical difficulties of moving a patient to a center that offers CPB, the high mortality and low chance of full neurologic recovery limit its application.

407

The use of CPB in the resuscitation of patients without a spontaneous circulation should be reserved for those who have suffered a *witnessed* cardiac arrest. Use of CPB following *unwitnessed* cardiac arrest is associated with unacceptably high mortality and cerebral morbidity.

The development of compact membrane oxygenators and disposable centrifugal blood pumps provides a means by which patients with acute cardiorespiratory failure can be sufficiently stabilized for transfer to a center offering ECMO support. In practice, however, veno-venous (rather than veno-arterial) ECMO is used for respiratory patients with preserved cardiac function.

Key points

- Induction of anesthesia and initiation of IPPV is hazardous in patients with large anterior mediastinal tumors.
- Maximal achievable flow rates during femoro-femoral bypass may be insufficient at normothermia.
- The use of CPB in the resuscitation of patients without a spontaneous circulation should be reserved for those who have suffered a *witnessed* cardiac arrest.

Further reading

Conacher ID. Dynamic hyperinflation – the anaesthetist applying a tourniquet to the right heart. *Br J Anaesth* 1998; **81**(2): 116–17.

Cardiovascular problems in the cardiac ICU

65

Trevor W. R. Lee and Jonathan H. Mackay

Hemodynamic instability following CPB is common. The goal of cardiovascular management in the ICU is to maintain adequate oxygen transport to end organs until complete recovery of cardiac function.

Postoperative circulation management

Preload optimization

The heart compensates for acute changes in venous return and end-diastolic volume (EDV) by varying the force and velocity of myocardial fiber shortening – the Frank–Starling relationship (Figure 4.2). The response to increasing preload can be thought of in three distinct phases (Table 65.1).

In health, preload optimization typically occurs with PAWP 10–15 mmHg. Many cardiac surgical patients have reduced LV compliance, which becomes further reduced by the effects of CPB and catecholamines. In these patients a higher PAWP (i.e. >15 mmHg) is often required to maintain adequate SV.

Rate, rhythm and contractility

Heart rate, rhythm and myocardial contractility are the major determinants of myocardial oxygen consumption (MVO_2). Myocardial ischemia is avoided by homeostatic mechanisms, which balance MVO_2 against CO and MAP. Because of its 30% augmentation of EDV, normal sinus rhythm (NSR) is desirable whenever possible. Atrial or atrioventricular pacing at 80–100 bpm can improve endocardial perfusion by shortening diastolic filling time and reducing EDV.

VF and unstable ventricular and supraventricular tachydysrhythmias should be immediately converted by either electrical or chemical cardioversion. Maintenance of normal or supranormal $[K^+]$ (i.e. 4.5–5.5 mmol l^{-1}) and $[Mg^{2+}]$ reduces ventricular irritability.

Table 65.1 The three phases of the response to increasing preload

1	Intact preload reserve	$\uparrow$ EDV $\rightarrow$ $\uparrow$ SV and $\uparrow$ CO
2	Preload optimization	$\uparrow$ EDV $\rightarrow$ CO unchanged
3	Exhausted preload reserve	$\uparrow$ EDV $\rightarrow$ $\downarrow$ CO and $\downarrow$ MAP

Table 65.2 Correction of hypovolemia and hypervolemia

Hypovolemia

Synthetic colloids (e.g. succinylated gelatin or hydroxyethylstarch) if [Hb] > 8.5 g dl^{-1}

Oxygen delivery maximized at hematocrit 24–30%

Hypervolemia

Diuretics $\downarrow$ intravascular volume by $\uparrow$ urine output and $\downarrow$ EDV by $\uparrow$ venous capacitance

Direct-acting vasodilators (e.g. nitroglycerin) $\uparrow$ venous capacitance

Enalaprilat, an angiotensin-converting enzyme inhibitor, is also a venodilator

An IV preparation is available for use

Venesection and erect posture

Cardiodepressant anti-dysrhythmics should be used with caution in patients with impaired myocardial function. Although amiodarone is the most commonly used anti-dysrhythmic in cardiac surgical patients, other classes of agent may be required for more complex or persistent rhythm abnormalities.

A hypercontractile ventricle, ejecting a maximal SV against a high afterload, does so at the expense of increased MVO_2. It is suggested that perioperative β-blockade improves long-term outcome in patients with coronary artery disease. The postoperative use of β-blockers in stable cardiac surgical patients is not uncommon.

Core Topics in Cardiac Anesthesia, Second Edition, ed. Jonathan H. Mackay and Joseph E. Arrowsmith. Published by Cambridge University Press. © Cambridge University Press 2012.

Table 65.3 Causes of increased afterload in the cardiac surgical patient

History of preoperative essential or secondary hypertension

Increased endogenous catecholamines released during CPB

Hypothermia

Emergence from anesthesia

Response to pain can lead to arteriolar vasoconstriction

Administration of exogenous vasoconstrictors

Afterload

Afterload can be viewed as the sum of external forces opposing ventricular ejection, of which SVR is one component. Laplace's law states that LV wall tension or stress is directly proportional to intracavity pressure and cavity radius, and inversely proportional to LV wall thickness (see Figure 31.2).

Depending on LV function, increased afterload (Table 65.3) may be associated with either hypertension or hypotension. Both can cause decreased coronary perfusion and systolic dysfunction. Uncontrolled hypertension can cause excessive surgical bleeding.

Common complications

Left ventricular dysfunction

Ventricular function is commonly depressed for 8–24 h following CPB. The ideal measure of LV performance, the slope of the end-systolic pressure–volume relationship (ESPVR), cannot easily be derived at the bedside. For this reason, surrogate measures of contractility (i.e. RA pressure, PAWP, MAP, PAP and CO) are used. Although echocardiography can be used to assess ventricular function, the findings are generally load-dependent (Figure 65.1).

Decreased contractility can be secondary to metabolic abnormalities, cardiodepressant agents, reperfusion injury and myocardial ischemia (coronary vasospasm, thrombosis or occlusion). The incidence of perioperative MI (often clinically silent) is thought to be ~5%. The diagnosis of MI in the post-CABG patient may be challenging (Table 65.4).

Before initiating inotropic therapy, all remediable factors (i.e. rate, rhythm, preload and afterload) should be addressed. Myocardial β-receptor desensitization and downregulation make the heart less sensitive to catecholamines. An understanding of the differential effects of inotropes on the heart and circulation, rapid assessment of response and

Table 65.4 Diagnosis of perioperative myocardial infarction

ECG	Difficult to interpret in perioperative period – particularly ST and T-wave alterations Reliance on Q-wave formation has a low sensitivity in this setting
CK-MB	Traditional enzyme marker used to confirm MI Found in skeletal muscle and atria Low specificity following cardiac surgery
Troponin I	Adenosine triphosphatase inhibitor of actin-myosin complex Higher sensitivity and specificity than CK-MB Levels >60 µmol l^{-1} correlate with both Q-wave MI and new RWMA

CK-MB, creatinine kinase MB (isoenzyme); TnI, troponin I; RWMA, regional wall motion abnormality.

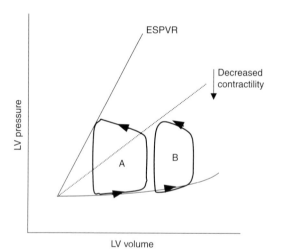

Figure 65.1 LV pressure–volume loops illustrating (A) the normal ventricle, and (B) the decrease in slope of the ESPVR line with decreased contractility. This decrease in contractility can also be accompanied by a decrease in SV, and an increase in LVEDP.

modification of therapy are probably more important than the order in which specific drugs are selected.

Since serum $[Ca^{2+}]$ may be reduced following CPB and the administration of citrated blood products, empirical $CaCl_2$ administration – which causes a transient increase in contractility and vascular tone – may be appropriate.

Mechanical support

In refractory LV failure or dysrhythmias – where inotropic, vasoactive and anti-dysrhythmic therapy is maximal – mechanical circulatory support may be necessary. The IABP decreases systolic LV wall tension (afterload reduced after balloon deflation) and improves coronary perfusion (diastolic aortic root pressure augmentation during balloon inflation). Contraindications to the IABP include femoral arterial and abdominal aortic disease, and moderate to severe aortic regurgitation. A mechanical ventricular assist device (VAD) may be required in intractable LV failure/dysrhythmia as a bridge to recovery or transplantation (see Chapter 57).

Right ventricular dysfunction

RV failure can be difficult to manage because of the dependence of LV filling on right-sided function. If RV output falls, LV filling and therefore LV output are reduced. The RV is extremely sensitive to increases in afterload (i.e. PVR). Reduced RV contractility or increased RV afterload results in increased RV wall tension and right heart distension. Isoproterenol or dobutamine are useful first-line agents, as they increase contractility while lowering PVR. Phosphodiesterase (PDE) inhibitors (e.g. enoximone and milrinone), which tend to cause less tachycardia than isoproterenol and dobutamine, are now commonly used to treat RV dysfunction. Although more effective in LV failure, the IABP may reduce RV afterload and improve coronary perfusion. Short-term use of a RV assist device (RVAD) may allow time for RV recovery.

Pulmonary hypertension

It is essential that primary and secondary pulmonary hypertension following CPB is identified and appropriately managed in the postoperative period. Reducing RV afterload can improve RV systolic performance and right heart CO. As an adjunct to milrinone, inhaled NO therapy has been shown to improve right-sided hemodynamics. When administered at 5–10 ppm it has been shown to reduce PVR. Epoprostenol (PGI_2), when given by IV infusion or an inhaled aerosol, is another agent that can be useful in reducing PA pressure. The usual initial dose for intravenous infusion is 2–5 ng kg^{-1} min^{-1}. Oral agents, such as sildenafil and bosentan, may be of use.

Pericardial tamponade

Pericardial tamponade is characterized by hypotension, tachycardia and elevated CVP. Although it typically occurs acutely within 24 h of cardiac surgery, it can develop chronically over several days. In tamponade, the decrease in the LV filling during inspiration is accentuated. The fall in SV produces a reflex increase in HR and myocardial contractility. Diagnostic clues include those described in Table 65.5.

In addition to detecting an obvious extracardiac collection, the most common TEE manifestation is collapse of right-sided chambers when their intracavity pressures

Table 65.5 Clinical signs suggestive of cardiac tamponade

Oliguria

Reduced or absent chest tube drainage

Pulsus paradoxus

Equalization of the RAP, PAD and PCWP

Loss of the y-descent in RAP and PCWP

Low-voltage ECG/electrical alternans pattern

Table 65.6 Resuscitation goals in cardiac tamponade

Preload	Elevated – avoid high PEEP
Heart rate	High – because of reduced SV
Rhythm	Sinus preferable but limited atrial kick
Systemic vascular resistance	High
Contractility	Normal or elevated

PEEP, positive end-expiratory pressure.

are at their lowest – i.e. the RV in early diastole and the RA in early systole. In the spontaneously breathing patient, transmitral E- and A-wave velocities are decreased during inspiration, with reciprocal changes in the right heart. Mechanical ventilation reverses this relationship (Figure 65.2). Management consists of resuscitation (Table 65.6) and prompt surgical drainage.

Postoperative atrial fibrillation

Atrial fibrillation and atrial flutter are the most common postoperative supraventricular tachydysrhythmias following cardiac surgery. New-onset AF occurs within 24–72 h of surgery in up to 30% of patients. Independent predictors of AF include age >65 years, hypertension, male sex, a previous history of AF and valve surgery. Patients undergoing heart transplantation or isolated CABG surgery have the lowest incidence of postoperative AF. Other factors that may contribute to AF include prolonged AXC time, pulmonary vein venting, perioperative pneumonia, COPD and prolonged postoperative mechanical ventilation.

Moderate-dose hydrocortisone therapy has also been shown to aid in the prevention of post-cardiac surgery atrial fibrillation. Multicenter studies examining the effect of methylprednisolone and dexamethasone in AF prophylaxis in cardiac surgery are currently under way.

Preoperative β-blockade and amiodarone therapy can reduce the incidence of AF following CABG. The POISE study demonstrated that, in non-cardiac surgical patients,

411

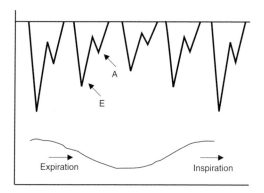

Figure 65.2 Pericardial tamponade physiology during positive-pressure ventilation: Mitral E wave velocity increases during the inspiratory phase and decreases during the expiratory phase.

Table 65.7 Simplified approach to hemodynamic management in the patient with optimal preload

↑ MAP and ↓ CO	Afterload is likely to be normal or high, and therapy with an inotrope plus a vasodilator, or with a PDE inhibitor might be considered
↓ MAP and ↑ CO	Afterload is probably low and a vasopressor should be considered
↓ MAP and ↓ CO	Contractility and afterload are reduced and therapy with both inotropes and vasopressors should be considered

metoprolol significantly reduced the risk of clinically important new AF. Other anti-dysrhythmic agents, such as calcium channel blockers and digoxin, are less effective as prophylactic regimes. IV magnesium administration and atrial pacing have also been shown to reduce the incidence of AF in some studies. Thoracic epidural anesthesia may also be of benefit.

In the absence of contraindications, all patients who develop AF should be anticoagulated within 24–48 h. Heparin is an appropriate first-line anticoagulant until therapeutic anticoagulation can be established with oral warfarin. Low-molecular-weight heparin (e.g. enoxaparin 1.5 mg kg^{-1} day^{-1}) may be used as an alternative. Aspirin therapy may be used in patients who cannot be warfarinized. If AF has persisted for more than 48 h and therapeutic anticoagulation has not been maintained, TEE should be performed to exclude the presence of LA thrombus. Electrical or chemical cardioversion to sinus rhythm is preferred, especially when patients are hemodynamically unstable, symptomatic or unable to receive anticoagulation. Where available, ibutelide and intravenous diltiazem may be of use. Otherwise, pharmacological ventricular rate control alone is acceptable in some cases. IV amiodarone is effective for both conversion to sinus rhythm and ventricular rate control, and can be easily converted to oral therapy. The need for anti-dysrhythmic therapy should be reviewed 6–8 weeks after surgery and discontinued if the patient is in sinus rhythm.

Simplified approach to hemodynamic management

Considering CO, MAP and PAWP in the patient with optimal preload simplifies hemodynamic management (Table 65.7).

Key points

- A PAWP >15 mmHg may be required following CPB.
- Increased afterload may cause hypertension or hypotension.
- Tamponade may be difficult to diagnose clinically and should be considered in all cases of hypotension/low CO following cardiac surgery.
- Intra-aortic balloon counterpulsation reduces cardiac chamber wall tension by systolic deflation and improves coronary blood flow by diastolic augmentation.
- AF should not be regarded as a benign condition after cardiac surgery.

Further reading

Dunning J, Treasure T, Versteegh M, Nashef SA. Guidelines on the prevention and management of de novo atrial fibrillation after cardiac and thoracic surgery. *Eur J Cardiothorac Surg* 2006; **30**(6): 852–72.

Maisel WH, Rawn JD, Stevenson WG. Atrial fibrillation after cardiac surgery. *Ann Intern Med* 2001; **135**(12): 1061–73.

Mangano DT, Layug EL, Wallace A, Tateo I. Effect of atenolol on mortality and cardiovascular morbidity after noncardiac surgery. Multicenter Study of Perioperative Ischemia Research Group. *N Engl J Med* 1996; **335**(23): 1713–20.

POISE Study Group. Effects of extended-release metoprolol succinate in patients undergoing non-cardiac surgery (POISE trial): a randomized controlled trial. *Lancet* 2008; **371**: 1839–47.

Slogoff S, Keats AS. Does perioperative myocardial ischemia lead to postoperative MI? *Anesthesiology* 1985; **62**(2): 107–14.

Solomon AJ, Greenberg MD, Kilborn MJ, Katz NM. Amiodarone versus β-blocker to prevent atrial fibrillation after cardiac surgery. *Am Heart J* 2001; **142**(5): 811–15.

66

Resuscitation after adult cardiac surgery

Jonathan H. Mackay

Defibrillation, ventilation, pacing and resuscitation are essential components of cardiac surgical care. The 2010 European Resuscitation Council (ERC) guidelines report the incidence of resuscitation as 0.7–2.9% after adult cardiac surgery. Overall in-hospital cardiac surgical mortality rates (>3.0%), together with the low prevalence of "do not attempt resuscitation" (DNAR) orders and the high proportion of treatable arrests in this population all suggest a higher true incidence of postoperative resuscitation. The most likely explanation for the discrepancy is that many resuscitation interventions are undertaken in house on the cardiac surgical ICU. As patients undergoing cardiac surgery become older and sicker, quality of resuscitation will continue to increase in importance. Conventional basic and advanced life support guidelines provide a useful framework but require modification in the cardiac surgical ICU setting. This chapter will highlight some of the key differences.

Resuscitation guidelines

Adult basic life support

Maintaining the circulation has been promoted ahead of airway management and breathing in recent adult basic life support (BLS) guidelines. The traditional Airway, Breathing, Circulation and Defibrillation ("ABCD" – or Accuse, Blame, Criticize and Deny in cardiac surgical mantra!) algorithm described in previous guidelines was replaced by Circulation, Airway and Breathing (i.e. "CAB"). In general, 30 chest compressions at a rate of 100–120 per min should now be given before any attempt to deliver rescue breaths. The efficacy of chest compressions can usually be

verified in ICU by studying the arterial pressure waveform. Interruptions to chest compressions should be minimized.

In situations where BLS is undertaken, the recommended ratio of chest compressions to ventilations is now 30:2. More chest compressions and fewer interruptions are achieved with this ratio than with the previously recommended 15:2 ratio. In the presence of a patent airway, effective chest compressions are considered more important than ventilation in the first few minutes of resuscitation. It should be borne in mind that coronary perfusion pressure progressively rises during chest compressions and rapidly falls with each pause for ventilation. Following a witnessed collapse in a patient with oxygenated arterial blood, the initial emphasis should normally be on chest compressions.

Because chest compressions may be injurious immediately following cardiac surgery, external cardiac massage is frequently deferred in cardiac ICU providing defibrillation or external pacing therapy can be delivered within 30–60 s. The rationale for this approach and modifications to the Advanced Life Support (ALS) algorithm are discussed later.

Adult advanced life support

Prompt and effective BLS and early defibrillation for shockable rhythms are the two most important interventions after cardiac arrest. The new 2010 Advanced Life Support (ALS) algorithm for the management of cardiac arrest in adults retains the shockable and non-shockable limbs (Figure 66.1). However, there are now significant differences in recommendations for defibrillation for shockable rhythms in cardiothoracic ICU.

Core Topics in Cardiac Anesthesia, Second Edition, ed. Jonathan H. Mackay and Joseph E. Arrowsmith. Published by Cambridge University Press. © Cambridge University Press 2012.

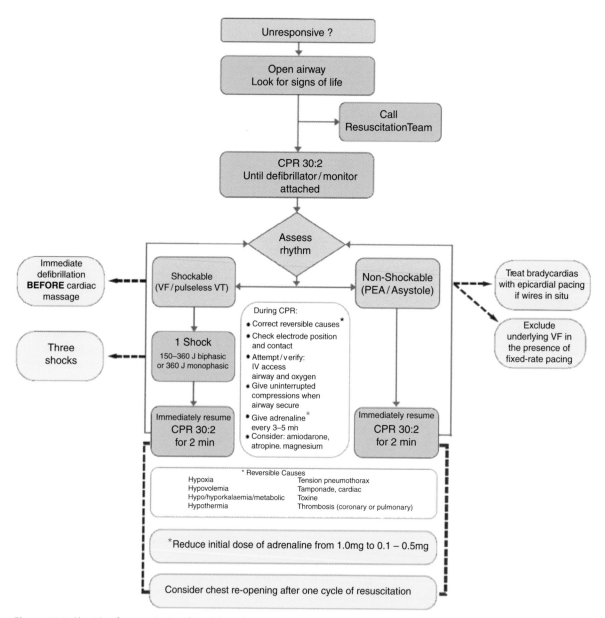

Figure 66.1 Algorithm for resuscitation after adult cardiac surgery. Six suggested modifications to the standard ALS algorithm are highlighted in the six bright yellow boxes to the sides and below. Therapeutic hypothermia may be considered after successful resuscitation. Adapted from the Resuscitation Council (UK) 2010 ALS algorithm.

Pulseless VT/VF

Pulseless VT and VF account for the majority of underlying dysrhythmias in patients who survive cardiac arrest in hospitals. For every minute the chances of successful defibrillation decline by 7–10%. Specialist cardiothoracic units should be capable of early detection, rapid defibrillation and superior outcomes. In the setting of the cardiac ICU, when external cardiac massage may be injurious, immediate defibrillation (i.e. "DCAB") should be the first-line response for all monitored in–hospital VF arrests.

Since 2005, a single shock (≥150 J biphasic or 360 J monophasic) has been recommended instead of three "stacked" shocks in general hospitals. Interruptions to CPR during delivery of three shocks and improved first shock efficacy of biphasic defibrillators

Table 66.1 An aide memoire to the causes of Pulseless electrical activity and asystole

The four "Hs"	The five "Ts"
Hypoxia	Tension pneumothorax
Hypovolemia	Tamponade
Hyperkalemia	Thromboembolic
Hypothermia	Therapeutic substances in overdose
	Toxic substances

were cited as reasons for the change. In practice, most cardiac surgical ICU and catheter laboratory staff were unconvinced by the evidence for single shocks and continued to deliver up to three stacked shocks in quick succession when treating VF. The authors of the 2010 guidelines recognized this and reverted to recommending three stacked shocks in quick succession for VF/VT arrests occurring in the cardiac catheter laboratory and cardiac surgical ICU. In addition, contrary to the latest guidelines, there is usually no need to commence chest compressions after a successful shock in invasively monitored cardiac surgical patients.

Non-VF/VT arrests

A heterogeneous group of conditions may present as non-VF/VT cardiac arrest (Table 66.1). Outcome is generally poor unless a reversible cause can be found and treated effectively. In the cardiac surgical ICU – where bleeding, hypovolemia and tamponade are all readily treatable, and where additional therapeutic options are available – outcomes are considerably better than in the general ICU population. Examination of trends in RA pressure, PAWP and airway pressure all provide useful pointers as to the likely etiology. Cessation of drainage from mediastinal drains does not exclude hemorrhage or tamponade as the drains may have become blocked. Although echocardiography is often very useful in the cardiac ICU, TEE may miss localized collections and thus delay re-operation. Patients with clinical signs suggestive of tamponade should be reopened even if the TEE is inconclusive.

When faced with an arrest of this type, it is essential to

- confirm that VF is not being missed and that ECG leads or pads are correctly attached
- treat bradycardia with epicardial pacing if wires are present

- exclude tension pneumothorax
- exclude underlying VF in the presence of fixed-rate pacing, and
- consider chest reopening if closed chest CPR is unsuccessful.

Symptomatic bradycardia is extremely common in the cardiac surgical ICU. ALS guidelines no longer recommend atropine as first-line treatment. In the cardiac surgical ICU, where tachycardia is equally undesirable, pacing (when possible) is the preferred option. If pacing is not an option (e.g. no wires *in situ* or failure to capture), isoproterenol or dopamine are often used. Management of asystole that fails to respond to pacing is an indication for prompt chest reopening.

Drugs in advanced cardiac life support

Although the use of vasopressors at cardiac arrests has become standard practice, proof of efficacy is limited. Epinephrine 1 mg is recommended every 3 min to improve coronary and cerebral perfusion. The American Heart Association has suggested that vasopressin may be used as an alternative to epinephrine. Clinical studies, however, have failed to demonstrate that either vasopressin or high-dose epinephrine (5 mg) offers any additional benefit.

On the cardiac surgical ICU it is entirely appropriate to modify the recommended pharmacological management of a monitored cardiac arrest. An α-agonist or smaller initial dosages of epinephrine (0.1–0.2 mg) may be administered to minimize the risk of hypertension and tachycardia following successful resuscitation. For patients with VF/VT arrests, it is standard practice to attempt at least three shocks before giving any epinephrine.

The evidence supporting the use of antiarrhythmic drugs in VF/VT was, until recently, surprisingly weak. Two studies of out-of-hospital VF/VT arrest demonstrated that the administration of amiodarone after three unsuccessful shocks increased the likelihood of survival to hospital admission. Significantly, neither study demonstrated that amiodarone improved survival to discharge. Despite this latter finding, amiodarone has now been promoted ahead of lidocaine in the VF/pulseless VT algorithm. A bolus of amiodarone 300 mg is recommended for VF/VT arrests that persist after three shocks but this should not delay surgical reopening (see below).

415

A further dose (150 mg) may be given for recurrent or refractory VF/VT, followed by an infusion of 900 mg over 24 h. Lidocaine can still be given for VF/VT if the patient has received amiodarone but the evidence supporting its efficacy is weak. Magnesium should also be considered if there is clinical suspicion of hypomagnesemia. Administration of sodium bicarbonate should be considered if arterial or mixed venous pH <7.1.

Airway and ventilation

The majority of patients will be intubated and mechanically ventilated. The inspired oxygen should be increased to 100% and positive end-expiratory pressure removed. Capnography often provides valuable information about endotracheal tube position and patency, ventilation and CO.

Chest reopening

Following surgery through a sternotomy, chest reopening is both a diagnostic and therapeutic option in the cardiac surgical ICU. In addition, chest reopening allows internal cardiac massage, which is considerably more effective than external chest compressions. Hemorrhage, tamponade, graft occlusion and graft avulsion are conditions likely to be remedied by this approach. Patients most likely to benefit are those with a surgically remediable lesion, those who arrest within 24 h of surgery, and those in whom the chest is reopened within 10 min of arrest. Delayed reopening or the finding of a problem that is not amenable to surgery (e.g. global cardiac dysfunction) is associated with a poor prognosis. The 2010 resuscitation guidelines confirm that chest reopening should be triggered by

- three failed shocks in VF/VT arrests (i.e. one resuscitation cycle)
- exclusion of reversible causes (e.g. tension pneumothorax) and failure of initial treatment for non-VF/VT arrest.

Chest reopening should not be used as a "last ditch" maneuver after a prolonged period of unsuccessful resuscitation. Although some units advocate initially stopping all infusions and syringe drivers to exclude iatrogenic drug administration errors, the majority tend to continue infusions unless there is a clinical suspicion of inadvertent vasodilator flushing being

responsible for loss of CO. Whichever policy is used, it is important to ensure that anesthesia and analgesia are restored prior to chest reopening.

Cardiopulmonary bypass

The reinstitution of CPB following emergency chest reopening may allow the resuscitation of a patient who would otherwise die. Hypothermic CPB restores organ perfusion, decompresses the heart, and allows the surgeon to consider all possible options in a more controlled setting. Valve replacement, repair of bleeding cannulation sites, graft revision and additional grafting may be undertaken with often surprisingly successful clinical outcomes. Whenever possible the patient should be transferred to the operating room before emergency reinstitution of CPB.

Late resuscitation on ICU

Patients with greater preoperative surgical risk, adverse intraoperative events and poor physiological state at the time of ICU admission are less likely to survive to hospital discharge. Similarly, refractory multi-system organ failure and recurrent nosocomial infection have been shown to be important determinants of mortality. For some patients, there comes a point when aggressive resuscitation is inappropriate and cardiopulmonary arrest becomes a terminal event. It is the duty of a doctor to identify these patients and to ensure that they are spared the indignity of futile interventions.

DNAR directives should be instituted if it is believed that death is inevitable and that CPR is unlikely to be successful. Sensible guidelines on implementation of DNAR orders can be found on the UK Resuscitation Council's website (http://www.resus.org.uk).

Resuscitation outside ICU
General ward or surgical floor

The management of a cardiac arrest outside the ICU differs little from a cardiac arrest on a general surgical or medical ward. Seemingly trivial symptoms and vague "early warning" signs should be taken seriously as they may herald a more sinister event. Although some arrests are unheralded, the majority of patients who arrest in the general ward setting display signs of physiological deterioration long before the event.

Early intervention seems intuitive and may reduce the incidence of cardiac arrests in the surgical ward setting. Early Warning Scores (EWS) are used to "track" patients' physiological status and "trigger" a response or intervention. Tracking the patient – the so-called "afferent limb" – involves either a single or multiple parameter scoring system. Single parameter scoring systems have limitations. Many of the suggested criteria for triggering a response are actually relatively late markers of physiological deterioration

Table 66.2 Suggested criteria for calling the Medical Emergency Team in a cardiothoracic hospital; oximetry is widely available and a potentially useful monitor in a cardiothoracic ward

Acute change	Physiology
Airway	Threatened
Breathing	All respiratory arrests Respiratory rate <5 or >36
Circulation	All cardiac arrests Pulse rate <40 or >140
Neurology	Fall in Glasgow Coma Scale (GCS) score >2 points
Renal	Urine output <0.5 ml kg h^{-1} for 2 consecutive hours
Oximetry	SpO$_2$ <90% regardless of FiO$_2$
Other	Patients giving cause for concern who do not meet above criteria

(Table 66.2). Aggregated weighted systems may provide earlier warning of deterioration and can be adapted for use in cardiothoracic wards (Table 66.3).

The use of medical emergency teams (MET) has been shown to reduce both the incidence and mortality from unexpected ward arrests in general hospitals. The effectiveness of the MET concept is significantly hampered by incomplete documentation of patient observations. Given the importance of respiratory rate and urinary output, recording of these values is often surprisingly poor.

The relative success of chest reopening following cardiac arrest on the ICU cannot be reproduced when chest reopening is undertaken on the ward or surgical floor. The proportion of surgically remediable causes of cardiac arrest decreases exponentially after surgery. As time passes thromboembolic phenomena and cardiac failure become more common than surgical bleeding or tamponade. Several case series have demonstrated the futility of chest reopening at the scene of arrest outside the ICU.

A small number of patients who sustain a *witnessed* arrest on the ward or surgical floor may benefit from chest reopening in the operating room. The decision to "scoop and run" is usually more difficult than the decision to reopen on the cardiac ICU. Whereas there is level-one evidence to support chest reopening in the cardiac ICU, the latest ERC guidelines do not specifically address the role of chest reopening for patients who arrest outside the cardiac

Table 66.3 Possible MEWS scoring system for wards in a cardiothoracic hospital

Score	Temp	AVPU[a] (CNS)	Resp rate	SATS on O$_2$	Heart rate (if β-blocked)	SYS BP	Urine output (ml kg^{-1} h^{-1})
3		U	≤8	<85	<40 (*<35*)	<70	Nil
2	≤35.0	P	9–10	85–89		71–80	<0.5
1	35.1–36.0	V		90–94	41–50 (*35–40*)	81–100	
0		A					
1	38.1–38.4	Confused or agitated	20–25		105–120 (*100–110*)		
2	≥38.5		26–34		121–135 (*111–130*)	>200	
3			>35		>135 (*>130*)		

[a] AVPU: A, alert and orientated; V, responds to voice, confused or agitated; P, responds to pain; U, unresponsive.
The total MEWS score is the additive score of the seven individual physiological scores.

Table 66.4 Factors influencing outcome from cardiac arrest and resuscitation on a ward

Geography	The geographical location and layout of cardiac surgical wards are important. Many patients understandably prefer to have their own room whilst staying in hospital. Given the lack of monitoring in some isolated rooms, cardiac patients may pay a heavy price for their privacy.
Training	Resuscitation training should place greater emphasis on the identification of the at-risk patient and prevention of cardiac arrests. Scenario-based training may be of value.
Prevention	Nowhere is the statement "Prevention is better than cure" more true than in the field of resuscitation. International studies have shown that many critically ill patients receive sub-optimal care on the general wards. Many terminal arrests on general wards are preceded by unrecognized or inadequately treated deterioration in their vital signs. Consideration should be given to the pre-emptive transfer of a deteriorating patient to the ICU. The appropriate use of DNAR orders significantly reduces the incidence of unexpected cardiac arrest.
Early detection	Outcomes from witnessed arrests are better than those where the initial arrest is undetected. With early detection, the proportion of primary VF/VT arrests is higher and time to defibrillation reduced.
Equipment	Automated external defibrillators (AEDs) are now increasingly being deployed in public sites. They are now so prevalent that BLS training is being extended to include teaching on the use of these straightforward devices. There is a strong argument for putting semi-automated defibrillators on general medical and surgical wards. AEDs for in-hospital use should include an ECG display and a manual override facility for use by the cardiac arrest team. Evidence suggests that biphasic defibrillation waveforms are superior to monophasic waveforms.

ICU. A scoop and run approach should be considered following:

1. A witnessed arrest
2. Unexpected arrest in a patient who had initially been making good progress
3. Tension pneumothorax considered and excluded
4. Non VF/VT arrest with a high index of suspicion of hypovolemia (major bleeding), tamponade, acute thromboembolism or air embolism
5. VF/VT arrests unresponsive to DC shocks that may have acute graft occlusion.

A patient's suitability for chest reopening and reinstitution of CPB should be considered after one cycle of CPR. The decision to scoop and run must be made early because time is of the essence. Good-quality chest compressions and ventilation must be maintained during transfer. Epinephrine 1 mg (or an alternative vasopressor) should be given every 3–5 min as per standard ALS guidelines rather than the reduced dosages recommended in cardiac surgical ICU for patients in the immediate post-operative period. It needs to emphasized that scoop and run will only be successful if both the heart and *brain* are successfully restored to normal or near-normal function.

Catheter laboratory arrests

VF/VT arrests during elective procedures in the catheter laboratory are invariably iatrogenic, typically amenable to very early defibrillation and associated with return of spontaneous circulation in >90% cases, and >80% chance of survival to discharge. Outcomes in patients undergoing primary percutaneous intervention, however, are less impressive. As discussed earlier, the 2010 ERC guidelines recommend administration of three stacked shocks in quick succession for VF/VT arrests occurring in the cardiac catheter laboratory. In cases of coronary dissection or other surgically amenable conditions, early consideration of transfer to the operating room and institution of CPB should be considered.

Post resuscitation care

Hypothermia

Two large multi-center studies, one in Europe and one in Australia, have demonstrated that mild hypothermia improves neurologic outcome in comatose patients successfully resuscitated following out-of-hospital VF arrest. At a time when the indications for therapeutic hypothermia are widening, it is perhaps underutilized in the cardiac surgical ICU. This may be due to concerns about arrhythmias, hypotension, coagulopathy and infection in the postoperative setting. Therapeutic hypothermia is discussed in Chapter 60.

Conclusion

Patients sustaining cardiac arrests in a cardiothoracic surgical unit are twice as likely to survive to hospital discharge as patients who arrest in a general hospital. The essential requirements for a good clinical outcome are early detection, effective BLS and early defibrillation.

Key points

- ALS algorithms require modification in the cardiac surgical ICU.
- Consider the possibility of underlying VF in "asystolic" arrests and paced patients with apparent pulseless electrical activity.
- Look for epicardial pacing wires in bradycardic arrests before giving atropine and epinephrine!

- The majority of cardiac arrests after cardiac surgery are heralded by symptoms and signs.

Further reading

Bernard S, Gray TW, Buist MD, *et al.* Treatment of comatose survivors of out-of-hospital cardiac arrest with induced hypothermia. *N Engl J Med* 2002; **346**: 557–63.

Dunning J, Fabbri A, Kolh PH, *et al.* Guideline for resuscitation in cardiac arrest after cardiac surgery. *Eur J Cardiothorac Surg* 2009; **36**(1): 3–28.

Mackay JH, Powell SJ, Osgathorp J, Rozario CJ. Six-year prospective audit of chest reopening after cardiac arrest. *Eur J Cardiothorac Surg* 2002; **22**: 421–5.

Soar J, Perkins GD, Abbas G, *et al.* European Resuscitation Council Guidelines for Resuscitation 2010 Section 8. Cardiac arrest in special circumstances: electrolyte abnormalities, poisoning, drowning, accidental hypothermia, hyperthermia, asthma, anaphylaxis, cardiac surgery, trauma, pregnancy, electrocution. *Resuscitation* 2010; **81**(10): 1400–33.

The hypothermia after cardiac arrest group. Mild therapeutic hypothermia to improve the neurological outcome after cardiac arrest. *N Engl J Med* 2002; **346**: 549–56.

Chapter

67

Respiratory complications

Florian Falter

Some degree of impairment of respiratory function occurs in all patients undergoing cardiac surgery. This ranges from transient problems, such as retained secretions and atelectasis, to overwhelming acute lung injury (ALI) and ARDS. The causes of respiratory complications following cardiac surgery are summarized in Table 67.1 A detailed pathophysiological discussion is beyond the scope of this chapter, which focuses on clinical management.

Respiratory failure

Acute respiratory failure is the inability to perform adequate intrapulmonary gas exchange causing hypoxia *with or without* hypercarbia. The accepted quantitative

Table 67.1 Causes of respiratory failure after cardiac surgery: the major determinant of pulmonary outcome following cardiac surgery is cardiac function

Central neurologic	CNS depressant drugs, CVA, pain
Spinal cord	Neuraxial anesthesia, trauma, ischemia
Peripheral neurologic	Trauma
Neuromuscular	NMBs, severe $\downarrow\downarrow$ K^+, Mg^{2+}, PO_4^{3-}, myasthenia gravis, starvation
Airway	Retained secretions, asthma
Chest wall	Flail chest, kyphoscoliosis, ankylosis
Pleural	Pneumothorax, pleural effusion
Lung	Smoking-related disease, atelectasis, pneumonia, aspiration, ARDS, PE
Cardiac	LVF, low cardiac output state, valve disease, tamponade, R→L shunt

NMB, neuromuscular blocker; LVF, left ventricular failure.

criteria for the diagnosis are PaO_2 <8.0 kPa (60 mmHg) whilst breathing air and $PaCO_2$ >6.5 kPa (49 mmHg) in the absence of primary metabolic alkalosis. Using this definition, however, many cardiac surgical patients have postoperative "respiratory failure" and yet make an uneventful recovery. In this setting the diagnosis of respiratory failure has to be made with reference to the patient's preoperative respiratory function, postoperative cardiac function, the effects of drugs and *trends* in RR, PaO_2 and PCO_2. The major determinant of pulmonary outcome following cardiac surgery is cardiac function.

Atelectasis

Atelectasis means "imperfect dilatation" of the lungs. This condition affects dependent areas of lung – particularly the left lower lobe following internal mammary artery harvest. The combined effects of anesthesia, mechanical ventilation and sternotomy reduce functional residual capacity (FRC), vital capacity and tidal volume (V_T). These effects may be compounded by diaphragmatic dysfunction caused by direct or thermal (cold) injury to the phrenic nerve. Recruitment maneuvers, such as PEEP and ensuring that the lungs are fully expanded prior to chest closure, may reverse some of the atelectasis that inevitably occurs during surgery. Postoperative atelectasis is best managed by adequate analgesia, physiotherapy and maneuvers such as intermittent positive-pressure breathing (IPPB), continuous positive airway pressure (CPAP), incentive spirometry and forced coughing.

The patient with poor gases

As many as 10% of cardiac surgical patients will have postoperative impairment of gas exchange that is sufficient to cause concern, prolong mechanical

Core Topics in Cardiac Anesthesia, Second Edition, ed. Jonathan H. Mackay and Joseph E. Arrowsmith. Published by Cambridge University Press. © Cambridge University Press 2012.

ventilation and delay discharge from ICU. Before escalating therapy it is essential to examine the patient, review the CXR and consider the problem in the context of the patient's preoperative respiratory status. As preoperative lung function tests and ABG analysis are not routinely undertaken in most units, preoperative oximetry and the results of the first ABG analysis after induction of anesthesia ($FiO_2 \approx 0.6$) can be used as a rough guide. By definition, the minority of patients who fail to improve with the passage of time, physiotherapy, mobilization, alveolar recruitment maneuvers and adequate analgesia satisfy the diagnostic criterion for ALI. A large proportion of these cases can be managed with CPAP or non-invasive ventilation (NIV). Pre-emptive (i.e. elective) tracheal intubation and mechanical ventilation should be considered in all patients with deteriorating pulmonary function and decreasing conscious level.

ALI and ARDS

Hypoxia with bilateral pulmonary infiltrates and a relatively low LA pressure following cardiac surgery used to be known as "pump lung". The clinical features, which resemble those of sepsis with severe hypoxemia, include increased PVR, increased vascular permeability, and elevated alveolar–arterial O_2 gradient. This ALI usually resolves within 48 h or progresses to ARDS (Table 67.2).

The features of ARDS are secondary to inflammatory damage to the pulmonary microvascular endothelium. The natural history of ARDS is classically divided into exudative and infiltrative phases, which progress to either recovery or fibrosis and scarring. The pattern of lung injury is typically heterogeneous, with the process sparing some areas and causing severe alveolar collapse and airway plugging in others.

The incidence of ARDS following CPB is reported to be as high as 2.5% in some series. Predisposing factors include redo cardiac surgery, hypotension, sepsis (both pulmonary and non-pulmonary) and

massive transfusion. The etiology and subsequent complications, rather than respiratory failure itself, dictate mortality from ARDS. Death is usually due to *multiple* organ dysfunction. The avoidance of CPB does not eliminate the risk of ALI or ARDS.

Management of ARDS
General measures

The management of ARDS is predominantly supportive. In the acute phase, efforts should be directed towards resuscitation, identification of the cause and prevention of further organ dysfunction. As a result of capillary leak and volume resuscitation, most patients are fluid over-loaded. Fluid restriction and forced diuresis often improve lung compliance and oxygenation. The potential benefits of this strategy however, have to be balanced against the consequences of vital organ hypoperfusion. In the setting of oliguria and impending renal failure, early institution of renal replacement therapy should be considered.

Ventilation

Progressive and potentially life-threatening hypoxia is the hallmark of ARDS. Most patients require mechanical ventilatory support until lung function improves. The combination of poor pulmonary compliance, ventilation–perfusion mismatch, pulmonary edema and heterogeneous alveolar infiltration make it impossible to select a ventilation strategy to suit all lung units.

Ventilation with large V_T (10–15 ml kg^{-1}) has been shown to be harmful in ARDS, resulting in ventilator-associated lung injury (VALI). The so-called "baby lung" concept describes the preferential ventilation of less diseased areas of lung resulting in excessive airway pressures (barotrauma) and over-distension (volutrauma) of areas of lung that were relatively healthy. Shear stress at the junctions between collapsed and aerated alveoli may cause alveolar rupture, leading to pneumothorax, pneumomediastinum and subcutaneous emphysema. Modern lung management strategies are based on pressure-controlled, small V_T (5–6 ml kg^{-1}) ventilation, optimal (best) PEEP, manipulation of the inspiratory: expiratory time ratio, permissive hypercarbia and patient posture.

Table 67.2 American–European consensus conference (AECC) definitions of acute lung injury (ALI) and the acute respiratory distress syndrome (ARDS)

ALI	PaO_2/FiO_2 <40 kPa (300 mmHg)
ARDS	Bilateral pulmonary infiltrates on CXR PAWP <18 mmHg PaO_2/FiO_2 <26 kPa (200 mmHg)

421

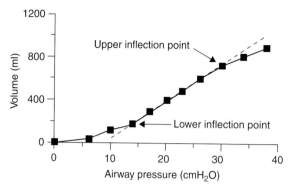

Figure 67.1 Determining the optimal level of PEEP. The lower inflection point represents the start of the part of the curve with the greatest compliance. The use of small tidal volumes prevents the pressure from exceeding the upper inflection point. PEEP has to be maintained just *above* the lower inflection point.

Pressure-controlled ventilation

Pressure-controlled ventilation (PCV) allows time-cycled, pressure-limited breaths to be delivered. Inspiratory V_T is determined by the preset pressure limit and pulmonary compliance, with gas flow being terminated as soon as this pressure is reached. The combination of decelerating flow and maintenance of airway pressure over time means that stiff lungs with a low static compliance and a long time constant are more likely to be inflated. Although PCV allows spontaneous ventilation, it is not particularly comfortable for the awake patient. Volume alarms require careful setting, as an abrupt fall in compliance will result in hypoventilation.

Pressure-support ventilation

Pressure-support ventilation (PSV), which supplements each spontaneous breath with gas flow until a preset airway pressure is reached, is a much more comfortable mode during weaning.

PEEP

PEEP increases FRC and redistributes extravascular lung water, which may in turn improve lung compliance and oxygenation. In the setting of pulmonary edema, CT has shown that within 30 min of the application of PEEP, there is an increase in lung cross-sectional area and a reduction in dependent lung density. The benefits of PEEP have to be set against impairment of venous return and the potential for barotrauma if the upper inspiratory pressure limit is not adjusted. The optimal level of PEEP can be estimated by reference to the inspiratory part of the pressure–volume curve (Figure 67.1).

Permissive hypercarbia

Permissive hypercarbia is the inevitable consequence of using PEEP and pressure-limited low V_T ventilation (i.e. deliberate alveolar hypoventilation). Although the highest tolerable $PaCO_2$ has not been defined, it has been said that $PaCO_2 > 10$ kPa (75 mmHg) represents "promiscuous" hypercarbia. The adverse effects of respiratory acidosis include hypoxia, myocardial depression, dysrhythmia, intracranial hypertension and an increased need for sedation. Over the course of several days, increased renal bicarbonate reabsorption generates a compensatory metabolic alkalosis. Neuromuscular blockade and dietary modification may have a marginal impact on metabolic CO_2 production.

Prone-position ventilation

Prone-position ventilation (PPV) has been shown to improve oxygenation in ARDS patients with severe hypoxia. Ventilation–perfusion mismatch in ARDS stems from the fact that pulmonary blood flow is directed by gravity to dependent areas of lung, which are collapsed and under-ventilated. The preferential ventilation of non-dependent areas of lung further compounds the situation during mechanical ventilation. Dependent areas of lung are, in effect, operating on the part of the pressure–volume curve (Figure 67.1) that lies *below* the lower inflection point. The net effect is an extracardiac shunt. The effects of PPV are:

(1) to redistribute blood flow from previously dependent areas of lung to previously non-dependent areas of lung, and

(2) to move previously dependent lung units up the pressure–volume curve.

The prone position should be maintained for as long as possible. Failure to respond to PPV should not preclude later attempts. Although studies of PPV have revealed improved oxygenation without hemodynamic compromise, no improvement in outcome has been demonstrated. Most deaths are caused by multiple organ dysfunction rather than acute hypoxia.

Adjuvant therapy

Pulmonary hypertension, due in part to hypoxic pulmonary vasoconstriction – a constant finding in ARDS, leads to worsening hypoxia. Inhaled pulmonary vasodilators (e.g. nitric oxide and prostacylin) offer some theoretical benefit. Although inhaled NO has been shown to improve oxygenation by >20% in two-thirds of patients, the effects are short-lived. Despite improving oxygenation without hemodynamic compromise, no randomized study has demonstrated improved survival in ARDS.

Peripheral, veno-venous ECMO has been used as rescue therapy for patients with life-threatening hypoxemia for over 30 years. It is indicated in patients with respiratory failure considered to have a reversible cause that is unresponsive to conventional therapy. It has taken the recent swine flu epidemics to raise the profile of ECMO. ICU survival rates of up to 45% have been reported. Despite improvements in extracorporeal technology, however, ECMO-associated complications such as intracranial hemorrhage remain a significant problem.

The use of extracorporeal technology to remove CO_2 in patients with deleterious hypercarbia remains controversial. The NovaLung iLA Membrane Ventilator® is a pump-less device that enables (typically femoral) arterio-venous CO_2 removal. The system incorporates a low-resistance, heparin-coated hollow-fiber diffusion membrane that effectively removes CO_2 using low blood flows of ~1 l min^{-1}. Unlike ECMO, however, the NovaLung provides limited oxygenation. The putative benefits are restoration of mild to moderate hypercarbia whilst reducing the risks of ventilator-associated barotrauma and volutrauma.

Tracheostomy

It is usual for ICU patients requiring long-term ventilatory support to undergo tracheostomy. There is a wide variation in practice and considerable debate about the optimal timing and operative technique. Improved patient cooperation and comfort, easier pulmonary toilet and reduced dead space are cited as reasons for early (i.e. <10 days) tracheostomy. In contrast, the long list of significant complications – particularly hemorrhage and infection – is often used to justify late (i.e. >14 days) tracheostomy. Institutional and personal preferences dictate whether open or percutaneous dilatational tracheostomy is performed.

Cardiovascular management

Both the underlying disease process and its treatment may compromise cardiovascular function. Increased PVR in ARDS leads to an increase in RV end-diastolic pressure and RV stroke work, and displacement of the interventricular septum. Continuous hemodynamic monitoring and assessment of end-organ function is

widely used. A disproportionate degree of hypoxia, in the absence of clinical and radiological signs, should trigger the echocardiographic exclusion of an intracardiac shunt. Despite continuing debate about the use of the PAFC in the general ICU, the device is still used in the setting of ARDS following cardiac surgery, where differentiation between ARDS and pulmonary edema is difficult.

Antimicrobial therapy

Infection may cause or complicate ARDS. As the typical radiological features of ARDS may mask the signs of intrathoracic infection (e.g. lung abscess and empyema) a high index of suspicion is required. CT is routinely used to exclude intrathoracic and intra-abdominal sepsis. Antimicrobial therapy, which initially may be empiric, should be guided by the patient's recent medical and surgical history and advice from local microbiologists.

Key points

- Respiratory failure is common after cardiac surgery.
- Treatment of ARDS is supportive and aims to avoid further organ dysfunction.
- Patients with ARDS tend to die from multiple organ failure.
- Lung-protective ventilation appears to be associated with significantly lower early mortality.
- Extra-corporeal support should be considered in patients with refractory hypoxemia.

Further reading

Bernard GR, Artigas A, Brigham KL, et al. The American-European Consensus Conference on ARDS. Definitions, mechanisms, relevant outcomes, and clinical trial coordination. *Am J Respir Crit Care Med* 1994; **149**(3 pt 1): 818–24.

Extracorporeal Life Support Organization ECMO Registry. http://www.elso.med.umich.edu.

Gattinoni L, Protti A, Caironi P, Carlesso E. Ventilator-induced lung injury: the anatomical and physiological framework. *Crit Care Med* 2010; **38**(10 Suppl): S539–48.

Kilpatrick B, Slinger P. Lung protective strategies in anaesthesia. *Br J Anaesth* 2010; **105**(Suppl 1): i108–16.

National Institute for Health and Clinical Excellence. *Extracorporeal membrane oxygenation for severe acute respiratory failure in adults.* Interventional procedure guidance 391. April 2011. http://www.nice.org.uk/guidance/ipg391.

423

Chapter

68

Gastrointestinal complications

Britta Millhoff and Paul Quinton

The reported incidence of gastrointestinal complications after cardiac surgery is low (<3%). However, the morbidity and mortality associated with GI complications are disproportionately high.

The pathogenesis of GI complications after cardiac surgery is multifactorial. Apart from the stress of major surgery, anesthesia, anticoagulation and hypothermia, cardiac surgery is associated with a reduction and redistribution in systemic blood flow. As a consequence, there may be a disparity between oxygen supply and demand in the mesenteric bed. CPB leads to a reduction in GI absorptive and barrier function through a combination of reduced mucosal blood flow, endothelial dysfunction and release of inflammatory mediators. Cardiac surgery without CPB, however, has a similar incidence of GI complications.

The mesenteric vasculature also lacks the autoregulation that maintains blood flow in other organs during periods of hypoperfusion. The increase in SVR during and after CPB, and the ensuing mesenteric vasoconstriction contribute to GI dysfunction.

Amongst the most common GI complications are bleeding and mesenteric ischemia (Table 68.1). A number of risk factors have been identified (Table 68.2). Despite improvements in perioperative care, anesthesia and operating techniques, the incidence of GI complications has not changed in recent years. This may, in part, be explained by the older surgical population and greater number of comorbidities.

The symptoms and signs of GI complications may be subtle; their onset is insidious and often masked by sedatives and analgesics. Transient, mild GI dysfunction after cardiac surgery, which is common, needs to be distinguished from more serious dysfunction requiring medical or surgical intervention. The lack of early signs and delayed diagnosis contributes to the high morbidity and mortality.

Table 68.1 Common gastrointestinal complications after cardiac surgery

Ileus

Hemorrhage

Mesenteric ischemia

Acute pancreatitis

Hepatic dysfunction

GI perforation

Cholecystitis

Postoperative ileus

A period of ileus is probably the most common GI complication after cardiac surgery. It is frequently a benign, self-limited problem, but occasionally it may reflect something more sinister. Simple ileus presents with large nasogastric aspirates, failure to absorb enteral feed and vomiting. This will usually improve spontaneously over a few days as the patient's condition improves. A plain abdominal radiograph may reveal distended loops of small or large bowel. Colonic distension (>10 cm in cross section) is associated with an increased risk of colonic rupture.

Contributing factors include gastric distension (possibly related to vagal injury), electrolyte disturbances ($\downarrow K^+$), hepatic or splanchnic congestion (systemic venous hypertension), inflammatory processes (e.g. cholecystitis, pancreatitis), retroperitoneal bleeding, pseudomembranous colitis, mesenteric ischemia and drugs (e.g. opioids).

Therapy should be directed at any identifiable precipitating process and preventing secondary complications. A nasogastric tube will prevent gastric distension until peristaltic activity returns. Prokinetics such as metoclopramide and erythromycin

Core Topics in Cardiac Anesthesia, Second Edition, ed. Jonathan H. Mackay and Joseph E. Arrowsmith. Published by Cambridge University Press. © Cambridge University Press 2012.

Table 68.2 Risk factors for GI complications after cardiac surgery

Demographic

Age >65 years
Poor nutritional status
History of peptic ulcer disease

Preoperative drugs

NSAIDs
Aspirin/clopidogrel/prasugrel
Corticosteroids
Warfarin

Type of surgery

Emergency operations (e.g. aortic dissection)
Redo operations
Valve operations
Combined procedures (e.g. valve and CABG)

Preoperative factors

Peripheral vascular disease
Renal insufficiency
Hepatic impairment
Preoperative LVEF <40%
Significant arrhythmia (e.g. AF)
Cardiogenic shock

Intraoperative and postoperative

Profound hypotension/hypoperfusion
Prolonged duration of CPB (>120 min)
Significant arrhythmia (e.g. AF)
Inotrope and vasoconstrictor therapy
IABP or TEE use
Hemorrhage and transfusion
Surgical re-exploration within 24 h
Respiratory failure – requiring prolonged ventilatory
support
Renal failure
Sternal/mediastinal infection

Table 68.3 Etiology of gastrointestinal bleeding during and after cardiac surgery

Upper	Esophagitis/variceal bleeding
	Gastritis/gastric ulceration/*H. pylori*
	Duodenitis/duodenal ulceration
Lower	Mesenteric ischemia/ischemic colitis
	Antibiotic-associated colitis – pseudomembranous colitis
	Hemorrhoids
	Tumors
	Diverticulosis
	Inflammatory bowel disease – Crohn's disease, ulcerative colitis
	Angiodysplasia – e.g. Heyde's syndrome (associated with aortic stenosis)

may be of use, even though the level of evidence supporting their use is low. In persistent cases a general surgical opinion should be sought. Failure to diagnose an incarcerated hernia, volvulus or obstruction secondary to adhesion bands has grave implications. Exploratory or diagnostic laparoscopy or laparotomy may be required.

Gastrointestinal hemorrhage

Hemorrhage from the GI tract accounts for 30–40% of all GI complications. In the majority of cases, bleeding arises in the upper GI tract, and is typically associated with ulceration or inflammation of the stomach and esophagus. Bleeding from the lower GI tract is very rare.

Histamine (H_2) receptor antagonists have reduced the incidence of GI hemorrhage worldwide and are routinely used for patients in intensive care who have not yet been established on full enteral nutrition. Whilst the practice of prescribing antacid prophylaxis has become routine in cardiac surgery, there still remains a lack of randomized controlled evidence to support this. This lack of evidence can perhaps be explained by the fact that during cardiac surgery the change of intragastric pH is not the only factor predisposing to upper GI hemorrhage. In fact mucosal hypoperfusion, inflammatory mediator release and anticoagulation or postoperative coagulopathy probably have a more significant role. That said, antacid prophylaxis in high-risk patients (e.g. the elderly, pre-existing ulcer disease, antiplatelet therapy, chronic dialysis) has been shown to reduce the incidence of upper GI hemorrhage. Enteral feeding, which stimulates GI tract activity and increases splanchnic blood flow, may also be effective at preventing ulceration. In the presence of critical splanchnic ischemia, however, enteral feeding may actually worsen the situation.

Although the clinical presentation may be dramatic – hematemesis, melena or rectal bleeding and hemodynamic collapse – tachycardia, uremia and anemia may be the only signs. Opinion varies as to when a patient should be referred for a gastroenterological assessment. Early diagnostic or therapeutic endoscopy is indicated in those patients least able to tolerate the hemodynamic instability associated with repeated episodes of bleeding. Current evidence suggests that rebleeding after therapeutic endoscopy, which occurs in up to 20% of cases, is best treated by further endoscopic intervention rather than surgery.

Proctoscopy, sigmoidoscopy or colonoscopy should be performed if upper GI endoscopy is negative or lower GI hemorrhage is suspected. In troublesome cases, mesenteric angiography or a radionuclide scan – performed while the patient is bleeding – allows identification of the bleeding vessel and permits embolization. Vasopressin and the somatostatin analog octreotide decrease splanchnic blood flow and may be beneficial in unrelenting hemorrhage. A selective arterial infusion of vasopressin may arrest hemorrhage in up to 90% of patients. The vast majority of patients respond to primary or secondary medical management. The proton pump inhibitors (e.g. omeprazole) have been shown to be effective in reducing further bleeding and the need for surgery in those with bleeding ulcers. Surgical intervention is required for patients who fail to respond to medical management. Surgery for intractable GI hemorrhage following cardiac surgery is associated with significant mortality.

Mesenteric ischemia

Up to a quarter of GI complications after cardiac surgery are related to mesenteric ischemia. Mesenteric ischemia in the setting of cardiac surgery is usually non-occlusive; due to low CO or prolonged CPB. Ischemia secondary to atherosclerotic embolism and arterial or venous thrombosis is less common. Persistent metabolic acidosis and worsening lactatemia may be the only suggestive signs in the sedated and ventilated patient. Abdominal pain is an inconsistent and often late symptom. In the context of multiple organ failure this is usually a terminal event.

Management is, in part, dictated by the severity and rate of progression of symptoms and signs. Mesenteric angiography may be used to exclude thromboembolism although the absence of vascular occlusion does not rule out ischemia. When combined with localized infusion of a vasodilator (e.g. papaverine) it may be therapeutic. The invasive nature of angiography and unfavorable predictive value mean that it is seldom used. Abdominal CT, which may reveal gut dilatation, gut wall thickening and gas in the intestinal wall and

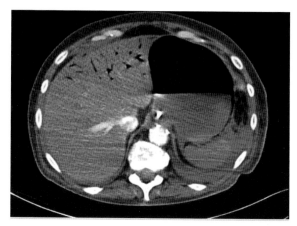

Figure 68.1 Gastrointestinal ischemia. Contrast-enhanced CT of a patient with severe atherosclerosis admitted with acute coronary syndrome and diffuse abdominal pain. Gas can be seen in the wall of the stomach and within the liver. There is also marked dilatation of the stomach (despite the presence of a nasogastric tube). The patient developed hypoglycemia and hyperlactatemia, and died of overwhelming sepsis and metabolic acidosis.

peritoneal fluid, is probably the investigation of choice (Figure 68.1). Diagnostic laparoscopy or laparotomy may be required in some patients.

The high mortality (50–100%) is partly explained by delays in diagnosis and the reluctance of surgeons to perform a laparotomy until the diagnosis is clear. Diagnosis is made more difficult by the fact that ileus, metabolic abnormalities (acidosis, hyperkalemia and leukocytosis) and radiological findings, such as dilated small bowel loops, are common in cardiac ICU patients. A high index of suspicion and a low threshold for an early laparotomy are the most important factors in reducing mortality.

Pancreatitis

Pancreatic cellular injury, indicated by transient pancreatic hyperamylasemia, is common after cardiac surgery. The etiology is believed to be pancreatic ischemia secondary to low cardiac output states and hypoperfusion; the vascular anatomy and high metabolic rate of the pancreas make it highly susceptible to hypoperfusion and inflammation. Profound hypothermia, high-dose thiopental, excessive administration of $CaCl_2$ (e.g. >800 mg m^{-2}) and transplant surgery may also result in pancreatic injury. In most patients symptoms of subclinical pancreatitis (e.g. anorexia, nausea, and ileus) are mild and resolve within a few days. The incidence of overt pancreatitis in this setting is around 3%. An elevated serum amylase concentration (>1000 IU l^{-1}) is diagnostic but has relatively low specificity (~70%). The simultaneous determination of serum pancreatic lipase increases both the sensitivity and specificity (90–95%). Pancreatic isoamylase and immunoreactive trypsin are more specific and sensitive markers of pancreatitis, but are less widely available. The serum amylase concentration does not appear to correlate with disease severity.

Management is largely supportive. The use of inhibitors of pancreatic autodigestion (e.g. glucagons, somatostatin, octreotide, anticholinergics) does not appear to greatly improve outcome. Anecdotal reports of improved outcome following hemofiltration have not been validated in randomized studies. The routine use of broad-spectrum antibiotics has, however, been shown to reduce the risk of infective complications and abscess formation, and significantly improves outcome from severe acute pancreatitis.

Uncomplicated acute pancreatitis is associated with 5–10% mortality, whereas the mortality from acute necrotizing pancreatitis is up to 50%. Untreated, a pancreatic abscess or infected pseudocyst is invariably fatal. Operative intervention carries a high mortality in acute pancreatitis and CT-guided percutaneous drainage of collections and abscesses is undertaken whenever possible. In aggressive forms of necrotizing pancreatitis, surgery may be the only means of saving the patient.

Hepatic dysfunction

Mild and transient elevation of the serum concentrations of hepatic enzymes without evidence of biliary obstruction is common after cardiac surgery. The most common causes are perioperative ischemia (despite the dual blood supply), hemolysis and transfusion. While hyperbilirubinemia occurs in 20% of patients, clinically obvious jaundice is rare and usually indicates other complications of cardiac surgery. Predictors of postoperative hyperbilirubinemia include elevated RA pressure, elevated preoperative bilirubin level and valve surgery. Significant hepatocellular damage is uncommon and progression to hepatitis and hepatic failure extremely rare. The presence of hepatic dysfunction usually indicates multiple organ system failure, which is associated with significantly increased mortality. Patients with severe preoperative liver dysfunction are at significant risk of hepatic failure, bleeding and infective complications after cardiac surgery. Worsening coagulopathy (rising prothrombin time) with persistent hypoglycemia is an ominous sign. Normal preoperative liver function tests do not preclude the development of significant postoperative hepatic dysfunction. Similarly, abnormal preoperative results do not identify every patient at risk.

Postoperative hepatic dysfunction in the presence of a low cardiac output state carries a poor prognosis. Frank hepatic necrosis is a recognized complication of cardiogenic shock. The only treatment options are supportive – improving cardiac performance and supplying adequate nutritional support. Laboratory tests of liver function (e.g. prothrombin time) are a useful barometer of treatment success.

The onset of hepatic dysfunction several days after surgery should trigger consideration of other causes such as drugs (particularly antibiotics), sepsis, viral hepatitis or cholestasis.

Cholecystitis

Cholecystitis after cardiac surgery accounts for 10–15% of GI complications and usually occurs in the absence of gallstones (i.e. acalculous). The pathogenesis of acalculous cholecystitis is multifactorial. It typically occurs in critically ill patients after major surgery and trauma. A combination of bile stasis, increased bile viscosity and drug-induced constriction of the ampoule lead to gall bladder distension and increased wall stress. Not infrequently, the symptoms and signs are vague and nonspecific, and may be masked by sedatives and analgesics. Ultrasound examination should be performed if symptoms persist or the clinical condition of the patient deteriorates. While supportive therapy alone may be adequate, percutaneous drainage should be considered in unstable patients. Delays in diagnosis and treatment undoubtedly contribute to the high mortality (~75%) associated with acute cholecystitis in this setting. Percutaneous cholecystotomy is recommended in the critically ill patient, whereas open or laparoscopic cholecystectomy is preferred in the more stable patient or in the presence of gangrene or perforation of the gallbladder. As with mesenteric ischemia, a high index of suspicion is required to make an early diagnosis. While the prognosis for cholecystitis in the setting of gallstones is good, the mortality associated with acalculous cholecystitis is high.

Perforation

Perforation may occur at any point in the GI tract. It may occur as the result of a pathological process (e.g. duodenal ulcer, diverticular disease) or a medical intervention (e.g. TEE, chest drain insertion, and sigmoidoscopy). While pneumoperitoneum (air under the diaphragm on a plain erect CXR) is normally diagnostic of abdominal viscus perforation, this is an unreliable sign in the setting of cardiac surgery. Air may be unintentionally introduced into the peritoneal cavity during sternotomy, mediastinal dissection or drain placement.

Esophageal perforation secondary to TEE is believed to have an incidence of 0.02% (i.e. 1 in 5000). Complications such as dysphagia, mucosal erosion and bleeding are considerably more common. While perforation may become immediately apparent *during* surgery (probe visible in chest), it is more commonly diagnosed postoperatively or even at autopsy.

Nutritional management

Most patients undergoing uncomplicated cardiac surgery do not appear to suffer any ill effects from a temporary interruption of their normal diet. Patients requiring prolonged intensive care and those who "fail to thrive" on the wards require dietetic assessment and nutritional support. Enteral (i.e. oral, nasogastric, nasojejunal) nutrition is preferred as there are few absolute indications for parenteral nutrition (e.g. intestinal obstruction, anatomical disruption, severe ischemia). In addition to the benefits of providing energy and protein, enteral nutrition improves splanchnic perfusion, maintains gut integrity (theoretically reducing bacterial translocation) and modulates the immune response. The early introduction of enteral nutrition after surgery is currently encouraged. The small intestine regains motor function within hours after surgery and thus makes jejunal feeding an attractive option.

Randomized controlled trials have demonstrated the benefits of oral feeding in mild to moderate pancreatitis and enteral (nasojejunal) feeding in severe pancreatitis. When compared to total parenteral nutrition, enteral feeding in this setting is associated with less pancreatic and systemic inflammation, a lower incidence of sepsis and multiple organ failure, a reduced requirement for operative intervention and

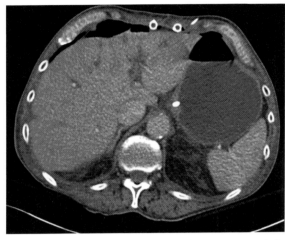

Figure 68.2 Abdominal CT in a patient with worsening metabolic acidosis and lactatemia after cardiac surgery. Two mediastinal drains are present. The stomach is markedly distended in spite of a nasogastric tube. There is free air in the upper abdomen around and beyond the lower mediastinal drains. The air also tracks along the falciform ligament. The appearances were reported as being suspicious for bowel ischemia. While the presence of free air may have been related to the drains, bowel perforation could not be excluded. No intra-abdominal pathology of viscus perforation was found at laparotomy and the patient made a full recovery.

significantly lower mortality. Nasojejunal feeding is well tolerated, as it usually does not stimulate pancreatic exocrine function in the same way that oral, gastric or duodenal feeding does.

Key points

- Despite the low reported incidence, morbidity and mortality associated with GI complications are disproportionately high.
- Mucosal ischemia secondary to splanchnic hypoperfusion is responsible for the majority of GI complications.
- Clinical signs and symptoms are often masked by sedatives and analgesics.
- A high index of suspicion and a low threshold for an early laparotomy is the most important factor in reducing mortality.

Further reading

Bavalia N, Anis A, Benz M, *et al.* Esophageal perforation, the most feared complication of TEE: early recognition by multimodality imaging. *Echocardiography* 2011; **28**(3): E56–9.

D'Ancona G, Baillot R, Poirier B, *et al.* Determinants of gastrointestinal complications in cardiac surgery. *Tex Heart Inst J* 2003; **30**(4): 280–5.

Filsoufi F, Rahmanian PB, Castillo JG, *et al.* Predictors and outcome of gastrointestinal complications in patients undergoing cardiac surgery. *Ann Surg* 2007; **246**(2): 323–9.

Mangi AA, Christison-Lagay ER, Torchiana DF, Warshaw AL, Berger DL. Gastrointestinal complications in patients undergoing heart operation: an analysis of 8709 consecutive cardiac surgical patients. *Ann Surg* 2005; **241**(6): 895–901.

Rodriguez R, Robich MP, Plate JF, Trooskin SZ, Sellke FW. Gastrointestinal complications following cardiac surgery: a comprehensive review. *J Card Surg* 2010; **25**(2): 188–97.

Sanisoglu I, Guden M, Bayramoglu Z, *et al.* Does off-pump CABG reduce gastrointestinal complications? *Ann Thorac Surg* 2004; **77**(2): 619–25.

Chapter

Renal complications

69

Shitalkumar Shah and William T. McBride

The overall incidence of postoperative acute renal failure (ARF) requiring renal replacement therapy (RRT) in the adult cardiac surgical population is ~5%. Despite the adoption of perioperative renoprotective strategies, reducing the incidence of this complication has proved an elusive goal. The reported incidence of ARF ranges from <1%, in patients with normal preoperative urea and creatinine concentrations, to >40% in patients with preoperative creatinine concentration >200 μmol l^{-1} (2.3 mg dl^{-1}). Although rarely the primary cause of death, ARF after cardiac surgery is associated with 50% mortality. Inevitably, renal dysfunction after cardiac surgery

significantly increases the length of ICU and hospital stay. The association between preoperative renal function and perioperative morality is clearly demonstrated in Figure 69.1 and Table 69.1. Postoperative renal impairment remains an independent risk factor of mortality after cardiac surgery regardless of the need for RRT. Available evidence suggests that preoperative preservation of glomerular filtration rate (GFR) reduces the impact of postoperative renal dysfunction on mortality. The additional costs associated with ARF are considerable, particularly as a small proportion of patients remain dependent on RRT after hospital discharge.

Table 69.1 Major studies showing renal dysfunction and mortality after cardiac surgery

| Reference | n | Renal dysfunction | | Dialysis outcome | |
		Incidence (%)	Mortality (%)	Incidence (%)	Mortality (%)/emphasis>
A	2417	7.7	19	1.4	40
B	2214	2.1	NR	1	30
C	31677	5.7	539	1.8	54

References: A, *Ann Intern Med* 1998; 128: 194–203; B, *Can J Cardiol* 2001; 17: 565–70; C, *Kidney Int* 2005; 67: 1112–9. NR, not reported.

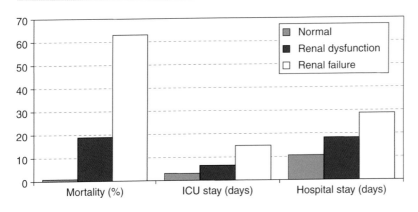

Figure 69.1 The influence of renal function on outcome from cardiac surgery. Data from the 1992–4 Multicenter Study of Perioperative Ischemia (McSPI) study – *Ann Intern Med* 1998; 128: 194–203. Renal dysfunction defined as [creatinine] >2 mg dl^{-1} (>177 μmol l^{-1}) or rise in [creatinine] > 0.7 mg dl^{-1} (>62 μmol l^{-1}). Renal failure defined as requirement for dialysis. A strikingly similar 30-day mortality was demonstrated in a prospective cohort study of 43 642 veterans who underwent CABG or valvular surgery between 1987 and 1994 – *Circulation* 1997; 95(4): 878–84.

Core Topics in Cardiac Anesthesia, Second Edition, ed. Jonathan H. Mackay and Joseph E. Arrowsmith. Published by Cambridge University Press. © Cambridge University Press 2012.

Table 69.2 Definitions of renal dysfunction, insufficiency and failure

Reference	Definition(s) used
Mangos (1995)	Postoperative *renal failure*: Doubling of serum creatinine to >1.5 mg dl^{-1} (>130 μmol l^{-1}) if preoperative creatinine <1.5 mg dl^{-1} (<130 μmol l^{-1}) OR rise of >1.1 mg dl^{-1} (>100 μmol l^{-1}) Postoperative *renal insufficiency*: a rise of serum creatinine >0.6 mg dl^{-1} (>50 μmol l^{-1})
Brivet (1996)	Severe ARF = a serum creatinine ≥3.5 mg dl^{-1} (≥310 μmol l^{-1}) ± BUN ≥100 mg dl^{-1} (≥36 mmol l^{-1}) OR an increase in creatinine or BUN to twice baseline level in patients with previous chronic renal insufficiency, defined as serum creatinine 1.7–3.4 mg dl^{-1} (150–300 μmol l^{-1})
Schneider (1996)	Clinically important ARF = an increase in serum creatinine >50% on first postoperative day and a serum creatinine >1.4 mg dl^{-1} (>120 μmol l^{-1})
Mangano (1998)	Postoperative *renal failure* = need for postoperative dialysis Renal *dysfunction* = serum creatinine >2 mg dl^{-1} (>177 μmol l^{-1}) and an increase of >0.7 mg dl^{-1} (>62 μmol l^{-1}). NB: excluded patients with preoperative renal failure, or renal dysfunction defined by a serum creatinine >2 mg dl^{-1} (>177 μmol l^{-1})
Osterman (2000)	Requirement for continuous veno-venous hemofiltration after CPB.

References: Mangos *et al. Aust NZ J Med* 1995; 25: 284–9. Brivet *et al. Crit Care Med* 1996; 24: 192–8. Schneider *et al. Anaesth Intensive Care* 1996; 24: 647–50. Mangano *et al. Ann Intern Med* 1998; 128: 194–203. Osterman *et al. Intensive Care Med* 2000; 26: 565–71.
BUN, blood urea nitrogen.

Definitions of renal failure

Until recently, there has been no universally recognized definition of ARF. While some have defined ARF as oliguria and an arbitrary increase (e.g. 50%) in creatinine concentration, others refer to this combination as "renal insufficiency or dysfunction" and reserve the term ARF for patients requiring RRT. Table 69.2 demonstrates some of the definitions of ARF used by investigators.

Nowadays the term ARF has been replaced by the term acute kidney injury (AKI). A consensus definition of AKI was proposed in 2002 by an international consensus conference of the Acute Dialysis Quality Initiative (ADQI). The RIFLE classification (**R**isk of renal dysfunction, **I**njury to the kidney, **F**ailure of kidney function, **L**oss of kidney function and **E**ndstage kidney disease) defines AKI according to changes in serum creatinine concentration and urine output (Figure 69.2).

Predictors of acute perioperative renal failure

A variety of perioperative factors have been shown to be associated with renal dysfunction after cardiac surgery (Table 69.3).

Mechanisms

The final common pathway of all renal insults is renal tubular cell death, by either apoptosis or necrosis. Patients with preoperative renal dysfunction are at increased risk from major complications, including major morbidity and the need for dialysis, but are not at a greater risk from renal injury relative to preoperative renal function. CPB may be injurious to kidneys as a result of loss of pulsatile blood flow; catecholamines and inflammatory mediators; arterial emboli; free hemoglobin, reduced renal blood flow (RBF) and reduced oxygen delivery secondary to hemodilution and hypotension. RBF during CPB is not autoregulated and varies with pump flow rate and systemic blood pressure. Moreover, perioperative LV dysfunction and low CO states compound the situation.

Hypoxia/hypotension

RBF accounts for ~20% of CO. A RBF of one liter per minute typically generates one millilitre of urine per minute. Renal oxygen delivery is huge (>80 ml min^{-1} 100 g^{-1}) and overall O_2 extraction is low (~10%). Paradoxically, the proximal tubules and medullary loops of Henle function in a hypoxic milieu and have little physiological reserve. The combination of the glomerular portal circulation and a vascular counter-current

431

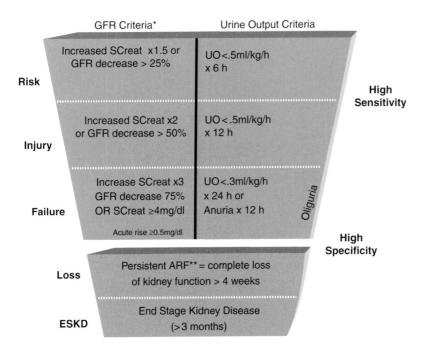

GFR Criteria*   **Urine Output Criteria**

Risk — Increased SCreat ×1.5 or GFR decrease > 25% | UO<.5ml/kg/h × 6 h   **High Sensitivity**

Injury — Increased SCreat ×2 or GFR decrease > 50% | UO<.5ml/kg/h × 12 h

Failure — Increase SCreat ×3 GFR decrease 75% OR SCreat ≥4mg/dl | UO<.3ml/kg/h × 24 h or Anuria × 12 h

Acute rise ≥0.5mg/dl

Oliguria

High Specificity

Loss — Persistent ARF** = complete loss of kidney function > 4 weeks

ESKD — End Stage Kidney Disease (>3 months)

Figure 69.2 The RIFLE (**R**isk of renal dysfunction, **I**njury to the kidney, **F**ailure of kidney function, **L**oss of kidney function and **E**nd-stage kidney disease) classification of ARF includes separate criteria for creatinine and urine output (UO). A patient can fulfill the criteria through changes in serum creatinine (SCreat) or changes in UO, or both. The criteria that lead to the worst possible classification should be used. Note that the F component of RIFLE is present even if the increase in SCreat is under three-fold as long as the new SCreat is greater than 4.0 mg dl^{-1} (350 μmol l^{-1}) in the setting of an acute increase of at least 0.5 mg dl^{-1} (44 μmol l^{-1}). The designation RIFLE-FC should be used in this case to denote "acute-on-chronic" disease. Similarly, when the RIFLE-F classification is achieved by UO criteria, a designation of RIFLE-FO should be used to denote oliguria. The shape of the figure denotes the fact that more patients (high sensitivity) will be included in the mild category, including some without actually having renal failure (less specificity). In contrast, at the bottom of the figure the criteria are strict and therefore specific, but some patients will be missed. Reproduced from Bellomo *et al. Crit Care* 2004; 8: R204. © 2004 Bellomo *et al.*; licensee BioMed Central Ltd.

reduces the PaO_2 of blood entering the medulla to 1–2 kPa (8–15 mmHg). For this reason renal tubules are especially vulnerable to hypoxia. The tone of renal blood vessels is controlled, at least in part, by the balance between the vasoconstrictive action of endothelin-1 (ET-1) and the vasodilator action of nitric oxide (NO) produced by endothelial nitric oxide synthetase (e-NOS). Hypoxia increases ET-1 expression and reduces e-NOS expression, thus compounding ischemic renal injury. In addition to this net vasoconstrictive effect, hypoxia increases levels of pro-inflammatory mediators within the kidney. Pro-inflammatory mediators also contribute to microcirculatory failure by further altering ET-1/e-NOS balance such that vasoconstriction may be maintained for several hours after normoxia is restored. Hence there is a localized pro-inflammatory response.

Inflammatory mediator/cytokine balance

Cellular inflammation plays an important role in the pathophysiology of postoperative renal dysfunction.

The systemic inflammatory response syndrome (SIRS) is induced by contact of cellular and humoral blood components with the CPB circuit, and is characterized by the activation of the clotting, kallikrein and complement systems.

The pro-inflammatory cytokine tumor necrosis factor alpha (TNF-α) causes direct damage to proximal tubular cells in vitro. Furthermore, systemic levels of the pro-inflammatory cytokine interleukin-8 (IL-8) have been found to correlate with increases in markers of subclinical tubular injury. The mechanism is thought to involve IL-8-mediated inflammatory infiltration of small renal vessels with a resultant reduction in oxygen delivery to vulnerable areas. In contrast, there is now evidence that the anti-inflammatory cytokine interleukin-10 (IL-10) has renoprotective properties. These findings suggest that the balance of pro- and anti-inflammatory cytokines is important for the preservation of renal function. In this context the use of corticosteroids in cardiac surgery is controversial.

Table 69.3 Risk factors for renal dysfunction and renal failure following cardiac surgery; post-renal causes of renal dysfunction should be excluded before attempting to differentiate between pre-renal and renal etiologies

Patient factors
Increasing age[a]
Diabetes[a]
Arterial hypertension/aortic atheroma
Preoperative MI/low CO states[a]
Preoperative creatinine >1.4 mg dl^{-1} (>130 μmol l^{-1})[a]
Renal tract obstruction/raised intra-abdominal pressure
Bladder outflow obstruction

Operative factors
Use of CPB and CPB duration/AXC time
Redo and emergency procedures
Valve and combined surgical procedures
Hyperglycemia[a]
Hemorrhage
Hemodilution/anemia
Infection/sepsis

Pharmacological
Contrast media
Loop diuretics
Non steroidal anti inflammatory drugs
Antimicrobials (aminoglycosides, amphotericin)
Cyclosporin

[a] Independent risk factors identified by the McSPI study.

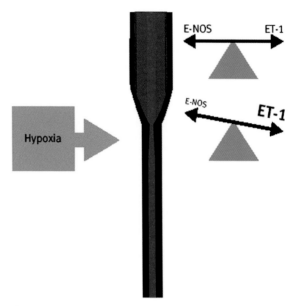

Figure 69.3 Diagrammatic representation of a renal medullary arteriole. At the top of the diagram the vessel is of normal caliber because vasoconstrictive ET-1 is in balance with vasodilatory e-NOS. Hypoxia alters this balance in favor of ET-1 leading to vasoconstriction, in turn jeopardizing renal perfusion (reproduced from McBride & Glillimand. *Surgery (Oxford)* 2009; 27(11): 480–5 with permission from Elsevier).

Prevention

Renal tubular injury has as its final common pathway apoptosis or necrosis secondary to the direct toxicity of inflammatory mediators or hypoxia due to imbalance of oxygen supply and demand. It follows that the twin approach of (1) reducing pro-inflammatory and other nephrotoxins together with (2) maintaining tubular oxygen supply above demand should minimize perioperative renal complications (Table 69.4).

Fluid and salt loading

The early restoration of renal perfusion in pure volume-responsive AKI (formerly termed pre-renal failure) should restore renal function. The maintenance of pre-load, CO and vital organ perfusion is a fundamental goal of cardiac anesthesia. The correction of hypovolemia is central to the prevention and progression of AKI in critically ill patients and should be undertaken before instituting any pharmacological intervention.

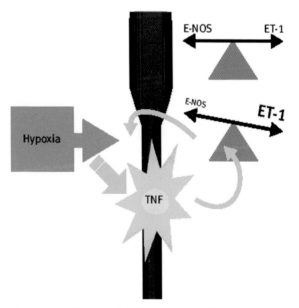

Figure 69.4 Hypoxic endothelium generates inflammatory mediators (e.g. tumor necrosis factor) which in turn exacerbate the ET-1/e-NOS imbalance such that vasoconstriction is maintained for several hours after normoxia is restored. Hence a transient period of hypotension leads to renal injury long after normotension is restored (reproduced from McBride & Glillimand. *Surgery (Oxford)* 2009; 27(11): 480–5 with permission from Elsevier).

Table 69.4 Preventing perioperative renal dysfunction

Reducing inflammatory or other toxins
  Withhold nephrotoxic drugs
  Maintain glycemic control in diabetic patients
  Avoid radiocontrast-induced nephropathy
  Treat sepsis
  Reduce CPB time as this will reduce CPB-related inflammatory mediators
  Recognize and treat rhabdomyolysis
  Retransfuse with washed mediastinal blood

Maintenance of tubular O_2 supply–demand balance
  Optimize volume status, cardiac output, and systemic arterial pressure
  Maintain adequate flow and mean systemic arterial pressure during CPB
  Avoid excessive hemodilution

Perfusion pressure

Renal perfusion pressure is the difference between MAP and IVC pressure. The use of vasopressors such as norepinephrine to increase MAP is controversial. Although norepinephrine undoubtedly raises MAP, a simultaneous increase in renal vascular resistance may actually reduce RBF. While norepinephrine may improve RBF, this is not always translated into an improvement in renal function.

Pharmacological

Pharmacological interventions to protect renal function have included diuretics, dopamine, fenoldopam, calcium antagonists, natriuretic peptides and *N*-acetylcysteine. Unfortunately the quality of the majority of clinical studies has been poor.

The use of loop diuretics is driven by the desire to convert oliguric AKI into non-oliguric AKI, on the grounds that the latter has a better prognosis. The risks of diuretic therapy include dehydration and direct nephrotoxicity. The logic underlying this approach is that loop diuretics disable the energy-dependent (i.e. $Na^+{:}K^+{:}Cl^-$ co-transport) tubular mechanisms that permit urine concentration and reduce renal oxygen demand. Without adequate fluid resuscitation, loop diuretics are ineffective in the prevention of AKI and may worsen tubular function.

Mannitol – an alcohol – is an osmotic agent that is freely filtered at the glomerulus and not reabsorbed by the renal tubules. Mannitol has a high diuretic potential and can markedly increase fluid flow rate in all nephron segments, including the proximal tubule. When administered early in the course of AKI, mannitol may flush out cellular debris and prevent tubular cast formation, which in turn may convert oliguric AKI into non-oliguric AKI. Conversion to non-oliguric AKI facilitates the management of fluid and electrolyte imbalance, drug therapy and nutritional needs of the patient. Whether this reduces the requirement for subsequent RRT is uncertain. Combining mannitol with a loop diuretic prevents compensatory increases in ion reabsorption in the loop of Henle. Mannitol is contraindicated in anuric patients.

Dopamine at low doses (i.e. <3 μg kg^{-1} min^{-1}) increases CO and RBF. Renal vasodilatation and the inhibition of tubular Na^+-K^+-ATPase result in increased GFR, urine volume and Na^+ excretion in healthy subjects. This "diuretic" effect has led to the widespread use of low-dose dopamine to prevent and treat ARF. In the setting of the general ICU, low-dose dopamine has no impact on peak serum creatinine concentration, the requirement for RRT, length of ICU stay or mortality. The authors of a meta-analysis, published in 2001, concluded "low-dose dopamine . . . should be eliminated from routine . . . use".

A recently published review concluded that, to date, no pharmacological renoprotective intervention in cardiac surgery has significantly reduced mortality. Only fenoldopam and atrial natriuretic peptide (ANP) have been shown to be renoprotective, reducing the need for RRT by 5% and 3.5%, respectively. Brain natriuretic peptide (BNP) reduces the incidence of AKI by 10% whereas dopamine actually causes a significant reduction in creatinine clearance.

Diagnosis

In clinical practice, renal function is typically assessed using hourly urine output and the serum concentrations of urea and creatinine. Unfortunately a seemingly adequate urine output (i.e. >0.5 ml kg^{-1} h^{-1}) and normal biochemical indices do not preclude renal dysfunction. Serum creatinine levels tend to remain normal until over 50% of renal tubular function is lost, and doubles with every subsequent halving of function. Despite their popularity, these traditional indices are not sensitive enough to detect the early stages of renal dysfunction. This has led to a search for more sensitive biomarkers.

Table 69.5 Urinary constituents used to measure renal injury or damage

Glomerular permea-selectivity	Albumin Transferrin Aspartate aminotransferase Immunoglobulin G
Tubular protein uptake	β_2-Microglobulin Retinol binding protein Ribonuclease
Proximal tubular brush border	Alanine aminopeptidase γ-Glutamyl transpeptidase
Proximal tubule	N-Acetyl β D-glucosaminidase (NAG) α-Glutathione S-transferase (α-GST)
Thick ascending limb	Tamm-Horsfall protein
Distal tubule	Π-Glutathione S-transferase

It is known that a number of kidney-specific enzymes are released into both blood and urine following renal injury, and that the detection of these may improve diagnosis and treatment (Table 69.5).

Cystatin C is a cysteine protease inhibitor produced at a constant rate and released into the bloodstream by all nucleated cells. It is freely filtered by the glomerulus due to its low molecular mass (13 kDa) and reabsorbed and metabolized in the proximal tubule. Serum cystatin C concentration does not depend on muscle mass, sex or age. Measuring serum cystatin allows earlier detection of renal impairment.

Human neutrophil gelatinase-associated lipocalin (NGAL), a 25 kDa protein covalently bound to gelatinase from human neutrophils, is usually barely detected in human tissues, including the kidney. NGAL appears to be an early biomarker for acute renal injury as increases in NGAL precede any increase of creatinine by 1–3 days.

Interleukin-18 concentrations in urine increase following renal injury in proportion to both the development and duration of perioperative renal dysfunction.

α-1-Microalbumin and *N-acetyl-β-glucosaminidase* (NAG) have been used as markers of renal glomerular and tubular damage. Alpha-1-microglobulin is freely filtered in the glomerulus and reabsorbed in the renal tubules. It is a sensitive marker for proximal tubular dysfunction and reversible tubular lesions even when no histological damage is detectable. NAG is a sensitive measure of renal tubular damage as it is present in the lysosomes of proximal tubular cells and is not filtered by the glomerulus due to its relatively high molecular weight (>130 kDa). Its increased elimination into the urine indicates renal tubular damage.

Glutathione S-transferases (GST) are selectively present in the proximal (GST-α) and distal tubule (GST-π). α-Glutathione S-transferase is detected in the urine after tubular damage, but not in the case of glomerular disorders. GSTs are thought to be very sensitive markers of renal tubular injury.

Kidney injury molecule 1 (KIM-1), a kidney-specific adhesion molecule, is detectable by immunochemistry (ELISA) in the urine of patients with established acute tubular necrosis. KIM-1 is expressed within 12 hours of an ischemic insult and represents proliferation of tubular cells to reconstruct a functional epithelium after ischemic/reperfusion injury.

Pre-existing renal impairment

Pre-existing renal dysfunction significantly increases operative risk – a creatinine concentration >200 μmol l^{-1} (>2.3 mg dl^{-1}) adds 2 points to the EuroSCORE. A number of issues are of importance to the anesthesiologist. It is essential that preoperative RRT does not remove excessive solute and render the patient hypovolemic. For this reason hemodialysis is usually discontinued and hypertonic peritoneal dialysis fluids avoided in the 12 hours before surgery. Unless the patient is truly anuric, a urethral catheter should be inserted.

The presence of a forearm arteriovenous fistula created for hemodialysis interferes with pulse oximetry and reduces the number of sites available for arterial and peripheral venous access. In addition, a fistula may represent a significant arteriovenous shunt, which may be worsened following the administration of vasoconstrictors. Occasionally a large fistula must be excluded from the circulation by ligation or application of proximal tourniquet.

Intraoperative "neutral balance" hemofiltration during CPB may delay the requirement for the reinstitution of RRT in the early postoperative period when anticoagulation may be undesirable. Although peritoneal dialysis avoids many of the potential

Table 69.6 Management of acute kidney injury after cardiac surgery

Exclude post-renal/obstructive etiology

Optimize circulation and renal perfusion pressure

Restrict fluid and K^+ intake

Discontinue nephrotoxic drugs

Reduce doses of drugs that accumulate in renal failure

Consider proton pump inhibitor for gastrointestinal prophylaxis

Exclude and aggressively treat any infection

Treat life-threatening hyperkalemia, acidosis and dysrhythmias

Slowly correct metabolic acidosis with isotonic bicarbonate

Consider early renal specialist advice

Table 69.7 Indications for renal replacement therapy

Hyperkalemia

Severe metabolic acidosis

Fluid overload

Severe uremia – encephalopathy, neuropathy or pericarditis

To facilitate enteral/parenteral feeding

To facilitate blood/blood product administration

Severe hyponatremia or hypernatremia

Hyperthermia

complications of hemofiltration, diaphragmatic splinting may lead to respiratory impairment.

Uremia-induced platelet dysfunction may lead to excessive perioperative bleeding. Platelet transfusion and desmopressin (DDAVP) may be of use in this group of patients.

Management

The treatment of patients with renal dysfunction and renal failure after cardiac surgery is largely supportive. In most centers management is expectant unless there is an indication for intervention or RRT. General measures are shown in Table 69.6.

RRT can be considered in three broad categories: peritoneal dialysis, intermittent hemodialysis and continuous veno-venous hemofiltration (CVVHF). Most adult patients developing renal failure after cardiac surgery are initially supported with CVVHF, whereas patients with pre-existing renal failure on established peritoneal dialysis may have this therapy reinstituted. Continuous hemodiafiltration, which achieves greater urea clearance, may be considered in patients who do not respond to hemofiltration. CVVHF requires insertion of a large-bore, double-lumen cannula specifically designed for CVVHF in the subclavian, internal jugular or femoral vein, and a degree of systemic anticoagulation. A continuous infusion of unfractionated heparin is used to maintain an ACT >200 s. Although numerous conditions contribute to the development of thrombocytopenia

during CVVHF, use of another anticoagulant (e.g. danaparoid, lepuridin) should only be considered if heparin-induced thrombocytopenia is suspected.

Key points

- Around 1 in 20 adult cardiac surgical patients require renal replacement therapy for acute postoperative renal failure.
- Postoperative renal impairment is an independent predictor of mortality after cardiac surgery regardless of the need for RRT.
- Acute renal hypoxia induces vasoconstriction that may be maintained for several hours after restoration of normoxia.
- No pharmacological renoprotective intervention in cardiac surgery has been shown to significantly reduce mortality.

Further reading

Bellomo R, Ronco C, Kellum JA, Mehta RL, Palevsky P. Acute renal failure – definition, outcome measures, animal models, fluid therapy and information technology needs: the Second International Consensus Conference of the Acute Dialysis Quality Initiative (ADQI) Group. *Crit Care* 2004; **8**(4): R204–12.

Chertow GM, Lazarus JM, Christiansen CL, *et al.* Preoperative renal risk stratification. *Circulation* 1997; **95**(4): 878–84.

Garwood S. Cardiac surgery-associated acute renal injury: new paradigms and innovative therapies. *J Cardiothorac Vasc Anesth* 2010; **24**(6): 990–1001.

Mangano CM, Diamondstone LS, Ramsay JG, *et al.* Renal dysfunction after myocardial revascularisation: risk factors, adverse outcomes and hospital resource utilisation. *Ann Intern Med* 1998; **128**(3): 194–203.

McBride WT, Allen S, Gormley SM, *et al.*
Methylprednisolone favourably alters plasma and
urinary cytokine homeostasis and subclinical renal
injury at cardiac surgery. *Cytokine* 2004; **27**(2–3): 81–9.

Moore E, Bellomo R, Nichol A. Biomarkers of acute kidney
injury in anesthesia, intensive care and major surgery:
from the bench to clinical research to clinical practice.
Minerva Anestesiol 2010; **76**(6): 425–40.

Patel NN, Rogers CA, Angelini GD, Murphy GJ.
Pharmacological therapies for the prevention of acute
kidney injury following cardiac surgery: a systematic
review. *Heart Fail Rev* 2011; **16**(6): 553–67.

Thakar CV, Worley S, Arrigain S, Yared JP, Paganini EP.
Influence of renal dysfunction on mortality after cardiac
surgery: modifying effect of preoperative renal function.
Kidney Int 2005; **67**(3): 1112–19.

Chapter 70

Neurologic complications

Rabi Panigrahi and Charles W. Hogue

Neurologic injury following cardiac surgery increases mortality and length of ICU and hospital stay, and reduces the likelihood of a return to independent living. Cardiac surgical patients are largely ignorant of this complication.

Manifestations

Brain injury following cardiac surgery ranges in severity from subtle changes in personality, behavior and cognitive function to fatal brain injury – the "cerebral catastrophe" (Table 70.1). In most cases a neurologic injury becomes evident as soon as the patient emerges from anesthesia. In a small number of patients, however, significant injury may develop following a "lucid interval" lasting several hours to several days after surgery.

Many neurologic injuries (e.g. visual field defects, tinnitus and ataxia) go unreported, uninvestigated and undocumented. Repeated prospective studies have shown that the measured incidence of neurologic injury increases with increased surveillance. Formal cognitive assessment, however, is labor-intensive and time-consuming. Investigational testing schedules are a compromise – short enough to ensure compliance, yet sufficient to assess a meaningful range of cognitive domains.

Mechanisms

Cerebral injury during cardiac surgery is primarily the result of cerebral embolism or cerebral hypoperfusion. The two mechanisms are not mutually exclusive. Neurologic injury may be worsened by exacerbation of ischemia/reperfusion injury by the systemic inflammation response that accompanies cardiac surgery.

The clinical manifestations of cerebral injury are dependent on both the anatomic location and

Table 70.1 Types and incidences of neurologic complications after cardiac surgery

Complication	Incidence (%)
Fatal brain injury	0.3
Non-fatal diffuse encephalopathy	
Delirium	8–32
Depressed conscious level	3
Behavioral changes	1
Cognitive impairment	
At hospital discharge	30–40
At 1 month after surgery	12–30
Seizures	
Choreoathetosis	0.3
Ophthalmological	
Visual field defects	25
Reduced visual acuity	4.5
Focal brain injury (Stroke)	1–3
Primitive reflexes	39
Spinal cord injury	0–0.1
Peripheral nerve injury	
Brachial plexopathy	7
Other peripheral neuropathy	6

magnitude of the ischemic lesion. A small internal capsule or brain stem infarct will result in an obvious neurologic deficit, whereas a considerably larger lesion in subcortical brain areas or the hippocampus might be manifest as a change in cognitive function.

Core Topics in Cardiac Anesthesia, Second Edition, ed. Jonathan H. Mackay and Joseph E. Arrowsmith. Published by Cambridge University Press. © Cambridge University Press 2012.

Brain imaging studies suggest that ~50% of strokes after cardiac surgery result from emboli. Cerebral microemboli, which can be detected (using carotid or transcranial Doppler sonography) in all patients subjected to CPB, have long been considered a significant cause of neurologic injury. There is an association between cognitive decline and intraoperative cerebral microembolic load. Air may reach the systemic circulation from the bypass circuit and as an unavoidable consequence of intracardiac procedures. Biological particles arise from the ascending aorta, components of the circulation and the operative site. Non-biological particles arise from the extracorporeal circuit, the cardiotomy reservoir, and from foreign material introduced into the operative site. Fatty material from the operative site, known to be returned with shed blood to the cardiotomy reservoir during CPB, is incompletely removed by arterial line filters and causes cerebral microembolism. It is believed that it is the composition rather than the absolute number of microemboli (i.e. air, fat, atheromatous debris) delivered to the cerebral circulation that dictates clinical consequences.

Risk factors

Patient factors, intraoperative factors and postoperative factors all contribute to the risk of perioperative neurologic injury (Table 70.2).

A multicenter study of over 2000 patients undergoing CABG identified 13 independent predictors of adverse neurologic outcome (Table 70.3). The overall incidence of neurologic injury was 6.1%. The incidences of type I (focal) and type II (diffuse) outcomes were 3.1% and 3.0% respectively.

Using the data obtained in this study, the Duke University group developed a model to predict the likelihood of neurologic injury after CABG. Using preoperative patient risk factors, the so-called Stroke Index allows rapid risk assessment (Figure 70.1).

Patient age

Age is probably the most robust predictor of morbidity and mortality after cardiac surgery. The relationship between age and risk is more a function of age-related comorbidities than age per se. The proportion of elderly patients presenting for cardiac surgery is steadily increasing.

Sex

Women are at greater risk of death and complications following cardiac surgery. Higher-risk profiles – rather than increased gender susceptibility – are the likely cause.

Diabetes mellitus

Diabetes is an independent risk factor for neurologic injury. Although hyperglycemia is known to worsen

Table 70.2 Putative risk factors for adverse neurologic outcome after cardiac surgery

Preoperative (patient) factors		Intraoperative factors	Postoperative factors
Demographic	**Medical history**		
Age	Cerebrovascular disease	Surgery type	Early hypotension
Gender	Diabetes mellitus	Aortic atheroma	Long ICU stay
Genotype	Cardiac function	Aortic clamp site	Renal dysfunction
Educational level	IABP use	Microemboli	Atrial fibrillation
	Alcohol consumption	Arterial pressure	
	Pulmonary disease	Pump flow	
	Hypertension	Temperature	
	Dysrhythmia	Hematocrit	
	Dyslipidemia	Use of DHCA	
	Diuretic use		

DHCA, deep hypothermic circulatory arrest.

Table 70.3 Adjusted odds ratios [95% confidence intervals] for type I (non-fatal stroke, TIA, stupor or coma at discharge, or death caused by stroke or hypoxic encephalopathy) and type II (new deterioration in intellectual function, confusion, agitation, disorientation, memory deficit or seizure without evidence of focal injury) adverse cerebral outcomes after CABG associated with independent risk factors

Risk factors	Type I outcomes	Type II outcomes
Proximal aortic atherosclerosis	4.52 [2.52–8.09]	
History of neurologic disease	3.19 [1.65–6.15]	
Use of IABP	2.60 [1.21–5.58]	
Diabetes mellitus	2.59 [1.46–4.60]	
History of hypertension	2.31 [1.20–4.47]	
History of pulmonary disease	2.09 [1.14–3.85]	2.37 [1.34–4.18]
History of unstable angina	1.83 [1.03–3.27]	
Age (per additional decade)	1.75 [1.27–2.43]	2.20 [1.60–3.02]
Admission systolic BP >180 mmHg		3.47 [1.41–8.55]
History of excessive alcohol intake		2.64 [1.27–5.47]
History of CABG		2.18 [1.14–4.17]
Dysrhythmia on day of surgery		1.97 [1.12–3.46]
Antihypertensive therapy		1.78 [1.02–3.10]

From Roach *et al.*, 1996.

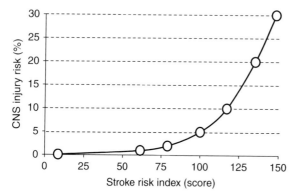

Risk factor	Score
Age	(Age – 25) X 1.43
Unstable angina	14
Diabetes mellitus	17
Neurologic disease	18
Prior CABG	15
Vascular disease	18
Pulmonary disease	15

Figure 70.1 Preoperative Stroke Risk Index for patients undergoing CABG. Arrowsmith *et al.*, 2000 – adapted from Newman *et al.*, 1996.

outcome from stroke, the greater incidence of hypertension, vascular disease and renal impairment in diabetics may partly explain this phenomenon.

Cerebrovascular disease

Patients with a history of symptomatic cerebrovascular disease are more likely to sustain neurologic injury. In patients with a history of stroke, the risk does not appear to decline over time. Patients undergoing cardiac surgery within 3 months of a focal event are more likely to extend the area of injury whereas patients with a remote stroke (i.e. >6 months) are more likely to have a stroke in a different vascular territory.

Aortic atheroma

The prevalence and severity of aortic atheroma increases with age. There is a strong association between proximal aortic atheroma and stroke following cardiac surgery. Surgical manipulation, cannulation and perfusion of the diseased aorta can liberate atheroemboli. Although TEE assessment is superior to digital palpation, the cannulation site is not usually visible. Epiaortic ultrasound represents the gold standard. Emerging evidence suggests that a change in surgical procedure, prompted by the detection of proximal aortic atheroma, improves neurologic outcome.

Procedure type

The risk of neurologic injury is, in part, dependent upon the type of surgery performed. Intracardiac and major vascular procedures carry the greatest risk – particularly when DHCA is employed. Combined procedures, such as CABG and MV surgery, carry a greater risk than isolated coronary, aortic or mitral surgery.

Conduct of CPB

Despite considerable research, the characteristics of "optimal" CPB perfusion remain to be defined. Profound hypotension combined with prolonged cerebral hypoperfusion is clearly injurious to the brain – particularly the watershed zones. Within the bounds of usual CPB conduct, however, pressure, flow rate and flow character appear to have little influence on neurologic outcome.

Hematocrit

A desire to reduce the use of homologous blood products has resulted in the tolerance of a lower hematocrit during cardiac surgery. In theory reduced oxygen-carrying capacity may expose the brain to hypoxia, particularly during rewarming and in the presence of significant cerebrovascular disease.

Temperature

Despite considerable research, the cardiovascular benefits and neurologic safety of so-called "normothermic" CPB have yet to be conclusively determined. Methodological shortcomings make it difficult to compare the conflicting conclusions of large studies conducted in this area. Any neuroprotection provided by hypothermia has to be weighed against adverse effects on hemostasis and the requirement for rewarming. Current temperature-monitoring methods (i.e. nasopharyngeal and bladder) may grossly underestimate brain temperature during rewarming. Rapid or excessive rewarming may cause cerebral metabolism to outstrip substrate delivery and exacerbate excitotoxic neuronal injury. Carefully conducted *and* monitored normothermic CPB reduces

the margin for surgical error and probably has little adverse influence on the brain.

Acid-base management strategy

The influence of pH management strategy during hypothermic CPB has been examined in a number of studies. When compared to pH-stat strategy, α-stat is associated with superior cognitive outcome. In patients undergoing DHCA, however, the use of the pH-stat strategy during cooling appears to improve neurologic outcome.

Dysrhythmia

Postoperative AF is associated with an increased risk of both stroke and cognitive dysfunction.

Improving outcome

Reducing the incidence and severity of neurologic injury requires identification of patients at increased risk, avoidance of factors known to cause neurologic injury (i.e. hypotension, hypoperfusion and emboli), detection of neuronal ischemia and avoidance of factors which exacerbate established injury.

Cerebral embolism
Arterial line filters

The use of arterial line filters (≤ 40 μm) during CPB reduces cerebral microembolism and is the standard of care in most centers.

Epiaortic ultrasound

Epiaortic ultrasound is more sensitive than either surgical palpation or TEE for detecting atheroma of the ascending aorta. Once identified, an atheromatous plaque should be avoided during aortic cannulation, aortic cross-clamping, and proximal CABG anastamoses.

Surgical technique

Surgical approaches for the patient with severe, diffuse aortic atheroma include off-pump surgery, cannulation of the axillary artery, use of a single AXC application technique, using induced VF arrest and replacement of the ascending aorta with DHCA.

Cell salvage

Lipid microemboli arising from the pericardial aspirate are not effectively removed from the circulation by existing arterial line or even leukocyte transfusion filters. Processing shed blood with a cell saver before return to the CPB circuit reduces the lipid content and may lead to a short-term improvement in cognitive function. One concern about this approach is the loss of platelets and coagulation factors into the discarded supernatant.

Carbon dioxide

Insufflating the operative field with CO_2 reduces the nitrogen content of any gaseous emboli that may enter the circulation. Because CO_2 is more soluble in blood than nitrogen, both the number and size of any microemboli reaching the brain are reduced. The practice has few risks and is probably justifiable despite the low level of evidence.

Avoiding CPB

Off-pump (OPCAB) surgery has been advocated as a way to reduce cerebral emboli and CPB-induced systemic inflammation. At the present time, prospective randomized studies have failed to demonstrate that avoiding CPB reduces the incidence of either stroke or cognitive dysfunction. Whether off-pump surgery is beneficial in high-risk patients has yet to be proven.

Cerebral perfusion

Cerebral injury resulting from hypoperfusion is a growing concern given the number of patients with pre-existing cerebral vascular disease. Studies employing preoperative brain imaging have demonstrated a high prevalence of ischemic lesions. In one MRI study, nearly two-thirds of postoperative strokes were found to have occurred in border zone arterial perfusion territories (i.e. watershed strokes). It was noted that a fall in MAP ≥ 10 mmHg from preoperative baseline during CPB increased the risk for watershed stroke nearly three-fold.

Perfusion pressure

Target perfusion pressure during CPB is empirically set at 50–60 mmHg. This practice is based in part on the fact that cerebral autoregulation remains intact during α-stat CPB. A MAP above the limit of autoregulation is considered undesirable because of increased cerebral embolic load and edema. Nevertheless a subgroup of patients with hypertension and cerebrovascular disease may have a higher upper autoregulation limit. Whether higher perfusion pressures (i.e. 60–80 mmHg) are associated with improved neurologic outcome remains controversial (see Chapter 63).

Hematocrit

Anemia is common in patients prior to cardiac surgery and worsened by hemodilution. The normal response to anemia is increased cerebral blood flow (CBF) and tissue O_2 extraction. As discussed above, an increase in CBF may be accompanied by an increase in microembolic load. Several retrospective studies have shown an independent link between low hematocrit during CPB and both stroke and mortality. In a randomized study of 107 elderly CABG patients, a target hematocrit of 15–18% was reported to be associated with a greater risk of cognitive dysfunction than a target hematocrit of 27%. Unfortunately there is little evidence that transfusion reverses this effect. Moreover, there is evidence to suggest that allogeneic transfusion increases both morbidity and mortality. The Society of Thoracic Surgeons and Society of Cardiovascular Anesthesiologists recommend that red cell transfusion is not indicated for a Hb >6 g dl^{-1} during CPB and >7 g dl^{-1} after surgery.

Monitoring

Near infrared spectroscopy (NIRS) may identify episodes of cerebral hypoxia that culminate in cognitive dysfunction or stroke. (See Chapter 26.) To date, no study using NIRS-directed interventions has been sufficiently powered to detect a statistically significant improvement in an isolated endpoint such as stroke and death.

Limiting ischemic injury

Areas of irreversible brain ischemia are invariably surrounded by tissue that is viable but vulnerable to further injury (the so-called ischemic penumbra). Limiting the extent of brain injury is directed at limiting propagation of the initial ischemic insult. Depolarization of ischemic neurons leads to excitatory neurotransmitter release and activation of cytotoxic pathways. These processes, which ultimately determine the eventual extent of neuronal injury, take place over 36–72 h. An understanding of the mechanisms of cerebral injury has revealed numerous potential therapeutic targets for cerebral protection.

Hypothermia

Experimentally, hypothermia protects against ischemic injury by reducing metabolic rate and the rate of release of the excitatory amino acids implicated in secondary neurotoxicity. Although the most common

Table 70.4 Summary of clinical trials evaluating pharmacological neuroprotection in patient undergoing cardiac surgery

Drug	Primary mechanism	Comments
Thiopental	$\downarrow$ CMRO$_2$	Contradictory findings from two clinical trials. Placebo controlled, double-blinded randomized studies of patients undergoing CPB using a membrane oxygenator, α-stat pH management and an in-line arterial filter showed no neuroprotective benefits
Propofol	$\downarrow$ CMRO$_2$	No evidence of neuroprotective efficacy in multicenter randomized, placebo-controlled study
Nimodipine	Ca^{2+} channel blocker	No evidence of neuroprotection in single center study but study terminated after interim analysis showed higher mortality in nimodipine-treated vs. control group
Prostacyclin	$\downarrow$ Platelet aggregation $\downarrow$ Inflammation	Small studies have failed to demonstrate improved cognitive outcomes 2 weeks after surgery compared with controls
GM1 ganglioside	$\downarrow$ EAA signaling	Small pilot trials failed to confirm neuroprotective efficacy in patients undergoing cardiac surgery
Remacemide	NMDA receptor antagonist	Improvement in some cognitive domains compared with placebo in randomized, double-blinded study of patients undergoing cardiac surgery. Confirmation needed before drug can be recommended
Pegorgotein	Antioxidant	Pilot study failed to show lower rates of cognitive dysfunction compared with placebo
Lidocaine	Na$^+$ channel blockade Membrane stabilization $\downarrow$ EAA release	Two randomized, double-blinded studies have failed to show improved cognitive outcome compared with placebo
Clomethiazole	GABA receptor agonist	Frequency of cognitive dysfunction no different to placebo in small single-center trial
Pexelizumab	$\downarrow$ C5a and C5b-9	Secondary analysis of data from multicenter study evaluating the drug for myocardial protection showed improvement in limited number of cognitive domains compared with placebo
Magnesium	Multiple mechanisms including $\downarrow$ Ca^{2+} entry and $\downarrow$ EAA signaling	Inconclusive results from several trials but single-center study showed lower rates of early cognitive dysfunction compared with placebo
Ketamine	NMDA receptor antagonist Inhibits apoptosis	Pilot studies suggest improved cognitive function and lower incidence of delirium after cardiac surgery compared with placebo
Erythropoietin	Anti-apoptotic growth factor	Single-center pilot study suggests improved cognitive function after cardiac surgery compared with placebo

CMRO$_2$, cerebral metabolic rate for oxygen; EAA, excitatory amino acid; GABA, γ-aminobutyric acid; NMDA, N-methyl D-aspartate.

method used for organ protection during CPB, there is scant evidence supporting hypothermia as a neuroprotectant during routine cardiac surgery. It is widely speculated that any benefits are negated by rewarming. (See Chapters 60 and 63.)

Normoglycemia

Prospective randomized trials of tight glycemic control during cardiac surgery have failed to demonstrate neurologic benefit. This is discussed further in Chapter 63.

Neuroprotective drugs

While each step in the "ischemic cascade" offers a potential target for pharmacologic intervention, it is unlikely that a single drug will prevent brain damage. Nevertheless, considerable effort has been expended in the search for neuroprotective drugs. Studies in cardiac surgery have largely been disappointing (Table 70.4). No drug is currently licensed for the prevention or treatment of neurologic injury associated with cardiac surgery.

Recommendations

Clinicians are accustomed to evaluating a broad range of evidence in making decisions regarding medical therapeutics and interventions. A structured, evidenced-based analysis of the literature is often employed to provide a structure to recommended treatments/interventions. Based on the above review, recommendations for cerebral protection during cardiac surgery using such an approach are listed in Table 70.5. These evaluations are based on data derived from human studies evaluating the primary outcome of clinical stroke and cognitive dysfunction.

Management

Diagnosis

The diagnosis of neurologic injury is made on the basis of clinical features. The degree of disability should be documented is a systemic and consistent fashion to permit serial assessment. The National Institutes of Health (NIH) Stroke Index provides a simple means of recording level of consciousness, orientation, response to commands, gaze, visual fields, facial movement, limb motor function, limb ataxia, sensory loss, aphasia, dysarthria and inattention.

Brain imaging is usually undertaken to document the presence and extent of intracranial pathology. Imaging occasionally influences management (i.e. subdural hematoma) and may guide decisions to withdraw treatment. Diffusion-weight MRI can be used to detect extracellular brain water (i.e. edema) several days before it becomes apparent on CT or conversional MRI.

Patients' subjective opinions of their cognitive function are usually inaccurate. Cognitive dysfunction, which is often reliably detected by the spouse or other close relative, may only become apparent after formal testing.

Table 70.5 Measures for reducing brain injury during cardiac surgery

Class I recommendations

A membrane oxygenator and an arterial line filter ($\leq$40 µm) should be used for CPB

Epiaortic ultrasound for detection of atherosclerosis of the ascending aorta

Avoid hyperthermia during and after CPB

Class IIa recommendations

A single aortic cross-clamp technique should be used for patients at risk of atheroembolism

During CPB in adults α-stat pH management should be considered

NIRS monitoring should be considered in high-risk patients

Class IIb recommendations

Arterial blood pressure should be kept >70 mmHg during CPB in high-risk patients

Intravenous insulin infusion should be given to keep serum glucose <8 mmol l^{-1} (<140 mg dl^{-1})

RBC transfusion should be considered in high risk patients with Hb $\leq$7 g dl^{-1} or at higher Hb if there is evidence of organ ischemia

Cardiotomy suction aspirate should be processed with a cell-saver device before returning the blood to the CPB circuit (blood aspirated from open cardiac chamber can be returned directly to the CPB circuit)

Treatment

The goals include prevention of secondary brain injury, recognition of pathology that may be amenable to early neurosurgical intervention, general supportive measures and prevention of secondary complications. These are summarized in Table 70.6.

Prognosis

One in four patients sustaining a stroke after cardiac surgery will have long-term disability. Prolonged depression of consciousness, coma and persistent vegetative state are associated with significant (>90%) mortality. The majority of patients with major brain injury succumb to the complications of extended ICU care or aspiration pneumonia. The pattern of neurologic recovery within the first 24–72 h is often an indicator of the eventual extent of recovery. Transient delirium and agitation – often considered a benign postoperative "inconvenience" – is known to be associated with prolonged hospital

Table 70.6 Treatment goals in established brain injury after cardiac surgery

Prevent secondary brain injury
  Maintain CO and cerebral oxygenation
  Consider therapeutic hypothermia
  Avoid hyperthermia and hyperglycemia
  Reduce brain swelling/raised intracranial pressure

Surgery
  Evacuation of subdural or intracranial hematoma
  Carotid or cerebral artery angioplasty
  Intracranial aneurysm coiling/clipping
  Ventriculostomy

General supportive measures
  Hydration and nutrition
  Prevention of pressure sores/contractures
  Antimicrobial therapy/thromboprophylaxis
  Rehabilitation, speech and language therapy

Specific drug therapy
  Seizures – phenytoin, valproic acid
  Muscle spasm – baclofen, tizanitidine, Botox
  Myoclonus – clonazepam, piracetam, levetiracetam
  Agitation – haloperidol, clonidine
  Depression – citalopram, fluoxetine, paroxetine
  Chronic pain – amitriptyline, gabapentin, pregabalin

stay, and significantly increased morbidity and mortality. Longitudinal studies have demonstrated that early preoperative cognitive dysfunction is an independent predictor of cognitive function, general health and employment status 5 years after surgery.

Key points

- Neurologic complications are common and often go undiagnosed.
- Neurologic complications increase mortality and length of hospital stay.
- Physical interventions such as arterial line filtration, cautious rewarming and α-stat blood gas management appear to improve neurologic outcome.
- Procedure modification and the use of novel devices and techniques may reduce neurologic injury.
- No drug is yet licensed specifically for neuroprotection during cardiac surgery.

Further reading

Arrowsmith JE, Grocott HP, Reves JG, Newman MF. Central nervous system complications of cardiac surgery. *Br J Anaesth* 2000; **84**: 378–93.

Grogan K, Stearns J, Hogue CW. Brain protection in cardiac surgery. *Anesthesiology Clinics* 2008; **26**: 521–38.

Hogue CW, Gottesman RF, Stearns J. Mechanisms of cerebral injury from cardiac surgery. *Critical Care Clinics* 2008; **24**: 83–98.

Hogue CW Jr, Palin CA, Arrowsmith JE. Cardiopulmonary bypass management and neurologic outcomes: An evidence-based appraisal of current practices. *Anesth Analg* 2006; **103**: 21–37.

Newman MF, Kirchner JL, Phillips-Bute B, *et al.* Longitudinal assessment of neurocognitive function after coronary-artery bypass surgery. *New Engl J Med* 2001; **344**: 395–402.

Newman MF, Wolman R, Kanchuger M, *et al.* Multicenter preoperative stroke risk index for patients undergoing coronary artery bypass graft surgery. Multicenter Study of Perioperative Ischemia (McSPI) Research Group. *Circulation.* 1996; **94**(9 Suppl): 1174–80.

Roach GW, Kanchuger M, Mora Mangano C, *et al.* Adverse cerebral outcomes after coronary artery bypass surgery. *New Engl J Med* 1996; **335**: 1857–63.

Infection

Margaret I. Gillham and Juliet E. Foweraker

Cardiac anesthesiologists need a working knowledge of antimicrobial prophylaxis for routine cardiac surgery, the management of serious surgical site infection, the prevention, diagnosis and treatment of endocarditis and the prevention and treatment of infection with multi-resistant micro-organisms.

Routine surgical prophylaxis

The primary aim of surgical prophylaxis is to reduce wound infection. Placebo-controlled trials have shown that the use of antibiotics such as flucloxacillin with activity against *Staphylococcus aureus* can significantly reduce the rate of infection following cardiac surgery. Antibiotic prophylaxis is also recommended for permanent pacemaker (PPM), implantable cardiac defibrillator (ICD) and ventricular assist device (VAD) implantation.

Following CABG surgery, Gram-negative bacilli (coliforms such *Escherichia coli*, *Klebsiella* species, *Enterobacter* species, and occasionally *Pseudomonas aeruginosa*) can also cause significant infection and are probably introduced during saphenous vein harvest. Prophylaxis for CABG surgery should therefore include antibiotics with activity against Gram-negative bacilli.

Some cardiac surgical centers use cephalosporins for prophylaxis against both Gram-positive and Gram-negative bacteria; however, gentamicin is active against a broader range of Gram-negatives. Furthermore, a cephalosporin is more likely to cause *Clostridium difficile* diarrhea than the combination of gentamicin and flucloxacillin. One dose of gentamicin is sufficient to maintain therapeutic levels throughout surgery and is unlikely to lead to nephrotoxicity or ototoxicity.

Patients who carry meticillin- (methicillin in the USA) resistant *Staph. aureus* (MRSA), whose MRSA

Table 71.1 Antibiotic regimes and typical adult doses

Antibiotic regime	Typical adult dose
Flucloxacillin + Gentamicin	1 g 6 hourly for 24 h (5 doses) 2 mg kg^{-1} as single dose
Cefuroxime	1.5 g pre-CPB and 1.5 g post-CPB, or 1.5 g pre-CPB and 750 mg 8 hourly
Vancomycin + Gentamicin	1 g pre-CPB and 1 g post-CPB 2 mg kg^{-1} as single dose

status is unknown or who have significant penicillin allergy should be prescribed vancomycin instead of either flucloxacillin or a cephalosporin. Erythromycin-resistant *Staph. aureus* is too prevalent for erythromycin or other macrolides (e.g. azithromycin, clarithromycin) to be recommended for routine prophylaxis.

Antibiotics should be given no earlier than 30 min before induction of anesthesia. For many general surgical procedures, single-dose prophylaxis is advocated, but this may not be appropriate for cardiac surgery, where there is some recent evidence that giving antibodies for at least 24 h is beneficial in prevention of sternal surgical site infection. Blood loss and hemodilution during CPB may significantly reduce antibiotic levels. If the drug has a short half-life (e.g. flucloxacillin) a second dose should be given after termination of CPB. Following the onset of CPB, vancomycin levels drop more than would be anticipated from hemodilution alone. For this reason a second dose of vancomycin should be given after CPB.

Other measures to reduce the risk of surgical site infection include preoperative bathing or showering, clipping hair from the surgical site on the day of surgery (avoiding the use of razors), solublized iodine

Core Topics in Cardiac Anesthesia, Second Edition, ed. Jonathan H. Mackay and Joseph E. Arrowsmith. Published by Cambridge University Press. © Cambridge University Press 2012.

(iodophor)-impregnated incision drapes, good oxygenation and perfusion during surgery and appropriate use of wound dressings. The UK National Institute for Health and Clinical Excellence (NICE) Clinical Guideline 74 (2008) gives further guidance on prevention of surgical site infection.

Mediastinitis

Deep sternal wound infection, osteomyelitis and/or mediastinitis are serious complications of cardiac surgery. Mediastinitis occurs in 1–2% of cardiac surgical patients and carries an overall mortality of 5%. Risk factors for both superficial and deep mediastinal infections include:

- diabetes mellitus
- re-sternotomy for hemorrhage
- bilateral mammary artery harvesting
- obesity
- renal failure.

The most likely causative agent is *Staph. aureus*, although streptococci (e.g. *Streptococcus pyogenes*) and coagulase-negative staphylococci may be implicated. Following CABG surgery, Gram-negative bacilli can cause deep infection, particularly when saphenous vein has been harvested.

Patients with mediastinal infection who require surgical re-exploration and debridement are invariably systemically unwell. Clinical features include fever, tachycardia, raised WBC and CRP, often with wound cellulitis and purulent discharge, wound breakdown or dehiscence. In addition to fever and general malaise there may be signs of pericardial tamponade or constriction, as well as cardiac, respiratory and renal dysfunction. Microbiological investigations should include culture of blood as well as fluids drained from the wound, pleurae or pericardium. A deep collection or mediastinitis should be considered when micro-organisms are cultured from blood, even if they are not cultured from the wound surface. Investigations should aim at excluding endocarditis, particularly in the presence of a prosthetic device (e.g. valve, PPM, ICD).

The management of mediastinitis typically involves surgical debridement, sternal rewiring and surgical drainage of infection, plus a prolonged course of antibiotics. Treatment with antibiotics should be continued for at least 4 weeks after the last debridement if there is sternal osteomyelitis.

Patients with apparently superficial infection may be found to have much more extensive infection at operation. The prudent anesthesiologist will arrange for postoperative admission to the ICU and prepare for the worst-case scenario!

Endocarditis prophylaxis

The NICE Clinical Guideline 64 (2008), *Prophylaxis against Infective Endocarditis*, lists the cardiac conditions that place a patient at increased risk of infective endocarditis:

- acquired valvular heart disease with stenosis or regurgitation
- valve replacement
- structural congenital heart disease, including surgically corrected or palliated structural conditions, but excluding isolated atrial septal defect, fully repaired ventricular septal defect or fully repaired patent ductus arteriosus, and closure devices that are judged to be endothelialized
- hypertrophic cardiomyopathy
- previous infective endocarditis.

This guidance is broadly similar to recommendations made in the 2008 update to the ACC/AHA 2006 *Guidelines for the Management of Patients With Valvular Heart Disease* (Table 71.2).

The common practice of using antibiotic prophylaxis for dentistry has been questioned. Recent studies have shown that bacteremia with oral micro-organisms occurs daily in association with chewing and tooth brushing, and epidemiological studies have shown a lack of association between endocarditis and prior dental treatment. International guidelines therefore advise that antimicrobial prophylaxis for endocarditis should no longer be given for dental or other procedures (GI, genitourinary and respiratory) unless there are signs of active infection, which should be treated effectively. While initially received with some scepticism, these new guidelines represent a significant change from recommendations presented in the first edition of this book. Patients at risk of endocarditis should be advised to maintain good oral health and any episode of infection (such as skin, urinary or dental sepsis) should be dealt with promptly. In hospital, the early diagnosis and treatment of infection including the removal of the source (such as an infected intravascular line) is crucial for the patient at risk of endocarditis.

Table 71.2 Updated ACC/AHA 2006 guidelines for infective endocarditis prophylaxis

Class	Recommendation
IIa	Prophylaxis against infective endocarditis is reasonable for the following patients at highest risk for adverse outcomes from infective endocarditis who undergo dental procedures that involve manipulation of either gingival tissue or the periapical region of teeth or perforation of the oral mucosa.
	Patients with prosthetic cardiac valve or prosthetic material used for cardiac valve repair (Level of Evidence: B)
	Patients with previous infective endocarditis (Level of Evidence: B)
	Patients with CHD (Level of Evidence: B)
	Unrepaired cyanotic CHD, including palliative shunts and conduits (Level of Evidence: B)
	Completely repaired congenital heart defect repaired with prosthetic material or device, whether placed by surgery or by catheter intervention, during the first 6 months after the procedure (Level of Evidence: B)
	Repaired CHD with residual defects at the site or adjacent to the site of a prosthetic patch or prosthetic device (both of which inhibit endothelialization) (Level of Evidence: B)
	Cardiac transplant recipients with valve regurgitation due to a structurally abnormal valve (Level of Evidence: C)
III	Prophylaxis against infective endocarditis is not recommended for nondental procedures (such as transesophageal echocardiogram, esophagogastroduodenoscopy, or colonoscopy) in the absence of active infection (Level of Evidence: B)

Table created from text presented in: *Circulation* 2008; 118(15): e523–661.

The individual at risk of infective endocarditis should receive standard prophylaxis for cardiac surgery. Dental hygiene should be reviewed before valve replacement and any source of recurrent infection at any body site should be treated.

The British Society for Antimicrobial Chemotherapy (BSAC) endocarditis working party has endorsed the NICE prophylaxis guidelines. The American Heart Association (2008) and the European Society of Cardiology (2009) continue to advocate antimicrobial prophylaxis for certain procedures, but only in patients at the highest risk of infective endocarditis.

Infective endocarditis

It may be difficult to make the diagnosis of endocarditis, and a high index of suspicion is required. Both pathological and clinical criteria are used. Pathological criteria include culture of micro-organisms from an intracardiac abscess or an embolized vegetation. A histological diagnosis may be made from a vegetation or intracardiac abscess. The presence of major and minor clinical criteria permits a clinical diagnosis of definite endocarditis to be made. Using the Duke clinical criteria, a diagnosis requires the presence of two major criteria, one major criterion and three minor criteria or five minor criteria (Table 71.3).

The AHA, European Cardiac Society (ECS) and BSAC have published guidelines for the treatment of infective endocarditis. The general principles are to use a prolonged course of a cidal antibiotic or an antibiotic combination. Drugs with a short half-life, such as the penicillins, are given at high dose and at frequent intervals to optimize pharmacokinetics and the pharmacodynamic interaction between drug and bacterium. The treatment for infective endocarditis should continue throughout valve surgery in addition to any antibiotics used for surgical prophylaxis. Modification of the antibiotic surgical prophylaxis regime may be necessary. As an example, if the patient has received benzylpenicillin or flucloxacillin preoperatively, an alternative agent such as vancomycin should be used for prophylaxis because of the risk of surgical site infection with resistant Gram-positive bacteria. If the patient is being treated for endocarditis with an antibiotic regime that includes gentamicin, serum levels must be monitored closely in the perioperative period to prevent nephrotoxicity.

Microscopy and culture of the resected valve is essential and may help guide the duration of antimicrobial treatment after surgery. Where a causative organism has not been identified preoperatively nor cultured from the excised valve, it may be helpful to look for evidence of microbial infection using polymerase chain reaction (PCR) amplification of bacterial and fungal ribosomal RNA genes.

449

Table 71.3 The Duke clinical criteria for the diagnosis of infective endocarditis

Major criteria	1	Positive blood cultures for infectious endocarditis; either typical micro-organisms consistent with infective endocarditis, or persistently positive blood cultures
	2	Evidence of endocardial involvement
		(a) Positive echocardiogram for endocarditis
		– Oscillating intracardiac mass – on valve or supporting structures, in path of regurgitant jet, or on implanted material
		– Abscess
		– New partial dehiscence of prosthetic valve
		(b) New valvular regurgitation (worsening or change of a pre-existing murmur is not sufficient for diagnosis)
Minor criteria	1	Predisposing heart condition or intravenous drug abuse
	2	Fever ≥38°C
	3	Vascular phenomena: major arterial emboli, septic pulmonary infarcts, mycotic aneurysm, intracranial hemorrhage, conjunctival hemorrhages, Janeway's lesions
	4	Immunological phenomena: glomerulonephritis, Osler's nodes, Roth's spots, positive rheumatoid factor
	5	Microbiological evidence: positive blood culture but not meeting major criteria, or serological evidence of active infection with organism consistent with infective endocarditis
	6	Echocardiographic findings consistent with infective endocarditis but not sufficient to meet major criteria

Clinical diagnosis = two major criteria, or one major criterion + three minor criteria, or five minor criteria.

Multi-resistant bacteria

The possibility that an infection could be caused by a multi-resistant organism should be borne in mind, particularly if the patient has been recently hospitalized. ICU patients are at particular risk if:

- they have been transferred from another center where an outbreak has occurred
- their ICU stay has been prolonged
- they have been exposed to multiple classes of antimicrobials.

Immunocompromised patients and those treated in renal, liver or hematology units are at even greater risk of infection with multi-resistant organisms. Prevention of infection relies on meticulous hand hygiene, isolation of infected or colonized patients and scrupulous environmental cleaning. Screening patients for the carriage of these organisms before surgery, on transfer from another ICU and on a weekly basis in ICU thereafter is advisable.

Methicillin-resistant *Staphylococcus aureus*

MRSA is resistant to all penicillins and cephalosporins. Many strains are also resistant to aminoglycosides (e.g. gentamicin) and quinolones (e.g. ciprofloxacin). Strains of MRSA appear no more pathogenic than drug-sensitive *Staph. aureus*. Infections, such as mediastinitis, osteomyelitis and infective endocarditis, can, however, be more difficult to treat. The treatment of choice for MRSA is a glycopeptide, such as vancomycin, both as treatment for proven MRSA infection and as part of empiric treatment of infection in MRSA carriers. Vancomycin is, however, not as effective an anti-staphylococcal agent for MRSA when compared with the use of flucloxacillin for a sensitive *Staph. aureus*. A second antimicrobial agent, such as rifampicin or fusidic acid, is therefore recommended for use in combination with vancomycin for deep MRSA infection. Many of the more recently introduced anti-MRSA antibiotics, such as linezolid, are bacteriostatic rather than bactericidal. An exception is daptomycin, but evidence of its effectiveness in mediastinitis and endocarditis is limited.

Spread of MRSA leads to more use of vancomycin and teicoplanin, which can select for vancomycin-resistant bacteria, for which there are few therapeutic options. Reduced vancomycin susceptibility can emerge during treatment and therefore it is advised to maintain an adequate trough vancomycin concentration (10–20 mg l^{-1}). High-level vancomycin-resistant *Staph. aureus* has been described in the USA but is fortunately rare.

MRSA is often carried as part of the normal flora on moist skin sites such as the anterior nares, throat, perineum and axillae. Systemic antibiotics do not achieve effective concentrations on body surfaces and have no effect on MRSA carriage, whereas topical agents (e.g. triclosan, chlorhexidine, mupirocin) may clear colonization. Every patient should be considered a potential MRSA carrier and the risk of spread can be reduced if staff wash hands or use a topical antiseptic after every contact with a patient or their immediate surroundings.

Patients who have been in hospital or institutional care are at increased risk of carrying MRSA. Many centers now screen all elective and emergency patients for MRSA before or at the time of admission to hospital. MRSA screening samples include swabs from carriage sites (nose, throat and perineum), sputum and wound sites, including line or drain insertion sites. Results of screening should be available within 24–48 h. Elective surgical patients can be screened in a pre-admission clinic and clearance of MRSA carriage using topical treatment should be attempted before cardiac surgery. Carriers of MRSA should be both isolated and barrier-nursed, and vancomycin should be included in their operative prophylaxis to prevent surgical site infection.

Nowadays there is a trend away from routine screening of staff. MRSA may be carried as part of the normal flora of a health care worker – usually in the nose. If their "practice" is good, they are unlikely to spread this to a patient unless they have a desquamating skin condition or an infected lesion. Screening of staff can lead to victimization of those who are carriers but not spreading organisms and conversely can cause complacency in those who are not carriers but do spread MRSA from patient to patient because they do not wash their hands.

Glycopeptide-resistant *Enterococcus* (GRE)

Enterococcus faecalis and *E. faecium* can become resistant to vancomycin or teicoplanin, leaving very few antibiotics available for treatment. GRE (also known as vancomycin-resistant *Enterococcus* or VRE) can be part of the gut flora and may be found on damaged skin sites such as wounds, drain sites and tracheal stomas. These bacteria are very hardy and survive well in the environment, therefore exemplary infection control practice is needed to stop spread. Fortunately, GRE are not very pathogenic and rarely cause infection even in the immunocompromised. When GRE is isolated from blood cultures, the likely source is an infected intravascular catheter, and removal of this is often sufficient to clear the bacteremia. GRE endocarditis can, however, be very difficult to treat. A patient infected with GRE should be barrier nursed where possible, although if access to a single-occupancy room is limited, priority should be given to carriers who are more likely to be a source of cross-infection, such as those with diarrhea, incontinence or colonized skin lesions. Vancomycin, teicoplanin and cephalosporin usage should be strictly controlled to discourage the emergence of GRE.

Multi-resistant Gram-negative bacilli

Multi-resistant Gram-negative bacilli are increasingly reported as a cause of hospital outbreaks of ventilator-associated pneumonia and infections of the urinary and biliary tracts. These organisms can spread between patients and survive for long periods in the environment. Control therefore relies on screening patients for carriage, isolation of infected patients and restricted use of broad-spectrum antibiotics.

Examples include coliforms that possess an extended spectrum β-lactamase (ESBL) which destroys penicillins and cephalosporins. In addition they often carry plasmids conferring resistance to other antimicrobials such as quinolones and gentamicin. Because of increasing prevalence of ESBL-producing bacteria, the carbapenems (e.g. meropenen, imipenem) are often used as empirical therapy of severe infections. However, in the last 3 years reports of carbapenem-resistant coliforms, particularly *Klebsiella pneumoniae*, have increased.

Epidemic strains of carbapenem- and multi-drug-resistant *Acinetobacter baumannii* have been described. There are few antimicrobial treatment options for infection and limited clinical data of effectiveness. Antibiotics such as tigecycline, colistin and amikacin have been used, either singly or in combination.

Clostridium difficile-associated diarrhea

Patients who acquire *C. difficile* gut colonization from the hospital environment and are then given antibiotics may go on to develop frank infection with *Clostridium difficile*. Additional risk factors include advanced age, serious underlying illness and infection with epidemic strains of *C. difficile*. The organism can spread on the hands of staff through contact with infected patients or the environment (e.g. floors, bedpans, toilets) contaminated with *C. difficile* spores which are resistant to drying and disinfection.

C. difficile-associated disease varies from asymptomatic colonization through mild self-limiting diarrhea to severe pseudomembranous colitis leading to colonic perforation and death. Diagnosis is made by testing feces for *C. difficile* toxins. More severe cases may need to be assessed by colonoscopy or abdominal CT.

Patients with suspected disease must be barrier nursed, especially when on an ICU. Mild disease may respond to discontinuing antibiotics, but more severe cases require treatment with metronidazole (IV or oral) or oral vancomycin. Intravenous vancomycin is ineffective in *C. difficile* infection.

Prevention involves restriction of antibiotic use (especially clindamycin, quinolones and cephalosporins), hand hygiene with soap and water rather than alcohol gel before and after patient contact, and enhanced environmental cleaning using a chlorine-based disinfectant.

Key points

- Surgical site infections following cardiac surgery can be difficult to treat – use of prophylactic antibiotics and compliance with additional measures to prevent infection are crucial.
- Early recognition and treatment of infection including the prompt removal of infected lines may help prevent endocarditis.
- Strains of MRSA appear no more pathogenic than drug-sensitive *Staphylococcus aureus*.

- Screening, hand hygiene, barrier nursing and appropriate use of antibiotics help prevent the spread of multi-resistant bacteria and *C. difficile*.

Further reading

Bonow RO, Carabello BA, Chatterjee K, *et al.* 2008 Focused update incorporated into the ACC/AHA 2006 guidelines for the management of patients with valvular heart disease: a report of the American College of Cardiology/American Heart Association Task Force on Practice Guidelines. *Circulation* 2008; **118**(15): e523–661.

British Society for Antimicrobial Chemotherapy guidelines on prevention and treatment of endocarditis and prophylaxis and treatment of Meticillin-Resistant Staphylococcus aureus (MRSA) infections (www.bsac.org.uk).

Department of Health and Health Protection Agency. *Clostridium difficile infection: how to deal with the problem.* 2009 (www.hpa.org.uk).

Durack DT, Lukes AS, Bright DK. New criteria for diagnosis of infective endocarditis: utilization of specific endocardiographic findings. *Am J Med* 1994; **96**(3): 200–9.

Mertz D, Johnstone J, Loeb M. Does duration of perioperative antibiotic prophylaxis matter in cardiac surgery? A systemic review and meta-analysis. *Ann Surg* 2011; **254**(1): 48–54.

National Institute of Health and Clinical Excellence. *Prophylaxis against infective endocarditis. Clinical Guideline* **64**. March 2008 (www.nice.org.uk/cg064).

National Institute of Health and Clinical Excellence. *Surgical site infection. Clinical Guideline* **74**. October 2008 (www.nice.org.uk/cg074).

Scottish Intercollegiate Guidelines Network. *Antibiotic Prophylaxis in Surgery.* 2008 (www.sign.ac.uk).

Regional anesthesia

Trevor W. R. Lee

The sympathetic stress response to surgery causes a multitude of adverse hemodynamic, metabolic, hematological, endocrine and immunological effects. In the setting of cardiac surgery, attenuation of pain and sympathetic autonomic activity has many theoretical attractions. The introduction of high-dose opioid techniques into cardiac anesthesia was based, in part, on the belief that they would inhibit the stress response. Failure to block the stress response completely, combined with equivocal evidence of clinical benefit and the need for prolonged postoperative mechanical ventilation, made the technique unpopular. The demonstration that thoracic sympathetic blockade improves blood flow in severely diseased coronary arteries and the emergence of less invasive cardiac surgical procedures and economic pressures have prompted renewed interest in regional anesthetic techniques.

Thoracic epidural anesthesia

The first description of the use of thoracic epidural anesthesia (TEA) for analgesia *after* cardiac surgery appeared in 1976. It was not until 1987, however, that the first report of epidural catheter insertion *before* cardiac surgery was published. In most published series the interspaces between C_7–T_1 and T_3–T_4 have been used for TEA. The higher approaches are technically easier, although it should be borne in mind that the ligamentum flavum in the thoracic region is thinner and more delicate than in the lumbar region. Most practitioners use a midline approach with the conscious patient sitting or lying. The method used to identify the epidural space varies. The avoidance of the "asleep" epidural in this setting is more a function of retaining the ability to assess the efficacy of the block *before* induction of anesthesia than a response

to concerns about medicolegal implications of neurologic injury.

Typical initial doses include 3 ml lidocaine 2% and 5 ml levobupivacaine 0.5% with or without fentanyl ~25 µg; repeated after 10 min, as necessary. Regardless of the epidural infusion recipe used, it is imperative that a bilateral T_1–T_5 dermatome block is present before proceeding. A continuous epidural infusion (e.g. levobupivacaine ~0.125% $\pm$ fentanyl 1–5 µg ml^{-1} $\pm$ clonidine 0.5 µg ml^{-1} at a rate of 4–10 ml h^{-1}) is then started during surgery and usually continued for up to 3 days. The synergy between agents of different classes (i.e. opioids and local anesthetics) permits the total dose and side effects of each to be reduced. Regular input from an acute pain management team maximizes epidural efficacy and allows early detection of adverse events.

The "pros" and "cons" of TEA in cardiac surgery are shown in Table 72.1.

TEA is almost invariably used as an adjunct to general anesthetic techniques tailored to early recovery and neurologic assessment. Recently some centers have been assessing the feasibility of using TEA as a sole anesthetic in beating heart surgery. Apart from showing that *it is possible* to rise to this fresh challenge and the associated publicity, it is difficult to think of any other reason why anyone would want to routinely perform cardiac surgery on awake patients. The additional anxiety for both patients and staff is unnecessary, spontaneous respiration with open pleura is physiologically undesirable, respiratory depression due to paralysis of diaphragm or thoracic musculature may occur and TEE is impossible. Common sense suggests that goals of anesthesia for cardiac surgery should include the prevention of unanticipated patient movement throughout the operation.

Core Topics in Cardiac Anesthesia, Second Edition, ed. Jonathan H. Mackay and Joseph E. Arrowsmith. Published by Cambridge University Press. © Cambridge University Press 2012.

Table 72.1 The "pros" and "cons" of thoracic epidural anesthesia and analgesia in cardiac surgery

Cardiac sympathetic blockade
Pro Unmyelinated sympathetic neurons very sensitive to local anesthetics
Blockade of sympathetic neurons from T_1–T_5
Dilatation of severely diseased coronary arteries
↓ Incidence of postoperative arrhythmias
↑ Myocardial contractility – remains unproven
Con Risk of hypotension
May inhibit sympathetic vasodilatation in normal coronary arteries

Attenuation of stress response
Pro Local anesthetics superior to epidural opioids alone
Attenuation of ↑ circulating catecholamine levels
BP and HR response to surgery blunted
Less effect on secondary metabolic, immune and hematological responses
Con Unequivocal evidence of stress response attenuation difficult to obtain

Analgesia
Pro Intense intraoperative and postoperative analgesia
Avoids adverse effects of parenteral narcotic analgesics
Early tracheal extubation and mobilization
Improved postoperative pulmonary function
Possible ↓ incidence of chronic pain syndromes
Con Unilateral block or missed segments render technique ineffective
Motor and proprioception block may limit mobilization

The insertion of an epidural catheter prior to full anticoagulation is less taboo than in the past. Emerging evidence suggests that those most likely to benefit are patients with borderline pulmonary function, opioid addicts and patients likely to be incompletely revascularized by surgery. Recently published prospective studies suggest that TEA is associated with a lower incidence of postoperative respiratory tract infection, supraventricular dysrhythmias and renal failure. No study yet published has had sufficient power to demonstrate any statistically significant reduction in perioperative mortality. Double-blind studies of TEA, with placement of a "non-therapeutic" epidural catheter in control group patients, have not been undertaken.

Spinal anesthesia

The first report of spinal anesthesia in cardiac surgery was published in 1980. In this report, as in the vast majority of subsequent publications, the agent used was preservative-free morphine sulfate. The potential benefits of spinal anesthesia in cardiac surgery are the same as those for TEA, although the risk of epidural hematoma is probably less. Unlike TEA, however, spinal anesthetic techniques in this setting have tended to be "single shot" and opioid-based. The limited duration of drug action dictates that lumbar puncture has to be performed shortly before heparinization. The major safety concerns therefore are respiratory depression and neuraxial bleeding, although pruritus, nausea, vomiting and urinary retention are usually more troublesome. The low lipid solubility of morphine results in delayed onset of analgesia and unpredictable effects. Although some investigators have demonstrated superior postoperative analgesia, others have reported either no benefit or delayed recovery. This may explain the failure of intrathecal morphine to attenuate the stress response to surgery.

In contrast, published investigations of intrathecal local anesthesia in cardiac surgery are scarce. In a retrospective study published in 1994, Kowalewski and colleagues reported that the combination of hyperbaric bupivacaine (30 mg) and morphine (0.5–1.0 mg) produced excellent postoperative analgesia compatible with same-day early tracheal extubation. More recently, Lee and colleagues have demonstrated that general anesthesia combined with intrathecal bupivacaine (37.5 mg) resulted in significant attenuation of the stress response and improved LV segmental wall motion. When compared to patients who had a "sham spinal", study patients had significantly lower serum levels of epinephrine, norepinephrine and cortisol, and significantly less atrial β-receptor dysfunction. Unfamiliarity with the technique and the perception of hemodynamic instability may limit widespread adoption of high-dose intrathecal bupivacaine and intrathecal morphine by cardiac anesthesiologists. Although hemodynamic instability is cited as one of the major risks of high spinal anesthesia, the physiological responses to total sympathectomy can be managed with small, titrated doses of intravenous vasoactive agents.

Table 72.2 Technique used for delivering a high or total-spinal anesthetic (Lee *et al.*, 2008)

Patient pre-medicated with oral diazepam (0.1 mg kg^{-1}) or oral gabapentin (1.5 mg kg^{-1})

Intravenous volume repletion and loading accomplished with synthetic colloid 500 ml

Lumbar spine is prepared and draped with the patient in the lateral decubitus position

25G pencil point spinal needle is used to administer the intrathecal blockade

Single-shot dose of 45 mg hyperbaric bupivacaine 0.75%, in combination with 2–3 µg kg^{-1} (maximum total dose 300 µg) of preservative-free spinal morphine injected into intrathecal space. Bevel of the spinal needle facing cephalad during injection may maximize local anesthetic spread

Operating table placed in <5° Trendelenburg, with the patient in supine position. A C8 or higher sensory block can take ~10 min to develop

Small doses of IV phenylephrine and ephedrine are used to maintain MAP >65 mmHg

General anesthesia induced, after complete cardiac sympathectomy achieved, using IV propofol 0.5–1.0 mg kg^{-1} and rocuronium 0.6–1.0 mg kg^{-1}. Intravenous narcotics may not be required for maintenance

To ensure amnesia and hypnosis, general anesthesia must be maintained at 0.5–1.0 MAC

Prior to chest closure, adjunctive analgesia can be provided using bilateral parasternal blocks

Prior to emergence, the patient is given IV morphine to achieve a respiratory rate between 15–20 bpm

Trachea extubated in operating room immediately after procedure

Neuraxial bleeding

There is little doubt that the uptake of neuraxial techniques in cardiac anesthetic practice has been slowed by "the ill-defined risk of permanent paraplegia in a fully anticoagulated, unconscious patient". For this reason, TEA and spinal anesthesia remain in the hands of enthusiasts. Questions commonly asked by anesthesiologists include those shown in Table 72.3.

It can be deduced from this list that the risks of neuraxial bleeding, epidural hematoma and permanent neurologic injury are foremost in anesthesiologists' minds. The absence of reported complications

Table 72.3 Questions frequently asked about the use of epidural anesthesia in cardiac surgery

1. What is the incidence of epidural-associated spinal hematoma?

2. Do normal laboratory coagulation test results give comfort that clotting is normal?

3. Do antiplatelet agents increase the risk of spinal hematoma?

4. How should patients taking oral anticoagulants be managed?

5. What is the safest epidural insertion–heparin administration interval?

6. What is the appropriate response to a "bloody tap" or "dural tap"?

7. Is there an "ideal" intervertebral space for epidural placement?

8. Does TEA make any difference to patient outcome?

in relatively small prospective series (i.e. <1000 patients) gives little cause for comfort – the so-called "zero numerator" problem. While estimates vary from 1:1500 to 1:150 000, data from neurologists and analysis of closed medicolegal claims may provide a more accurate measure of the true incidence of epidural hematoma. In the context of the major risks of cardiac surgery (i.e. death and stroke), the risk of epidural-related paraplegia is very small.

In calculating the predicted risk, Ho *et al.* used existing published data to estimate the minimum and maximum risk of hematoma formation following instrumentation for cardiac surgery. The incidence of a clinically significant spinal hematoma was estimated to be 1:220 000–1:3600 after spinal anesthesia and 1:150 000–1:1500 after TEA for cardiac surgery. In 2010, Horlocker *et al.* published guidelines on the use of neuraxial techniques in patients receiving antiplatelet agents and low-molecular-weight heparin. Current recommendations suggest the avoidance of regional anesthesia if potent antiplatelet drugs (e.g. thienopyridine derivatives) have been used within 7 days, in the case of clopidogrel, or 10–14 days, in the case of ticlopidine. Neuraxial anesthesia is contraindicated in fully anti-coagulated patients. In the event of a "bloody tap", it is recommended that the institution of therapeutic heparinization be delayed by at least 1 h, in order to reduce the relative risk of subsequent complications.

The higher risk of hematoma formation following TEA may explain the preference for spinal anesthesia and analgesia for cardiac surgery in some institutions. The use of small-gauge needles and the avoidance of catheter insertion/removal are believed to reduce the risk of epidural hematoma after spinal anesthesia.

Patient refusal, local or systemic infection, decompensated AS and coagulopathy are regarded as absolute contraindications to neuraxial blockade. In practice, coagulopathy means a platelet count $<100 \times 10^9 \ l^{-1}$, INR >1.2 or APTT >45 s. Most patients undergoing elective cardiac surgery will be asked to discontinue aspirin and other antiplatelet agents 5–10 days before surgery. The magnitude of any additional epidural-related risk, directly attributable to concurrent antiplatelet therapy, is unknown. Oral anticoagulation should be stopped 3–4 days before surgery and normalization of the INR confirmed. Patients who cannot have their oral anticoagulation safely withdrawn before surgery should not have TEA. Opinion regarding the minimum safe interval between epidural catheter insertion and the administration of unfractionated heparin varies from 1 to 12 h.

The optimal management of a bloody tap is unknown. Practices vary from the extreme; abandoning TEA and postponing surgery for 24 h, to resiting the epidural and continuing with the surgical procedure. The latter approach is based on the belief that blood clots in 10–12 min and that heparin is not thrombolytic. Due to the theoretical risk of bleeding following removal of the epidural catheter, the procedure is usually performed after normalization of coagulation has been confirmed by laboratory tests. In patients receiving unfractionated heparin, the epidural catheter is typically removed not less than 4 h after discontinuing the infusion or 1 h before any dose of low-molecular-weight heparin. In some centers, the institution of oral anticoagulation is delayed until after the epidural catheter has been removed.

The neurologic sequelae that may accompany a spinal hematoma range from vague sensory and motor symptoms to dense paraplegia or even quadriplegia. The presence and extent of any neurologic deficit may only be apparent after discontinuation of the block and removal of the epidural catheter. If there is any doubt, CT or MRI must be undertaken urgently and neurosurgical advice sought. Failure to make the diagnosis and institute management will rightly draw criticism.

Parasternal and paravertebral blockade

Although used routinely in some centers, parasternal blockade following cardiac surgery is poorly represented in the literature. Prior to skin closure, preservative-free isobaric bupivacaine 0.25% with or without epinephrine (total volume 40–50 ml) is injected along the sternal borders, deep to the posterior intercostal membrane, to block the anterior cutaneous branches of the intercostal nerves for 6–10 h. The technique may be considered in the patient with abnormal coagulation.

Paravertebral blockade is most commonly used to provide analgesia during and after thoracic surgery. Paravertebral blockade for cardiac surgery is used far less frequently. The paravertebral space lies just anterior to the parietal pleural of the lung, and posterior to the intercostal intimus muscle. Small-bore catheters are usually placed percutaneously, by "walking" a large bore epidural needle off the superior aspect of the transverse process of the thoracic vertebra (T3–T5). As with TEA, a "loss of resistance" technique is used to identify the paravertebral space. Boluses of local anesthetic (e.g. 5–10 ml bupivacaine 0.5%) are followed by an infusion (e.g. 6–8 ml h^{-1} bupivacaine 0.1%). A unilateral approach may be used for minimally invasive cardiac surgery via anterior short thoracotomy. Although continuous paravertebral blockade provides good analgesia and facilitates early tracheal extubation, difficulty identifying and catheterizing the paravertebral space and a definite failure rate limit its applicability.

Key points

- Cardiac sympathetic blockade, profound postoperative analgesia and attenuation of the stress response *may* improve patient outcome.
- The emergence of less invasive cardiac surgical procedures has prompted renewed interest in regional techniques.
- Although no longer taboo, the ill-defined risk of paraplegia in unconscious anticoagulated patients has deterred the majority of anesthesiologists from using TEA in cardiac surgical patients.
- The optimal management strategy for the "bloody tap" is unknown.
- Prospective, randomized, multicenter studies are required to demonstrate that TEA or spinal anesthesia are superior to combined α- and β-adrenergic blockade.

Further reading

Canto M, Sanchez MJ, Casas MA, Bataller ML. Bilateral paravertebral blockade for conventional cardiac surgery. *Anaesthesia* 2003; **58**: 365–70.

Chaney MA. Intrathecal and epidural anesthesia and analgesia for cardiac surgery. *Anesth Analg* 2006; **102**(1): 45–64.

Ho AM, Chung DC, Joynt GM. Neuraxial blockade and hematoma in cardiac surgery: estimating the risk of a rare adverse event that has not (yet) occurred. *Chest* 2000; **117**(2): 551–5.

Horlocker TT, Wedel DJ, Rowlingson JC, *et al*. Regional anesthesia in the patient receiving antithrombotic or thrombolytic therapy: American Society of Regional Anesthesia and Pain Medicine Evidence-Based Guidelines (Third Edition). *Reg Anesth Pain Med* 2010; **35**(1): 64–101.

Lee TWR, Jacobsohn E. Spinal anesthesia in cardiac surgery. *Tech Reg Anesth Pain Manag* 2008; **12**(1): 54–6.

Svircevic V, van Dijk D, Nierich AP, *et al*. Meta-analysis of thoracic epidural anesthesia versus general anesthesia for cardiac surgery. *Anesthesiology* 2011; **114**(2): 271–82.

Chapter

73

Pain management after cardiac surgery

Siân I. Jaggar and Amod Manocha

The prospect of sternotomy and the real possibility of disability or death give cardiac surgical patients a high expectation of postoperative pain and an understandable degree of apprehension. New procedures and surgical approaches present fresh challenges in acute pain management. The rational application of effective management strategies requires an understanding of pain pathophysiology. The importance of adequately treating postoperative pain is widely recognized and led to a campaign for the "pain score" to be designated the fifth vital sign.

The incidence of acute pain following major surgery is under-reported. Up to one in five patients experience severe pain or inadequate pain relief. Severe chronic pain affects 2–4% of patients 1 year after cardiac surgery.

Routine cardiac surgery produces a combination of somatic and visceral pain. (Table 73.1) Commonly used incisions include cervical, thoracic and lumbar dermatomes. (Figure 73.1)

Basic pain physiology

Teleologically, pain acts as a stimulus for protective reflexes generating withdrawal and avoidance responses. However, it is important to recognize that pain and nociception are different:

- Nociception describes the complex neural processes – transmission, transduction and

Table 73.1 Types and sources of pain following cardiac surgery

Superficial
   Skin incisions
   Drain and cannulation sites

Musculoskeletal
   Sternal and costal fractures
   Sternoclavicular and acromioclavicular joints
   Costovertebral and cervicothoracic zygoapophyseal
   joints

Visceral
   Pericardium
   Pleura
   Myocardium (ischemia)
   Diaphragm

Neurologic
   Peripheral nerve (e.g. radial, saphenous) injury
   Nerve entrapment
   Nerve plexus (e.g. brachial) injury

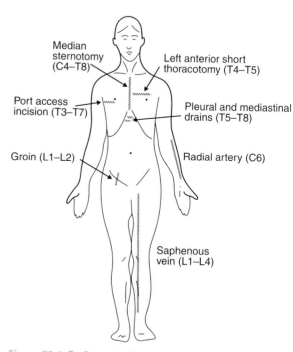

Figure 73.1 Cardiac surgical incisions and corresponding dermatomes.

458   *Core Topics in Cardiac Anesthesia, Second Edition*, ed. Jonathan H. Mackay and Joseph E. Arrowsmith. Published by Cambridge University Press. © Cambridge University Press 2012.

Table 73.2 Summary of characteristics of principle pain fiber type

	Aβ-fibers	Aδ-fibers	C-fibers
Threshold	Low	Medium	High
Axon diameter	6–14 μm	1–6 μm	0.2–1.0 μm
Myelination	Yes	Thinly	None
Conduction velocity	36–90 m s^{-1}	5–36 m s^{-1}	0.2–1.0 m s^{-1}
Receptive field size	Small	Small	Large
Pain quality	Touch	Sharp – first pain	Dull – second pain

modulation – that convey sensory information from peripheral tissues to the CNS. It is now clear that nociception cannot be explained in terms of simple rigid mechanisms. Rather it is plastic; changing with time and previous experience.

- Pain, by contrast, involves an unpleasant sensory and emotional experience (in addition to mere neural processing). It is what the patient says it is.

Surgical trauma triggers the production of inflammatory mediators capable of activating and modulating nociceptor responses. These mediators act on cation channels either directly (e.g. protons), or indirectly by modulating the activity of G-protein-coupled receptors (e.g. bradykinin) and neurotrophin receptors (e.g. nerve growth factor). Some mediators (e.g. ATP, glutamate) have both direct and indirect effects. An understanding of the molecular mechanisms by which these mediators elicit an action potential may provide new therapeutic targets.

Once induced, nociceptor impulses are transmitted to the dorsal horn (DH) of spinal cord via first-order neurons:

- very fast Aβ fibers – conducting touch
- fast Aδ fibers – causing sharp localized pain
- slow C fibers – producing dull poorly localized pain.

From the DH, impulses are transmitted via second-order neurons to the mid-brain. The majority of these second-order neurons decussate before ascending via spinothalamic pathways. Fibers from the midbrain project into the sensory cortex via the third-order neurons, where the perception of pain occurs. Pain perception is subject to historical alteration and the balance between ascending noxious impulses and inhibitory impulses both within the CNS and descending in the spinal cord. Pathological changes in these pathways are thought to be responsible for the development of chronic pain. A simplified illustration of the neural pathways involved in nociception is shown in Figure 73.2.

Pain from different anatomic structures is associated with different types of pain – reflecting the differing pathways of the nociceptive impulse conduction.

Somatic pain

Somatic pain can be superficial or deep, arising from skin, muscle and bone. Stimulation of free dermal nerve endings causes *superficial pain*, which is sharp and well localized because of the high density of neurons (e.g. pain associated with sternal skin incision). *Deep somatic pain*, in contrast, is dull and poorly localized (e.g. pain originating from muscles damaged during saphenous vein harvesting).

Visceral pain

Visceral pain arises from deep, internal tissues and is typically diffuse, poorly localized and associated with autonomic disturbances such as nausea and sweating. In comparison with somatic structures, the viscera have relatively fewer Aδ and C fibers, with afferents travelling via the autonomic nervous system – the vagus nerve, cervical ganglia and upper five thoracic ganglia. Within the spinal cord these autonomic afferents share ascending pathways with their somatic counterparts. This convergence of information at a spinal level explains the referred pain often associated with the visceral pain. Visceral pain is usually referred to the dermatome that shares the same embryonic origin, for example myocardial pain is often referred to the neck and arm.

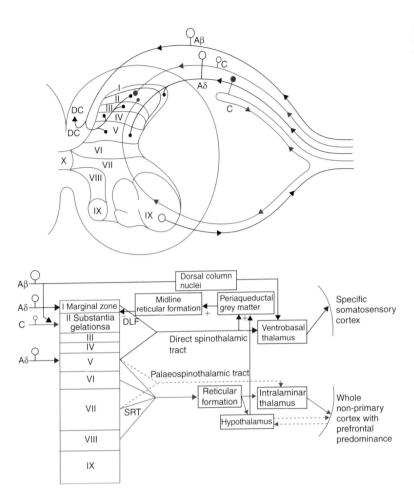

Figure 73.2 Central nociceptive and antinociceptive pathways. DLF, dorsolateral fasciculus; SRT, spinoreticular tract.

Neuropathic pain

Neuropathic pain (also known as neuralgia) arises as a consequence of nerve damage and is often accompanied by dysasthesia, allodynia and hyperalgesia. One of the mechanisms involved is thought to be the over-expression of neural ion channels following trauma.

Acute pain management

It has been repeatedly demonstrated that healthcare providers underestimate both the severity and deleterious effects of pain. Moreover, they overestimate both the efficacy and potential side-effects of analgesics.

Patients also often contribute to under-treatment of their pain because of worries about analgesic dependency and side-effects. Patient counseling (by trained staff) regarding postoperative pain therapy is an essential element of pre-assessment.

Simple measures go a long way to enhancing patient comfort. This includes attention to posture, maintaining diurnal rhythm, avoiding unpleasant noise and providing supplemental analgesia before mobilization.

Rationale

Pain is a normal response to trauma and some effects may be beneficial. Uncontrolled pain is associated with an increase in both morbidity and mortality.

Practical considerations

The philosophy of acute pain management can be considered under four headings:

1. *Prevention* – attention to patient positioning, choice of incision(s) and operative technique.
2. *Pre-emptive analgesia* – prevention of neuronal plasticity (e.g. opioids, N-methyl-D-aspartate receptor antagonists).

Table 73.3 Advantages and disadvantage of pain after cardiac surgery

System	Advantages	Disadvantages
Cardiovascular	Avoids bradycardia	↑ HR and ↑ SVR ↑ O_2 demand with ↓ supply, resulting in ischemia and dysrhythmias
Respiratory	Avoids ↓ respiratory rate and potential ↑ in $PaCO_2$	↑ Respiratory rate and ↓ tidal volume → ↑ work of breathing Atelectasis Ineffective cough Retention of secretions
Central nervous system	Heightened awareness	Exhaustion, disorientation and agitation ↓ Satisfaction
Peripheral nervous system		↑ Incidence chronic pain
Gastrointestinal		Nausea, vomiting and anorexia
Other		Hypercoagulability, with ↑ risk of DVT and graft failure Electrolyte imbalance with ↑ risk arrhythmias Hyperglycemia and immunosuppression with ↑ risk infection Increased length of stay

3. Depression and reversal of afferent-induced changes in the excitability of central neurons (e.g. opioids).
4. Breaking the vicious cycle of the physiological response to pain.

Some aspects of postoperative pain are preventable. Positioning the arms at the sides in internal, rather than external, rotation reduces the incidence of shoulder pain. Similarly, bony fractures and excessive sternal retraction, particularly during internal mammary artery harvesting, should be avoided. The use of endoscopic techniques for saphenous vein and radial artery harvesting may reduce the extent of incisional pain.

In conventional cardiac surgery it is virtually impossible to provide pain relief with local or regional techniques alone (Figure 73.1). For this reason, nurse-controlled IV morphine infusions have been the mainstay of postoperative analgesia since the early days. Balanced or "multimodal" analgesia can be achieved by combining an opioid with regular doses of a NSAID and paracetamol (acetaminophen).

Whenever possible, staff should be conscious of a patient's level of analgesia before embarking on potentially painful interventions or procedures. The pain associated with chest drain removal, physiotherapy and mobilization may be the only memory a patient has of the first postoperative day.

Despite abundant evidence of the safety of NSAIDs, the routine perioperative use of NSAIDs in cardiac surgical patients remains controversial. In the absence of any specific contraindication to their use, valid concerns about excessive surgical bleeding, renal dysfunction and GI hemorrhage in an elderly population mean that NSAIDs are usually withheld until at least the second postoperative day. In many centers NSAIDs are reserved for patients with pleural and pericardial pain. The theoretical advantages of selective cyclooxygenase II (COX-II) inhibitors (e.g. parecoxib, valdecoxib) in the setting of cardiac surgery have not been realized. Recent studies suggest an increase in the risk of major adverse cardiovascular events, such as MI, PE and stroke. Current evidence suggests that COX-II inhibitors should not be given to patients with severe coronary artery disease and those undergoing CABG surgery.

Occasionally, when severe acute pain does not respond to this traditional multimodal analgesic approach, chronic pain management techniques and early referral to a pain specialist should be considered. Local and regional techniques, transcutaneous

461

electrical nerve stimulation (TENS), acupuncture and adjunctive agents (e.g. α_2 agonists, γ-aminobutyric acid (GABA) agonists, gabapentin, pregabalin, amitriptyline, NMDA anatagonists) may be effective.

Chronic pain management

Pain at an operative site that persists for more than 3 months can be defined as chronic. Using this definition, the incidence of chronic pain after cardiac surgery may be >30% – far more common than most cardiac anesthesiologists appreciate. The most common site of chronic pain after cardiac surgery is the sternum. Other sites include shoulders, back, neck and conduit harvest sites. Pain at more than one site is common.

Chronic sternotomy pain

Chronic post-sternotomy pain is defined as new-onset, non-cardiac, thoracic pain after sternotomy. The reported incidence varies widely (21–56%); probably as a result of heterogeneity in both the definition of pain and patient populations, as well as the retrospective nature of most investigations. Younger patients seem to be at greater risk. As with acute pain, the cause of persistent pain after sternotomy is multifactorial and may result from:

- surgical tissue destruction, including rib fractures and intercostal nerve trauma
- scar formation
- infection at sternal or conduit harvest site
- presence of stainless-steel sutures
- costochondral separation.

Saphenous neuralgia

The saphenous nerve is the terminal sensory branch of the femoral nerve (L2–L4), supplying the skin of the antero-medial aspect of the leg. It is closely related to the great saphenous vein and the continuity of the nerve and its branches is at risk during any surgical procedure in this region. Saphenous neuralgia describes a symptom complex which includes anesthesia to both light touch and pin prick, combined with hyperesthesia and pain in the distribution of the saphenous nerve.

Rationale

Although mild persistent chest pain is common after sternotomy, it does not usually interfere with daily life. Patients who report chronic post-sternotomy and post-saphenectomy pain, however, have measurably lower quality of life. Unfortunately many studies evaluating outcome from cardiac surgery have not included chronic pain as an end-point.

Risk factors

Overwhelming evidence suggests that poorly treated severe acute postoperative pain is associated with a high incidence of chronic postoperative pain. Known risk factors are shown in Table 73.4, although it is possible that some patients are simply more susceptible to both acute and chronic postoperative pain.

Table 73.4 Risk factors for chronic pain after cardiac surgery

Age <60 years

Internal mammary artery harvesting

Body mass index >25 kg m^{-2}

Preoperative angina pectoris

Pre-existing arthritis

Female sex

Poor perioperative analgesia

Practical considerations

The approach to the cardiac surgical patient with chronic pain is no different from that to any patient with chronic pain. The principal aims are to identify the type of pain (i.e. musculoskeletal or neuropathic), exclude the presence of a new diagnosis (e.g. recurrent angina, arthritis, cervical spondylosis, myeloma) and formulate a treatment plan. A careful history should be taken using the patient's own words to describe their symptoms and the impact that they have on their quality of life. It is important to document any exacerbating and relieving factors, and to review the effect of previous therapies. It is essential to consider the possibility of coexisting depression and substance abuse.

In addition to pharmacological therapy, consideration should be given to psychological support (e.g. cognitive behavioral therapy), physiotherapy and graded physical exercise, adjuvant therapies such as local anesthetic infiltration, nerve blocks (e.g. intercostal) and regional techniques (e.g. epidural), and complementary therapies (e.g. TENS, acupuncture).

Table 73.5 Drug therapy in chronic pain

Antidepressants	Amitriptyline	25–50 mg at night
	Nortriptyline	10–25 mg at night
	Imipramine	20–100 mg
	Paroxetine	40 mg daily
	Citalopram	40 mg daily
	Fluoxetine	20 mg daily increasing to a maximum of 60 mg daily
Antiepileptics	Sodium valproate	100 mg TDS increasing to a maximum of 2400 mg daily in divided doses. Maximum effect probably achieved at 200 mg TDS
	Carbamazepine	200 mg TDS increasing to 400 mg TDS Maximum daily dose: 1600 mg
	Gabapentin	100 mg TDS increasing to a maximum of 3600 mg daily. Maximal effect probably achieved at 400 mg TDS
	Pregabalin	50 mg TDS increasing to a maximum of 600 mg daily
Antispasmodics	Baclofen	5 mg TDS increasing to a maximum of 100 mg daily
	Dantrolene	25 mg daily increasing to 100 mg QDS
	Piracetam	2.4 g TDS increasing to 20 g daily
NSAIDs[a]	Ibuprofen	200 mg TDS increasing to 600 mg QDS
	Diclofenac	150 mg daily as slow release preparation
COX-II inhibitors[a]	Rofecoxib	25–50 mg OD
	Celecoxib	100 mg BD increasing to 200 mg BD
Opioids	Codeine	30–60 mg QDS
	Dihydrocodeine	30–60 mg QDS
	Morphine	10–20 mg BD as slow release preparation (i.e. MST)
	Oxycodone	10 mg BD as modified release preparation
	Fentanyl	2–100 µg h^{-1} (transcutaneous delivery)
	Buprenorphine	5–70 µg h^{-1} (transcutaneous delivery)
Others	Paracetamol	1 g QDS
	Tramadol	50–100 mg BD increasing to 100 mg QDS
	Clonidine	50 µg BD increasing to 75 µg BD
	Ketamine	Continuous subcutaneous infusion
	Capsaicin	Topical 0.075% cream
	Magnesium	
	Corticosteroids	

[a] NSAIDs and COX-II inhibitors should not be used in patients with severe coronary artery disease or those who have undergone CABG survey.
OD, once daily; BD, *bis die* = twice daily; TDS, *ter die sumendus* = three times daily; QDS, *quater die sumendus* = four times daily.

Chronic refractory angina

As many as 10% of patients undergoing coronary angiography will be found to have coronary anatomy that is amenable to neither percutaneous nor surgical revascularization. When angina occurs in spite of maximal medical therapy the condition is termed chronic refractory angina (CRA) – a neuropathic pain syndrome. Myocardial ischemia leads to a chronic elevation of sympathetic tone, which in turn leads to a vicious cycle of myocardial oxygen imbalance and

myocardial dystrophy. Patients with CRA rapidly become incapacitated by their symptoms and require frequent hospital admissions. Therapeutic interventions have included transmyocardial and percutaneous laser revascularization, high thoracic epidural analgesia and electrical spinal cord stimulation (SCS).

SCS has been shown to produce a more homogeneous pattern of coronary blood flow in patients with myocardial ischemia. This redistribution of coronary blood flow may explain the subsequent increase in

Table 73.6 Care pathway in chronic refractory angina

1	Counseling	Explain management plan Provide advice on diet, smoking, physical activity, etc. Agree a realistic treatment contract
2	Rehabilitation	Exercise. Relaxation training
3	Cognitive therapy	Cognitive behavioral therapy Consider formal psychological assessment
4	TENS	May be used with permanent pacemakers
5	Temporary sympathectomy	Stellate ganglion block T3/4 paravertebral block in stages High thoracic epidural
6	SCS	Alternative to redo surgery in some high-risk patients
7	Opioids	Transdermal, oral, epidural or intrathecal[a]
8	Destructive sympathectomy[a]	Surgical – open or thoracoscopic Phenol – rarely used
9	Laser revascularization[a]	Open (transmyocardial) or percutaneous Efficacy unproven – consider as part of clinical trial
10	Transplantation	If other indications are present (see Chapter 44) Angina alone is not an indication

Adapted from the recommendations of The National Refractory Angina Centre, Liverpool, UK. http://www.angina.org.
[a] It is recommended that use of intrathecal opioids, destructive sympathectomy and laser revascularization be confined to patients enrolled in clinical studies.

effort tolerance in the face of unchanged total coronary blood flow. Although it has been suggested that SCS alters the balance between sympathetic and parasympathetic tone, patients show no change in HR variability.

Key points

- Cardiac surgical patients worry about death, disability and postoperative pain.
- An understanding of the pathophysiology of acute and chronic pain allows rational management strategies to be developed.
- Inadequate control of acute pain is associated with increased morbidity and mortality.
- A multimodal approach to analgesia provides the best results
- Spinal cord stimulation in chronic refractory angina may reduce the frequency of hospital readmission and improve quality of life.

Further reading

Andréll P, Yu W, Gersbach P, et al. Long-term effects of spinal cord stimulation on angina symptoms and quality of life in patients with refractory angina pectoris – results from the European Angina Registry Link Study (EARL). *Heart* 2010; **96**(14): 1132–6.

Ho SC, Royse CF, Royse AG, Penberthy A, McRae R. Persistent pain after cardiac surgery: an audit of high thoracic epidural and primary opioid analgesia therapies. *Anesth Analg* 2002; **95**(4): 820–3.

Holdcroft A, Jaggar S (Eds.). *Core Topics In Pain*. Cambridge: Cambridge University Press; 2005.

Lahtinen P, Kokki H, Hynynen M. Pain after cardiac surgery: a prospective cohort study of 1-year incidence and intensity. *Anesthesiology* 2006; **105**(4): 794–800.

Meyerson J, Thelin S, Gordh T, Karlsten R. The incidence of chronic post-sternotomy pain after cardiac surgery – a prospective study. *Acta Anaesthesiol Scand* 2001; **45**(8): 940–4.

Reimer-Kent J. From theory to practice: preventing pain after cardiac surgery. *Am J Crit Care* 2003; **12**(2): 136–43.

Hematological problems

Joseph E. Arrowsmith and Jonathan H. Mackay

Patients with hematological conditions or restrictive religious beliefs may require cardiac surgery. Uncommon problems require advanced warning, a review of current literature and recommendations, formulation of a detailed management plan and specialist hematological advice.

Increased bleeding tendency

Antiplatelet therapy

Aspirin, the thienopyridines (clopidogrel, prasugrel) and the glycoprotein (GP-IIb/IIIa) antagonists (abciximab, eptifibatide and tirofiban) improve outcome in acute coronary syndromes. The small numbers of patients who subsequently require emergency surgery are at increased risk of major perioperative bleeding as a result of their exposure to these drugs (Table 74.1). It is essential therefore, that the cardiac anesthesiologist be aware of the differences between them and the implications of their use.

The observation that cytochrome P450 polymorphism may underlie clopidogrel resistance has, in part, led to the introduction of prasugrel. In the TRITON-TIMI-38 study, the combination of prasugrel and aspirin was found to significantly reduce the combined rate of death from cardiovascular causes, non-fatal MI or nonfatal stroke in patients with acute coronary syndromes compared to the combination of clopidogrel and aspirin. Although there was no difference in mortality there was a significantly greater incidence of serious and fatal bleeding in prasugrel-treated patients.

While the impact of aspirin and thienopyridines on perioperative blood loss and transfusion requirements remains unclear, there is little doubt that the GP-IIb/IIIa antagonists have a much greater

Table 74.1 Characteristics of commonly used antiplatelet drugs

Aspirin	Impair ability of platelets to synthesis and release thromboxane
Clopidogrel **Plavix**®	Irreversibly inhibits ADP-induced platelet aggregation Half-life of main metabolite 8 h Excreted in urine and feces Platelet function normalizes ~5 days after discontinuation
Prasugrel **Effient**® **Efient**®	A prodrug. Irreversibly inhibits ADP-induced platelet aggregation Half-life of main metabolite 7 h Platelet function normalizes 5–9 days after discontinuation
Abciximab **Reopro**®	Non-selective monoclonal antibody Duration of platelet inhibition 24–48 h
Eptifibatide **Integrilin**®	Cyclic heptapeptide Duration of platelet inhibition 2–4 h Renal excretion. No active metabolites
Tirofiban **Aggrastat**®	Synthetic non-peptide Duration of platelet inhibition 4–8 h Renal excretion. No active metabolites

potential for causing problems. Where possible, it is recommended that surgery be delayed 12–24 h following abciximab exposure and 4–6 h following eptifibatide or tirofiban. In the Evaluation Prevention of Ischemic Complications (EPIC) study, patients undergoing CABG surgery following abciximab treatment were twice as likely to have major bleeding and three times more likely to die than patients given placebo. Bleeding complications following eptifibatide and tirofiban treatment are far less common.

Core Topics in Cardiac Anesthesia, Second Edition, ed. Jonathan H. Mackay and Joseph E. Arrowsmith. Published by Cambridge University Press. © Cambridge University Press 2012.

Severe, GP-IIb/IIIa antagonist-induced thrombocytopenia occurs in 0.1–0.5% patients.

The mainstay of treatment for excessive perioperative bleeding is platelet transfusion. Prophylactic platelet transfusion should be considered in abciximab-treated patients. Most anesthesiologists give platelets empirically following CPB. Some anesthesiologists regard GP-IIb/IIIa antagonist exposure as an indication to reduce the dose of heparin administered before CPB, aiming for a celite-ACT of 400 s. The role of off-pump coronary surgery has yet to be evaluated in this setting.

Thrombocytopenia

A low circulating platelet count usually indicates an increased tendency towards bleeding. Thrombocytopenia may be primary (idiopathic) or secondary (fictitious, dilutional, drug-induced, paraneoplastic, post-infectious and immuno-deficient). Idiopathic thrombocytopenia (ITP), which is three times more common in women, is a diagnosis of exclusion. Maintenance therapy typically comprises intermittent courses of corticosteroids with or without plasmapheresis, γ-globulin or immunosuppresssion.

While mild degrees of thrombocytopenia are relatively common in patients following cardiac surgery, it is important to identify those with type II heparin-induced thrombocytopenia (HIT) – a paradoxical *procoagulant* state defined as a platelet count $<100 \times 10^9 \, l^{-1}$ in association with immunoglobulin (Ig) G or IgM antibodies against the heparin–platelet factor 4 (PF4) complex. Paradoxically, patients with type II HIT are at significant risk of thromboembolic occlusion of medium and large vessels by platelet aggregates. Further doses of heparin should not be administered and the drug should be considered an allergen until after the disappearance of circulating anti-heparin–PF4 antibodies.

HIT is principally a clinical diagnosis. Supporting laboratory evidence has low positive predictive value and may take 24–72 h to obtain. Patients with known type II HIT present a considerable problem when considering anticoagulation for CPB. Although plasma exchange may be considered, surgery should be postponed until heparin can be given safely. Alternatively, anticoagulation with danaparoid, hirudin, lepirudin, bivalirudin, argatroban or prostacyclin may be considered. These agents are discussed in Chapter 11.

Hemophilia

Deficiency of either factor VIII (hemophilia A or classic hemophilia) and factor IX (hemophilia B or Christmas disease) are sex-linked recessive disorders that significantly increase the risk of excessive perioperative bleeding. Cardiac surgery in hemophiliacs requires considerable planning and close liaison with the local hemophilia service. Perioperative management comprises the administration of exogenous plasma-derived or recombinant anti-hemophilic factors and regular functional assays to assess circulating levels. Patients with factor VIII or factor IX inhibitors may be particularly difficult to manage.

von Willebrand's disease

von Willebrand's disease (vWD) consists of dysfunction or deficiency of von Willebrand factor (vWF), a multimeric plasma protein, and a variable degree factor VIII deficiency. It may be congenital (autosomal dominant or recessive) or acquired (e.g. hypothyroidism, Wilm's tumor, rheumatoid arthritis, systemic lupus erythematosus, renal disease and paraneoplastic), and affects females as well as males. Patients with mild forms of the disease respond to desmopressin (DDAVP), which increases circulating levels of vWF–antigen and factor VIII coagulant protein.

Increased thrombotic tendency

Antiphospholipid syndrome

This autoimmune condition, characterized by arterial and venous thrombosis, affects 2% of the general population and 7% of hospitalized patients. These patients are at risk of recurrent vascular occlusive disease (CVA, migraine, DVT) and cardiac manifestations (valve pathology, coronary artery disease, intracardiac thrombosis, pulmonary hypertension). Paradoxically, antiphospholipid (APL) antibodies act as in vitro (so-called "lupus") anticoagulants: interfering with laboratory tests of coagulation (i.e. prolonged APTT) without protecting the patient from in vivo thrombosis. The problem for the anesthesiologist is that an ACT >450 s may not represent adequate anticoagulation for CPB. Given that a blood heparin concentration of 3–4 units ml^{-1} is adequate for CPB, it has been suggested that the preoperative construction of a heparin–celite-ACT response

Table 74.2 Blood conservation strategies in Jehovah's Witness patients undergoing cardiac surgery

Preoperative	Anemia	Consider iron, folate, and erythropoietin
	Anticoagulation	Early withdrawal of antiplatelet agents and warfarin. Switch to unfractionated heparin if necessary
	Patient size	Anticipate hemodilution effect of CPB
Anesthetic	ANH	10–15 ml kg^{-1} from large-bore central line
	Pharmacologic	Consider antifibrinolytic
Bypass	Blood salvage	Needs preoperative discussion with patient
Surgical	Technique	Meticulous attention to hemostasis
Postoperative	Bleeding	Early re-exploration
	Severe anemia	↑ Risk multi-organ failure and infection
	Renal failure	Consider peritoneal dialysis

curve permits known whole-blood heparin concentrations to be correlated with ACTs.

Thrombophilia

The term thrombophilia encompasses a number of inherited hypercoagulable states.

Factor V Leiden

Factor V Leiden (FVL) polymorphism is the most common thrombophilia, affecting up to 5% of Caucasians. The substitution of glutamine for arginine-506 produces a variant that is resistant to activated protein C (APC). Affected individuals typically present with deep vein thrombosis, pulmonary embolism, stroke and recurrent miscarriage. Homozygotes are at significantly greater (10–20 times) risk of these complications than heterozygotes. FVL appears to protect cardiac surgical patients from blood loss and transfusion. FVL should be considered when a Caucasian patient below the age of 45 presents with a thrombotic event, or in any person with a family history of venous thrombosis. The diagnosis is usually confirmed by comparing the impact of APC on either the APTT or Russell's viper venom test time. Antifibrinolytic agents should be used with caution. In a study of 14 patients with symptomatic FVL undergoing cardiac surgery, there was a very high incidence of fatal and nonfatal thromboembolic events in the perioperative period and during 3 year follow-up. Continuation of perioperative oral anticoagulation was safe and prevented perioperative thromboembolic events in three patients.

Protein S and C deficiency

Protein S is a vitamin K-dependent plasma glycoprotein synthesized in endothelium where it functions as a non-enzymatic cofactor to protein C in the inactivation of Factors Va and VIIIa.

Hereditary protein S deficiency may be quantitative or qualitative. Homozygous forms are incompatible with life. In contrast, acquired protein S deficiency may be due to vitamin K deficiency, warfarin, pregnancy, liver disease or HIV infection. Vitamin K deficiency or warfarin-induced protein S deficiency impairs the coagulation system (factors II, VII, IX and X) and predisposes to *bleeding* rather than thrombosis. Protein S deficiency is the underlying cause of a small proportion of cases of disseminated intravascular coagulation, DVT and PE. Protein S deficiency is associated with graft occlusion following CABG surgery and an eight-fold increase in thromboembolic complications.

Antithrombin deficiency

Antithrombin (AT) is a serine protease inhibiting glycopeptide of hepatic origin that inactivates several enzymes in the coagulation system. AT deficiency may be defined as the failure of 500 units kg^{-1} unfractionated heparin to prolong the ACT to >480 s. A reduction in AT activity to 40–70% of normal occurs in congenital AT deficiency (incidence ~1:1000). These patients typically present with spontaneous thromboembolic phenomena and recurrent miscarriage. Acquired AT deficiency is a common sequel of heparin administration. Patients with AT

467

levels <70% of normal may be difficult to anticoagulate prior to CPB. Therapeutic options in this situation include administration of AT concentrate (expensive), FFP or red cells, which usually contain sufficient AT to prolong the ACT.

Cold agglutinins

IgG or IgM antibodies that induce erythrocyte or platelet aggregation under hypothermic conditions are termed cold agglutinins. The diagnosis is suggested by unexpectedly high arterial-line pressures during hypothermic CPB and massive hemolysis during rewarming. In known cases blood temperature must be maintained above the critical agglutination threshold. For this reason hypothermic CPB and cold cardioplegic solutions are best avoided. Preoperative corticosteroid therapy and plasmapheresis have been used to reduce cold antibody titers. The differential diagnosis includes other causes of hemolysis during CPB.

Hemoglobin S disease

Patients with sickle cell trait or sickle cell disease are at increased risk of microvascular occlusion during cardiac surgery. All patients in "at-risk" groups who are unaware of their phenotype should be tested before cardiac surgery. Heterozygotes are unlikely to undergo sickling unless exposed to profound hypoxia (SaO_2 <40%) or hypothermia. In contrast, homozygotes tend to sickle at SaO_2 <85% and may develop potentially lethal thrombosis during CPB. In addition, autosplenectomy renders patients susceptible to infection with encapsulated bacteria and renal tubular dysfunction impairs their ability to concentrate urine. Preoperative transfusion and exchange transfusion are used to reduce the level of hemoglobin SS (Hb-SS) to <30%. Hypoxia, acidosis, hypovolemia and hypothermia should be avoided.

Miscellaneous

Heparin or protamine allergy

True allergy to these agents is fortunately rare but may cause considerable problems. Some of the alternative therapies are discussed in Chapter 11. Patients with severe fish allergy confirmed by intradermal (skin-prick) testing should probably not receive protamine.

The Jehovah's Witness

The refusal of Jehovah's Witness (JW) patients to accept allogenic blood products or stored autologous blood increases the risks of cardiac surgery. Preoperative anemia should be corrected, and antiplatelet agents and anticoagulants discontinued at an early stage. Iron and recombinant erythropoietin are often administered if the hemoglobin concentration is <13 g dl^{-1}.

Most JW patients accept cell salvage and acute normovolemic hemodilution (ANH) providing the removed blood maintains in contact throughout surgery (Table 74.2). ANH theoretically reduces the number of RBCs lost during surgery. Platelets and clotting factors in the sequestered blood are protected from damage during CPB.

Key points

- Uncommon hematological problems require specialist advice.
- Heparin-induced thrombosis produces a paradoxical procoagulant state.
- Acquired AT deficiency is a common sequel of heparin administration.
- Most Jehovah's Witness patients accept acute normovolemic hemodilution.

Further reading

Boehrer JD, Kereiakes DJ, Navetta FI, Califf RM, Topol EJ. Effects of profound platelet inhibition with c7E3 before coronary angioplasty on complications of coronary bypass surgery. EPIC Investigators. Evaluation Prevention of Ischemic Complications. *Am J Cardiol* 1994; **74**(11): 1166–70.

Riess FC. Anticoagulation management and cardiac surgery in patients with heparin-induced thrombocytopenia. *Semin Thorac Cardiovasc Surg* 2005; **17**(1): 85–96.

Weiss S, Nyzio JB, Cines D, *et al.* Antiphospholipid syndrome: intraoperative and postoperative anticoagulation in cardiac surgery. *J Cardiothorac Vasc Anesth* 2008; **22**(5): 735–9.

Wiviott SD, Braunwald E, McCabe CH, *et al.* Prasugrel versus clopidogrel in patients with acute coronary syndromes. *N Engl J Med* 2007; **357**(20): 2001–15.

Cardiovascular disease and non-cardiac surgery

75

Hans-Joachim Priebe

Magnitude of the problem

Underlying cardiovascular disease (CVD) is a potentially modifiable risk factor that contributes significantly to perioperative morbidity and mortality. Major non-cardiac surgery is associated with a 0.5–1.5% incidence of perioperative cardiac death and a 2.0–3.5% incidence of major cardiovascular complications (non-fatal cardiac arrest, non-fatal myocardial infarction (MI), heart failure, clinically relevant arrhythmias, stroke). Depending on patient age and the type of surgery, the prevalence of CVD in patients undergoing non-cardiac surgery ranges from <5% to 70%. The prevalence is greatest in patients aged >70 years undergoing major vascular surgery. Reducing perioperative and long-term morbidity and mortality requires preoperative identification of patients with, or at risk of having, CVD and risk-modifying perioperative management.

Preoperative cardiac risk assessment

A thorough history and physical examination remain the best means of identifying the patient at increased perioperative cardiac risk. Risk factors known to independently influence cardiac outcome should be sought (Table 75.1).

Cardiac risk indices

Cardiac risk indices incorporate clinical factors that independently predict cardiac outcome. The most commonly used is the Lee Revised Cardiac Risk Index (RCRI) (Table 75.1).

The *Guidelines for Preoperative Cardiac Risk Assessment and Perioperative Cardiac Management in Non-Cardiac Surgery* published in 2009 by the European Society of Cardiology (ESC) recommend the use of clinical risk indices for postoperative assessment (class

Table 75.1 Independent predictors of perioperative cardiovascular complications

Lee, 1999 (RCRI)	Kheterpal, 2009
High-risk surgery	Emergency surgery
History of ischemic heart disease	Previous cardiac intervention
History of congestive heart failure	Active congestive heart failure
History of cerebrovascular disease	Cerebrovascular disease
Preoperative treatment with insulin	Age >68 years
Preoperative serum creatinine concentration >177 µmol l^{-1} (2.0 mg dl^{-1})	BMI >30 kg m^{-2}
	Hypertension
	Duration of surgery ≥3.8 h
	PRBC transfusion ≥1 unit

From: Lee *et al.* (1999) and Kheterpal *et al.* (2009).
RCRI, Revised Cardiac Risk Index; BMI, body mass index; PRBC, packed red blood cells.

of recommendation I, level of evidence B) and the Lee RCRI for perioperative risk stratification (class I, level A). See Appendix 1 for definitions of class of recommendation and level of evidence.

Despite the strong ESC recommendation, cardiac risk indices have limitations. The Lee RCRI was introduced more than a decade ago and includes only preoperative predictors of outcome. A more recently published study failed to confirm that all of the Lee RCRI risk factors were independent predictors of

Core Topics in Cardiac Anesthesia, Second Edition, ed. Jonathan H. Mackay and Joseph E. Arrowsmith. Published by Cambridge University Press. © Cambridge University Press 2012.

Table 75.2 Risk classes and incidence of cardiac complications

Risk class	Risk factors	Lee, 1999 (RCRI)		Kheterpal, 2009		
		n	% (95% CI)	n	%	HR (95% CI)
I	0	2/488	0.4 (0.05–1.5)	5/2222	0.2	–
II	1	5/567	0.0 (0.3–2.1)	13/2531	0.5	2.3 (0.8–6.4)
III	2	17/258	6.6 (3.9–10.3)	25/1885	1.3	6.0 (2.3–15.6)
IV	≥3	12/109	11.0 (5.8–18.4)	40/1102	3.6	16.7 (6.6–42.4)

From: Lee et al. (1999) and Kheterpal et al. (2009).
RCRI, Revised Cardiac Risk Index; CI, confidence interval; HR, hazard ratio.

outcome, and identified additional independent pre-operative and intraoperative predictors of outcome (Table 75.1). If confirmed in other studies, the validity of the Lee RCRI will need to be reassessed. The large overlap between the 95% confidence intervals of risk classes (Table 75.2) means that they are of limited value for the prediction of individual perioperative cardiac risk, and are better suited for comparing cardiac risk in different populations.

Cardiac risk assessment algorithm for non-cardiac surgery

The ESC guidelines recommend a systematic, step-wise approach to preoperative cardiac risk assessment is recommended for individual risk assessment (Figure 75.1). The extent of preoperative cardiac evaluation will depend on the urgency of the procedure, and on patient and surgical characteristics.

Step 1: Assess the urgency of the surgical procedure. In the case of emergency/urgent surgery, no additional preoperative cardiac evaluation or treatment is possible. In the case of elective surgery, proceed to step 2.

Step 2: Establish the presence of active cardiac conditions. If present (Table 75.3), these conditions require preoperative assessment and treatment according to relevant national or international guidelines (e.g. ESC, American Heart Association, AHA; American College of Cardiology, ACC). Subsequent management (delay, modification or cancellation of the planned procedure) will depend on test results and the response to treatment. If no active cardiac conditions are present, proceed to step 3.

Step 3: Assess surgical risk. If surgical risk of perioperative cardiac death and MI is low (i.e. <1%; Table 75.4), surgery can usually be performed without additional cardiac testing. If the planned surgical procedure carries an intermediate (1–5%) or high (>5%) risk, proceed to step 4.

Step 4: Assess the patient's functional capacity. In case of intermediate- or low-risk surgery (Table 75.4), functional capacity (Table 75.5) should be assessed. Assessment of functional capacity is probably the most important step in the entire risk assessment algorithm. A questionnaire can be used to estimate the number of metabolic equivalents of task (METs) the patient is able to generate in daily life (1 MET ≈ oxygen consumption of 3.5 ml kg^{-1} min^{-1}).

Even in patients with IHD, the ability to generate > 4 METs in daily life (as indicated by confirmatory answers to the respective questions) generally implies a good perioperative prognosis and surgery can be performed as planned without additional cardiac testing. In patients with documented IHD or cardiac risk factors, preoperative initiation of statin therapy and a titrated low-dose beta-blocker regimen can be considered. If functional capacity is ≤ 4 METs or unknown, however, proceed to step 5.

Step 5: Re-assess surgical risk. As patients with reduced functional reserve carry an increased perioperative cardiac risk, re-assessment of the cardiac risk of the surgical procedure (Table 75.4) is recommended in patients with unknown or a functional capacity of ≤ 4 METs. Such patients may undergo intermediate-risk surgery without additional cardiac testing. In this case, optimal cardiovascular medication should be ensured and a baseline ECG obtained in patients with cardiac risk factors. If high-risk surgery is planned, proceed to step 6.

Step 6: Assess cardiac risk factors. The ESC algorithm states that in patients with up to two clinical cardiac risk factors (Table 75.6), surgery can be performed

as planned after optimization of cardiovascular medication.

Step 7: Consider non-invasive testing. Because of the uniformly low positive predictive values of cardiac stress tests, they are strongly recommended only in patients with three or more clinical risk factors scheduled for high-risk surgery (i.e. open aortic or open lower extremity arterial surgery) (Table 75.4).

Step 8: Interpret test results. Risk assessment and subsequent management depend on the degree of stress-induced myocardial ischemia (Figure 75.2). If cardiac stress testing shows no or only mild stress-inducible myocardial ischemia, the ESC guidelines do not make additional invasive testing mandatory, but recommend to start therapy with statins and titrated low-dose beta-blockers.

Patients with extensive stress-inducible myocardial ischemia present a challenge. On the one hand, even optimal medical treatment will not necessarily provide

Table 75.3 Active or unstable cardiac conditions[a]

Unstable angina pectoris

Acute heart failure

Significant cardiac arrhythmias

Symptomatic valvular heart disease

Recent MI[b] and residual myocardial ischemia

[a] Conditions for which the patient should undergo evaluation and treatment before non-cardiac surgery.
[b] A MI within 30 days, according to the universal definition of MI.
Based on guidelines published by the American College of Cardiologists, American Heart Association and European Society of Cardiology.

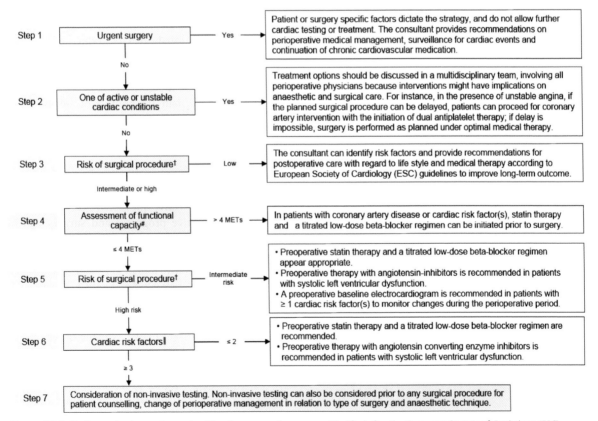

Figure 75.1 Cardiac evaluation and care algorithm for non-cardiac surgery. Modified after the European Society of Cardiology (ESC) algorithm for preoperative cardiac risk assessment and management. MET = metabolic equivalent task. † See Table 75.4 for risk of surgical procedure. # See Table 75.5 for assessment of functional capacity. || See Table 75.6 for cardiac risk factors.

Table 75.4 Surgical risk estimates*

Low risk (<1%)

Endoscopic procedures
Superficial procedures (e.g., reconstructive)
Eye, dental, endocrine, breast surgery
Minor gynaecologic, urologic and orthopedic surgery

Intermediate risk (1–5%)

Vascular (peripheral arterial angioplasty, carotid
endarterectomy, endovascular aneurysm repair)
Head and neck surgery
Intraperitoneal and intrathoracic
Major orthopedic surgery (e.g., major hip and spine
surgery)
Major urological surgery (e.g. prostatectomy)
Lung/kidney/liver transplantation

High risk (>5%)

Aortic surgery (open)
Major peripheral vascular surgery
Emergent major operation particularly in elderly
Anticipated prolonged surgical procedures associated
with large blood loss and/or fluid shifts

* Combined incidence of cardiac death and non-fatal MI within
30 days of surgery. Patients undergoing low risk procedures do
not generally require further preoperative cardiac testing. Based
on guidelines published by the American College of Cardiologists,
American Heart Association and European Society of Cardiology.

Table 75.6. Cardiac risk factors

History of angina pectoris

History of myocardial infarction

History of heart failure

History of stroke/transient ischemic attack

Diabetes mellitus requiring treatment with insulin

Renal dysfunction (serum creatinine concentration
> 170 μmol/l (2.0 mg/dl) or a creatinine clearance
of < 60 ml/min

sufficient cardioprotection. On the other hand, preoperative prophylactic coronary revascularization usually does not improve perioperative outcome in this patient population. Under these circumstances, a highly individualized approach is required. The very high cardiac risk of the planned surgical procedure needs to be balanced against the possible harms of not performing surgery (e.g. risk of rupture of an abdominal aneurysm). If there is an indication for coronary revascularization,

Table 75.5 Estimated energy requirements for various activities

	Can you . . .
1 METs	. . . take care of yourself?
	. . . eat, dress, or use the toilet?
	. . . walk indoors around the house?
	. . . walk a block or two on level ground at 2–3 miles h^{-1} (3.2–4.8 km h^{-2})?
	. . . do light work around the house like dusting or washing dishes?
4 METs	. . . climb a flight of stairs or walk up a hill?
	. . . walk on level ground at 4 miles h^{-1} (6.4 kph)?
	. . . do heavy work around the house (e.g., scrubbing floors)?
	. . . participate in moderate recreational activities (e.g., dancing, doubles tennis)?
>7 METs	. . . run at 5 mph (8 km h^{-2})?
	. . . participate in strenuous sports (e.g., swimming, singles tennis, skiing)?

Derived from the Duke Activity Status Index (DASI; Hlatky et al., 1989)
and approximate metabolic equivalents of task (METs).

the angiographic findings, patient preference, and the anticipated time interval between coronary revascularization and surgery will influence the method of coronary revascularization (Figure 75.2).

Preoperative cardiac testing
Non-invasive cardiac testing

Resting electrocardiography:

- is recommended for patients with one or more risk factors who are scheduled for intermediate or high-risk surgery (I, B);
- should be considered in patients with one or more risk factors who are scheduled for low-risk surgery (IIa, B);
- may be considered in patients with no risk factor(s) who are scheduled for intermediate-risk surgery (IIb, B);
- is not recommended in patients with no risk factor scheduled for low-risk surgery (III, B).

Other non-invasive tests are performed to identify the presence of myocardial ischemia and document ventricular and valvular function. As the positive predictive values of resting echocardiography, resting myocardial imaging techniques and cardiac stress tests (exercise ECG, stress echocardiography, stress myocardial imaging) for perioperative cardiac events

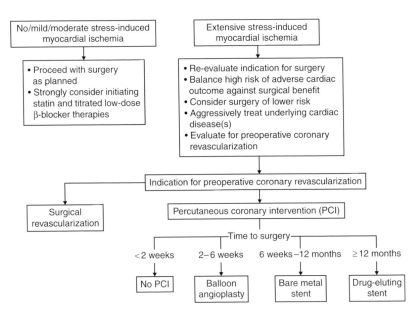

Figure 75.2 Evaluation and care algorithm according to non-invasive cardiac stress test results.

are very low (i.e. likely absence of perioperative cardiac events despite abnormal test result), the indications for performing these tests are very restrictive.

Resting echocardiography:

- is recommended in patients with severe valvular heart disease (I, C);
- should be considered for left ventricular (LV) assessment in patients with known or suspected valvular heart disease (IIa, C);
- should be considered for LV assessment in patients scheduled for high-risk surgery (IIa, C);
- is not recommended for assessment of LV function in asymptomatic patients (III, B).

Cardiac stress testing:

- is recommended in patients with three or more clinical risk factors scheduled for high-risk surgery (I, C);
- may be considered in patients with one or two clinical risk factors scheduled for high-risk surgery (IIb, B);
- may be considered in patients scheduled for intermediate risk surgery (IIb, C);
- is not recommended in patients scheduled for low-risk surgery (III, C).

Invasive cardiac testing

Coronary angiography

As coronary angiography in cardiovascular high-risk patients carries the potential for life-threatening complications, and as there is no convincing evidence that

preoperative coronary revascularization reliably improves perioperative outcome, the indications for preoperative coronary angiography are restrictive and identical to those in the non-operative setting. Preoperative coronary angiography merely to confirm the existence of coronary artery disease is rarely indicated.

Before performing a preoperative coronary angiography, it should be clear beforehand that the patient is a potential candidate for subsequent preoperative coronary revascularization, which necessitates a prior detailed discussion of the implications of preoperative coronary revascularization (e.g., possible postponement of surgery and need for anti-platelet therapy) between medical care givers and the patient. If the patient is a potential candidate for preoperative coronary revascularization, preoperative angiography

- is recommended in patients with acute ST-elevation myocardial infarction (STEMI), with non-ST-elevation MI (NSTEMI) and unstable angina pectoris, and with angina pectoris not controlled with adequate medical therapy (I, A);
- may be considered in cardiac stable patients undergoing high-risk (IIb, B) and intermediate-risk surgery (IIb, C);
- is not recommended in cardiac stable patients undergoing low-risk surgery (III, C).

If the coronary anatomy found on subsequent coronary angiography fulfils the indication(s) for coronary revascularization, consultation between

473

cardiologist, surgeon, anesthesiologist and patient is required to determine the most appropriate method of coronary revascularization (i.e. surgical vs. percutaneous intervention; if interventional, balloon angioplasty vs. bare metal stenting vs. drug-eluting stenting) (Figure 75.2).

Cardiac biomarkers

IHD and myocardial disease are frequently accompanied by increased plasma concentrations of C-reactive protein (CRP), and of brain natriuretic peptide (BNP) and NT-proBNP, reflecting the considerable inflammatory component associated with cardiovascular disease and increased myocardial wall stress, respectively. The results of several recent systematic reviews and meta-analyses and observational studies have shown that elevated preoperative serum concentrations of high-sensitivity CRP and BNP or NT-proBNP are powerful, independent predictors of adverse postoperative short- and intermediate-term cardiac outcome in major non-cardiac surgery. In addition, preoperative measurements of these biomarkers provide additive prognostic information for major adverse cardiac events and mortality after high-risk surgery. However, the cut-off concentrations of CRP and of BNP and NT-proBNP associated with adverse outcome varied tremendously between studies, indicating that we are far from knowing what a "normal" preoperative concentration of these biomarkers might be. Measurements of these biomarkers may be helpful in improving individual risk assessment by increasing the uniformly low positive predictive values of clinical scoring systems and of preoperative cardiac stress tests, by possibly being able to estimate the severity of an underlying cardiac condition (particularly in patients with low or unknown functional capacity), and in deciding on the need for additional cardiac assessment.

It is undecided whether postponement of surgery for treatment of the underlying cardiovascular disease until normalization or at least improvement of the concentrations of these biomarkers will improve perioperative outcome. According to the ESC guidelines preoperative measurement of plasma concentrations of BNP and NT-proBNP should be considered to obtain independent prognostic information for perioperative and late cardiac events in high-risk patients (IIa, B). Routine measurements of cardiac biomarkers (BNP, NT-proBNP, cardiac troponins) are not recommended (III, C).

Preoperative coronary revascularization

Despite numerous publications and respective guidelines and recommendations, the issue of preoperative coronary artery revascularization remains highly controversial, mostly because findings of randomized and non-randomized trials have been contradictory. Numerous variables must be expected to affect the impact of preoperative coronary artery revascularization on perioperative cardiac outcome. They include morbidity and mortality associated with coronary angiography and revascularization, especially in cardiac high-risk patients, underlying cardiac risk (high- vs. intermediate-risk findings on cardiac stress tests; high- vs. intermediate-risk coronary anatomy), surgical risk (high- vs. intermediate risk surgery), indication for coronary artery revascularization (prophylactic to "get the patient through surgery" vs. class IA indication; for symptoms vs. for prognosis; class I vs. class II recommendation), type of coronary artery revascularization (interventional vs. surgical), completeness of coronary artery revascularization, and, possibly most importantly, perioperative management of anti-ischemic, plaque-stabilizing and anti-platelet medication. In general, because of lack of clear evidence for an outcome benefit of preoperative coronary artery revascularization, and the risk associated with coronary artery revascularization in general, the indications for preoperative coronary artery revascularization should be handled very restrictively and are, in general, the same as those in the non-surgical setting. Therefore, preoperative coronary artery revascularization:

- is recommended in patients with acute coronary syndrome (in all patients with STEMI; in patients with NSTEMI at high risk, such as elevated serum troponin concentration and ST-segment depression at baseline, ongoing symptoms, high thrombotic risk, advanced age, diabetes mellitus; all I, A);
- is recommended in patients with stable angina pectoris or silent ischemia *and* left main coronary artery stenosis > 50% (I, A), any proximal left anterior descending coronary artery stenosis > 50% (I, A), two- or three-vessel coronary artery disease with impaired LV function (I, B), documented LV ischemic area > 10% (I, B), single remaining patent vessel with > 50% stenosis and impaired LV function (I, C);
- can be considered in patients with persistent signs of extensive ischemia or a high cardiac risk scheduled for high-risk vascular surgery (IIb, B).

However, in this high-risk patient population the ultimate decision has to be based on individual assessment of medical and surgical short- and long-term prognosis, and on informed patient consent based on such assessment. If preoperative coronary revascularization is to be performed, it must be remembered that the surgical procedure needs to be postponed for at least 2 weeks after balloon angioplasty, 3 months after placement of a bare-metal stent and 12 months after placement of a drug-eluting stent.

Specific diseases

Coronary artery disease

The majority of perioperative MIs occur in myocardium supplied by coronary arteries that have been previously determined by angiography to have only mild or moderate luminal stenoses. This indicates that plaque transformation (i.e. from stable to vulnerable) can be acute and helps to explain the observation that chronic, stable coronary atherosclerosis can transform into acute, potentially life-threatening coronary events at any time. The perioperative period induces large, unpredictable and unphysiological changes in sympathetic tone, cardiovascular performance, coagulation and inflammatory responses. These changes induce, in turn, unpredictable alterations in plaque morphology, function and progression. Simultaneous perioperative alterations in homeostasis and coronary plaque characteristics may trigger a mismatch between myocardial oxygen supply and demand. If not alleviated in time, these will ultimately result in MI, irrespective of etiology (morphologically, hemodynamically, inflammatory or coagulation-induced).

The etiology of perioperative MI (PMI) remains poorly understood, but is certain to be multifactorial. Existing data are inconclusive and do not unequivocally demonstrate whether long-duration subendocardial myocardial ischemia or acute coronary occlusion due to plaque disruption or thrombosis is the primary mechanism of PMI. This uncertainty is to be expected considering the enormous structural and functional diversity of coronary atherosclerosis, the unpredictability of plaque progression and vulnerability, and the remaining methodological problems of reliably detecting and diagnosing perioperative myocardial ischemia and PMI.

With the many diverse factors involved in the etiology of PMI, it is highly unlikely that one single intervention will successfully improve cardiac outcome following non-cardiac surgery. A multi-factorial, step-wise approach is indicated (Figure 75.1). Two principal strategies have been employed in an attempt to reduce the incidence of PMI and other adverse cardiac events; cardioprotective pharmacological treatment and preoperative coronary revascularization. Perioperative plaque stabilization by pharmacological means (e.g. statins, aspirin, β-blockers) is probably more effective in the prevention of PMI than an increase in myocardial oxygen supply (by coronary revascularization) or a reduction in myocardial oxygen demand (by β-blockers or α_2-agonists).

Hypertension

Hypertension is generally no longer considered an independent predictor of adverse perioperative cardiac outcome in non-cardiac surgery. The findings of a recent study suggesting otherwise await validation. Consequently, delaying surgery in patients with uncontrolled hypertension in order to initiate or optimize antihypertensive medication is not evidence-based. However, the presence of end-organ dysfunction and accompanying cardiovascular pathology needs to be ruled out. If present, and particularly when accompanied by additional risk factors, the patient's medical condition requires closer assessment. In each individual case, the potential benefit of delaying surgery to allow optimization of medical therapy must be weighed against the inconveniences and risks of delaying surgery.

In long-term untreated hypertensive patients, in whom the autoregulatory pressure–flow curve is right-shifted, acute aggressive preoperative control of blood pressure may cause complications. Even treated hypertensive patients have persistent impairment of vasomotor tone exposing them to the risks of both hypertensive and hypotensive episodes. With the arguable exception of angiotensin-converting enzyme (ACE) inhibitors and angiotensin-II-receptor blockers, antihypertensive medication should be continued until the morning of surgery.

Valvular heart disease

As patients with valvular heart disease (VHD) are, in general, at increased risk of perioperative cardiac complications during non-cardiac surgery, echocardiography should be considered in all patients with suspected VHD (IIa, B). In all patients with severe VHD, clinical and echocardiographic evaluation

475

should be performed (I, C) and, if indicated, appropriately treated preoperatively.

Aortic stenosis

Of all of the types of VHD, severe AS (AV orifice area <1 cm^2 or <0.6 cm^2 m^{-2}) carries the greatest perioperative cardiovascular morbidity and mortality. The key factors in preoperative decision-making are the urgency of the surgical procedure, the severity of AS and the clinical condition of the patient.

In the setting of urgent non-cardiac surgery, close and intensive hemodynamic monitoring is essential because coronary perfusion is critically dependent on diastolic arterial pressure. Asymptomatic patients with severe AS usually tolerate low to intermediate-risk surgery. If scheduled for high-risk surgery, patient evaluation by a specialist is advisable. Independent predictors of outcome in asymptomatic patients with severe AS in the non-operative setting are female sex, peak transvalvular velocity and BNP concentration.

Symptomatic patients with severe AS and certain asymptomatic patients with severe AS scheduled for high-risk surgery are candidates for valve replacement. AVR should preferably be performed before non-cardiac surgery. If preoperative conventional AVR is contraindicated (unacceptably high risk due to serious comorbidity, patient refusal, relative urgency of surgery), careful perioperative hemodynamic management is imperative, only vital surgery should be performed, and preoperative balloon aortic valvuloplasty or transcatheter valve implantation should be considered.

Mitral stenosis

In patients with non-critical MS (MV orifice area >1.5 cm^2) and in patients with critical MS (MV orifice area <1.5 cm^2) with systolic PA pressure <50 mmHg, non-cardiac surgery is relatively safe and preoperative valve replacement rarely indicated. Asymptomatic patients with critical MS and a systolic PA pressure >50 mmHg and symptomatic patients may benefit from preoperative MVR or percutaneous mitral commissurotomy, especially when scheduled for high-risk surgery. Control of HR and volume status, maintenance of sinus rhythm and effective prophylaxis against thromboembolism are mandatory in this patient population.

Aortic and mitral valve regurgitation

In general, chronic valvular regurgitation is better tolerated than stenosis. In non-cardiac surgery, the perioperative cardiac risk is acceptably low in asymptomatic patients, even in the presence of severe AR or MR (as defined by ESC and AHA guidelines), as long as LV function is preserved. By contrast, symptomatic patients or asymptomatic patients with poor LV function (LV ejection fraction $<30\%$) should undergo only essential surgery.

Status post valve replacement

In the absence of clinically relevant valvular or ventricular dysfunction, non-cardiac surgery following correction of VHD carries little additional risk. Following implantation of a prosthetic valve, perioperative modification of the usual anticoagulation regimen is often required. This usually involves temporary discontinuation of oral anticoagulants and bridging with intravenous or subcutaneous unfractionated heparin or subcutaneous low-molecular-weight heparin. In patients undergoing non-cardiac surgery at risk of bacteremia, antibiotic prophylaxis against infective endocarditis needs to be started according to national and international guidelines (see Chapter 71).

Heart failure

Heart failure is a major independent predictor of adverse perioperative cardiac outcome in non-cardiac surgery. It carries a greater perioperative risk than IHD. The perioperative prognostic value of heart failure with preserved LV ejection fraction (previously referred to as diastolic heart failure) remains to be determined. Current ESC guidelines recommend comparable perioperative management in patients with impaired and preserved LV systolic function.

Patients with suspected or known heart failure should undergo preoperative evaluation by a specialist to assess the severity of the disease and to ensure optimal medical therapy. The findings on stress echocardiography and the serum concentration of BNP or NT-proBNP may be used for risk stratification.

Heart failure patients are invariably on multiple chronic medications, including ACE-inhibitors, angiotensin-II-receptor blockers, β-blockers, aldosterone antagonists and diuretics. Medication-associated side effects (mostly electrolyte disturbances, renal insufficiency, intraoperative therapy-resistant hypotension) are common. As there is evidence that perioperative use of ACE-inhibitors, β-blockers, statins and aspirin improves outcome in patients with LV dysfunction undergoing major vascular surgery, perioperative continuation of such therapy is recommended.

Patients with well-controlled heart failure are, nevertheless, at increased risk of developing acute postoperative heart failure as a result of exposure to various perioperative stressors (e.g. anemia, hypervolemia, tachycardia, neuroendocrine stress responses to surgery). The diagnosis may be difficult to make because the etiology and symptoms often differ from the non-operative setting. A high suspicion for the development of postoperative heart is thus warranted in patients with a history of heart failure.

Cerebrovascular disease

Cerebrovascular disease is the third leading cause of death in developed countries. The reported incidence of perioperative stroke is 0.08–0.7% in general surgery, and 1–5% in peripheral and carotid artery surgery. A history of recent stroke or TIA is the strongest predictor of perioperative stroke. If present, additional preoperative cerebrovascular assessment is indicated. According to the new ESC guidelines, routine preoperative screening for symptomatic or asymptomatic carotid artery stenosis may be considered (IIb, C). Routine preoperative treatment of carotid stenosis before non-cardiac surgery is not evidence-based. In cases where there is >70% carotid lumen narrowing, antiplatelet therapy or surgery is recommended (I, A).

Preoperative discontinuation of anticoagulants or antiplatelet drugs is associated with an increased risk of perioperative stroke and should thus be avoided whenever possible. Contrary to common belief, most perioperative strokes are not associated with perioperative hypotensive episodes and appear to occur despite intact cerebral autoregulation. Cerebral ischemia and emboli, rather than hemodynamic compromise, account for most perioperative strokes. Nevertheless, avoiding unphysiological decreases in blood pressure, particularly in hypertensive patients and in patients at increased risk of perioperative stroke, is advisable. There is suggestive evidence that individually defined blood pressure targets and control of body temperature and blood glucose concentration reduce the perioperative risk of stroke.

General management strategy

The following 10 management steps are recommended:
1. Identify the patient at increased perioperative risk.
2. Perform preoperative cardiac risk assessment.
3. Perform appropriate preoperative cardiac testing.
4. Ensure optimal pharmacological therapy.
5. Continue cardiac medication until the time of surgery (with the possible exception of ACE inhibitors and angiotensin-II-receptor blockers in the treatment of hypertension).
6. Define pathophysiology of underlying cardiovascular disease.
7. Set hemodynamic goals.
8. Select anesthetic method and drugs to achieve set hemodynamic goals.
9. Select type and duration of hemodynamic monitoring (based on likely incidence, type, severity, time of occurrence, and severity of potential hemodynamic complication).
10. Be prepared to acutely treat hemodynamic complications.

Key points

- The risk of perioperative cardiovascular complications depends on the urgency of surgery, the presence of active cardiac conditions, the magnitude of surgery and the patient's functional capacity.
- In patients at increased perioperative cardiac risk, systematic preoperative cardiac risk assessment is imperative to guide appropriate perioperative management.
- Additional preoperative cardiac testing should only be performed if the results are likely to affect overall management.
- Knowledge of the pathophysiology of cardiovascular disease is of the utmost importance, as it determines all aspects of perioperative management.

Further reading

Biccard BM, Rodseth RN. A meta-analysis of the prospective randomised trials of coronary revascularisation before noncardiac vascular surgery with attention to the type of coronary revascularisation performed. *Anesthesia* 2009; **64**: 1105–1.

Buellesfeld L, Windecker S. Transcatheter aortic valve implantation: the evidence is catching up with reality. *Eur Heart J* 2011: **32**: 133–7.

Choi J-H, Cho DK, Song Y-B, *et al.* Preoperative NT-proBNP and CRP predict perioperative major cardiovascular events in non-cardiac surgery. *Heart* 2010; **96**: 56–62.

Fleisher LA, Beckman JA, Brown KA, *et al.* ACC/AHA 2007 Guidelines on Perioperative Cardiovascular Evaluation and Care for Noncardiac surgery: executive summary: a report of the American College of Cardiology/American Heart Association Task Force on Practice Guidelines (Writing Committee to Revise the 2002 Guidelines on Perioperative Cardiovascular Evaluation for Noncardiac Surgery). *Circulation* 2007; **116**(17): e418–99.

Goei D, Hoeks SE, Boersma E, *et al.* Incremental value of high-sensitivity C-reactive protein and N-terminal pro-B-type natriuretic peptide for the prediction of postoperative cardiac events in noncardiac vascular surgery patients. *Coron Art Dis* 2009; **20**: 219–24.

Hammill BG, Curtis LH, Bennett-Guerrero E, *et al.* Impact of heart failure on patients undergoing major noncardiac surgery. *Anesthesiology* 2008; **108**(4): 559–67.

Hlatky MA, Boineau RE, Higginbotham MB, *et al.* A brief self-administered questionnaire to determine functional capacity (the Duke Activity Status Index). *Am J Cardiol.* 1989; **64**(10): 651–4.

Kheterpal S, O'Reilly M, Englesbe M, *et al.* Preoperative and intraoperative predictors of cardiac adverse events after general, vascular, and urological surgery. *Anesthesiology* 2009; **110**(1): 58–66.

Landesberg G, Beattie WS, Mosseri M, *et al.* Perioperative myocardial infarction. *Circulation* 2009; **119**(22): 2936–44.

Lee TH, Marcantonio ER, Mangione CM, *et al.* Derivation and prospective validation of a simple index for prediction of cardiac risk of major noncardiac surgery. *Circulation* 1999; **100**(10): 1043–9.

Monin J-L, Lancellotti P, Monchi M, *et al.* Risk score for predicting outcome in patients with asymptomatic aortic stenosis. *Circulation* 2009; **120**(1): 69–75.

Mythen M. Pre-operative coronary revascularisation before non-cardiac surgery: think long and hard before making a pre-operative referral. *Anaesthesia* 2009; **64**: 1048–50.

Poldermans D, Bax J, Boersma E, *et al.* Guidelines for pre-operative cardiac risk assessment and perioperative cardiac management in non-cardiac surgery. *Eur Heart J* 2009; **30**(22): 2769–812.

Priebe H-J. Preoperative cardiac management of the patient for non-cardiac surgery: an individualized and evidence-based approach. *Br J Anaesth* 2011; **107**(1): 83–96.

Ryding A, Kumar S, Worthington A, Burgess D. Prognostic value of brain natriuretic peptide in noncardiac surgery: a meta-analysis. *Anesthesiology* 2009; **111**(2): 311–19.

Voûte MT, Winkel TA, Poldermans D. Optimal medical management around the time of surgery. *Heart* 2010; **96**: 1842–8.

Wong EYW, Lawrence HP, Wong DT. The effect of prophylactic coronary revascularization or medical treatment on patient outcomes after noncardiac surgery – a meta analysis. *Can J Anesth* 2007; **54**(9): 705–17.

Zahn R, Gerckens U, Grube E, *et al.* Transcatheter aortic valve implantation: first results from a multi-centre real-world registry. *Eur Heart J* 2011; **32**: 198–204.

Appendix 1: Classification of recommendations

Size of treament effect

SIZE OF TREATMENT EFFECT →

	CLASS I *Benefit > > > Risk* Procedure/Treatment **Should** be performed/ administered	**CLASS IIa** *Benefit > > Risk* *Additional studies with focused objectives needed* **IT IS REASONABLE** to perform procedure/administer treatment	**CLASS IIb** *Benefit ≥ Risk* *Additional studies with broad objectives needed; additional registry data would be helpful* Procedure/Treatment **MAY BE CONSIDERED**	**CLASS III** *Risk ≥ Benefit* Procedure/treatment should **NOT** be performed/administered **SINCE IT IS NOT HELPFUL AND MAY BE HARMFUL**
LEVEL A Multiple populations evaluated* Data derived from multiple randomized clinical trials or meta-analyses	■ Recommendation that procedure or treatment is useful/effective ■ Sufficient evidence from multiple randomized trials or meta-analyses	■ Recommendation in favor of treatment or procedure being useful/effective ■ Some conflicting evidence from multiple randomized trials or meta-analyses	■ Recommendation's usefulness/efficacy less well established ■ Greater conflicting evidence from multiple randomized trials or meta-analyses	■ Recommendation that procedure or treatment is not useful/efective and may be harmful ■ Sufficient evidence from multiple randomized trials or meta-analyses
LEVEL B Limited populations evaluated* Data derived from a single randomized trial or nonrandomized studies	■ Recommendation that procedure or treatment is useful/effective ■ Evidence from single randomized trial or nonrandomized studies	■ Recommendation in favor of treatment or procedure being useful/effective ■ Some conflicting evidence from single randomized trial or nonrandomized studies	■ Recommendation's usefulness/efficacy less well established ■ Greater conflicting evidence from single randomized trials or nonrandomized studies	■ Recommendation that procedure or treatment is not useful/effective and may be harmful ■ Evidence from single randomized trial or nonrandomized studies
LEVEL C Very limited populations evaluated* Only consensus opinion of experts, case studies, or standard of care	■ Recommendation that procedure or treatment is useful/effective ■ Only expert opinion, case studies, or standard or care	■ Recommendation in favor of treatment or procedure being useful/effective ■ Only diverging expert opinion, case studies, or standard of care	■ Recommendation's usefulness/efficacy less well established ■ Only diverging expert opinion, case studies,or standard of care	■ Recommendation that procedure or treatment is not useful/effective and may be harmful ■ Only expert opinion, case studies,or standard of care
Suggested phrases for writing recommendations⁺	should is recommended is indicated is useful/effective/beneficial	is reasonable can be useful/effective/beneficial is probably recommended or indicated	may/might be considered may/might be reasonable usefulness/effectiveness is unknown/unclear/uncertain or not well established	is not recommended is not indicated should not is not useful/effective/beneficial may be harmful

ESTIMATE OF CERTAINTY (PRECISION) OF TREATMENT EFFECT (vertical axis label)

Appendix 2: Conversion factors for SI and traditional units

Parameter	Traditional unit	SI unit	To convert Trad → SI	To covert SI → Trad
Albumin	g/dl	g/l	× 10	× 0.1
Bilirubin	mg/dl	µmol/l	× 17.104	× 0.0585
Calcium	mg/dl	mmol/l	× 0.2495	× 4.008
Chloride	mg/dl	mmol/l	× 0.2821	× 3.5453
Cholesterol	mg/dl	mmol/l	× 0.026	× 38.66
Creatinine	mg/dl	µmol/l	× 88.402	× 0.0113
Digoxin	µg/l	nmol/l	× 1.28	× 0.781
Fibrinogen	mg/dl	g/l	× 0.01	× 100
Glucose	mg/dl	mmol/l	× 0.0555	× 18.016
Hemoglobin	g/dl	mmol/l	× 0.6206	× 1.611
Lactate	mg/dl	mmol/l	× 0.111	× 9.008
Magnesium	mg/dl	mmol/l	× 0.4113	× 2.4312
Phosphate	mg/dl	mmol/l	× 0. 3229	× 3.0974
Potassium	mg/dl	mmol/l	× 0.2557	× 3.9102
Sodium	mg/dl	mmol/l	× 0.435	× 2.2989
Total protein	g/dl	g/l	× 10	× 0.1
Triglycerides	mg/dl	mmol/l	× 0.0114	× 87.5
Urea (BUN)	mg/dl	mmol/l	× 0.3651	× 2.808
Urea	mg/dl	mmol/l	× 0.1665	× 6.006

Core Topics in Cardiac Anesthesia, Second Edition, ed. Jonathan H. Mackay and Joseph E. Arrowsmith. Published by Cambridge University Press. © Cambridge University Press 2012.

Appendix 3: The phonetic and surgical alphabets

Letter	Phonetic	Surgical	Letter	Phonetic	Surgical
A	Alpha	Accuse	N	November	Niggle
B	Bravo	Blame	O	Oscar	Ostracize
C	Charlie	Criticize	P	Papa	Penalize
D	Delta	Deny	Q	Quebec	Quarrel
E	Echo	Extort	R	Romeo	Ridicule
F	Foxtrot	Flagellate	S	Sierra	Slander
G	Golf	Gouge	T	Tango	Terrorize
H	Hotel	Harass	U	Uniform	Undermine
I	India	Incite	V	Victor	Violate
J	Juliet	Jibe	W	Whiskey	Waste
K	Kilo	Kick	X	X-ray	X-ray (lost swab)
L	Lima	Libel	Y	Yankee	Yank
M	Mike	Maim	Z	Zulu	Zap

Core Topics in Cardiac Anesthesia, Second Edition, ed. Jonathan H. Mackay and Joseph E. Arrowsmith. Published by Cambridge University Press. © Cambridge University Press 2012.